CHECK YOUR HEALTH KNOWLEDGE

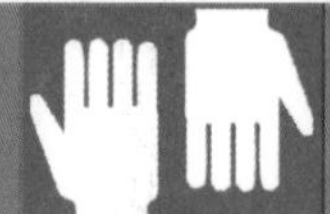

TRUE FALSE 16. About as many people are injured because of seatbelt use as are protected by seatbelts.

TRUE FALSE 17. Alcohol is an important contributor to both intentional and unintentional injuries.

TRUE FALSE 18. "No pain, no gain," is true for receiving health benefits from exercise.

TRUE FALSE 19. The lower a person's cholesterol, the lower his or her risk of dying.

TRUE FALSE 20. Eating a high-protein diet is important for good health.

TRUE FALSE 21. Totally eliminating alcohol from one's life is a healthy choice.

TRUE FALSE 22. People who experience chronic pain have underlying psychological disorders that are the real basis of their pain problem.

TRUE FALSE 23. Men are more likely than women to develop heart disease.

TRUE FALSE 24. African Americans are more likely than European Americans to develop and to die of heart disease.

TRUE FALSE 25. Both positive and negative events may produce stress.

TRUE FALSE 26. Psychologists have found that lack of will power is the primary reason why smokers cannot quit.

TRUE FALSE 27. Sugar pills (placebos) can boost the effectiveness of both psychological and medical treatments.

TRUE FALSE 28. People with a minor illness are about as likely as people with a serious illness to seek medical treatment.

TRUE FALSE 29. People who live with a smoker have about the same risk for cancer and heart disease as do smokers.

TRUE FALSE 30. Sick people who have a lot of friends usually live longer than sick people who have no close friends.

The answers to these questions appear throughout the book, but you may also find a key on the Web site for this book: **www.psychology.wadsworth.com/brannon_5e**

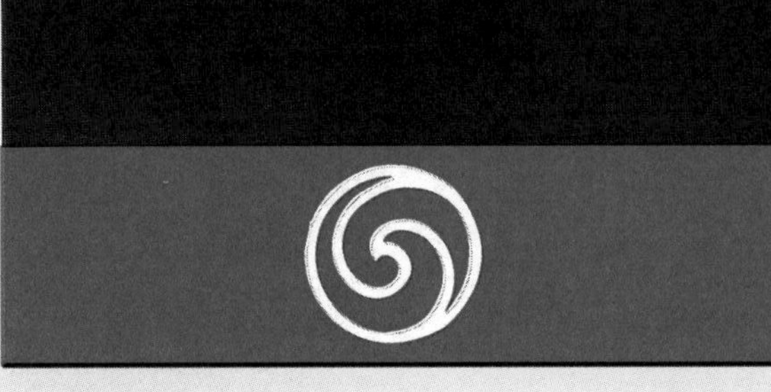

Health Psychology:

An Introduction to Behavior and Health

5th edition

LINDA BRANNON
McNeese State University

JESS FEIST
McNeese State University

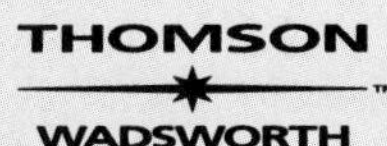

Australia • Canada • Mexico • Singapore • Spain
United Kingdom • United States

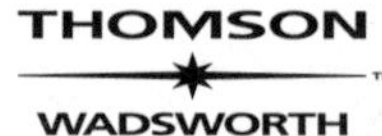

Psychology Editor: Michele Sordi
Assistant Editor: Jennifer Wilkinson
Editorial Assistant: Chelsea Junget
Technology Project Manager: Darin Derstine
Marketing Manager: Chris Caldeira
Marketing Assistant: Laurel Anderson
Advertising Project Manager: Brian Chaffee
Project Manager, Editorial Production: Paul Wells
Print/Media Buyer: Rebecca Cross
Permissions Editor: Elizabeth Zuber
Production Service: Carlisle Publishers Services
Text Designer: Andrew Ogus
Photo Researcher: Mary Reeg
Copy Editor: Jane Parrigin
Illustrator: Carlisle Communications, Ltd.
Cover Designer: Todd Damotte, Rokusek Design, Inc.
Cover Image: Copyright 2003 Rokusek Design, Inc.
Cover Printer: Phoenix Color Corp
Compositor: Carlisle Communications, Ltd.
Printer: Phoenix Color Corp

Printed in the United States of America
1 2 3 4 5 6 7 07 06 05 04 03

For more information about our products, contact us at:
Thomson Learning Academic Resource Center
1-800-423-0563
For permission to use material from this text, contact us by:
Phone: 1-800-730-2214
Fax: 1-800-730-2215
Web: http://www.thomsonrights.com

Library of Congress Control Number: 2003100989
Student Edition: ISBN 0-534-50600-3

Wadsworth/Thomson Learning
10 Davis Drive
Belmont, CA 94002-3098
USA

Asia
Thomson Learning
5 Shenton Way #01-01
UIC Building
Singapore 068808

Australia/New Zealand
Thomson Learning
102 Dodds Street
Southbank, Victoria 3006
Australia

Canada
Nelson
1120 Birchmount Road
Toronto, Ontario M1K 5G4
Canada

Europe/Middle East/Africa
Thomson Learning
High Holborn House
50/51 Bedford Row
London WC1R 4LR
United Kingdom

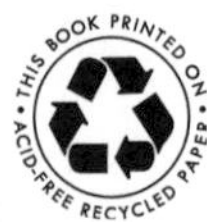

Brief Contents

Part I
Foundations of Health Psychology

Part II
Stress, Pain, and Coping

Part III
Behavior and Chronic Disease

Part IV
Behavioral Health

Part V
Looking toward the Future

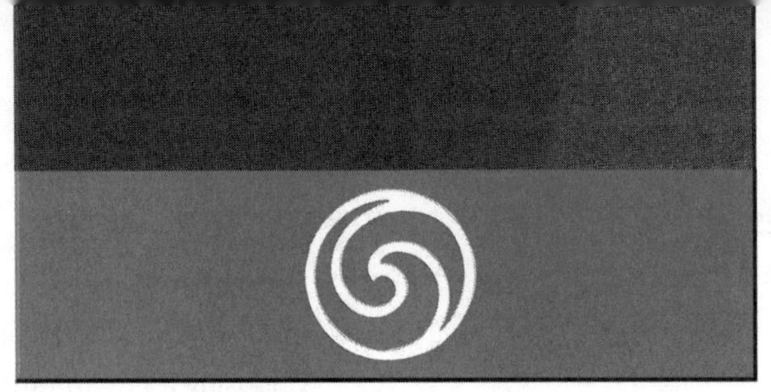

Contents

Part II

Stress, Pain, and Coping

Chapter 5
Defining and Measuring Stress 97

Chapter 6
Understanding Stress and Disease 126

Chapter 7
Understanding Pain 153

Chapter 8
Coping with Stress and Pain 186

Part III

Behavior and Chronic Disease

Chapter 9
Cardiovascular Disease 215

Chapter 10
Behavioral Factors in Cancer 249

Chapter 11 Living with Chronic Illness 276

Part IV

Behavioral Health

Chapter 12 Preventing Injuries 308

Chapter 13
Smoking Tobacco 345

Chapter 14
Using Alcohol and Other Drugs 381

Chapter 15
Eating to Control Weight 419

Chapter 16
Exercising 453

Part V

Looking toward the Future

Chapter 17
Future Challenges 483

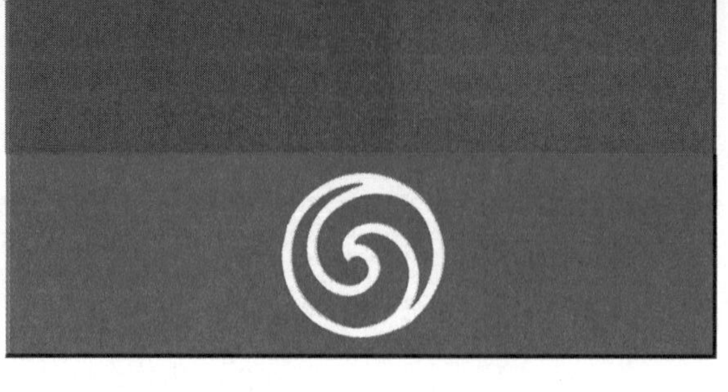

Preface

At the beginning of the 20th century, most serious diseases were caused by contact with viruses and bacteria. People had little individual responsibility for preventing diseases because these microorganisms were nearly impossible to avoid. Today, most serious diseases and disorders occur as the result of individual behaviors—or failures to behave. As health and disease became more closely linked to behavior, psychology—the science of behavior—became involved in many health-related issues. This involvement led to the birth and development of *health psychology,* the scientific study of behaviors that relate to health enhancement, disease prevention, safety, and rehabilitation.

As the profession of health psychology emerged and grew, a need for a comprehensive undergraduate textbook became apparent. Several such books—including the first edition of *Health Psychology: An Introduction to Behavior and Health*—came onto the market. Most of these early attempts failed to find the core of undergraduate health psychology. With its emphasis on the science and its accessibility to students, *Health Psychology: An Introduction to Behavior and Health* was an exception: it not only found that core, it helped define it.

Our purpose in writing the fifth edition of *Health Psychology: An Introduction to Behavior and Health* was to present students with a readable text that will help them keep up to date with the crucial research on behavior and health. To that end, we have written the fifth edition in a more concise style and have added tables and figures to further enhance students' learning.

The Fifth Edition

We have organized the fifth edition of *Health Psychology: An Introduction to Behavior and Health* into five parts. Part 1, which includes the first four chapters, lays a solid foundation in research and theory for understanding subsequent chapters; Part 2 deals with stress, pain, and coping; Part 3 discusses heart disease, cancer, and other chronic diseases; Part 4 includes chapters on safety, tobacco use, drinking alcohol, eating and weight control, and physical activity; and Part 5 looks toward future challenges in health psychology.

What's New?

Readers of earlier editions of *Health Psychology: An Introduction to Behavior and Health* will notice a completely new two-color design in the fifth edition that enhances the text's accessibility and visual impact, and a more concise and accessible writing style with more selective examination of research studies. In addition, the present edition introduces a number of new topics and expanded coverage of many more.

Added material includes new boxes on:

- the health benefits of attending college
- the ethics of placebo treatment
- the dangers of being in a hospital
- the risks of not complying to a placebo prescription
- the stress created by the September 11 attacks on the World Trade Center and the Pentagon
- the possibility of increasing one's lifespan by religious involvement
- the association between heart disease and hair loss
- the advantages of physical activity throughout the lifespan
- the validity of the old adage, "Moderation in all things"

Other new or reorganized topics within the chapters include:

- a description of the complex and troubled health care system in the United States
- personality factors that influence adherence
- relationship, family, workplace, and community conditions that lead to stress
- a description of cytokines, the chemical messengers secreted by cells in the immune system
- psychological factors in the experience of pain
- an updated classification of headaches and new information on their physiology
- personal strategies for coping
- emotional disclosure as a coping strategy
- emotional responses and emotional support for cancer patients
- a discussion of genetic factors in cancer
- a new section on asthma
- added coverage on Type 2 diabetes
- added information on childhood obesity and its health effects
- information on genetic factors in alcohol use
- the role of advertising in cigarette consumption
- a discussion of body image and its role in eating disorders

Topics that received elaboration or expansion include:

- ethnicity and cultural diversity
- the placebo effect
- barriers to receiving medical care
- genetics of Alzheimer's disease
- strategies for staying safe
- smoking as a means of weight control at different ages
- benefits of moderate drinking
- the relationship between leptin and body weight
- the increasing levels of obesity in the United States
- problems of the escalating costs of medical care

New Comprehensive Health Knowledge Quiz

Located on the inside front cover endsheets, this new Health Knowledge Quiz for the first day of class prompts students to consider myths and facts of health behavior. Answers to the Health Quiz are posted on the book web site.

What Has Been Retained?

We have retained several of the popular existing features, each of which was developed to stimulate critical thinking and to facilitate learning. These features include (1) Chapter-Opening Questions, (2) a "Check Your Health Risks" box in most chapters, (3) a "Would You Believe . . .?" box in each chapter, and (4) a "Becoming Healthier" feature. The purpose of these features is to actively engage readers in the process of acquiring health-related information that will enhance their personal well-being.

Questions and Answers Each chapter begins with a series of *Questions* that are designed to organize the chapter, preview the material, and enhance active learning. As each chapter unfolds, answers to these questions are revealed through a discussion of relevant research findings. At the end of each major topic, an *In Summary* section offers a succinct summary of that topic. Then, at the end of the chapter, *Answers* to the chapter-opening questions appear. This *preview, read, and review* method facilitates learning and improves recall.

Check Your Health Risks At the beginning of most chapters, a "Check Your Health Risks" box personalizes material in that chapter. Each box consists of several health-related behaviors or attitudes that readers should check before looking at the rest of the chapter. After checking the items that apply to them and then becoming familiar with the chapter's material, readers can develop a more research-based understanding of their health risks.

Would You Believe Boxes We have kept the popular "Would You Believe" boxes, adding nine new ones and deleting several old ones. Each box begins with the question "Would You Believe" and then highlights a particularly intriguing finding in health research. These boxes are designed to explore some preconceived notions and to challenge students to take an objective look at issues that previously they may have seen from a nonscientific viewpoint.

Becoming Healthier Embedded in most chapters is a "Becoming Healthier" box with advice on how to use the information in the chapter to acquire a healthier lifestyle. Although some people may not agree with all of these recommendations, each is based on the most current available research findings. We believe that if you follow these guidelines, you will increase your chances of a long and healthy life.

Other Changes and Additions

We have made a number of subtle changes in this edition that we believe make it an even stronger book than its four predecessors. More specifically, we

- deleted several hundred old references and exchanged them for over 600 recent ones
- reorganized many of the chapters to improve the flow of information
- added several new tables and figures to aid students' understanding of difficult concepts
- strengthened the emphasis on the biopsychosocial approach to health psychology, examining issues and data from a biological, psychological, and social viewpoint
- recognized and emphasized gender issues whenever appropriate
- retained our emphasis on theories and models that strive to explain and predict health-related behaviors

InfoTrac College Edition

This edition also includes a strategy for searching **InfoTrac College Edition,** which is available as a bonus to students who purchase *Health Psychology: An Introduction to Behavior and Health,* fifth edition, published by Wadsworth Publishing Company. We include a list of keyword search terms at the end of each chapter. Using these keyword search terms gives users access to thousands or articles and additional material related to the chapters. This database is directly accessible to students with Internet service, creating an easy way for students to successfully negotiate the Internet.

To access InfoTrac College Edition, enter http://www.infotrac-college.com as the address. The screen that appears will have a box to enter a password that adopters and students receive. Once you enter a valid password, you can perform a keyword search using the suggested terms at the end of each chapter. In addition, InfoTrac College Edition offers search capabilities by subject, and each article includes a linking function that allows users to find additional related publications. This innovative service can introduce students to the Internet or allow experienced users to hone their search skills.

Writing Style

We believe strongly in a readable and engaging writing style, and with each edition, we have worked to improve our connection with readers. Although this edition frequently explores complex issues and difficult topics, we use clear, concise, and comprehensible language as well as an informal writing style. The book is designed for upper-division undergraduate students and should be easily understood by those with a minimal background in psychology and biology. Health psychology courses typically draw students from a variety of college majors, necessitating the inclusion of some elementary material that may be repetitive to some students. For other students, this material will fill in the background they need to comprehend the information within the field of health psychology.

Technical terms appear in **boldface type,** and a definition usually appears at that point in the text. These terms also appear in an end-of-book glossary.

Instructional Aids

Besides a glossary, we have supplied several other features to help both students and instructors. These include stories of people whose behavior typifies the topic, frequent summaries within each chapter, and annotated suggested readings.

Stories

A story from real life appears at the beginning of each chapter—except the first and final ones. The purpose of the stories is to illustrate the topics for that chapter, using real people as examples. Because these people are never perfect examples, we have often been asked why we included features and behaviors that may seem to run counter to what usually happens. The stories are not perfect examples because they come from real people, whereas the typical case is an average of many individuals. We have never invented any specific characteristics for these people but have reported these cases as they are, hoping that their stories will help students personalize the chapter's scientific information. Each story matches research findings in some ways but not others; we hope this imperfection will illustrate to students that real people do not fit the statistical profiles in every way.

We would like to thank the people who shared details of their lives with us so that we could write these stories. We have changed some details of their lives to protect their privacy, but we have preserved those details of their stories that relate to their health and behavior.

Within-Chapter Summaries

Rather than waiting until the end of each chapter to present a lengthy chapter summary, we have placed shorter summaries at key points within each chapter. In general, these summaries correspond to each major topic in a chapter. We believe these shorter, more frequent summaries will keep readers on track and promote a greater understanding of the chapter's content.

Annotated Suggested Readings

At the end of each chapter are three or four annotated suggested readings that students may wish to examine. We chose these readings for their capacity to shed additional light on major topics in a chapter. Most of these suggested readings are quite recent, but we have also selected several that have lasting interest. We have included only those readings that are intelligible to the average college student and that are accessible in most college and university libraries.

Study Guide

We have authored the study guide for the fifth edition of *Health Psychology: An Introduction to Behavior and Health* because we feel that a study guide written by the textbook's authors provides students with a more accurate and meaningful account of the contents of the text. Like the textbook, the study guide is divided into 17 chapters. Each chapter of the study guide begins with a challenge to students to "Fill in the Rest of the Story," a feature that should facilitate learning through active participation.

In addition, the study guide contains a variety of *test questions* and a "Let's Get Personal" feature that provides students an opportunity to integrate health information into their personal lives. We believe these features will help students organize their study methods and will also enhance their chances of achieving their best scores on class quizzes.

Instructor's Manual

This edition of *Health Psychology: An Introduction to Behavior and Health* is accompanied by a comprehensive instructor's manual. Each chapter begins with a *lecture outline,* designed to assist instructors in preparing lecture material from the text. Many instructors will be able to lecture strictly from these notes; others will be able to use the lecture outline as a framework for organizing their own lecture notes.

A test bank of nearly 1,300 *multiple-choice test items* makes up a large section of each chapter of the instructor's manual. We wrote these test items. Some of these items are factual, some are conceptual, and others ask students to apply what they have learned. These test items will reduce instructors' work in preparing tests. Each item, of course, is marked with the correct answer.

We have added *True/False questions* to this edition of the Instructor's Manual for Health Psychology. Instructors now have a choice among 10 of these items per chapter. We also included *essay questions* for each chapter, along with an outline answer of the critical points that should appear in answers to these questions.

Each chapter also includes *suggested activities.* These activities vary widely—from video recommendations to student research to classroom debates. We have tried to include more activities than any instructor can feasibly assign during a semester to give instructors a choice of activities.

The growing availability of electronic resources prompted us to include a *Surf the Net* activity. In this section, we suggest online activities, including Web sites that are relevant to each chapter. This activity supplements Wadsworth's InfoTrac College Edition, expanding the electronic resources students may use to explore health-related topics.

New Instructor's Resource CD-ROM with Biology Animations

This exciting new CD-ROM includes figures from the book in PowerPoint format, plus animations of biological/physiological processes that make difficult, abstract concepts easier to understand.

MyCourse 2.1

Whether you want only the easy-to-use tools to build an online course or the content to furnish it, MyCourse 2.1 offers you a simple solution for a custom Web site that allows you to assign, track, and report on student progress, load your syllabus, and more. Contact your local Wadsworth representative for details.

Acknowledgments

Many people have contributed to the completion of this book, and we wish to express our gratitude. First, we thank Patrick Moreno, who has acted as adviser and librarian. His untiring efforts to make the book better have made the book better.

Next, we acknowledge the considerable assistance of the staff at the McNeese library, whose help has been essential for the completion of this project. Brantley Cagle and Jeannie Brock have been especially helpful—each has exhibited outstanding skill and constant good humor in acquiring material for our use.

In addition, we would like to thank the people at Wadsworth for their assistance. Michele Sordi served as editor for the fifth edition, and we are grateful for her helpful suggestions for improving this book. Marianne Taflinger supervised two prior editions and helped shape the book in many ways. Chris Caldeira, Marketing Manager, Jennifer Wilkinson, Assistant Editor, Chelsea Junget, Editorial Assistant, Laurel Anderson, Marketing Assistant, Darin Derstine, Managing Technology Project Manager, Paul Wells, Production Project Manager, and Vernon Boes, Art Director have also provided excellent support in the preparation of this edition. We are also indebted to a number of reviewers who read all or parts of the manuscript for this and earlier editions. We are grateful for the valuable comments of the following reviewers:

Richard Lazarus, University of California, Berkeley (deceased)

Ralph Paffenbarger, Jr., Stanford School of Medicine

Paul B. Paulus, University of Texas, Arlington

David Abwender, SUNY Brockport

Bruce Bartholow, University of North Carolina, Chapel Hill

Jerusha Detweiler-Bedell, Lewis and Clark College

Nancy Dye, Humboldt State University

Sussie Eshun, East Stroudsburg University

Regan Gurung, University of Wisconsin, Green Bay

Susan Johnson, University of North Carolina, Charlotte

Authors typically thank their spouses for being understanding, supportive, and sacrificing. We thank our spouses, Barry Humphus and Mary Jo Feist, because they were understanding, supportive, and sacrificing. But they have given much more than the traditional emotional support. Both have made contributions that have helped to shape the book. In addition to his creative contributions to the book, Barry provided generous, patient, live-in, expert computer consultation that proved essential in the preparation of the manuscript, and Mary Jo has made suggestions on style and content.

About the Authors

Linda Brannon and Jess Feist are both Professors in the Department of Psychology at McNeese State University in Lake Charles, Louisiana. Linda joined the faculty at McNeese after receiving her doctorate in human experimental psychology from the University of Texas at Austin, and Jess came to McNeese after receiving his doctorate in counseling from the University of Kansas. Jess and Linda have each been selected to receive the annual Distinguished Faculty Award from McNeese State University.

In the early 1980s, Linda and Jess became interested in the developing field of health psychology, which led to their co-authoring the first edition of this book. They have watched the field of health psychology emerge and grow, and the subsequent editions of the book reflect that growth and development.

Their interests converge in the area of health psychology but diverge in other areas of psychology. Jess carries his interest in personality theory to his authorship of *Theories of Personality,* co-authored with his son Greg Feist. Linda's interest in gender and gender issues led her to publish

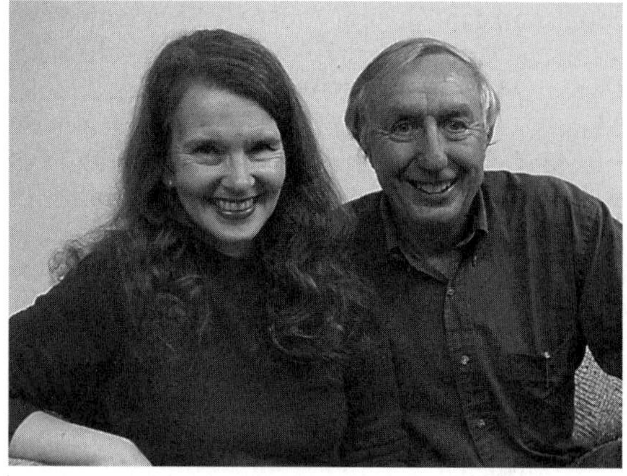

Gender: Psychological Perspectives, and she is also co-author of *Psychology,* which is an introductory psychology textbook.

When he relaxes from his writing and teaching duties, Jess plays golf, gardens, and jogs. Linda is also a jogger, but not as enthusiastic about it (or as good at it) as Jess. Linda would rather watch movies than jog.

1

Introducing Health Psychology

CHAPTER OUTLINE

The Changing Field of Health

Psychology's Involvement in Health

QUESTIONS

This chapter focuses on two basic questions:

1. How have views of health changed?

2. What is psychology's involvement in health?

Before beginning this chapter, please take the time to complete the "Check Your Health Knowledge" questionnaire found on the inside front cover. The answers to questions 1, 2, and 3 appear in this chapter, and those answers differ from many people's expectations. Indeed, misconceptions concerning health information are common, which means that students have trouble answering these health questions accurately.

The Changing Field of Health

A century ago, most people in the United States had views of disease and health that were similar to those who answered "True" to question 1 on the questionnaire on the inside front cover; they saw health as the absence of disease. However, the diseases that were most common 100 years ago differed from the picture of illness today. In the early 1900s, people's diseases were largely the result of contact with impure drinking water, contaminated foods, or sick people. Once they were ill, people were expected to seek medical care to be cured, but medicine had few cures to offer. The duration of most diseases—such as typhoid fever, pneumonia, and diphtheria—was relatively short; a person either died or got well in a matter of weeks. People felt very limited responsibility for contracting a disease because they believed it was impossible to avoid a contagious disease. That situation has changed.

During the 20th century, health in the United States changed in several important ways. First, the leading causes of death changed from infectious diseases to those that relate to unhealthy behaviors and lifestyle. Second, the escalating cost of medical care rose sharply, spotlighting the importance of educating people about how health-related behaviors could lower their risk of becoming ill. Third, a new definition of health emerged, one that regarded health as the presence of positive well-being, not merely the absence of disease. Fourth, some people in the health care field began to advocate a broader perspective of health and disease, questioning the usefulness of the traditional biomedical model.

Patterns of Disease and Death

The 20th century brought about monumental changes in the patterns of disease and death in the United States. During the first 95 years of that century, the major causes of death shifted from infectious diseases such as influenza, pneumonia, tuberculosis, and diphtheria to **chronic diseases,** such as heart disease, cancer, and other disorders that develop and then persist or recur over a long period of time. Then, during the last few years of the 20th century, deaths from chronic diseases—those related to unhealthy lifestyles and behaviors—began to *decrease* while deaths from diseases not closely related to lifestyles and behaviors began to *increase.*

Causes of Death Chronic diseases are not new, of course, but the proportion of people who die of them has changed dramatically since 1900. Figure 1.1 reveals important differences in the leading causes of death in the United States as recorded in 1900 and 2000. In 1900, the majority of deaths were from diseases that were rooted in public or community health problems, such as pneumonia, tuberculosis, and diarrhea. Currently, most deaths are attributable to diseases associated with individual behavior and lifestyle. Heart disease, cancer, stroke, chronic lower respiratory diseases (including emphysema and chronic bronchitis), unintentional injuries, diabetes, suicide, and cirrhosis of the liver have been linked to cigarette smoking, alcohol abuse, unwise eating, stress, and sedentary lifestyle. As Robert Sapolsky (1998, p. 2) said, "we are now living well enough and long enough to slowly fall apart."

However, a closer look at recent data indicates a *decrease* in mortality from diseases associated largely with individual behavior and lifestyle. Of the top 15 causes of death in the United States, 9 had lower mortality rates in

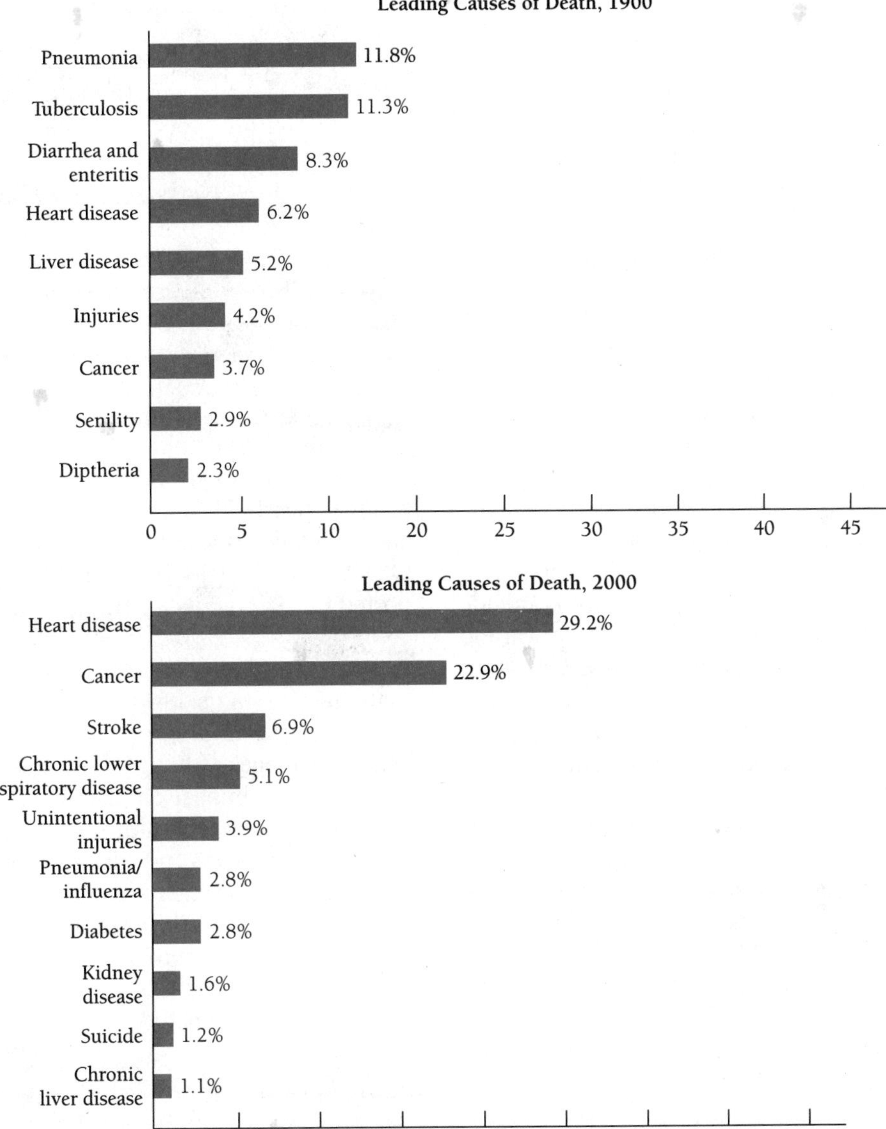

Figure 1.1 Leading causes of death, United States, 1900 and 2000.

Sources: "Healthy people, 2010," 2000, by U.S. Department of Health and Human Services, Washington, DC: U.S. Government Printing Office; and "Deaths: Preliminary data for 2000," 2001, by A. M. Minino & B. L. Smith, National Vital Statistics Report, *vol. 49 no. 12, pp.14–17.*

2000 than in 1999. Of these 9 diseases, all have at least some behavior component. For example, from 1999 to 2000, homicide decreased 7%, followed in order by unintentional injuries (accidents), heart disease, suicide, stroke, chronic lower respiratory disease, chronic liver disease and cirrhosis, cancer, and diabetes. In contrast, the causes of death that increased from 1999 to 2000 had a smaller behavior component. These diseases included Alzheimer's disease, influenza and pneumonia, kidney disease, and septicemia, or blood infection (Hoyert, Freedman, Strobino, & Guyer, 2001).

These data suggest that the causes of death that are decreasing, such as homicide and unintentional injuries, are those associated with mortality among young and middle-aged people, whereas those that are increasing, such as Alzheimer's disease, influenza, and pneumonia, are more likely to strike older people. Thus, the ranking of causes of death for the entire population may not reflect any specific age group. For example, cardiovascular disease (which includes heart disease and stroke) and cancer account for about 60% of all deaths in the United States, but they are not the leading cause of death for young people. For individuals between 15 and 24 years of age, unintentional injuries are the leading cause of death. These injuries account for almost 44% of the deaths in this age group, homicide for about 15%, and suicide for 12.5% (Minino & Smith, 2001). As Figure 1.2 reveals, other causes of death account for much smaller percentages of deaths among adolescents and young adults than unintentional injuries, homicide, and suicide.

For adults 25 to 44 years old, the picture is somewhat different. Unintentional injuries are also their leading cause of death, but they account for only less than half as many deaths in this age group as for 15- to 24-year-olds. Cancer is the cause of death for almost 16% of people in this age group, followed closely by heart disease. As Figure 1.2 shows, suicide and homicide account for substantially smaller percentages of deaths in people 25 to 44, but HIV is much higher for this age group (Minino & Smith, 2001).

Ethnicity, Income, and Disease In the United States, ethnic background is strongly related to health and life expectancy. Question 2 from the quiz at the beginning of this chapter asked if the United States is among the top 10 nations in the world in terms of life expectancy. If African Americans and European Americans in the United States were considered to be different nations, European America would have a higher ranking, indicating a longer life expectancy. However, even European America would not be in the top 10; that ranking would be 12th in the world in terms of life expectancy. African America has a much shorter life expectancy; that ranking would be 33rd in the world (Dwyer, 1995). Thus, neither ethnic group ranks as high as nations such as Japan and Canada in terms of longevity.

The dramatic difference between Whites and African Americans does not apply to Hispanic Americans, although they have socioeconomic disadvantages similar to African Americans (CDC, 2001d). Those disadvantages include poverty and low educational level, both of which have health consequences. Less than 10% of European Americans live below the poverty level, whereas nearly 30% of both African Americans and Hispanic Americans do (USDHHS, 2000). One study (Abdel-Ghany & Wang, 2001) reported that people who have low educational levels are less likely than other people to have health insurance, and another study (Shi, 2001) found that minority status, low income, and poor health are all related to a low probability of adequate health coverage. Although these economic differences have an impact on health and health care, the reasons for the health discrepancy between Hispanic Americans and African Americans must have other origins and remain poorly understood.

Access to health insurance and medical care are not the only factors that make poverty a health risk. Indeed, the health risks associated with poverty begin before birth. With no prenatal care, poor mothers, especially teen mothers, are more likely to deliver low-birth-weight babies, who are more likely than normal-birth-weight infants to die (Hoyert et al., 2001). Also, pregnant women living below the poverty line are more likely than other pregnant women to be physically abused and to deliver babies who suffer the consequences of prenatal child abuse (Zelenko, Lock, Kraemer, & Steiner, 2000).

Income level is strongly related to health, not only at the poverty level but at higher income levels as well. Within any income group, such as the middle class, those at higher levels have better health and lower mortality than those at lower

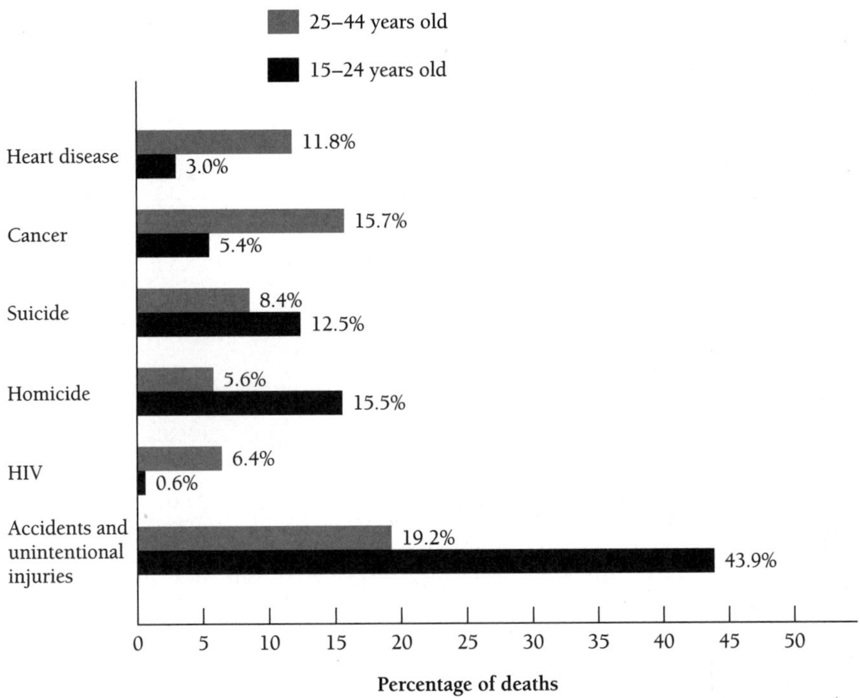

Figure 1.2 Leading causes of death among adults, 15 to 24 versus 25 to 44, United States, 2000.

Source: "Deaths: Preliminary data for 2000, 2001," by A. M. Minino and B. L. Smith, 2001, National Vital Statistics Report, *vol. 49, no. 12, pp. 25–26.*

levels, but the reasons for this relationship remain unclear. One possibility is the relation of income to educational level, which, in turn, is related to occupation, social class, and ethnicity. In addition, low educational level is related to behaviors that increase health risks such as smoking, eating a high-fat diet, and maintaining a sedentary lifestyle; that is, the higher the educational level, the less likely people are to engage in unhealthy behaviors (Lantz et al., 1998). Thus, the possibilities for influence are numerous, and the mechanisms that underlie the relationship of health to income, ethnicity, educational level, and social class remain to be clarified.

Changes in Life Expectancy During the 20th century, life expectancy rose dramatically in the United States and other industrialized nations. In 1900, life expectancy was 47.3 years (USBC, 1975), whereas today it is nearly 77 years (United States Department of Health and Human Services [USDHHS], 2000). In other words, infants born today can, on average, expect to live more than a generation longer than their great-great-grandparents born at the beginning of the 20th century.

What factors have accounted for the 30-year increase in life expectancy during the 20th century? Question 3 from the quiz at the beginning of this chapter asked if advances in medical care were responsible for this increase, but other factors are more important. The control of many infectious diseases through widespread vaccination as well as safer drinking water and milk supplies were the most important changes. A healthier lifestyle also contributed, as did more efficient disposal of sewage, and better nutrition. The contribution of medical advances such as antibiotics and advanced surgical technology, efficient paramedic teams, and more

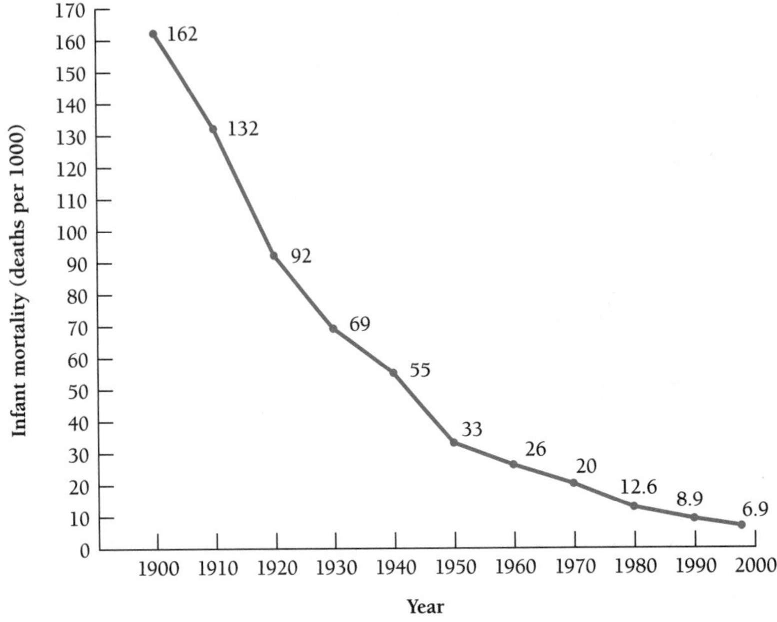

Figure 1.3 Decline in infant mortality in the United States, 1900 to 2000 (rates per 1,000).

Source: Data from "Annual summary of vital statistics: 2000," 2001, by D. L. Hoyert, M. A. Freedman, D. M. Strobino, & B. Guyer, Pediatrics, 108, *1241–1255; and* Historical Statistics of the United States: Colonial Times to 1970, *1975, by U.S. Bureau of the Census, Washington, DC: U.S. Government Printing Office, p. 60.*

skilled intensive care personnel played a relatively minor role in increased life expectancy.

Although these advances helped extend lives, the single most important contributor to the increase in life expectancy was the lowering of infant mortality. When infants die before their first birthday, these deaths lower the population's average life expectancy much more than the deaths of middle-aged or elderly people. Thus, decreasing deaths at a young age can have a substantial statistical impact. As Figure 1.3 shows, a dramatic decline in infant death rates occurred between 1900 and 2000. Unfortunately, this benefit did not apply equally to all ethnic groups. African American infants are nearly three times as likely as European American infants to die in infancy—14.0 per 1,000 births versus 5.7. Again, Hispanic Americans have about the same rate of infant mortality as do European Americans, despite having the disadvantages of lower educational levels and higher rates of poverty than European Americans.

Escalating Cost of Medical Care

The second major change within the field of health has been the escalating cost of medical care. These costs, of course, have some relationship to increased life expectancy: as people live to middle and old age, they tend to develop chronic diseases that require extended (and often expensive) medical treatment. People who die at age 65 have an average lifetime expenditure for medical costs of about $31,000, whereas those who live to age 90 have an average lifetime cost of about $200,000, an increase due largely to increases in nursing home costs (Spillman & Lubitz, 2000). Thus, the increasing life expectancy, in the absence of a healthier old age, will continue to contribute to medical costs.

In the United States, medical costs have increased at a much faster rate than inflation. Between 1960 and 1995, these costs represented a larger and larger proportion of the gross domestic product (GDP). Since 1995, however, the pro-

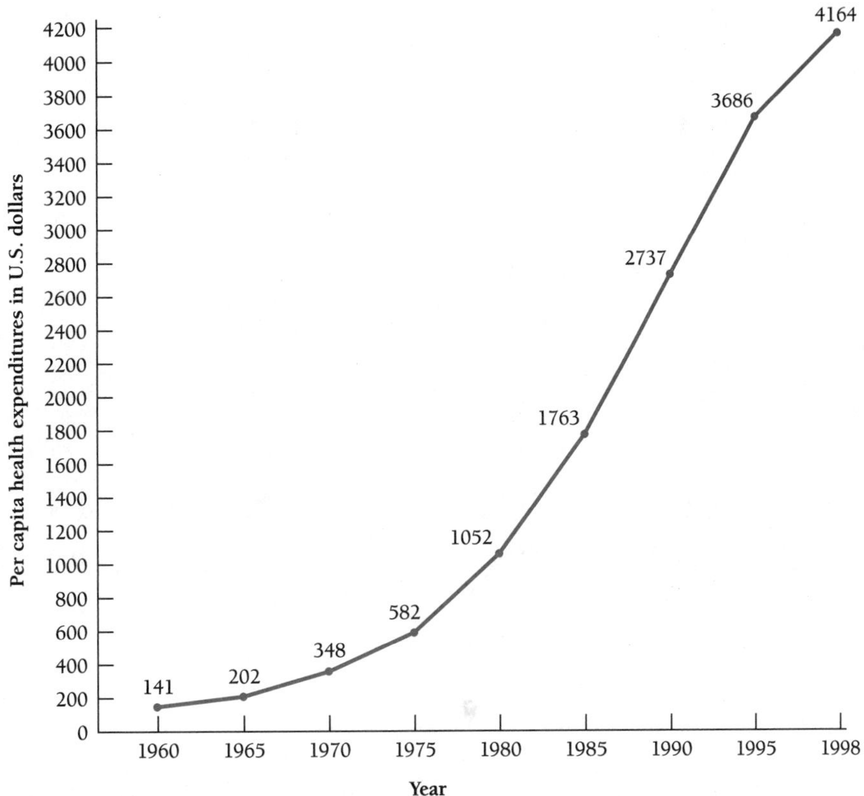

Figure 1.4 Per capita health expenditures, United States, 1960 to 1998.

Source: Data from Health, United States, 2001, *2001, by National Center for Health Statistics, Hyattsville, MD: U.S. Government Printing Office, p. 327.*

portion of medical care costs to the GDP has leveled off at about 13%. Nevertheless, this percentage of the GDP is greater than that of any other country, with only Germany and Switzerland spending more than 10% of their GDP on medical care. Figure 1.4 shows that from 1975 to 1998, the total yearly cost of health care increased from $582 to $4,164 per person, a jump of more than 600% and a much faster annual increase than that reported for the years 1960 to 1975 (National Center for Health Statistics, 2001).

Although medical treatment during the 20th century has performed nearly miraculous cures for some individuals, the mounting monetary costs of medical miracles militate against the traditional philosophy of health, which emphasizes diagnosis, treatment, and cure. Expensive medical procedures such as heart surgery, hemodialysis, and high-technology imaging techniques contribute substantially to the rising cost of health care in the United States, even though they are used with only a relatively small proportion of the population.

Curbing mounting medical costs requires a greater emphasis on the early detection of disease and on changes to a healthier lifestyle and to behaviors that help prevent disease. For example, early detection of high blood pressure, high serum cholesterol, and other precursors of heart disease allows these conditions to be controlled, thereby decreasing the risk of serious disease or death. Screening people for risk is preferable to remedial treatment because chronic diseases are quite difficult to cure and living with chronic disease decreases quality of life. Avoiding disease by adopting a healthy lifestyle is even more

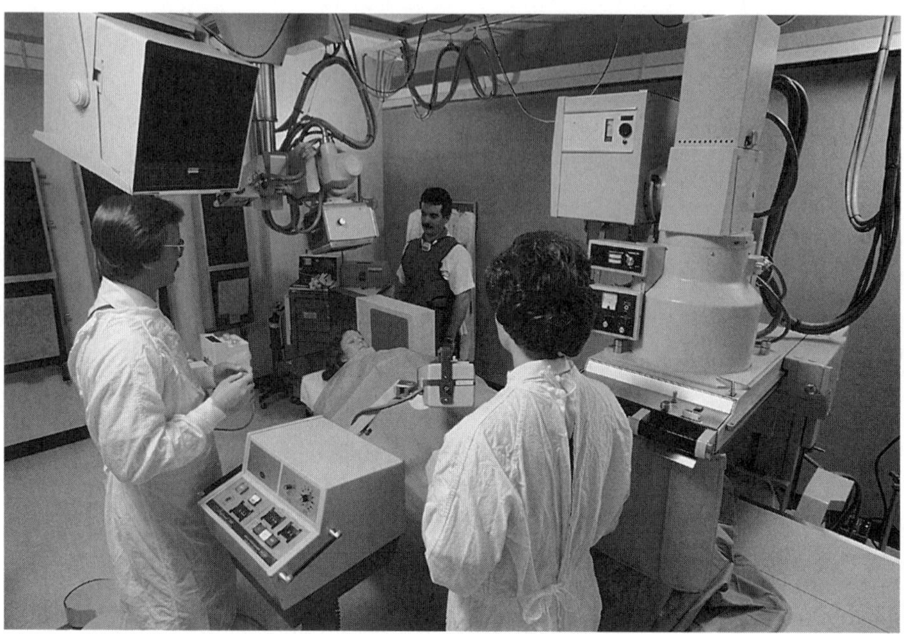

Corbis

Technology in medicine is one reason for escalating medical costs.

preferable to treating diseases or screening for risks. Staying healthy is typically less costly than becoming sick and then getting well. Thus, prevention of disease through a healthy lifestyle, early detection of symptoms, and reduction of health risks have all become part of the changing philosophy within the health care field.

What Is Health?

What does it mean to be healthy? Question 1 from the questionnaire on the inside front cover asked if health is an absence of disease. Is it more complex? Is health the presence of some positive condition? Is health a single condition, or is it multidimensional?

According to George Stone (1987), definitions of health fall into two categories: those that portray health as an ideal state and those that portray health as movement in a positive direction. The first definition implies that any disease or injury is a deviation from good health and that the ideal state can be restored by removing the disease or disability. With this limited definition of health, a blind concert violinist would not be healthy, despite his or her accomplishments, productivity, and contribution to society. The second definition avoids this problem by considering health as a direction on a continuum. This definition implies that movement toward greater health is better than movement in the opposite direction. But because health is multidimensional, all aspects of living—biological, psychological, and social—must be considered. By this definition, a scientist who disregards personal safety or physical health to search for a cure for contagious disease would be moving away from biological health but toward social and perhaps psychological health.

One part of good health, in Stone's view, is improved biological functioning, such as normal blood pressure, superior cardiac output, a high level of respiratory volume, and the ability to withstand stress, infection, and physical injury. Stone proposed that the psychological manifestation of health is a subjective feeling of well-being. Social manifestations of health include the capacity for high levels of social productivity and low demands on the health care system.

Has the definition of health varied over time or over different cultures? Table 1.1 summarizes the

TABLE 1.1 *Definitions of Health Held by Various Cultures*

Culture	Time Period	Health Is
Prehistoric	10,000 BCE	endangered by spirits that enter the body from outside
Babylonians and Assyrians	1800–700 BCE	endangered by the gods, who send disease as a punishment
Ancient Hebrews	1000–300 BCE	a gift from God, but disease is a punishment from God
Ancient Greeks	500 BCE	a holistic unity of body and spirit
Ancient China		a balance of the forces of nature
Galen in Ancient Rome	130 CE–200 CE	the absence of pathogens, such as bad air or body fluids, that cause disease
Early Christians	300 CE–600 CE	not as important as disease, which is a sign that one is chosen by God
Descartes in France	1596–1650	a condition of the mechanical body, which is separate from the mind
Vichow in Germany	late 1800s	endangered by microscopic organisms that invade cells, producing disease
Freud in Vienna	late 1800s	influenced by emotions and the mind
World Health Organization	1946	"a state of complete physical, mental, and social well-being"

definitions that people in various cultures and during different times have held regarding health. In 1946, the United Nations established the World Health Organization (WHO) and wrote into the preamble of its constitution a modern, Western definition: "Health is a state of complete physical, mental and social well-being, and not merely the absence of disease or infirmity." This definition clearly affirms that health is a positive state.

Changing Models of Health

Throughout the 20th century, the biomedical model allowed medicine to conquer or control many of the diseases that once ravaged humanity. The **biomedical model** is the perspective that considers disease to be a simple, almost mechanistic result of exposure to a specific **pathogen,** a disease-causing organism. This view spurred the development of synthetic drugs and medical technology, which in turn engendered the belief that many diseases could be cured. However, the belief that a disease is traceable to a specific agent places more focus on disease than on health. In addition, this biomedical model defined health exclusively in terms of the absence of disease.

Although the biomedical model of disease has been the predominant view in medicine, an alternative model has evolved, one that advocates a *holistic* approach to medicine. This holistic model considers social, psychological, physiological, and even spiritual aspects of a person's health. While conceding that the biomedical model has been responsible for much progress in the treatment of disease, a few physicians, many psychologists, and some sociologists have become dissatisfied with the biomedical model and have begun to question its usefulness in dealing with the current patterns of disease and death.

Dissatisfaction, however, is not sufficient to prompt a shift to a newer model. An alternative model must have the power of the old model plus the ability to solve problems that the old model has failed to solve. In the health field, this alternative model is called the **biopsychosocial model,** the approach to health that includes biological, psychological, and social influences. The biopsychosocial model has at least two advantages over the older biomedical model; first, it incorporates not only biological conditions but also psychological and social factors, and second, it once again views health as a positive condition.

Although the biomedical model was the dominant view of medicine during the 20th century, before 1900, most physicians held a view of disease that emphasized the patient more than the symptoms. Joseph Matarazzo (1994), a pioneer in the development of health psychology, argued that before the widespread use of drugs, a compassionate, empathic bedside manner was about all that physicians had to offer patients. He also contended that the relatively recent explosion of scientific knowledge in such areas as biology, physiology, chemistry, and microbiology has produced several generations of physicians who know little about that type of bedside manner.

In Summary

Four major trends have changed the field of health care in the past century. One trend is the changing pattern of disease and death in the United States and other industrialized nations. Chronic diseases have replaced infectious diseases as the leading causes of death and disability. These chronic diseases include heart disease, stroke, cancer, emphysema, and adult-onset diabetes, all of which have causes that include individual behavior.

The increase in chronic disease has contributed to a second trend: the escalating cost of medical care. Costs for medical care rose dramatically between 1975 and 1995, but more recently, they have shown some stability in relation to the gross domestic product. Much of this cost is due to a growing elderly population and innovative but expensive medical technology as well as to inflation.

A third trend is the changing definition of health. Many people continue to view health as the absence of disease, but a growing number of health care professionals view health as a state of positive well-being. To accept this definition of health is to reconsider the biomedical model that has dominated health.

The emergence of the biopsychosocial model of health is the fourth trend that has changed the health care field. Rather than defining disease as the simple presence of pathogens, the biopsychosocial model emphasizes positive health and sees disease, particularly chronic disease, as resulting from the interaction of biological, psychological, and social conditions.

Psychology's Involvement in Health

Although chronic diseases have many causes, no one seriously disputes the evidence that individual behavior and lifestyle are strongly implicated in their development. Because most chronic diseases stem at least partly from individual behavior, psychology—the science of behavior—has become involved in health care.

A large part of psychology's involvement in health care is a commitment to keeping people healthy rather than waiting to treat them after they become ill. Psychology shares this role with medicine and other health care disciplines, but unlike medicine (which tends to study specific diseases), psychology contributes certain broad principles of behavior that cut across specific diseases and specific issues of health. Among psychology's contributions to health care are techniques for changing behaviors that have been implicated in chronic diseases. In addition to changing unhealthy behaviors, psychologists have also used their skills to relieve pain and reduce stress, improve compliance with medical advice, and help patients and family members live with chronic illnesses.

Psychology in Medical Settings

Psychology has been involved with people's physical health almost from the beginning of the 20th century. In 1911, the American Psychological Association (APA) convened a panel to discuss the role of psychology in medical education. Psychologists of the time agreed that medical students would profit from instruction in psychology and recommended psychology as part of premedical training or the medical school curriculum. As reasonable as this proposal now seems, most medical

WOULD YOU BELIEVE

College Is Good for Your Health

Would you believe that attending college may be good for your health? Many college students may find it difficult to believe that college improves their health. To the contrary, college seems to add stress, offer opportunities for drugs use, and limit the time available for eating a healthy diet, exercising, and sleeping. How could going to college possibly be healthy?

College students may not follow all recommendations for leading a healthy life, but people who go to college have lower death rates than those who do not enroll. This advantage applies to both women and men and to infectious diseases, chronic diseases, and unintentional injuries (NCHS, 2001). Education provides an overall health advantage: People who graduate from high school have lower death rates than those who do not, but going to college offers much more protection. For example, people with less than a high school education died at a rate of 561 per 100,000; those who graduated from high school showed a rate of 465 per 100,000, but people who attended college had a death rate of only 223 per 100,000. That is, people who have attended college showed a death rate of less than half that of high school graduates.

What factors contribute to this health advantage for people with more education? People who attend college, and especially those who graduate from college, have higher average incomes than those who do not, and thus they are more likely to have access to health care. In addition, educated people are more likely to be informed consumers of health care, gathering information on their diseases and potential treatments. Education is also associated with a variety of health-related habits that are positively related to good health and long life. For example, people with a college education are less likely than others to smoke or use illicit drugs (Johnston, O'Malley, & Bachman, 2001), and they are more likely to eat a low-fat diet and to exercise. Examining both financial and behavioral differences related to education, a group of Dutch researchers (Schrijvers, Stronks, van de Mheen, & Mackenbach, 1999) attempted to determine which set of factors was most influential for the health difference in educational level. This analysis indicated that the financial factors were somewhat more important than the behavioral ones, but it is almost impossible to separate these two categories of influences. That is, people who are employed with few financial problems are also more likely to exercise, maintain a healthy weight, and not smoke. Thus, people who attend college acquire many resources that are reflected in their lower death rate—income potential, health knowledge, attitudes about the importance of health, and positive health habits.

schools failed to pursue the recommendation. The APA again broached the topic in 1928 and once more in 1950, but medical schools implemented few changes during that time. According to a 1913 survey of medical schools, only 27% of those with academic affiliations collaborated with psychology departments (Franz, 1913).

During the 1940s, medical training typically incorporated the study of psychological factors as they relate to disease, but this training was usually conducted by physicians and was limited to the medical specialty of psychiatry. Before 1950, only a handful of psychologists were employed in medical schools (Matarazzo, 1994), and the duties of most of those were limited largely to teaching. A few of these clinical psychologists provided psychological services, such as testing and psychotherapy for patients with emotional problems, but few were involved in research. Also, psychologists seldom collaborated with medical specialists other than psychiatrists. That relationship between psychology and psychiatry can be summarized by saying, "Behavioral science and psychiatry was a good marriage . . . until the behavioral scientists were sought out by other medical departments such as family medicine, pediatrics, internal medicine, and preventive medicine for clinical and research collaboration" (Pattishall, 1989, p. 45). As psychology became more widespread in medical training and as the

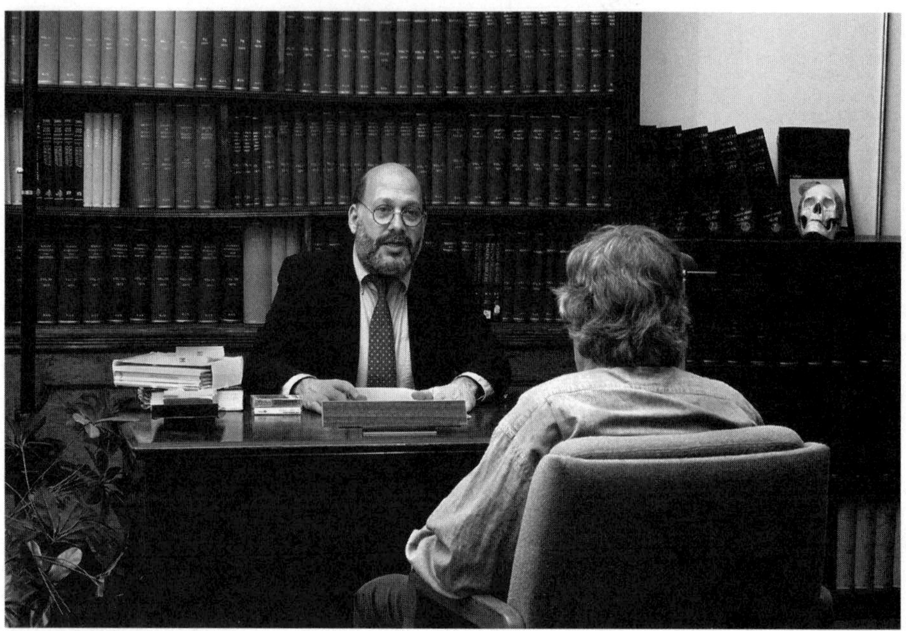
Corbis

By the 1990s psychologists had become staff members of many hospitals.

research base increased to give behavioral science academic credibility, psychology's role in medicine began to expand.

Behavioral science became part of the curriculum in most medical schools in the 1960s, when many new medical schools were established and new curricula for these schools were developed. Matarazzo (1994) estimated that the number of psychologists who held academic appointments on medical school faculties nearly tripled from 1969 to 1993. By the beginning of the 21st century, psychologists had made significant progress in their efforts to gain greater acceptance by the medical profession (Pingitore, Scheffler, Haley, Seniell, & Schwalm, 2001). A 2001 meeting of the APA Council of Representatives reported three recent gains for psychologists working in medical settings. First, the American Medical Association (AMA) has accepted several new categories for health and behavior. These new categories—implemented in 2002—permit psychologists to bill for services for patients with physical diseases; second, Medicare's Graduate Medical Education program now accepts psychology internships; and third, The World Health Organization is working with the APA to adopt a new diagnostic system for biopsychosocial disorders (Thorn & Saab, 2001). In summary, the role of psychologists in medical settings has expanded beyond traditional mental health problems to include procedures and programs to help people stop smoking, eat a healthy diet, exercise, adhere to medical advice, reduce stress, control pain, live with chronic disease, and avoid unintentional injuries.

The Rise, Decline, and Fall of Psychosomatic Medicine

The notion that psychological and emotional factors can contribute to physical ailments can be traced to the days of Socrates and Hippocrates. Early humans saw disease as spiritual as well as physical, and many cultures in ancient history included psychological and social factors in their views of disease. In the 18th century, a German professor named Gaub anticipated the biopsychosocial approach to disease and health when he wrote, "The reason why a sound body becomes ill or an ailing body recovers very often lies in the mind" (as cited in Fritz, 2000, p. 8).

Psychosomatic medicine continued to find a fertile field in the popular theories of Sigmund Freud, who emphasized the importance of unconscious psychological factors in the development of physical symptoms. But Freud's methods relied on clinical experience and intuitive hunches that were largely unverified by laboratory research. The research base for psychosomatic medicine began with Walter Cannon's observation in 1932 that physiological changes accompany emotion (Kimball, 1981). Cannon's research demonstrated that emotion can cause physiological changes that might be related to the development of physical disease; that is, emotion can cause changes, which in turn, may cause disease. From this finding, Helen Flanders Dunbar (1943) developed the notion that habitual responses, which people exhibit as part of their personalities, are related to specific diseases. In other words, Dunbar hypothesized a relationship between personality type and disease. A little later, Franz Alexander (1950), a one-time follower of Freud, began to see emotional conflicts as a precursor to certain diseases.

Unfortunately, these views led others to begin seeing specific illnesses as "psychosomatic." These illnesses included such disorders as peptic ulcer, rheumatoid arthritis, hypertension, asthma, hyperthyroidism, and ulcerative colitis. Many lay people began to look at these psychosomatic disorders as not being "real" but merely "all in the head." Coupled with this oversimplified belief were the modern medical advances that led many in the health care field to neglect the mind–body continuum and to concentrate on powerful remedies for specific diseases. These remedies included penicillin, antibiotics, insulin, and vaccines (Fritz, 2000). With such effective medical procedures available, many physicians and other health care providers began to lose sight of the psychological and social concomitants of disease. Others, however, have supported a newer kind of psychosomatic medicine, one that sees disease as being linked to a complex of biological, psychological, and social factors. Thus, this newer psychosomatic medicine holds that many diseases flow from some combination of genetics, physiology, social support, personal control, stress, compliance, personality, poverty, ethnic background, and cultural beliefs. We discuss each of these factors in subsequent chapters.

The Emergence of Behavioral Medicine

From the remnants of the old psychosomatic medicine emerged two new and interrelated disciplines—*behavioral medicine* and *health psychology*.

A 1977 conference at Yale University led to the definition of a new field, **behavioral medicine,** defined as "the interdisciplinary field concerned with the development and integration of behavioral and biomedical science knowledge and techniques relevant to health and illness and the application of this knowledge and these techniques to prevention, diagnosis, treatment and rehabilitation" (Schwartz & Weiss, 1978, p. 250).

This definition indicates that behavioral medicine is designed to integrate medicine and the various behavioral sciences, especially psychology. The goals of behavioral medicine are similar to those in other areas of health care: improved prevention, diagnosis, treatment, and rehabilitation. Behavioral medicine, then, attempts to use psychology and the behavioral sciences in conjunction with medicine to promote health and treat disease. Chapters 3 through 11 cover topics in behavioral medicine.

The Emergence of Health Psychology

At about the same time that behavioral medicine was given life, a new discipline called *behavioral health* began to emerge. Behavioral health emphasizes the enhancement of health and the prevention of disease in healthy people rather than the diagnosis and treatment of disorders in sick people. Behavioral health includes such concerns as injury prevention, cigarette smoking, alcohol use, diet, and exercise, topics we discuss in Chapters 12 through 16.

Behavioral health has not continued to develop as a strong, formal discipline, and its goals have largely been incorporated by a new field called **health psychology,** the branch of psychology that concerns individual behaviors and lifestyles affecting a person's physical health. Health psychology includes psychology's contributions to the enhancement of health, the prevention and treatment of disease, the identification of health risk factors, the improvement of the health care system, and the shaping of public opinion with regard to health. More specifically, it involves the application of psychological principles to such physical health areas as lowering high blood pressure, controlling cholesterol, managing stress, alleviating pain, stopping smoking, and moderating other risky behaviors, as well as encouraging regular exercise, medical and dental checkups, and safer behaviors. In addition, health psychology helps identify conditions that affect health, diagnose and treat certain chronic diseases, and modify the behavioral factors involved in physiological and psychological rehabilitation. As such, health psychology interacts with both biology and sociology to produce health- and disease-related outcomes (see Figure 1.5). Note that neither psychology nor sociology contribute directly to outcomes; only biological factors contribute directly to physical health and disease.

A Brief History of Health Psychology As an identifiable area, health psychology received its first important impetus in 1973, when the Board of Scientific Affairs of the American Psychological Association (APA) appointed a task force to study the potential for psychology's role in health research. Three years later, this task force (APA, 1976) reported that few psychologists were involved in health research and that research conducted by psychologists in the area of health was not often reported in the psychology journals. However, the report envisioned a future in which health psychology might help to enhance health and prevent disease.

In 1978, the American Psychological Association established Division 38, Health Psychology, as "a scientific, educational, and professional organization for psychologists interested in (or working in) areas at one or another of the interfaces of medicine and psychology" (Matarazzo, 1994, p. 31). Four years later, in 1982, the journal *Health Psychology* began publication as the official journal of Division 38. Currently, health psychology is not only a well-established division within the American Psychological Association but is also recognized by the American Psychological Society, another powerful professional organization, one that emphasizes research over clinical practice.

Health Psychology's Position within Psychology In 2001, the APA membership voted to change its bylaws and to include the term "health" in its mission statement. This statement now reads: "The objects of the American Psychological Association shall be to advance psychology as a science and profession and as a means of promoting health and human welfare . . ." (Thorn & Saab, 2001).

Health psychologists are first and foremost psychologists, with the same basic training as any other psychologists. This training core was determined by the landmark Boulder Conference of 1949, which established psychology as both a scientific discipline and a practicing profession. From that time, every doctoral program within a department of psychology has offered nearly the same core of generic course work for psychologists. Along with the core courses required of all psychologists, health psychologists take courses in such fields as biostatistics, epidemiology, physiology, biochemistry, and cardiology. Like other psychologists, health psychologists rely on and contribute to the basic core of psychological research and then apply this knowledge to a particular field of specialization. In other words, health psychologists are psychologists first and specialists in health second. According to Matarazzo (1987b), "psychology" is the *noun* that identifies the subject matter; and "health" is the *adjective* that describes the client, problem, or setting to

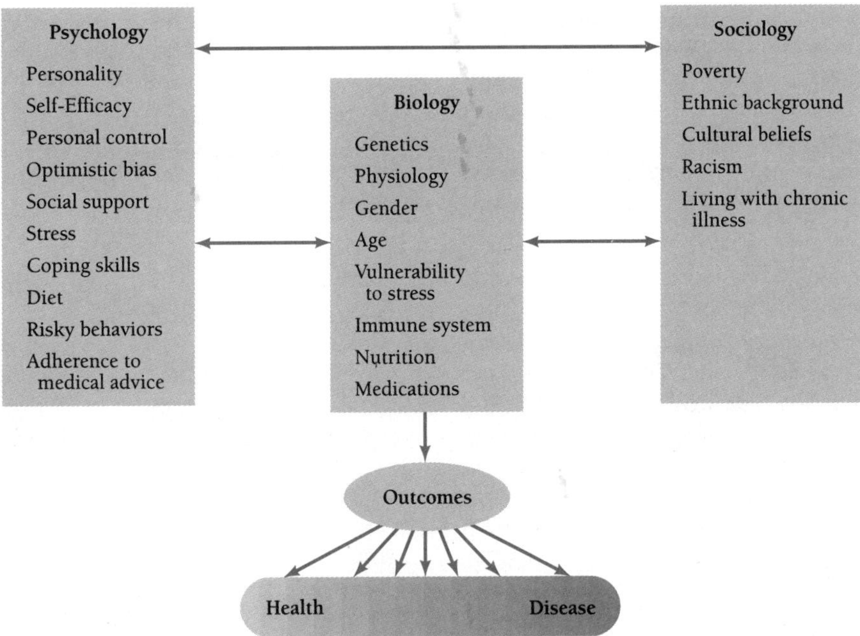

Figure 1.5 The biopsychosocial model. Biological, psychological, and sociological factors interact to produce health or disease.

which psychology is applied. Like other fields of psychology, health psychology applies the principles of generic psychology to a particular area. Health psychology does not exist as a profession separate from generic psychology; rather it applies both research knowledge and clinical experience to the science and profession of generic psychology.

Health psychology has clearly emerged as a unique profession, having met six criteria for a separate profession. First, it has founded its own national and international associations; second, it has established a number of its own journals in addition to *Health Psychology;* third, it has received acknowledgment from professionals in other fields of psychology that its subject matter, methods, and applications are different from theirs; fourth, health psychology has set up postdoctoral training specific to health psychology and distinct from other fields of psychology; fifth, it has received recognition from the American Board of Professional Psychology; and sixth, it has been recognized by the American Psychological Association Commission on the Recognition of Specialties and Proficiencies in Professional Psychology (Belar, 1997; Matarazzo, 1987b; Thorn & Saab, 2001). In addition, health psychology is becoming recognized within medical schools, schools of public health, universities, and hospitals.

In Summary

Psychology's involvement in health dates back to the beginning of the 20th century, but at that time, few psychologists were involved in medicine. The psychosomatic medicine movement sought to bring psychological factors into the understanding of disease, but that view gave way to the biopsychosocial approach to health and disease. By the 1970s, psychologists had begun to develop research and treatment aimed at chronic disease and health promotion; this research and treatment led to the founding of two new fields, behavioral medicine and health psychology.

Behavioral medicine is concerned with applying the knowledge and techniques of behavioral research to physical health, including prevention, diagnosis, treatment, and rehabilitation. Health psychology overlaps behavioral medicine, and the two professions have many common goals. However, behavioral medicine is an interdisciplinary field, whereas health psychology is a specialty within the discipline of psychology that is concerned with issues of physical health. Health psychology strives to enhance health, prevent and treat disease, identify risk factors, improve the health care system, and shape public opinion regarding health issues.

Answers

This chapter addressed two basic questions:

1. How have views of health changed?

Views of health are changing, both among health care professionals and among the general public. Several trends have prompted these changes, including (1) the changing pattern of disease and death in the United States from infectious diseases to chronic diseases; (2) increasing medical costs that, until recently, represented a progressively larger percentage of gross domestic product for the United States; (3) growing acceptance of a view of health that includes not only the absence of disease but also the presence of positive well-being; and (4) an emerging new biopsychosocial model of health that departs from the traditional biomedical model and the psychosomatic model by including not only biochemical abnormalities but also psychological and social conditions.

2. What is psychology's involvement in health?

Psychology has been involved in health almost from the beginning of the 20th century. During those early years, however, only a few psychologists worked in medical settings and most were considered adjuncts rather than full partners with physicians. Psychosomatic medicine emphasized psychological explanations of certain somatic diseases and increased the need for psychologists in the health field. By the 1960s and early 1970s, psychology and other behavioral sciences were beginning to play a role in the prevention and treatment of chronic diseases and in the promotion of positive health, giving rise to two new fields: behavioral medicine and health psychology.

Behavioral medicine is an interdisciplinary field concerned with applying the knowledge and techniques of behavioral science to the maintenance of physical health and to prevention, diagnosis, treatment, and rehabilitation. Behavioral medicine, which is not a branch of psychology, nonetheless overlaps with health psychology, a division within the field of psychology. Health psychology uses the science of psychology to enhance health, prevent and treat disease, identify risk factors, improve the health care system, and shape public opinion with regard to health.

Suggested Readings

Landrine, H. & Klonoff, E. A. (2001). Cultural diversity and health psychology. In A. Baum, T. A. Revenson, & J. E. Singer (Eds.). *Handbook of Health Psychology* (pp. 851–891). Mahwah, NJ: Erlbaum. In this chapter, Hope

Landrine and Elizabeth Klonoff summarize the health beliefs and practices of each of the major ethnic groups in the United States.

Matarazzo, J. D. (1994). Health and behavior: The coming together of science and practice in psychology and medicine after a century of benign neglect. *Journal of Clinical Psychology in Medical Settings, 1,* 7–39. Matarazzo covers many of the same issues discussed in this chapter; in addition, he briefly discusses some examples of misbehaviors, such as smoking, overeating, and living a hostile lifestyle.

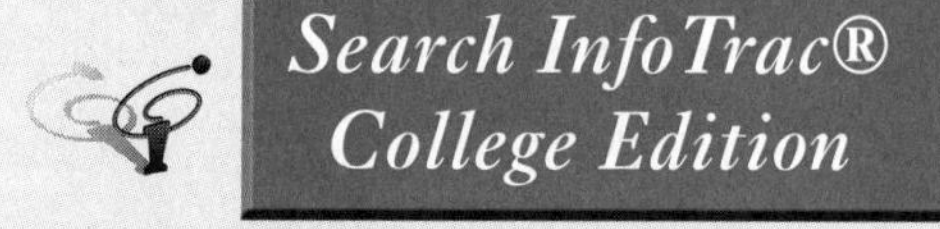

Search these terms to learn more about topics in this chapter:

- Life expectancy and United States
- Life expectancy and demographic aspects
- Disease and 20th century
- Infant mortality and demographic aspects
- Life expectancy and income
- Socioeconomic status and disease
- Culture and medicine and disease
- Biomedical model
- Biopsychosocial and health

2

Conducting Health Research

The Story of Diane

CHAPTER OUTLINE

The Placebo in Treatment and Research

Research Methods in Psychology

Research Methods in Epidemiology

Determining Causation

Research Tools

QUESTIONS

This chapter focuses on five basic questions:

1. What is a placebo and how does it affect research and treatment?
2. How has psychology contributed to health?
3. How has epidemiology contributed to health?
4. How can scientists determine if a behavior causes a disease?
5. How do theory and measurement contribute to health psychology?

The Story of Diane

Diane, a 22-year-old college senior, wanted to quit smoking but did not know how to stop. Her roommate, who was enrolled in a health psychology class, told Diane that smoking was one of the topics included in the course and advised Diane to talk to the professor. When Diane visited the health psychology professor, she asked her to recommend a therapist to hypnotize her so she could quit smoking.

The professor asked Diane why she wanted to use hypnosis rather than some other smoking cessation program, and Diane replied that she had enrolled in a group class in hypnosis 2 years earlier and had quit smoking for almost a year. The professor explained that hypnosis has a number of uses and can be effective for some problems but that hypnosis is not very useful in helping people quit smoking. Nevertheless, Diane believed that hypnosis had been successful for her once and that it would be successful a second time. She did not see her resumption of smoking as a failure of the hypnotherapy; instead, she blamed herself and the stresses in her life for her return to smoking.

Diane insisted that hypnosis was the technique she wanted despite the professor's argument that research had not shown hypnosis to be an effective treatment for smoking. Research evidence did not impress Diane; her personal experience was more important than results from scientific studies. She was convinced that hypnosis would work for her, even if it did not work for other smokers.

Like many people, Diane was relying more on personal experience than research evidence. She believed that her own observations were more valid (especially for her) than research conducted on large groups of people. She did not see that her own biases were interfering with her judgment of the value of hypnosis—that is, Diane had trouble accepting the value of scientific research on a personal level. She had, however, accepted the idea that smoking was dangerous to her health, and she acknowledged that the evidence for this belief also had come from research. Like many people, Diane chose what research to accept and what to ignore.

This chapter looks at the way scientists work, emphasizing psychology from the behavioral sciences and epidemiology from the biomedical sciences. These two disciplines share some methods for investigating health-related behaviors, but the two areas also have their own unique contributions to scientific methodology. Before we begin to examine the methods that psychologists and epidemiologists use in their research, we need to consider what the professor was trying to explain to Diane—that any success with hypnosis might have been due to the **placebo effect,** an effect that is due to expectation rather than to effects of the treatment.

The Placebo in Treatment and Research

Diane had difficulty accepting the notion that the success of her first attempt to quit smoking was probably not due to any specific aspect of hypnosis but may have been the result of her expectations for success. Like many people receiving treatment, Diane benefited from her positive expectations. However, these same expectations can become a disadvantage to scientists trying to evaluate the effectiveness of treatments. Thus, the placebo effect may be helpful to an individual but complicate the job of researchers. That is, it can have treatment benefits but research drawbacks.

A **placebo** is an inactive substance or condition that has the appearance of an active treatment and that may cause participants in an experiment to improve or change behavior due to their belief in the placebo's efficacy. This belief is capable of causing effects separate from any influence of the treatment itself. People act in the ways that they *think* they should, which are influenced by their personal and cultural histories of treatment (Moerman, 2002). In addition, receiving treatment may elicit responses that people have associated with such procedures. That

CHECK YOUR BELIEFS
About Health Research

Check the items that are consistent with your beliefs.

- ☐ 1. Placebo effects can influence both psychological and physical disorders.
- ☐ 2. Pain patients who expect a medication to relieve their pain often experience a reduction in pain after taking a "sugar pill."
- ☐ 3. Personal testimonials are a good way to decide about treatment effectiveness.
- ☐ 4. Newspaper reports of scientific research give an accurate picture of the importance of the research.
- ☐ 5. Information from longitudinal studies is generally more informative than information from the study of one person.
- ☐ 6. All scientific methods yield equally valuable results, so the research method is not important in determining validity of results.
- ☐ 7. Studies with nonhuman subjects can be just as important as those with human participants in determining important health information.
- ☐ 8. Results from experimental research are more likely than results from observational research to suggest a causal relationship.
- ☐ 9. Valuable research is done by people outside the scientific community, but scientists try to discount the importance of such research.
- ☐ 10. Scientific breakthroughs happen every day.
- ☐ 11. Each new report of health research seems to contradict previous findings, so there is no way to use this information to make good personal decisions about health.

Items 1, 2, 5, and 8, are consistent with sound scientific information, but each of the other items represent a na¨ve or unrealistic view of research that can make you an uninformed consumer of health research. Information in this chapter will help you become more sophisticated in your evaluation of and expectations for health research.

is, through classical and operant conditioning, people learn to anticipate certain effects of the treatment (Christensen, 2001). Thus, both expectancy and learning contribute to the placebo effect.

Treatment and the Placebo

The potency of "sugar pills" has long been known. Henry Beecher (1955) observed the effects of people's beliefs and concluded that the therapeutic effect of the placebo was substantial—about 35% of patients showed improvement. However, Judith Turner and her colleagues (Turner, Deyo, Loeser, Von Korff, & Fordyce, 1994) reviewed more than 200 articles dealing with the placebo effect on pain and found that some improvement rates were higher than 35%, but some were lower. For example, some researchers (Kirsch, Moore, Scoboria, & Nicholls, 2002) argued that the placebo effect is responsible for up to 80% of the effectiveness of antidepressant drugs. Both physician and patient expectations can produce reductions in pain, but most physicians greatly underestimate the power of the placebo effect. This effect is related to the reputation of the physician, the expense of treatment, the culture in which treatment occurs, and the attention, interest, and concern shown by the physician (Moerman, 2002).

Placebos are also capable of producing adverse effects, called the **nocebo effect** (Turner et al., 1994). Nearly 20% of healthy volunteers given a placebo in a double-blind study experienced some negative effect as a result of the nocebo effect. The presence of negative effects demonstrates that the placebo effect is not merely improvement but includes any change resulting from receiving a treatment.

The association of the placebo effect with "sugar pills" has led many people to believe that placebo cures are not "real" and that they cure only psychological conditions that have no physical basis. However, placebos have been found to reduce or cure a remarkable range of disorders and symptoms, including insomnia, low back pain, burn pain, headache, asthma, hypertension, anxiety, and Parkinson's disease (Fuente-Fernández et al., 2001; Hrøbjartsson & Gøtzsche, 2001). People who respond positively to drug treatment tend to be the same ones who respond to placebo treatment, and researchers are beginning to establish that the underlying physiological mechanisms for placebo responses are the same as for drug treatments (Amanzio & Benedetti, 1999). In addition, drugs that block the action of analgesic drugs also block the placebo response to analgesic drugs (Benedetti & Amanzio, 1997). These results provide strong evidence that the placebo effect is physiologically real.

The form of placebo medications can affect their potency (Shapiro, 1970). Injections are more powerful than pills. Very large and very small pills are perceived as stronger than medium-sized ones. Colored pills are more effective than plain white pills; capsules produce stronger effects than tablets; brand-name drugs are believed to be better than generics. The improvements are sometimes the same as those caused by physiologically active drugs and other specific medical treatments. Indeed, in most situations involving medical treatment, patients' improvements may be a combination of treatment plus the placebo effect (Christensen, 2001).

When patients' positive expectations increase their chances for improvement, the placebo is a valuable adjunct in counseling and other treatment conditions. Because improvement is the goal of treatment, *any* factor that enhances effectiveness is a bonus. The underlying causes for improvement are the concern of researchers more than practitioners. Therefore, the placebo effect may be considered a positive factor in medical and behavioral therapies, as it was for Diane. Indeed, Diane's belief in the effectiveness of this therapy might lead her to change her behavior, even if hypnosis were ineffective as a therapy for smoking.

Placebo-induced cures are indistinguishable from improvements that occur as a result of other treatments. A cure is a cure, and the method of cure makes no difference to the well-being of patients. Placebo effects are a tribute to the ability of humans to heal themselves, and practitioners can enlist this ability to help patients become more healthy (Ezekiel & Miller, 2001).

Research and the Placebo

The pain-relieving or antidepressant properties of the placebo may be a plus for treatment, but its effects present problems in evaluating a treatment's effectiveness. For a treatment to be judged effective, it must show a higher rate of effectiveness than that produced by a placebo. This standard calls for researchers to use at least two groups: one that receives the treatment and another that receives a placebo. Both groups must have equal expectations concerning the effectiveness of the treatment. In order to create equal expectancy, not only must the participants be ignorant of who is getting a placebo and who is getting the treatment, but the experimenters who dispense both conditions must also be "blind" as to which group is which. The arrangement in which neither participants nor experimenters know about treatment conditions is called a **double-blind** design. As the Would You Believe . . . ? box points out, this design strategy presents ethical dilemmas.

Psychological treatments such as counseling, hypnosis, biofeedback, relaxation training, massage, and a variety of stress and pain management techniques also produce expectancy effects. That is, the placebo effect also applies to research in psychology, but double-blind designs are not so easy to perform with these treatments. Placebo pills can look the same as pills containing an active ingredient, but this situation is more difficult to arrange for behavioral treatments because

WOULD YOU BELIEVE

Providing Ineffective Treatment Is Considered Ethical

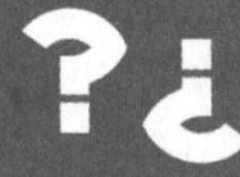

Would you believe that it is ethical for researchers to treat people with techniques that they know to be bogus? To conduct studies on the effectiveness of treatment, researchers need to provide conditions that allow them to establish that effectiveness, but the placebo effect complicates this process. In controlling for participants' expectancies, researchers typically use a double-blind design in which neither the participants nor the experimenters know which participants are in the new treatment group and which are in the placebo group. This arrangement places some participants in a group that receives a placebo, which is an ineffective treatment.

Health care providers are supposed to act in the best interest of their patients, yet the demands of research with new treatments require placebo control designs to demonstrate that new treatments are more effective than a placebo. These two goals seem to be contradictory. How do researchers reconcile this ethical difficulty?

Part of the answer to that question lies in the rules governing research with human participants (APA, 1992). Providing an ineffective treatment—or any other treatment—is ethical if participants know about the risks before they agree to participate in the study. This element of research procedure is known as *informed consent* and stipulates that participants must be informed of factors in the research that may influence their willingness to participate before they consent to participate. Informed consent does not mandate that researchers tell participants exactly what will happen to them, but participants must know about the risks so that they can decide if they want to participate or to withdraw.

When participants in a clinical trial agree to take part in the study, they receive information about the possibility of being assigned to a group that receives a placebo as well as learning about the risks associated with the treatment. Those participants who find the chances of receiving a placebo unacceptable may refuse to participate in the study.

Both participants and researchers in clinical trials must keep in mind that research to develop new treatments is not the same as receiving medical treatment (Horng & Miller, 2002). Health care providers who treat people are ethically obligated to provide the best care that they can. When researchers conduct studies to develop new treatments, they are doing research that may not benefit all participants.

A dramatic example of this conflict—and an example of the placebo effect—comes from a study testing the effectiveness of two different types of arthroscopic knee surgery for osteoarthritis and contrasting each with placebo surgery (Moseley et al., 2002). This study included a placebo group that received sham knee surgery; that is, 60 of the 180 participants underwent a procedure that involved anesthesia and incisions to the knee but no arthroscopic procedure. These patients had experienced pain serious enough to prompt them to seek surgery for their knee problems. In addition, they experienced the risks associated with a surgical procedure, yet they received only sham surgery. This research was ethical because the researchers were careful to let participants know that they were in a research study, allowed those who did not wish to participate to decline (44% did so), and explained the possibility that participants might receive sham surgery. The results indicated that the placebo surgery was as effective as either of the other two types of arthroscopic surgery in relieving knee pain. In this study, the placebo surgery appears to have done no harm to participants. Even if the study had indicated an advantage for the surgical procedures that the placebo group did not receive, the careful use of the informed consent would make the use of placebo surgery ethically acceptable.

the providers always know when they are providing a sham treatment. In these studies, researchers use a **single-blind design** in which the participants do not know if they are receiving the active or inactive treatment, but the providers are not blind to treatment conditions. In single-blind designs, the control for expectancy is not as complete as in double-blind designs, but creating equal expectancies for participants is usually the more important control feature.

In Summary

A placebo is an inactive substance or condition having the appearance of an active treatment. It may cause participants in an experiment to improve or change behavior due to their belief in the placebo's effectiveness and their prior experiences with receiving treatment. Although placebos can have a positive effect from the patient's point of view, they are a continuing problem for the researcher. In general, a placebo's effects are estimated at about 35%; its effects on reducing pain may be higher, whereas its effects on other conditions may be lower. Placebos have been known to influence a wide variety of disorders and diseases, and they can even cause dependence.

Experimental designs that measure the efficacy of an intervention, such as a drug, typically use a placebo so that people in the control group (who receive the placebo) have the same expectations for success as do people in the experimental group (who receive the active treatment). Drug studies are usually double-blind designs, meaning that neither the participants nor the people administering the drug know who receives the placebo and who receives the active drug. Researchers in psychological treatment studies are often not "blind" concerning the treatment, but participants are, creating a single-blind design for these studies.

Research Methods in Psychology

Although Diane was aware of much of the data linking cigarette smoking to heart disease and cancer, she chose to ignore the research on the ineffectiveness of hypnosis as a means of quitting smoking. Instead, she believed the unfounded claims that hypnosis was a simple and painless way to stop smoking. Much unfounded information on health-related behaviors comes from individuals and organizations trying to sell a product. Fortunately, scientists have discovered a vast body of health-related information that is relatively objective and free from self-serving claims. This information has been produced by researchers trained in the behavioral and biomedical sciences who typically are associated with universities and research hospitals. Because these men and women use the methods of science in their work, evidence usually accumulates gradually over an extended period of time. Dramatic breakthroughs are rare.

When scientists are familiar with each other's work, use controlled methods of collecting data, keep personal biases from contaminating results, make claims cautiously, and are able to replicate their studies, evidence is more likely to be evolutionary than revolutionary. Claims to the contrary are most often motivated by financial or other personal interests.

The news media are in the business of getting peoples' attention, so the headlines and news coverage of health information are often misleading. And, of course, commercial advertisements that champion their product as a revolutionary new cure for insomnia, an effortless way to eat all you desire and still lose weight, a simple way to stop smoking, or a food that protects you against cancer or heart disease either are not using or are distorting scientific evidence when they make their claims.

Like many people, Diane was concerned about her health. She not only wanted to quit smoking, but she tried to exercise regularly, watch her diet, and avoid too much stress. But how do people, such as Diane, know that these health practices will indeed contribute to better health? What is the source of health information? Who conducts the basic research that suggests which behaviors are healthy and which are harmful?

Much health-related information comes from studies conducted by behavioral and biomedical scientists using a variety of research methods. The choice of methods depends in large part on what questions the scientists are trying to answer. Because heart disease is the leading cause of death among women and men in every ethnic group in the United States (Landrine & Klonoff, 2001), we have chosen to look at this disease from a variety of research methods, each of which adds to an understanding of heart disease.

As the scientific study of behavior, psychology has made several important contributions to the understanding of those behaviors and lifestyles that relate to health and illness, including heart disease. First, psychology has provided a variety of techniques for changing behaviors that have been implicated in heart disease. Second, psychology is committed to keeping people healthy rather than waiting to treat them after they become ill. Third, psychology has a long history of developing reliable and valid measuring instruments for assessing factors related to heart disease. Fourth, psychologists have constructed and used theoretical models to explain and predict those behaviors associated with heart disease. Fifth, psychology has contributed a solid foundation of scientific methods for studying such behaviors.

When researchers are interested in what factors predict or are related to either disease or healthy functioning, they use correlational studies; when they want to compare people across different age groups, they rely on cross-sectional studies; when they desire information on stability or instability of health status or some other characteristic over a period of time, they use longitudinal studies; and when they wish to compare one group of participants with another, they can use either experimental designs or ex post facto designs. Correlational studies, cross-sectional studies, longitudinal investigations, experimental studies, and ex post facto designs, then, are all methods from the discipline of psychology that have application in the field of health.

Correlational Studies

Correlational studies yield information about the degree of relationship between two variables, such as body fat and heart disease. Correlational studies *describe* this relationship and are, therefore, a type of **descriptive research** design. Although scientists cannot determine causal relationships through a single descriptive study, the degree of relationship between two factors may be exactly what a researcher wants to know.

To assess the degree of relationship between two variables (such as waist circumference and cardiovascular risk factors), the researcher measures each of these variables in a group of participants and then calculates the **correlation coefficient** between these measures. The computation yields a number that varies between − 1.00 and + 1.00. Positive correlations occur when the two variables increase or decrease together. Negative correlations occur when one of the variables increases as the other decreases. Correlations that are closer to 1.00 (either positive or negative) indicate stronger relationships than do correlations that are closer to 0.00. Small correlations—those less than 0.10—can be *statistically significant* if they are based on a very large number of scores. However, such small correlations, though not random, offer the researcher very little ability to predict scores on one variable from knowledge of scores on the other variable.

Correlation allowed a group of researchers (Waldstein, Burns, Toth, & Poehlman, 1999) to determine the relationship between waist circumference and a group of cardiovascular risk factors in elderly African American women and men. The study showed significant correlations between waist size and systolic blood pressure, diastolic blood pressure, and heart rate. These results suggest that waist circumference is related to known risk factors for cardiovascular disease and therefore waist size itself is a risk factor for heart disease. (A **risk factor** is any characteristic or condition that occurs with greater frequency in people with a disease than in people free from that disease.)

Cross-Sectional and Longitudinal Studies

Researchers use two approaches to study developmental issues. **Cross-sectional studies** are those conducted during only one point in time, whereas **longitudinal studies** follow participants over an extended period. In a cross-sectional design, the investigator studies a group of people from at least two different age groups to determine the possible differences between the groups for some variable of interest, such as degree of blockage of coronary arteries, systolic blood pressure, cholesterol level, or other measures.

Longitudinal studies can yield information that cross-sectional studies cannot because they assess the same people over time, which allows researchers to identify developmental trends and patterns. However, longitudinal studies have one obvious drawback: They take time. The time factor usually makes longitudinal studies more costly than cross-sectional studies, and they frequently require a large team of researchers.

Cross-sectional studies have the advantage of speed, but they have a disadvantage as well. Cross-sectional studies compare two separate groups of individuals, which makes them incapable of revealing information about changes in people over a period of time. For example, a cross-sectional study of blood pressure in children (Guerra, Ribeiro, Duarte, & Mota, 2002) showed that 13-year-olds had higher blood pressure readings than 8-year-olds. Such information does not demonstrate that blood pressure levels go up as children become older (the 8-year-olds may have lower blood pressure when they are 13). Only a longitudinal study, looking at the same people over a long period of time, can show the developmental trend that blood pressure increases with age.

A longitudinal study of blood pressure changes during childhood (Whincup, Cook, Papacosta, & Walker, 1995) showed that blood pressure increases with age. This study concentrated on children with low birth weights, looking for increases in blood pressure that might relate to the development of heart disease during adulthood. The study included measurements of a group of children once when they were between ages 5 and 7 and again when they were between 9 and 11 years old. The results indicated that blood pressure increased in these children, with greater increases for systolic than diastolic blood pressure and greater increases for girls than boys. The findings from this study may be restricted to children whose birth weight was low, but the results show a developmental trend toward higher blood pressure with age, even during childhood. Furthermore, this study helped explain the nature of the link between low birth weight and cardiovascular disease, which earlier studies had found.

Experimental Designs

Correlational studies, cross-sectional designs, and longitudinal studies all have important uses in psychology, but none of them is able to determine causality. Sometimes psychologists want information on the ability of one variable to cause or directly influence another. Such information requires a well-designed experiment.

An experimental design consists of a comparison of at least two groups, often referred to as an experimental group and a control group. The participants in the *experimental group* must receive treatment identical to that of participants in the control group except that those in the experimental group receive one level of the **independent variable,** whereas people in the *control group* receive a different level. The independent variable is the condition of interest, which the experimenter systematically manipulates to observe its influence on behavior—that is, on the **dependent variable.** The manipulation of the independent variable is a critical element of experimental design because this manipulation allows researchers to control the situation by choosing and creating the appropriate levels. In addition, good experimental design requires that experimenters assign participants to the experimental or control group randomly to ensure that the groups are equivalent at the beginning of the study.

Often the experimental condition consists of administering a treatment, whereas the control condition consists of withholding that treatment and perhaps receiving some sort of placebo. If manipulation of the independent variable causes a change in the dependent variable, which can be evaluated by contrasting the experimental and control groups, the independent variable has a cause-and-effect relationship with the dependent variable.

For example, Andrew Steptoe and his colleagues (Steptoe, Doherty, Kerry, Rink, & Hilton, 2000) conducted an experiment to determine the effectiveness of behavioral counseling (independent variable) in lowering dietary fat intake (dependent variable) and other risk factor for heart disease. Participants were patients with one or more known risk factors for cardiovascular disease, such as smoking, high cholesterol, or having a combination of high body fat and a sedentary lifestyle. The experimenters divided the participants into two groups—an experimental group that received behavioral counseling and a control group that received standard advice regarding dietary fat. The counselors in the experimental condition were nurses trained in brief behavioral counseling methods that emphasized patients' readiness to change their diets. They also focused on patients overcoming barriers to change and maintaining change in the presence of obstacles. Nurses working with the control group emphasized the standard health-promotion procedures that encouraged patients to lower their dietary fat consumption.

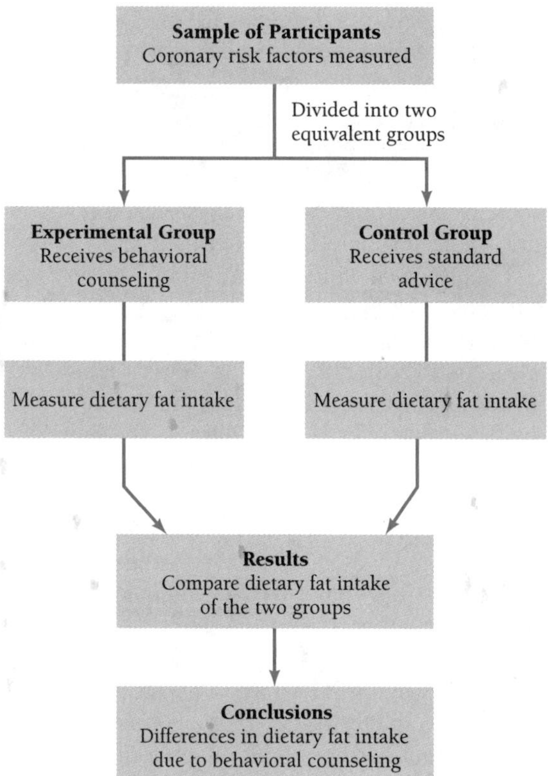

Figure 2.1 Example of an experimental method.

Results indicated that a behavioral counseling program was more effective than standard advice in lowering dietary fat intake in patients with one or more risk for cardiovascular disease. Because the two groups were equal in all respects except the behavioral counseling program, any posttest differences between the two groups in consumption of dietary fat can be attributed to differences in the experimental condition. Such an experimental design allows investigators to speak of causation or at least of probable causes of changes in diet. Figure 2.1 shows a typical experimental design comparing an experimental group with a control group, with counseling as the independent variable and dietary fat as the dependent variable.

Experimental designs with health outcomes pose ethical problems because of the requirement for randomly assigning participants to groups. For example, it would be ethically unacceptable to either prevent or require participants to smoke, live a sedentary lifestyle, or eat a high-fat diet. One strategy to avoid this ethical dilemma is to use nonhuman animals rather than human participants. One such study (Kramsch, Aspen, Abramowitz, Kreimendahl, & Hood, 1981) investigated the effects of exercise (independent variable) on serum cholesterol levels, **atherosclerosis** (narrowing of the arteries), and sudden death from heart failure (dependent variables) in monkeys fed a high-fat diet. The researchers randomly divided 27 monkeys into three groups. All animals were fed a very high-fat diet, but those in the two control groups were permitted little exercise, whereas those in the experimental group were forced to run on a treadmill for 1 hour, three times a week. After 3 1/2 years, monkeys in the exercise group had the same total cholesterol levels as the sedentary monkeys, but they had higher levels of "good" cholesterol, lower levels of "bad" cholesterol, and less atherosclerosis. In addition, the only monkeys that died suddenly were the sedentary ones. This study demonstrated that exercise can protect against coronary risk factors in monkeys; it could also suggest similar results for humans, if one is willing to generalize from monkeys to humans.

Ex Post Facto Designs

Ethical restrictions or practical limitations prevent researchers from manipulating many variables, which means that experiments are not possible, but this restriction does not prevent all research on such variables. When researchers are prevented by either ethical or practical restrictions from manipulating variables in a systematic manner, they sometimes rely on ex post facto designs.

Ex post facto designs, which are one of several types of quasi-experimental studies, resemble experiments in some ways but differ in others. Both types of studies involve contrasting groups to determine differences, but ex post facto designs do not involve the manipulation of independent variables. Instead, researchers choose a variable of interest and select participants who differ on this variable, called a **subject variable.** Both experiments and ex post facto studies involve the measurement of dependent variables. For example, researchers might study dietary fat (subject variable) and level of atherosclerosis (dependent variable) by selecting a group of participants who already eat a high-fat diet and choosing a comparison group of people who eat a diet lower in fat to determine differences in atherosclerosis.

The comparison group in an ex post facto design is not an equivalent control group because these participants were assigned to the groups because of the diet they ate rather than randomly. Variables other than diet may also differ between the groups, such as exercise, weight, cholesterol levels, or smoking. The existence of these other differences means that researchers cannot pinpoint the subject variable as the cause of differences in atherosclerosis between the groups. However, findings about differences in level of atherosclerosis between the two groups can yield useful information, making this type of study a choice for many investigations.

Ex post facto designs are quite common in health psychology because researchers are often interested in investigating variables they cannot manipulate. For example, one study (Colhoun, Rubens, Underwood, & Fuller, 2000) examined the signs of heart disease in people between the ages of 30 and 40 years old, divided according to their occupational and educational levels. To conduct this study, the researchers tested the amount of calcification of the arteries that supply blood to the heart in 149 men and women and also asked these participants to report their occupation and whether or not they were full-time students when they were 19 years old. The researchers used occupation to divide participants into contrast groups based on occupational status (subject variable) and found that participants classified as manual working class had higher levels of artery disease than other classifications. The results also revealed that artery disease progress differed by educational level (another subject variable); people who were still going to school at age 19 had healthier arteries more than 10 years later. This ex post facto study showed that two subject variables differentiated between groups in terms of a physical condition that relates to the development of heart disease.

Ex post facto designs allow comparisons between or among groups, but they do not permit researchers to determine that one variable *causes* changes in another variable. In the study on occupational and educational level, for example, the researchers could not conclude that occupational or educational level caused the difference in artery disease, but the study does provide information about occupational and educational status as a risk for coronary artery disease.

In Summary

We have seen that health psychology has benefited from several psychology research methods, including correlational studies, cross-sectional and longitudinal studies, experimental designs, and ex post facto studies. Correlational studies indicate the degree of association between two variables, but they can never show causation. Cross-sectional studies investigate a group of people at one point in time, whereas longitudinal studies follow the participants over an extended period of time. Although longitudinal studies may yield more useful results than cross-sectional studies, they are more time consuming and expensive. With experimental designs, researchers manipulate the independent variable so that any resulting differences between experimental and control groups can be attributed to their differential exposure to the independent variable. Experimental studies typically include a placebo given to people in a control group so that they will have the same expectations as people in the experimental group. Ex post facto studies are similar to experimental designs in that researchers compare two or more groups and then record group differences in the dependent variable.

Research Methods in Epidemiology

In addition to contributions from psychology methods, the field of health psychology has profited from medical research, especially the research of epidemiologists. **Epidemiology** is a branch of medicine that investigates factors contributing to increased health or the occurrence of a disease in a particular population (Beaglehole, Bonita, & Kjellström, 1993). Epidemiology literally means the study of (*logos*) what is among (*epi*) the people (*demos*).

Epidemiology is among the oldest branches of medicine, having its origins in ancient Greece and Babylon when observers first began to compare people who had a particular disease or characteristic to those who did not (Lilienfeld & Lilienfeld, 1980). However, epidemiology did not evolve as a science until the 19th century, when infectious diseases such as cholera, smallpox, and typhoid fever threatened the lives of millions of people. Many of these infectious diseases were controlled or conquered largely through the work of the epidemiologists who gradually and laboriously identified their causes. With the increase in chronic diseases during the 20th century, epidemiologists continued to make fundamental contributions to health by identifying those behaviors and lifestyles that were related to heart disease, cancer, and other chronic diseases. For example, epidemiology studies were the first to detect a relationship between the behavior of smoking and heart disease.

Two important concepts in epidemiology are prevalence and incidence. **Prevalence** refers to the proportion of the population that has a particular disease at a specific time; **incidence** measures the frequency of *new cases* of the disease during a specified period, usually 1 year (Ahlbom & Norell, 1990). With both prevalence and incidence, the number of people in the population at risk is divided into either the number of people with the disease (prevalence) or the number of new cases in a particular time frame (incidence). The prevalence of a disease may be quite different from the incidence of that disease. For example, the prevalence of hypertension is much greater than the incidence because people can live for years after a diagnosis. In a given community, the annual incidence of hypertension might be 0.025, meaning that for every 1,000 people in that community, 25 people per year will receive a diagnosis of high blood pressure. But because hypertension is a chronic illness, the prevalence in that community will be far more than 25 per 1,000. On the other hand, for a disease such as influenza with a relatively short duration (due either to the patient's rapid recov-

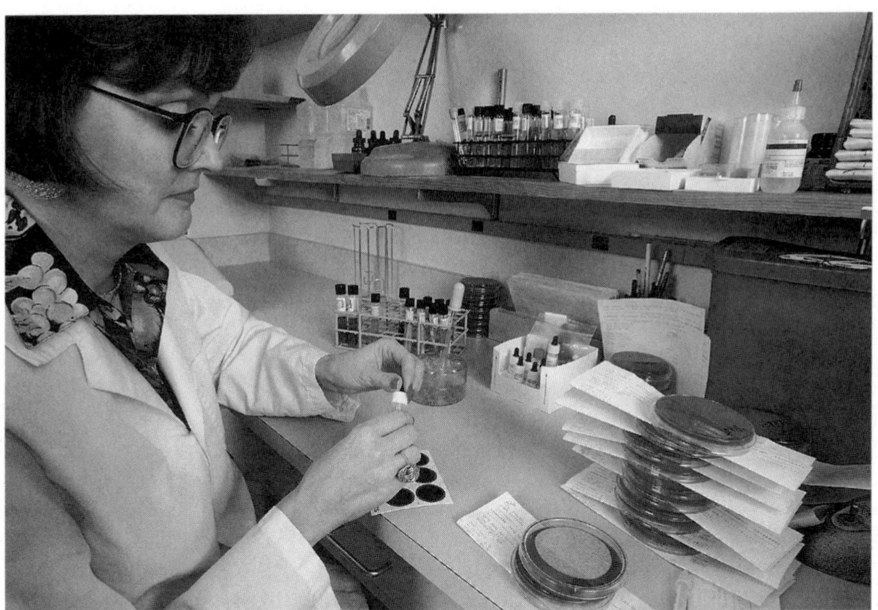

One purpose of epidemiological research is to determine the origins of a disease.

ery or quick death), the incidence per year will exceed the prevalence at any specific time during that year.

Research in epidemiology uses three broad methods: (1) observational studies, (2) randomized, control trials, and (3) natural experiments. Each method has its own requirements and yields specific information. Although epidemiologists use some of the same methods and procedures employed by psychologists, their terminology is not always the same. Figure 2.2 lists the broad areas of epidemiological study and shows their approximate counterparts in the field of psychology.

Observational Methods

Epidemiologists use observational methods to look at and analyze the occurrence of a specific disease in a given population. These methods do not show causes of the disease, but researchers can draw inferences about possible factors that relate to the disease. Observational methods are similar to correlational studies in psychology; both show an association between two or more conditions, but neither can be used to demonstrate causation.

Two important types of observational methods are prospective studies and retrospective studies. **Prospective studies** begin with a population of disease-free participants and follow them over a period of time to determine whether a given condition, such as cigarette smoking, high blood pressure, or diet is related to a later condition, such as heart disease or death. For example, one prospective study (Oomen et al., 2000) looked at the relationship between eating fish and subsequent death from heart disease. The researchers measured fish consumption of a large **cohort** (a group of participants starting an experience together) of Finnish, Italian, and Dutch men 50 to 69 years old who were free from coronary heart disease at the beginning of the study. After 20 years, about 17% of the participants had died of coronary heart disease. After controlling for age, body mass index, smoking, and food intake, the investigators found no significant relationship between either total fish consumption or

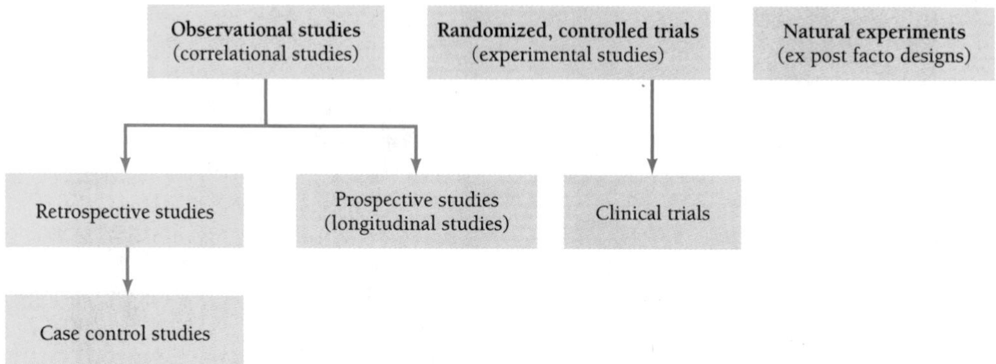

Figure 2.2 Research methods in epidemiology, with their psychology counterparts in parentheses.

lean fish consumption and death from heart disease. However, the results showed an inverse relationship between eating fatty fish and death from heart disease; that is, men in these three countries who ate large amounts of fatty fish, compared with those who ate very little or none, had lower rates of heart disease mortality. Prospective studies, such as this one, are longitudinal, making them equivalent to longitudinal studies in psychology: both provide continuing information about a group of participants and both take a long time to complete.

In contrast, **retrospective studies** use the opposite approach; they begin with a group of people already suffering from a particular disease or disorder and then look backward for characteristics or conditions that marked them as being different from people who do not have that problem. This approach has an advantage over prospective studies in that it need not take as much time or expense. One retrospective study (Sacco et al., 2001) investigated whether or not high-density lipoprotein cholesterol (HDL), which is known to protect against heart disease, might also protect people against stroke. The researchers began by selecting an ethnically diverse group of older stroke victims, that is, patients who already had experienced a stroke, and compared them with a stroke-free group of participants who were similar on such variables such as age, gender, and ethnic background. The results showed that in each ethnic group, the higher the HDL, the less likely people would have a stroke. These findings strongly suggest that high-density lipoprotein may offer some protection against stroke. Retrospective studies such as this one are also referred to as **case-control studies** because cases (people affected by stroke) were compared with controls (people not affected).

Randomized, Controlled Trials

A second type of epidemiological study—the randomized, controlled trial—is equivalent to experiments in psychology. With a randomized, controlled trial, researchers randomly assign participants to either a study group or a control group, thus making the two groups equal on all pertinent factors except the variable being studied. (In psychology this would be called the independent variable.) Researchers must also control variables other than the variable being studied to prevent these variables from affecting the outcome. A randomized, control trial, as with the experimental method in psychology, must avoid the problem of **self-selection**; that is, it must not permit participants to choose whether to be placed in the experimental group or the control group; assignment to groups must be random.

An example of a randomized, controlled trial was the part of the Women's Health Initiative that tested the effectiveness of hormone-replacement therapy in preventing heart disease (Writing Group for the Women's Health Initiative Investigators, 2002). This study was a randomized, controlled trial in which over 16,000 healthy postmenopausal women were divided into groups randomly. One group received pills that were a combination of estrogen and progestin, and the other group received a placebo. The researchers were primarily interested in the effects of hormone-replacement therapy on the development of heart disease, which they measured as cardiovascular disease deaths and nonfatal heart attacks. The study was supposed to continue for 8 1/2 years but the investigators terminated it after about 5 years because the results indicated that hormone-replacement therapy *increased* rather than decreased the risk for heart disease. That is, those women who received hormone-replacement therapy showed increased incidence of heart attacks and cardiovascular disease deaths. This randomized, controlled trial demonstrated that hormone-replacement therapy for postmenopausal women presents more health risks than health benefits.

A research design that tests the effects of new drugs or medical treatment is called a *clinical trial.* Many clinical trials are randomized, controlled trials because the random assignment and control of other variables are design features that allow researchers to determine that the new treatment is effective. For example, in a clinical trial to test the efficacy of a cholesterol-lowering drug, participants with high serum cholesterol are randomly assigned to one of two groups—the group that receives the active drug or a control group that receives a placebo pill. Because the two groups are similar in all other pertinent aspects, any differences between the two groups in subsequent total cholesterol levels could be attributed to the differences in treatment. Such a randomized, placebo-controlled trial would require a double-blind design in which neither the participants nor the people who administer the drugs would know which pills contained the active ingredient and which were placebos. All drugs approved by the U.S. Food and Drug Administration (FDA) must first undergo extensive clinical trials of this nature.

Randomized, placebo-controlled, double-blind trials are often regarded as the zenith of the hierarchy of research designs. They are commonly used to measure the effectiveness of new drugs but are also used to assess the efficacy of various psychological and educational interventions. However, John Concato and his colleagues (Concato, Shah, & Horwitz, 2000) presented some evidence that well-designed observational studies are capable of providing the same level of information yielded by randomized, controlled trials. Concato et al. looked at five recent major medical journals and found 99 studies that evaluated five different treatments. For each treatment, there were several observational studies and several randomized, controlled trials. Results from the observational studies and the randomized, controlled trials were quite similar, indicating that observational studies do not overestimate the size of the treatment effect and can provide the same information as randomized, controlled trials. Moreover, these researchers concluded that observational studies have the advantage of being cheaper and easier to conduct.

Natural Experiments

A third area of epidemiological study is the natural experiment, in which the researcher can only select the independent variable, not manipulate it. Natural experiments are similar to the ex post facto designs used in psychology and involve the study of natural conditions that provide the possibility for comparison.

When two similar groups of people naturally divide themselves into those exposed to a pathogen and those not exposed, natural experiments are possible. The German blockade of the Russian city of Leningrad (now St. Petersburg) during World War II provided the circumstances for a natural experiment on the effects of prenatal malnutrition on the development of heart disease. Malnutrition was widespread during the blockade, which lasted 872 days, significantly affecting birth weights for babies born during this time of famine. Previous findings that low birth weight is related to the development of heart disease during adulthood prompted researchers (Stanner et al., 1997) to compare babies born during the blockade to those born earlier and thus not exposed to prenatal malnutrition. The results of this natural experiment showed that, although the experience of prenatal malnutrition produced changes in cells in the heart, it did not increase the chances for heart disease during adulthood. Therefore, the increased risk of heart disease in low-birth-weight children is not due to prenatal malnutrition.

This natural experiment differs from case-control studies in that it began by examining all the adults who were born at a specific place and in a specific time period rather than testing only those with disease, and it differs from randomized, controlled trials in that the researchers selected the participants rather than manipulating conditions. In a true randomized, controlled trial, researchers would assign participants to prenatal nutrition conditions, but of course, ethical considerations prevent researchers from depriving pregnant women of food to examine the effects on the offsprings' heart disease. Natural experiments have a long tradition in epidemiology, going back at least to 1848 and the classical natural experiment in London by John Snow.

Two Examples of Epidemiological Research

Epidemiology provides useful techniques for taking a first look at a health-related problem. Two examples of these techniques are the pioneering work of John Snow in London and the ongoing Alameda County Study in California.

The Pioneering Work of John Snow A dramatic example of how epidemiologists function is the work of John Snow, the brilliant English epidemiologist and anesthetist and one of the founding members of the London Epidemiological Society. During the 1848 outbreak of cholera in London, Snow made careful observations of the distribution of cholera deaths in the southern section of the city. At that time, two different companies supplied drinking water to the residents of south London. The water mains of the two companies were interwoven so that residences on the same side of the street received their water from two separate sources. One water company pumped its water from a polluted area of the Thames River; the other had recently relocated its pumps to a less polluted area. Snow noted which houses received water from each company and calculated that the cholera death rate was more than five times higher in homes receiving their water from the Thames than in homes receiving water from the other south London company. He then compared both sets of death rates with those from the rest of London. Snow observed that the pattern of cholera deaths closely paralleled the distribution of polluted water. In 1855, without yet understanding the specific organism responsible for cholera, Snow published a report in which he suggested the existence of a cholera "poison" and expressed his views that the disease was spread through drinking water. He also devised an ingenious plan of intervention: he simply turned off the source of polluted water. Not until 30 years later did Robert Koch isolate the cholera bacterium, thus establishing the essential validity of Snow's views.

Snow had identified a risk factor for a deadly disease; he had not discovered a specific cause. During the last half of the 20th century, epidemiological work has shifted from tracking infectious diseases to discovering factors associated with positive health or with chronic diseases, but the procedures are quite like Snow's. Identifying these factors does not prove causation, but it is a necessary first step leading to the control or eradication of a particular disease.

The Alameda County Study The Alameda County Study is an ongoing prospective study of a single community to identify health practices that may protect against death and disease. We have seen that epidemiologists identify risk factors by studying large populations over some period of time and by sifting out behavioral, demographic, or physiological conditions that show a relationship to subsequent disease or death.

The Alameda County Study began as an attempt to identify the health practices and social variables that relate to mortality from all causes. In 1965, epidemiologist Lester Breslow and his colleagues from the Human Population Laboratory of the California State Department of Public Health began a survey of a sample of all the households in Alameda County (Oakland), California. After determining the number of adults living at these addresses, the researchers sent detailed questionnaires to each resident 20 years of age or older. Usable returns were eventually received from nearly 7,000 people. Among other questions, these participants answered questions about seven basic health practices: (1) getting 7 or 8 hours of sleep daily, (2) eating breakfast almost every day, (3) rarely eating between meals, (4) drinking alcohol in moderation or not at all, (5) not smoking cigarettes, (6) exercising regularly, and (7) maintaining weight near the prescribed ideal.

At the time of the original survey in 1965, only cigarette smoking had been implicated as a health risk. Evidence that any of the other six practices predicted health or mortality was quite tenuous. Because several of these practices require some amount of good health, it was necessary to investigate the possibility that original health status might confound subsequent death rates. To control for these possible confounding effects, the Alameda County investigators asked residents about their disabilities, acute and chronic illnesses, physical symptoms, and current levels of energy.

A follow-up 5 1/2 years later (Belloc, 1973) revealed that Alameda County residents who practiced six or seven of the basic health-related behaviors were far less likely to have died than those who practiced zero to three. This decreased mortality risk was independent of their 1965 health status, thus suggesting that healthy behaviors lead to lower rates of death.

In 1974, investigators conducted a major follow-up of living participants and also surveyed a new sample to determine whether the community in general had adopted a healthier lifestyle between 1965 and 1974 (Berkman & Breslow, 1983; Wingard, Berkman, & Brand, 1982). The 9-year follow-up determined the relationship between mortality and the seven health practices, considered individually as well as in combination. Five of the health practices predicted mortality rates independent of participants' use of preventive health services and their physical health in 1965. Cigarette smoking, lack of physical activity, and alcohol consumption were strongly related to mortality, whereas obesity and too much or too little sleep were only weakly associated with increased death rates. As it turned out, skipping breakfast and snacking between meals were not significantly related to mortality.

Men who practiced zero to two health-related behaviors were nearly three times more likely to have died than were those who engaged in four to five of the behaviors. For women, the effect was even more dramatic: When compared to women who practiced four or five of these behaviors, those who engaged in zero to two were over three times more likely to have died. Moreover, the number of close social relationships also predicted mortality: people with few social contacts were two and a half times more likely to have died than were those with many such contacts (Berkman & Syme, 1979).

If some health practices are inversely related to *mortality,* then a second question would be how these same factors relate to *morbidity* or disease. A condition that predicts death need not also predict disease. Many disabilities, chronic illnesses, and illness symptoms do not inevitably lead to death. Therefore, it is important to know whether basic health practices and social contacts predict later physical health. Stated another way: Do health practices merely contribute to survival time, or do they also raise an individual's general level of health?

To answer this question, researchers (Camacho & Wiley, 1983; Wiley & Camacho, 1980)

BECOMING AN INFORMED READER OF HEALTH-RELATED RESEARCH

How can you judge the worth of the abundance of health-related information you read or hear? Several questions serve as criteria for evaluating such information.

1. Is the information based solely on testimonials of "satisfied" consumers, with financial gain an obvious motive?
2. Is the information based on studies conducted by trained scientists who are affiliated with universities, research hospitals, or governmental agencies? Useful information does not typically spring from secret sources.
3. Is the information generally consistent with previous research? Dramatic breakthroughs and isolated evidence are rare in science.
4. Have the research findings been replicated by other researchers? Valid evidence should emerge from different laboratories.
5. Is the information based on studies using many participants? Information from small studies is usually less reliable than that from large-scale studies.
6. Conversely, is the information based on huge studies or **meta-analyses** involving hundreds of thousands of people? With very large samples, even tiny differences can be statistically significant and can thus appear important even though they have little practical significance or ability to predict health outcomes for a single individual.
7. Is the information based on correlational or experimental studies? Correlational studies cannot prove causation.
8. If the information comes from an experimental design, did the researchers control for the placebo effect?
9. Have the researchers reached conclusions that are consistent with their data?
10. Are the participants representative of some identified population?
11. Did the researchers use reliable and valid measures of the independent and dependent variables?
12. If the design is experimental, did the experimenters assure that the control and experimental groups were alike on everything except the independent variable?
13. If the design is prospective or retrospective, did the researchers adequately control for smoking, diet, exercise, and other possible confounding variables?

studied a subset of the original sample of Alameda County participants. In addition to the five health practices that related to mortality, this investigation included a Social Network Index that combined marital status, contacts with friends and relatives, and membership in church and other organizations. Each of the five health behaviors as well as the Social Network Index were related to changes in health. More specifically, (1) both former smokers and nonsmokers had better health than smokers; (2) moderate drinkers were healthier than either heavy drinkers or abstainers; (3) people who slept 7 or 8 hours per night did better than those who got either more or less sleep; (4) both men and women who engaged in high levels of physical activity were healthier than their more sedentary counterparts; (5) normal-weight people achieved higher health status than either overweight participants (30% or more above desirable weight) or underweight individuals (10% or more below desirable weight); and (6) people who scored high on the Social Network Index were healthier than those who received a low rating.

Interestingly, the Social Network Index showed that marriage did not have equal effects on the health of men and women. With both men and women, individuals who were formerly

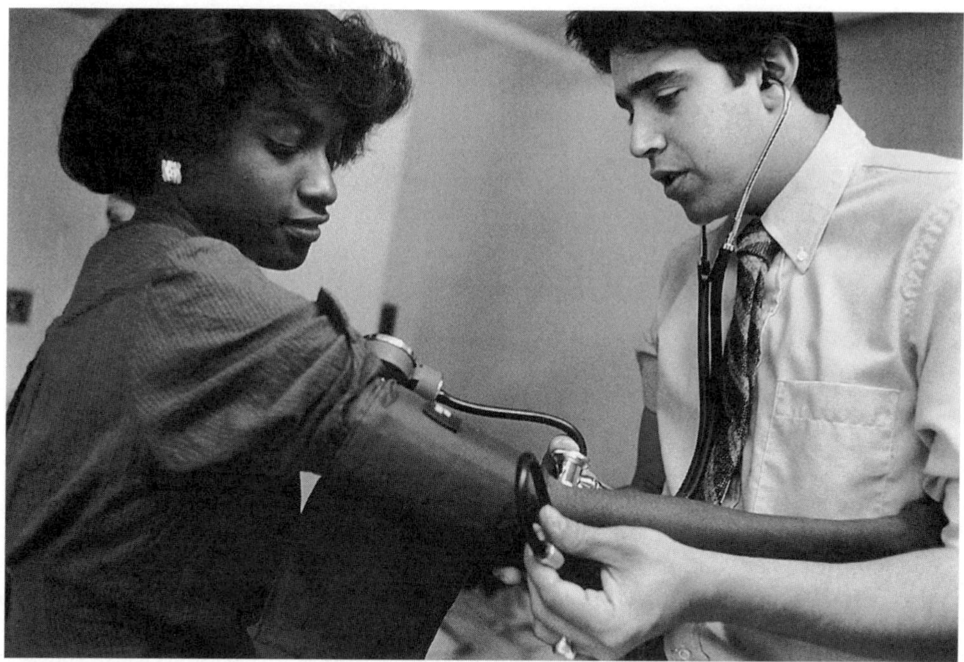

Blood pressure is a risk factor for cardiovascular disease, indicating that people with high blood pressure are at elevated risk but not that high blood pressure causes cardiovascular disease.

married—separated, divorced, or widowed—had greater negative changes in health, but women who had never been married were much healthier than were men who had never married. Never-married men had slightly negative health scores compared with married men, but never-married women had considerably higher health scores than either married or formerly married women. Marriage, it seems, provides health benefits to men, but the single life is apparently healthier for women.

In Summary

In order to investigate those factors that contribute either to health or to the frequency and distribution of a disease, epidemiologists use scientific methods that are quite similar to those used by psychologists. Among these methods are observational studies, randomized, controlled trials, and natural experiments. Observational studies, which are similar to correlational studies, can be either retrospective or prospective. (Retrospective studies begin with a group of people already suffering from a disease and then look for characteristics of these people that are different from those of people who do not have that disease, whereas prospective studies are longitudinal designs that follow the forward development of a group of people). Randomized, controlled trials are similar to experimental designs in psychology. Clinical trials, a common type of randomized, controlled trials, are typically used to determine the effectiveness of new drugs, but they can be used in other controlled studies. Natural experiments, which are similar to ex post facto studies, are used when naturally occurring conditions allows for comparisons.

Epidemiologists frequently use the concepts of risk factor, prevalence, and incidence. A risk factor is any condition that occurs with greater frequency in people with a disease than it does in people free from that disease. Prevalence refers to the proportion of the population that has a particular disease at a specific time, whereas incidence measures the frequency of new cases of the disease during a specified period of time.

Determining Causation

We have seen that both prospective and retrospective studies can identify risk factors for a disease, but they do not demonstrate causation. Obesity, hypertension, high total cholesterol, and cigarette smoking, for example, are all demonstrated risk factors for coronary artery disease (CAD). People with one or more of these risks are more likely than people with none of these risks to develop heart disease. However, some people with no known risks will develop heart disease and some people with multiple risks may never have CAD. This section looks at the risk factor approach as a means of suggesting causation and then examines evidence that cigarette smoking *causes* disease.

The Risk Factor Approach

The risk factor approach was popularized by the Framingham Heart Study (Dawber, 1980; Voelker, 1998), a large-scale epidemiology investigation that began in 1948 and included more than 5,000 men and women in the town of Framingham, Massachusetts. From its early years and continuing to the present, this study has allowed researchers to identify such risk factors for cardiovascular disease (CVD) as serum cholesterol, gender, high blood pressure, cigarette smoking, and obesity. These risk factors do not necessarily cause cardiovascular disease, but they are related to it in some way. Obesity, for example, may not be a direct cause of heart disease, but it is generally associated with hypertension, which is strongly associated with cardiovascular disease. Because obesity is related to a known risk factor, it too is a relative risk factor for CVD.

Relative risk must be distinguished from absolute risk. **Relative risk** (RR) refers to the ratio of the incidence (or prevalence) of a disease in an exposed group to the incidence (or prevalence) of that disease in the unexposed group. The relative risk of the unexposed group is always 1.00, so that an RR of 1.50 indicates that the exposed group is 50% more likely to develop the disease in question than the unexposed group. A relative risk of 0.70 means that the rate of disease in the exposed group is only 70% of the rate in the unexposed group. **Absolute risk** refers to the person's chances of developing a disease or disorder independent of any risk that other people may have for that disease or disorder. For example, cigarette smokers have a relative risk of about 9.0 for dying of lung cancer (Lubin, Blot, et al., 1984), meaning that they are nine times more likely to die of lung cancer than nonsmokers. However, a smoker's absolute risk of dying of lung cancer in any one year is only about 0.001, or about 1 in 1,000, a very low absolute risk. Over a lifetime of 50 years as a smoker, the absolute risk would be .05, or one chance in 20 that this smoker will die of lung cancer. However, this same smoker has various levels of absolute risk of dying from a number of other cigarette-related diseases, including other cancers and cardiovascular disease. Considering all these risks, a long-time smoker has about a 50% chance of dying from smoking and about a 50% chance of dying from some other cause (Centers for Disease Control and Prevention [CDC], 1993).

A further illustration comes from comparing the risk that cigarette smokers have of dying from cardiovascular disease with their risk of dying from lung cancer. Smokers have a relative risk of only about 2.0 for dying from cardiovascular disease (1993) but about 9.0 for dying from lung cancer. Nevertheless, because heart disease is far more common than lung cancer, smokers have a higher absolute risk of dying from CVD than they have of dying from lung cancer. More specifically, about 150,000 smokers die each year from CVD, but only about 120,000 die from lung cancer (CDC, 2002). When a disease is very rare, a person may have an extremely high relative risk for that disease but only a small absolute risk.

Although risk factors do not derive from experimental studies, they can determine the *probability* that a person will develop a particular disease. Not all cigarette smokers will develop heart disease, but if you smoke, you are about twice as likely to die of cardiovascular disease than if you do not smoke (CDC, 1993). Clearly, smoking cigarettes places one at risk for developing CVD. In a similar fashion, high cholesterol levels, high blood pressure, obesity, and stress are all risk factors for cardiovascular disease, but there is no *experimental* evidence that any of these conditions *cause* coronary heart disease or stroke.

Cigarettes and Disease: Is There a Causal Relationship?

In 1994, representatives from all the major tobacco companies came before the United States Congress House Subcommittee on Health to defend charges that cigarette smoking causes a variety of health problems, including heart disease and lung cancer. The crux of their argument was that no scientific study had ever proven that cigarette smoking causes heart disease or lung cancer in humans. Technically, their contention was correct, because only experimental studies can absolutely demonstrate causation, and no such experimental study has ever been or ever will be conducted on humans.

During the past 50 years, however, researchers have used nonexperimental studies to establish a link between cigarette smoking and several diseases, especially cardiovascular disease and lung cancer. Accumulated findings from these studies present an example of how researchers can use those nonexperimental studies to make deductions about a causal relationship. In other words, experimental and randomized, controlled studies are not required before scientists can infer a causal link between the independent variable (smoking) and the dependent variables (heart disease and lung cancer). Epidemiologists draw conclusions that a causal relationship exists if certain conditions are met (Beaglehole, Bonita, & Kjellström, 1993; Susser, 1991). Using their criteria, does sufficient evidence exist to infer a cause-and-effect relationship between cigarette smoking and heart disease and lung cancer?

The first criterion is that a *dose-response relationship must exist* between a possible cause and changes in the prevalence or incidence of a disease. A **dose-response relationship** is a direct, consistent association between an independent variable, such as a behavior, and a dependent variable, such as a disease. In other words, the higher the dose, the higher the death rate. A body of research evidence (Doll & Hill, 1956; USDHHS, 1990) has demonstrated a dose-response relationship between both the number of cigarettes smoked per day and the number of years one has smoked and the subsequent incidence of heart disease and lung cancer.

Second, the prevalence or incidence of *a disease should decline with the removal of the possible cause.* Research (Ben-Shlomo, Smith, Shipley, & Marmot, 1994; Kawachi et al., 1993; USDHHS, 1990) has consistently demonstrated that quitting cigarette smoking lowers one's risk of cardiovascular disease and greatly decreases one's risk of lung cancer. Moreover, quitting adds years to one's life (Fielding, 1985). People who continue to smoke continue to have increased risks of these diseases.

Third, the *cause must precede the disease.* Cigarette smoking almost always precedes incidence of disease. (We have little evidence that people tend to begin cigarette smoking as a means of coping with heart disease or lung cancer.)

Fourth, *a cause-and-effect relationship between the condition and the disease must be plausible*; that is, it must be consistent with other data and it must make sense from a biological viewpoint. Although scientists may not completely understand the exact mechanisms responsible for the effect of cigarette smoking on the cardiovascular system and the lungs, such a physiological connection is plausible. It is not necessary that the underlying connection between a behavior and a disease be known, only that it be a possibility. The existence of experimental evidence demonstrating that smoking causes lung cancer and heart disease in nonhuman animals adds to this plausibility.

Fifth, *research findings must be consistent.* For 50 years, evidence from ex post facto and correlational studies, as well as from various epidemiological studies, has demonstrated a strong and consistent relationship between cigarette smoking and disease. As early as 1956, British researchers Richard Doll and A. B. Hill noted a straight linear relationship between average number of cigarettes smoked per day and death rates from lung cancer. Although a positive correlation such as this is not sufficient to demonstrate causation, hundreds of additional correlational and ex post facto studies since that time have yielded overwhelming evidence to suggest that cigarette smoking causes disease.

Sixth, the *strength of the association between the condition and the disease must be relatively high.* Again, research has revealed that cigarette smokers have about a two-fold risk for cardiovascular disease (CDC, 1993) and are nine times more likely than nonsmokers to die of lung cancer (Lubin, Blot, et al., 1984). Because other studies have found comparable relative risk figures, epidemiologists accept cigarette smoking as a causal agent for both CVD and lung cancer.

The final criterion for inferring causality is the *existence of appropriately designed studies.* Although no experimental designs with human participants have been reported on the relationship between cigarettes and disease, well-designed observational studies can yield the same results as experimental studies (Concato et al., 2000), and a large number of these observational studies have consistency revealed a close association between cigarette smoking and both cardiovascular disease and lung cancer.

Because each of these seven criteria are clearly met by a preponderance of evidence, epidemiologists are able to discount the argument of tobacco company representatives that cigarette smoking has not been proven to cause disease. When evidence is as overwhelming as it is in this case, scientists infer a causal link between cigarette smoking and a variety of diseases, including heart disease and lung cancer. Criteria for determining causation are summarized in Table 2.1.

In Summary

A risk factor is any characteristic or condition that occurs with greater frequency in people with a disease than it does in people free from that disease. Although the risk factor approach alone cannot determine causation, epidemiologists use several criteria for determining a cause-and-effect relationship between a condition and a disease: (1) A dose-response relationship must exist between the condition and the disease; (2) the removal of the condition must reduce the prevalence or incidence of the disease; (3) the condition must precede the disease; (4) the causal relationship between the condition and the disease must be physiologically plausible; (5) research data must consistently reveal a relationship between the condition and the disease; (6) the strength of the relationship between the condition and the disease must be relatively high; and (7) the relationship between the condition and the disease must be based on well-designed studies. When all seven of these criteria are met, scientists can infer a cause-and-effect relationship between an independent variable (such as smoking) and a dependent variable (such as heart disease or lung cancer).

Research Tools

Psychologists frequently rely on two important tools to conduct research: theoretical models and psychometric instruments. Many, but not all, psy-

TABLE 2.1 *Criteria for Determining Causation Between a Condition and a Disease*

1. A dose-response relationship exists between the condition and the disease.
2. Removal of the condition reduces the prevalence or incidence of the disease.
3. The condition precedes the disease.
4. A cause-and-effect relationship between the condition and the disease is physiologically plausible.
5. Relevant research data consistently reveals a relationship between the condition and the disease.
6. The strength of the relationship between the condition and the disease is relatively high.
7. Studies revealing a relationship between the condition and the disease are well designed.

chology studies are driven by a theoretical model and are attempts to test hypotheses suggested by that model. Also, many psychology studies rely on measuring devices to assess behaviors, physiological functions, attitudes, abilities, personality traits, and other independent and dependent variables. This section provides a brief discussion of these two tools.

The Role of Theory in Research

As the scientific study of human behavior, psychology shares with other disciplines the use of scientific methods to investigate natural phenomena. The work of science is not restricted to research methodology; it also involves constructing theoretical models to serve as vehicles for making sense of research findings. Health psychologists have developed a number of models and theories to explain health-related behaviors and conditions, such as stress, pain, smoking, alcohol abuse, and unhealthy eating habits. To the uninitiated, theories may seem impractical and superfluous, but scientists regard them as practical tools that give both direction and meaning to their research.

Scientific **theory** has been defined as "a set of related assumptions that allow scientists to use logical deductive reasoning to formulate testable hypotheses" (Feist & Feist, 2002, p. 4). Theories have an interactive relationship with scientifically derived observations. A theory gives meaning to observations, and observations in turn fit into and alter the theory erected to explain these observations. Theories, then, are dynamic and become more powerful as they expand to explain more and more relevant observations.

Near the beginning of this cycle, when the theoretical framework is still rudimentary and not yet sufficiently comprehensive to explain a large number of observations, the term **model** is more appropriate than theory. In practice, however, *theory* and *model* are sometimes used interchangeably.

The role of theory in health psychology is basically the same as it is in any other scientific discipline. First, a useful theory should generate research—both descriptive research and hypothesis testing. The goal of descriptive research is to expand the existing theory. This type of research deals with measurement, labeling, and categorization of observations. A useful theory of psychosocial factors in heart disease, for example, should generate a multitude of investigations that describe the psychological and social factors of people who have been diagnosed with heart disease. On the other hand, hypothesis testing is not specifically carried out to expand the theory but rather to contribute valid data to the body of scientific knowledge. Again, a useful theory of psychosocial factors in heart disease should stimulate the formulation of a number of hypotheses that, when tested, produce a greater understanding of the psychological and social conditions that relate to heart disease. Results of such studies would either support or fail to support the existing theory; they ordinarily do not enlarge or alter it.

Second, a useful theory should organize and explain the observations derived from research and make them intelligible. Unless research data are organized into some meaningful framework, scientists have no clear direction to follow in their pursuit of further knowledge. A useful theory of the psychosocial factors in heart disease, for example, should integrate what is currently known about such factors and allow researchers to frame discerning questions that stimulate further research.

Third, a useful theory should serve as a guide to action, permitting the practitioner to predict behavior and to implement strategies to change behavior. A practitioner concerned with helping others change health-related behaviors is greatly aided by a theory of behavior change. For instance, a cognitive therapist will follow a cognitive theory of learning to make decisions about how to help clients and will thus focus on changing the thought processes that affect clients' behaviors. Similarly, psychologists with other theoretical orientations rely on their theories to supply them with solutions to the many questions they confront in their practice.

Theories, then, are useful and necessary tools for the development of any scientific discipline. They generate research that leads to more knowledge, organize and explain observations, and help the practitioner (both the researcher and the clinician) handle a variety of daily problems, such as predicting behavior and helping people change unhealthy practices. Later chapters discuss several theoretical models that are frequently used in health psychology.

The Role of Psychometrics in Research

From the work of Sir Francis Galton (1879, 1883) during the 19th century until the present time, psychology has developed a close relationship with the measurement of human abilities and behaviors. Indeed, one of psychology's most important contributions to behavioral medicine and behavioral health is its sophistication in assessment techniques. Nearly every important issue in health psychology demands the measurement of the phenomenon under investigation. Psychologists have reacted to this demand by constructing a number of instruments to assess such behaviors and conditions as stress, pain, hostility, eating habits, and personal hardiness.

For these or any other measuring instruments to be useful, they must be both *reliable* (consistent) and *valid* (accurate). The problems of establishing reliability and validity are critical to the development of any measurement scale.

Establishing Reliability The **reliability** of a measuring instrument is the extent to which it yields consistent results. In health psychology, reliability is most frequently determined by comparing scores on two or more administrations of the same instrument (*test-retest reliability*) or by comparing ratings obtained from two or more judges observing the same phenomenon (*interrater reliability*).

Reliability is most frequently expressed in terms of either correlation coefficients or percentages. The correlation coefficient, which expresses the degree of correspondence between two sets of scores, is the same statistic used in correlational studies. High reliability coefficients (such as 0.80 to 0.90) indicate that participants have obtained nearly the same scores on two administrations of a test. Percentages can be used to express the degree of agreement between the independent ratings of observers. If that agreement between two or more raters is high (such as 85% to 95%), then the instrument is capable of eliciting nearly the same ratings from two or more interviewers.

Establishing reliability for the numerous assessment instruments used in health psychology is obviously a formidable task, but it is an essential first step in developing useful measuring devices.

Establishing Validity A second step in constructing assessment scales is to establish their validity. Measuring scales may be reliable and yet lack validity, or accuracy. **Validity** is the extent to which an instrument measures what it is designed to measure.

Psychologists determine the validity of a measuring instrument by comparing scores from that instrument with some independent or outside criterion—that is, a standard that has been assessed independently of the instrument being validated. In health psychology, that criterion is often some future event, such as a diagnosis of heart disease. An instrument capable of predicting who will receive such a diagnosis and who will remain disease free is said to have *predictive validity.* For example, life events scales (see Chapter 5) have been used to measure stress and to predict future mortality or morbidity. For such a scale to demonstrate predictive validity, it must be administered to participants who are currently free of disease. If people who score high on the scale eventually have higher rates of death or disease than participants with low scores, then the scale can be said to have predictive validity; that is, it differentiates between participants who will remain disease free and those who will die or become ill.

In Summary

The work of scientists is aided by two important tools—useful theories and accurate measurement. Useful theories (1) generate research, (2) predict and explain research data, and (3) help the practitioner solve a variety of problems. Accurate psychometric instruments are both reliable and valid. Reliability is the extent to which an assessment device measures consistently, and validity is the extent to which an assessment instrument measures what it is supposed to measure.

Answers

This chapter addressed five basic questions:

1. What is a placebo and how does it affect treatment and research?

A placebo is an inactive substance or condition that has the appearance of the independent variable and that may cause participants in an experiment to improve or change behavior due to their belief in the placebo's efficacy. In other words, a placebo is any treatment that is effective because of a patient's beliefs that it will be effective and their previous experiences with treatment.

The therapeutic effect of placebos is generally judged to be about 35%, but that rate varies with many conditions, including treatment setting and culture. Placebos have been known to be effective in a wide variety of situations, such as lowering blood pressure, curing insomnia, reducing low back pain, attenuating burn pain (but not the tissue damage), alleviating headache, reducing asthma attacks, diminishing anxiety, and decreasing symptoms of Parkinson's disease. Placebos can also produce adverse effects and are then called nocebos.

The positive effects of placebos are usually beneficial to patients, but they create problems for researchers attempting to determine the efficacy of the treatment. Experimental designs that measure the effectiveness of the treatment intervention balance that intervention against a placebo so that people in the control (placebo) group have the same expectations as do people in the experimental (treatment intervention) group. Experimental studies frequently use designs in which the participants do not know which treatment condition they are in (single-blind design) or a design in which neither the participants nor the people administering the treatment know who receives the placebo and who receives the treatment intervention (double-blind design).

2. **How has psychology contributed to health?** Psychology has made at least five important contributions to health. First, is its long tradition of techniques to change behavior; second is an emphasis on health rather than disease; third is the development of reliable and valid measuring instruments; fourth is the construction of useful theoretical models to explain health-related research; and fifth are various research methods used in psychology. This chapter is concerned mostly with the fifth contribution.

   The variety of research methods used in psychology include (1) correlational studies, (2) cross-sectional studies and longitudinal studies, (3) experimental designs, and (4) ex post facto designs. Each of these makes its own unique contribution to the understanding of behavior and health. Correlational studies indicate the degree of association or correlation between two variables, but by themselves, they cannot be used to determine a cause-and-effect relationship. Cross-sectional studies investigate a group of people at one point in time, whereas longitudinal studies follow the participants over an extended period. In general, longitudinal studies are more likely to yield useful and specific results, but they are more time consuming and expensive than cross-sectional studies. With experimental designs, researchers manipulate the independent variable so that any resulting differences between experimental and control groups can be attributed to their differential exposure to the independent variable. Ex post facto designs are similar to experimental designs in that researchers compare two or more groups and then record group differences in the dependent variable. However, in the ex post facto study, the experimenter merely selects a subject variable on which two groups have naturally divided themselves rather than creating differences through manipulation.

3. **How has epidemiology contributed to health?** Modern epidemiology began making significant contribution to health during the 19th century when it helped conquer such infectious diseases as cholera, smallpox, and typhoid fever. During the 20th century, epidemiology continued to provide basic research that uncovered risk factors for heart disease, cancer, and other lethal and chronic diseases.

   Many of the research methods used in epidemiology are quite similar to those used in psychology. Epidemiology uses at least three basic kinds of research methodology: (1) observational studies, (2) randomized, controlled trials, and (3) natural experiments. Observational studies, which parallel the correlation studies used in psychology, are of two types: retrospective and prospective. Retrospective studies are usually case-control studies that begin with a group of people already suffering from a disease (the cases) and then look for characteristics of these people that are different from those of people who do not have that disease (the controls). Prospective studies are longitudinal designs that follow the forward development of a population or sample. Randomized, controlled trials are similar to experimental designs in psychology. With both studies, researchers manipulate the independent variable to determine its effect on the dependent variable. Randomized, controlled trials are capable of demonstrating cause-and-effect relationships. The most common type of randomized, controlled trials are clinical trials, which are frequently used to measure the efficacy of medications. Natural experiments, which are similar to ex post facto studies, involve selection rather than manipulation of the independent variable.

   Epidemiology has also contributed the concepts of risk factor, prevalence, and incidence. A risk factor is any characteristic or condition that occurs with greater frequency in people with a disease than it does in people free from that disease. Prevalence is the proportion of the population that has a particular disease at a specific time; incidence measures the frequency of new cases of the disease during a specified time.

4. **How can scientists determine if a behavior causes a disease?** Seven criteria are used for determining a cause-and-effect relationship between a condition and

a disease: (1) A dose-response relationship must exist between the condition and the disease; (2) the removal of the condition must reduce the prevalence or incidence of the disease; (3) the condition must precede the disease; (4) the causal relationship between the condition and the disease must be physiologically plausible; (5) research data must consistently reveal a relationship between the condition and the disease; (6) the strength of the relationship between the condition and the disease must be relatively high; and (7) the relationship between the condition and the disease must be based on well-designed studies.

5. **How do theory and measurement contribute to health psychology?**
   Theories are important tools used by scientists to (1) generate research, (2) predict and explain research data, and (3) help the practitioner solve a variety of problems. Health psychologists use a variety of measurement instruments to assess behaviors and theoretical concepts. To be useful, these psychometric instruments must be both reliable and valid. Reliability is the extent to which an assessment device measures consistently, and validity is the extent to which an assessment instrument measures what it is supposed to measure.

Suggested Readings

Morgan, W. P. (1997). Methodological considerations. In W. P. Morgan (Ed.), *Physical activity and mental health* (pp. 3–32). Washington, DC: Taylor & Francis. In this chapter, William Morgan offers an insightful review of the methodological problems involved in discovering evidence for a link between physical activity and psychological health, but his recommendations can be extended to the association between any health-related behavior and its consequence.

Sandler, D. P. (2000). John Snow and modern-day environmental epidemiology. *American Journal of Epidemiology, 152,* 1–3. In this short article, Dale Sandler argues that, although science is important in shaping government attitude, social forces such as committee involvement of residents living near environmental hazards may be more important in changing laws.

Susser, M. (1991). What is a cause and how do we know one? A grammar for pragmatic epidemiology. *American Journal of Epidemiology, 133,* 635–648. Since the 1950s, epidemiologists have developed ways of showing causality in nonexperimental designs, and in this practical article, Susser presents criteria for making these causal inferences.

Vaillant, G. E. (2002). *Aging well: Surprising guideposts to a happier life from the landmark Harvard Study of Adult Development.* Boston: Little Brown. For readers interested in longitudinal studies, George Vaillant provides an interesting look at health-related factors of three superlong studies: the Harvard Study of Adult Development (average date of birth, 1921); Gluecks' nondelinquent inner-city boys (average date of birth, 1930); and the women in Terman's gifted children's study (average date of birth, 1911).

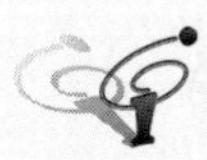

Search InfoTrac College Edition

Search these terms to learn more about topics in this chapter:

Placebo effect and health	Health research and methods
Medical research and media	Research technique and health

3

Seeking Health Care

The Story of Jeff

CHAPTER OUTLINE

Adopting Health-Related Behaviors

Seeking Medical Attention

Receiving Health Care

QUESTIONS

This chapter focuses on three basic questions:

1. Why do people adopt health-related behaviors?
2. What factors are related to seeking medical attention?
3. What problems do people encounter in receiving medical care?

The Story of Jeff

While playing a game of half-court basketball, Jeff jammed his right hand on the backboard and felt an immediate pain. However, he continued playing, as minor injuries were merely "part of the game." For the rest of the day, his hand continued to hurt, and he had difficulty writing, eating, or using the hand for other tasks. The next day, Jeff's hand was somewhat discolored and quite swollen. To reduce the swelling, he wrapped an ice pack around the hand for 20 to 30 minutes two or three times that day. Still, Jeff continued with his daily activities as well as he could, believing that the swelling would soon disappear. On the third day, however, his hand was no better, so he decided to seek advice. But the advice he sought was not from a physician or other health practitioner; rather, it was from two colleagues at his law office, neither of whom had any medical training. Both colleagues advised Jeff to have his hand x-rayed to learn whether it was broken. Still, Jeff hesitated. He feared that taking time to be x-rayed and to see a doctor would be both inconvenient and expensive.

When he finally decided that an X ray was warranted, Jeff went to a local imaging center that specialized in X rays. The person at the imaging center informed Jeff that his hand could not be x-rayed there unless a physician referred him. Indeed, she seemed shocked that anyone would come to the imaging center without a physician's referral. So Jeff, an intelligent attorney with little understanding of how to seek health care in this instance, called his internist and asked her to order an X ray. The internist ordered the X ray and also referred Jeff to an orthopedic specialist, whom he saw the next day. Results of his X ray revealed a broken metacarpal, a bone in the hand between the wrist and the fingers. The orthopedist placed Jeff's hand in a cast and told him to wait 6 weeks before playing any more basketball or using his right hand for nearly anything else.

Why was Jeff reluctant to seek medical care? Why was the pain he experienced not sufficient to prompt him to go to the doctor? Why did he ask the opinion of people with no medical training before getting advice from a trained professional?

Adopting Health-Related Behaviors

Like Jeff, most people in the world value health and want to avoid disease and disability. Nevertheless, many people do not behave in ways that maximize health and minimize disease and disability. Why do some people, such as Jeff, seem to behave unwisely on issues of personal health? Why do others seek medical treatment when they are not ill? What explains people's reluctance to believe that their own risky behaviors are unsafe and their willingness to believe that those same behaviors place other people in jeopardy? No final answers to these questions are possible at this point, but psychologists have formulated several theories or models in the attempt to predict and to make sense of behaviors related to health. This chapter looks briefly at some of these theories as they relate to health-seeking behavior, whereas Chapter 4 examines theory-driven research about people's adherence to medical advice.

Theories of Health-Protective Behaviors

In Chapter 2, we said that useful theories (1) generate research, (2) organize and explain observations, and (3) guide the practitioner in predicting behavior. Health psychologists frequently use theoretical models to meet each of these criteria. These models include the health belief model, which originally grew out of the work of Geoffrey Hochbaum (1958) and his colleagues at the Public Health Service; the theory of reasoned action by Martin Fishbein and Icek Ajzen (Ajzen & Fishbein, 1980; Fishbein & Ajzen, 1975); the concept of planned behavior, which Ajzen developed as an alternative to the theory of reasoned action (Ajzen, 1985, 1991);

CHECK YOUR HEALTH RISKS

Check the items that apply to you.

- ☐ 1. If I feel well, I believe that I am healthy.
- ☐ 2. I see my dentist twice yearly for regular checkups.
- ☐ 3. The last time I sought medical care was in a hospital emergency room.
- ☐ 4. If I had a disease that would be a lot of trouble to manage, I would rather not know about it until I was really sick.
- ☐ 5. I try not to allow being sick to slow me down.
- ☐ 6. If I don't understand my physician's recommendations, I ask questions until I understand what I should do.
- ☐ 7. I think it's better to follow medical advice than to ask questions and cause problems, especially in the hospital.
- ☐ 8. When facing a stressful medical experience, I think the best strategy is to try not to think about it and hope that it will be over soon.
- ☐ 9. When I have severe symptoms, I try to find out as much information as possible about my medical condition.
- ☐ 10. I believe that if people get sick, it is because they were due to get sick, and there was nothing they could have done to prevent their sickness.
- ☐ 11. I'm a smoker who knows that smoking can cause heart disease and lung cancer, but I believe that other smokers are much more likely than me to get these diseases.
- ☐ 12. In order not to frighten patients faced with a difficult medical procedure, it is best to tell them that they won't be hurt, even if they will.

Items 2, 6, and 9 represents healthy attitudes or behaviors, but each of the other items relate to conditions that may present a risk or lead you to less effective health care. As you read this chapter, you will see the advantages of adopting healthy attitudes or behaviors to make more effective use of the health care system.

and the precaution adoption process model of Neil Weinstein (1988). In Chapter 4, we look at the behavioral model, self-efficacy theory, and the transtheoretical model and see their application of adherence to medical advice.

The Health Belief Model Since the early work of Geoffrey Hochbaum (1958), several versions of the *health belief model* (HBM) have been devised. The one that has attracted the most attention and generated the most research is that of Marshall Becker and Irwin Rosenstock (Becker & Rosenstock, 1984; Rosenstock, 1990).

Like all health belief models, the one developed by Becker and Rosenstock assumes that beliefs are important contributors to health-seeking behavior. This model includes four beliefs that should combine to predict health-related behaviors: (1) perceived *susceptibility* to disease or disability, (2) perceived *severity* of the disease or disability, (3) perceived *benefits* of health-enhancing behaviors, and (4) perceived *barriers* to health-enhancing behaviors, including financial costs.

Each of these factors played a part in Jeff's decision to seek assistance after he hurt his hand. At first, Jeff did not believe that his injury was serious or that he was vulnerable to disability. Thus, he saw little benefit in going to a doctor, an action that would have taking him away from his work as an attorney. After two of his colleagues expressed their belief that his injury might be serious, and after two days of eating, driving, writing, and dressing with his left hand, Jeff changed his beliefs and subsequently sought medical attention. Unlike most people who seek health care, financial cost was not a serious barrier to Jeff, whose most serious obstacle was lack of information about the health care system.

The health belief model corresponds with common sense. When people perceive that they are susceptible to a severe illness and can benefit from their ability to overcome barriers to good health, they should be guided by their own self-interest and actively seek health care. Common sense, however, does not always predict health-related behaviors. Research on the health belief model has been extensive, but results of that research generally suggests that a health belief model that includes only susceptibility, severity, benefits, and barriers does not predict health-related behaviors as well as models that include such additional variables as perceived health risks, optimism, personal control, ethnic background, and having a regular place to go for health care.

Perceived health risks may override perceived benefits to prevent people from seeking health care or adopting a healthy lifestyle. For example, women 70 years old and older reported that they feared adopting a physical activity program because it would be a risk to their heart (Cousins, 2000). Most of these women recognized the potential health benefits of exercise but worried that vigorous physical activity might lead to a heart attack, and this fear presented a barrier for them.

A second factor that affects people's beliefs about health care is their level of optimism, a variable not included in the original health belief model. Some research (Clarke, Lovegrove, Williams, & Machperson, 2000) has found that both women and men who knew about the severity and their personal susceptibility to cancer as well as the benefits and barriers of cancer screening had an unrealistic optimism that was more influential than the four HBM variables. That is, the women optimistically believed that a mammogram was not worth the trouble and the men had the same optimistic belief that prostate screening was unnecessary because cancer happened to other people and not to them.

A third factor that might mitigate the four elements of the health belief model is perceived personal control. A study of intentions of undergraduate students to engage in AIDS-preventive behaviors (Smith & Stasson, 2000) found that perceived behavioral control—the level of control people believe they have over their own behavior—was stronger than any of the elements of the HBM in predicting intention to use condoms and to discuss AIDS information with a partner.

A fourth factor, and one frequently more powerful than the components of the HBM, is ethnic background. For example, a prospective study (Hyman, Baker, Ephraim, Moadel, & Philip, 1994) showed that being an African American woman—rather than a European American woman—was a better predictor of mammography use than any of the four elements of the health belief model. (**Mammography** is an X-ray technique for detecting breast cancer before it can be seen or felt.) Poverty also plays a powerful part in seeking health care. People who lack monetary resources and/or insurance are less likely to seek help when they are sick or disabled. Having a regular place to go for health care and having a physician who recommends screening tests are better predictors of who will seek health care than the combined factors of the health belief model (Aiken, West, Woodward, & Reno, 1994).

How can the health belief model be improved to better predict who will seek health care? One approach would be to construct an instrument that would consider unrealistic optimism and irrational beliefs about the risk of health care procedures. A group of researchers (Christensen, Moran, & Wiebe, 1999) has attempted to solve this problem by developing the Irrational Health Belief Scare (IHBS), an instrument that has moderate reliability and validity for measuring health-related cognitive distortions. The scale consists of 20 hypothetical health-related scenarios and asks participants to rate their attitudes toward each situation on a 5-point scale from "not at all like I would think" to "almost exactly what I would think." To date, little research has been reported on the IHBS.

In summary, studies that have showed the strongest predictive value of the HBM generally used an expanded version of the model, including perceived personal control, perceived risks, intentions to behave, perceived social norms, and **self-efficacy,** or the belief that one is capable of performing the behaviors that will produce desired outcomes. For this reason, some researchers (e.g., Poss, 2000) have combined aspects of the health belief model with concepts from other models, including the theory of reasoned action.

The Theory of Reasoned Action The *theory of reasoned action* (Ajzen & Fishbein, 1980; Fishbein & Ajzen, 1975) assumes that people are quite reasonable and make systematic use of information when deciding how to behave. Moreover, they "consider the implications of their actions before they decide to engage or not engage in a given behavior" (Ajzen, 1985, p. 5). In addition, the theory of reasoned action assumes that behavior is directed toward a goal or outcome and that people freely choose those actions that they believe will move them in the direction of that goal. They can also choose not to act, if they believe that such an action would move them away from their goal, as when Jeff decided not to seek immediate medical attention because he believed that a cast on his hand would hamper his regular work routine.

The immediate determinant of behavior is the *intention* to act or not to act. Intentions, in turn, are shaped by two factors. The first is a personal evaluation of the behavior—that is, one's *attitude toward the behavior.* The second is one's perception of the social pressure to perform or not perform the action—that is, one's *subjective norm.* One's attitude toward the behavior is determined by beliefs that the behavior will lead to positively or negatively valued outcomes. One's subjective norm is shaped by one's perception of the evaluation that a particular individual (or group of individuals) places on that behavior and one's *motivation* to comply with the norms set by that individual (or group of individuals). In predicting behavior, the theory of reasoned action also considers the relative weight of personal attitudes measured against subjective norms (see Figure 3.1).

In predicting whether Jeff, with a painful, discolored, and swollen hand, will seek medical attention, the theory of reasoned action relies on several pieces of information. First, does Jeff believe that going to the doctor's office is related to his goal of a healthy hand? Second, how strong is his belief that other people expect him to seek medical attention balanced against his need to comply with others' expectations? The answer to the first question reveals Jeff's attitude toward seeking medical assistance, and the answer to the second question suggests the level of social pressure on him to seek assistance. These two answers reflect his attitude toward seeking medical care and his subjective norm about seeking care. Because Jeff's attitudes and his subjective norms were initially in conflict, his early intention was somewhat mixed, making prediction of his behavior difficult. Nevertheless, the theory of reasoned action has the potential to make valid predictions when investigators accurately measure both the strength of a person's attitude toward a behavior and the person's need to conform to social norms.

Does the theory of reasoned action predict health-seeking behavior? In general, researchers have found the theory to be useful for predicting safe and unsafe health-related behaviors, including use of mammograms and condoms and driving while intoxicated. In the study on mammograms (Montano, Thompson, Taylor, & Mahloch, 1997), low-income women were questioned regarding their attitude, subjective norms, intentions, and previous use of mammography. All basic components of the theory of reasoned action were significantly related to intention to get a mammogram, and intention predicted use of mammography.

The theory of reasoned action also predicts intentions to use condoms. Two groups of researchers (Albarracin, Fishbein, Johnson, & Muellerleile, 2001; Sheeran & Taylor, 1999) conducted meta-analyses of 67 studies on the efficacy of the theories of reasoned action and planned behavior to predict use of condoms. The earlier analysis (Sheeran & Taylor, 1999) revealed small correlations between intentions to

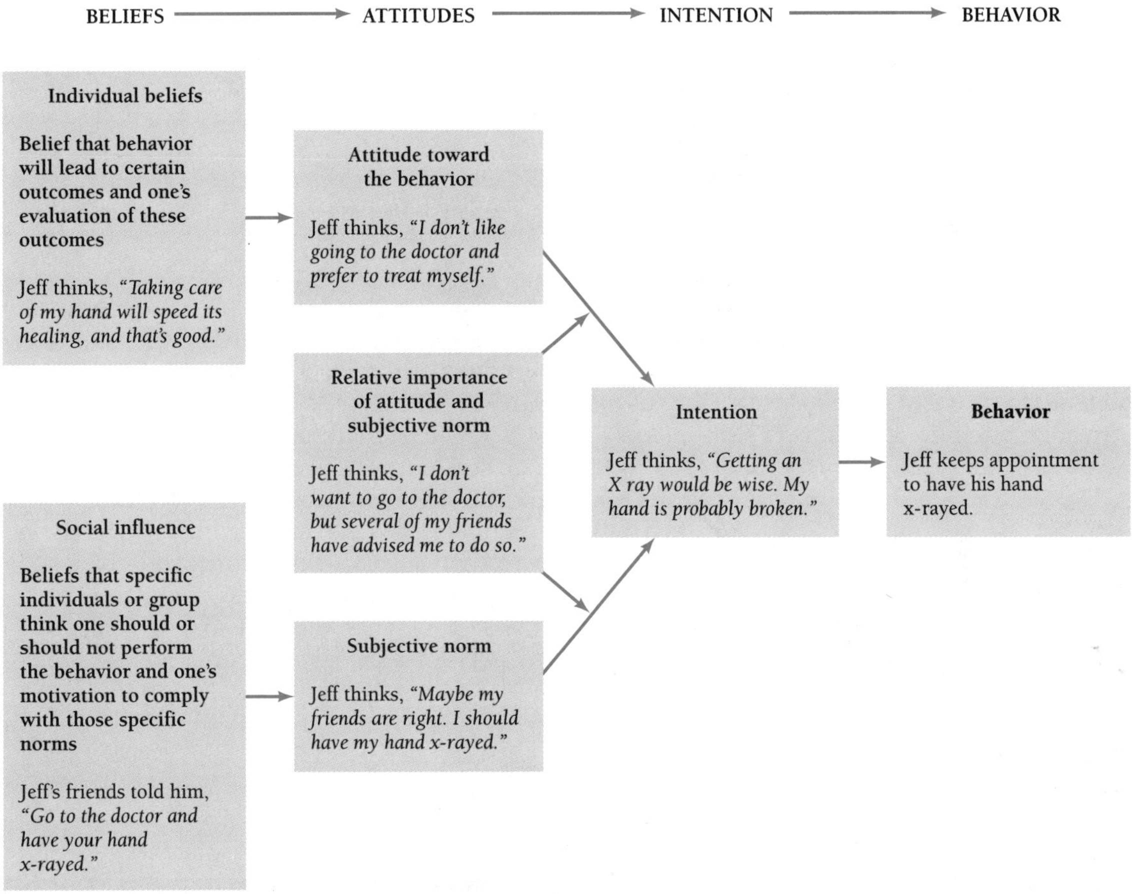

BELIEFS → ATTITUDES → INTENTION → BEHAVIOR

Individual beliefs

Belief that behavior will lead to certain outcomes and one's evaluation of these outcomes

Jeff thinks, *"Taking care of my hand will speed its healing, and that's good."*

Attitude toward the behavior

Jeff thinks, *"I don't like going to the doctor and prefer to treat myself."*

Relative importance of attitude and subjective norm

Jeff thinks, *"I don't want to go to the doctor, but several of my friends have advised me to do so."*

Social influence

Beliefs that specific individuals or group think one should or should not perform the behavior and one's motivation to comply with those specific norms

Jeff's friends told him, *"Go to the doctor and have your hand x-rayed."*

Subjective norm

Jeff thinks, *"Maybe my friends are right. I should have my hand x-rayed."*

Intention

Jeff thinks, *"Getting an X ray would be wise. My hand is probably broken."*

Behavior

Jeff keeps appointment to have his hand x-rayed.

Figure 3.1 Theory of reasoned action applied to health-seeking behavior.

Source: Adapted from Understanding Attitudes and Predicting Social Behavior *(p. 8) 1980, by I. Ajzen and M. Fishbein, Englewood Cliffs, NJ: Prentice-Hall. Copyright 1980 by Prentice-Hall, Inc. Reprinted by permission.*

use condoms and demographic variables, sexual experience, personality traits, knowledge about AIDS, and perceived threat of the disease. However, this analysis yielded medium to strong relationships between intention to use condoms and both attitudes and subjective norms, two components of the theory of reasoned action. The second analysis (Albarracin et al., 2001) included 96 studies and also found moderate to strong support for each of the components of the theory of reasoned action to predict condom use; that is, attitudes and subjective norms predicted intentions, and intentions in turn were moderately correlated with use of condoms.

These and other studies have found the theory of reasoned action to be at least as adequate as the health belief model in explaining and predicting health-seeking behaviors. Key elements in the theory of reasoned action seem to be attitudes toward the behavior and subjective norms, both of which relate to the intention to perform a behavior.

The Theory of Planned Behavior Ajzen has extended the theory of reasoned action to include the concept of perceived behavioral control, an extension he calls the *theory of planned behavior.* The primary difference between the theory of

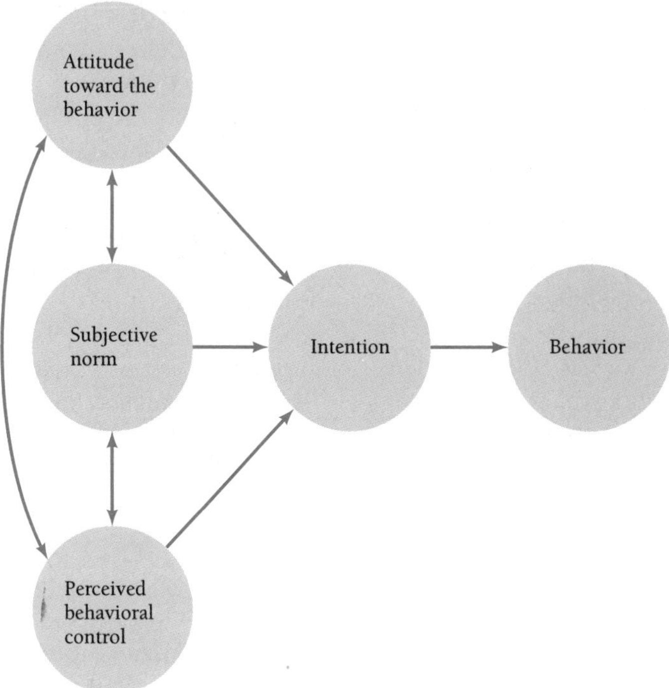

Figure 3.2 Theory of planned behavior.

Source: From "The theory of planned behavior." by I. Ajzen, 1991, Organizational Behavior and Human Decision Processes, 50, *(p. 182). Reprinted by permission of Academic Press.*

reasoned action and the theory of planned behavior is the latter's inclusion of the *perception of how much control* people have over their behavior (Ajzen, 1985, 1988, 1991). The more resources and opportunities people believe they have, the stronger are their beliefs that they can control their behavior. Figure 3.2 shows that predictions of behavior can be made from knowledge of (1) people's attitude toward the behavior, (2) their subjective norm, and (3) their perceived behavioral control. All three components interact to shape people's intentions to behave. Perceived behavioral control is the ease or difficulty one has in achieving desired behavioral outcomes; it reflects both past behaviors and perceived ability to overcome obstacles. The theory assumes that people who believe they can easily perform a behavior are more likely to *intend* to perform that behavior than people who believe they have little control over performing that behavior.

The theory of planned behavior has been used to predict a wide variety of health-related issues, including having unprotected sex. The two studies cited earlier (Albarracin et al., 2001; Sheeran & Taylor, 1999), supporting the ability of the theory of reasoned action to predict condom use, also looked at perceived behavioral control—the added ingredient to the theory of planned behavior. The results were somewhat mixed. The earlier study (Sheeran & Taylor, 1999) found that perceived behavioral control was positively related to intentions to use condoms and added significantly to the effects of attitudes and subjective norms. However, the second study (Albarracin et al., 2001) found that although perceived behavioral control was positively related to intentions, it did not add significantly to the other components of the theory of planned behavior. A third study with college students (Conner & Flesch, 2001) found that all components of the theory of planned behavior—including perceived behavioral control—predicted intentions to use condoms during casual sex. In this study, alcohol was added to the scenario and, along with the availability of condoms, it increased students' intentions to engage in casual sex.

Other research has demonstrated that the theory of planned behavior has at least moderate ability to predict intentions of young people to purchase and use the illicit drug ecstasy (Orbell, Blair, Sherlock, & Conner, 2001), to smoke cigarettes (Maher, & Rickwood, 1997), and to engage in health-related behaviors such as breast self-examination, testicular self-examination, and dental flossing (McCaul, Sandgren, O'Neill, & Hinsz, 1993).

The Precaution Adoption Process Model Neil Weinstein (2000) has criticized other theoretical models for their narrow focus on people's perceived *severity* and perceived *susceptibility* of a disease or disorder and for ignoring people's transition from one stage to another in their readiness to adopt health-related behaviors. His *precaution adoption process model* (Weinstein, 1988) assumes that when people begin new and relatively complex behaviors aimed at protecting themselves from harm, they go through several *stages of belief* about their personal susceptibility. People do not move inevitably from lower to higher stages, and they may even move backward, as when a person who previously had considered stopping smoking abandons that consideration.

Weinstein's precaution adoption process model holds that people move through seven stages in their readiness to adopt a health-related behavior (see Figure 3.3). In stage 1, people have not heard of the hazard and thus are unaware of any personal risk. In stage 2, they are aware of the hazard and believe that others are at risk, but they hold an **optimistic bias** regarding their own level of risk. Stage 3 people acknowledge their personal susceptibility and accept the notion that precaution would be personally effective, but they have not yet decided to take action.

Stages 4 and 5 are critical. In stage 4, people decide to take action, whereas in the parallel stage 5, people decide that action is unnecessary. Some people who branch off to stage 5 may later return to stage 4 and decide to take appropriate action. In stage 6, people have already taken the precautions aimed at reducing risks. Stage 7 involves maintaining the precaution, if needed. Maintenance would be unnecessary in the case of a lifetime vaccination, but it is essential for smoking cessation or dietary changes. Before people take action, they must first perceive that the relative benefits of the precaution outweigh its costs.

Although Weinstein's notion of optimistic bias has generated substantial research, his more global concept of the precaution adoption process model has attracted less attention from researchers. One study (Blalock et al., 1996) of 35- to 45-year-old women reported that this model was useful in predicting calcium consumption and weight-bearing exercise, two behaviors recommended to reduce the risk of osteoporosis. These researchers found that: (1) the women's stages of change paralleled their knowledge of and attitude toward osteoporosis; (2) Weinstein's stages of change were related to the women's perceived benefits of exercise and calcium consumption as well as to the inconvenience of these two behaviors; (3) women at the different stages differed in their requests for information on osteoporosis, with those at the higher stages wanting to know more about the illness; and (4) contrary to expectations, women who had given up exercise and stopped taking extra calcium had more favorable attitudes toward those two behaviors than some of the other women. Although these findings offer support for the precaution adoption process model, little research on Weinstein's total theory has been reported in recent years.

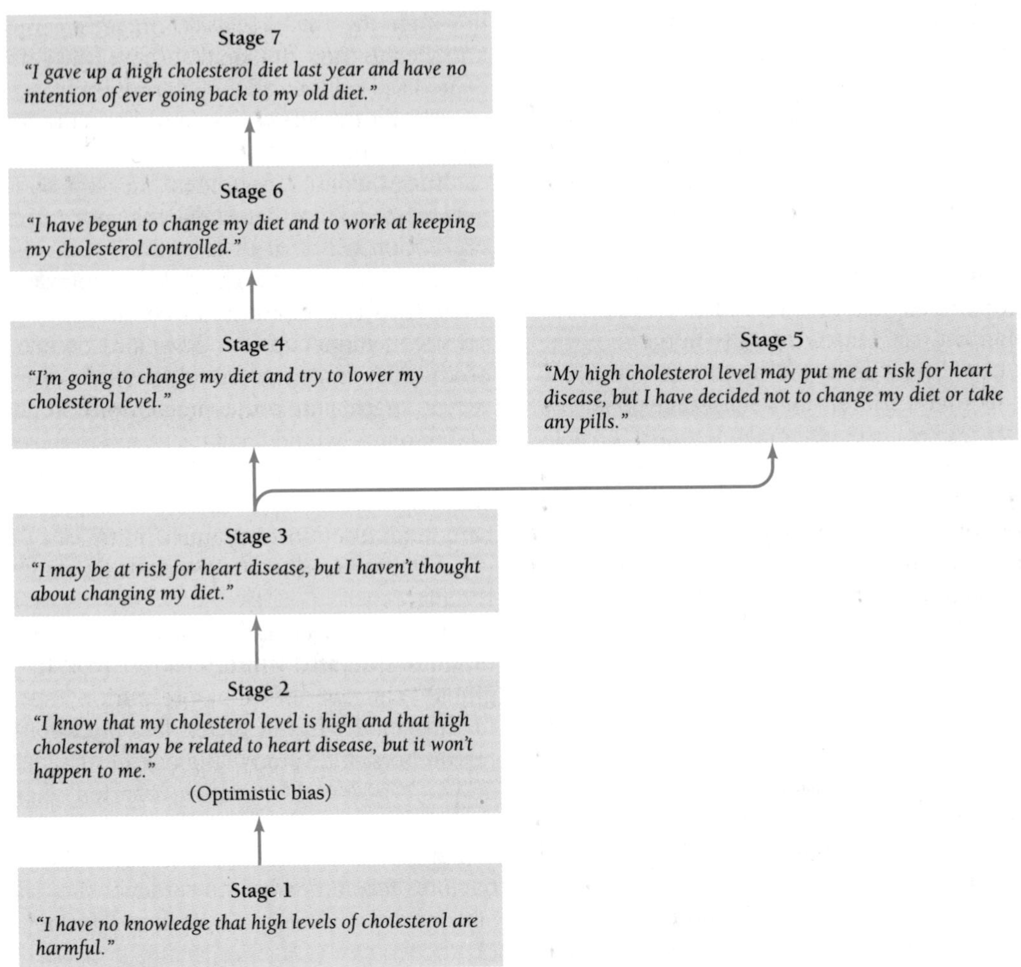

Figure 3.3 Weinstein's seven stages of the precaution adoption process model.

Critique of Health-Related Theories

In Chapter 2, we said that a useful theory should (1) generate significant research, (2) organize and explain observations, and (3) help the practitioner predict and change behaviors. How well do these health-related theories meet these three criteria? First, the older theories—namely, the health belief model, the theory of reasoned action, and self-efficacy theory—have all produced substantial amounts of research, and the newer models show promise of stimulating additional research. In addition, all these models are able to do better than chance in explaining and predicting behavior, and they generally are more accurate than demographic factors in predicting health-related behaviors.

Despite some modest success of health-related theories, a need still exists for models that more accurately differentiate between people who will seek medical attention and those who will not in a variety of health-related situations. One review of the effectiveness of the health belief model, the theory of reasoned action, the theory of planned behavior, and self-efficacy theory as they applied to cardiovascular disease risk reduction found weaknesses in each of the models (Fleury, 1992). This review looked at 10 studies that used the health belief model and concluded that, at best, this model has yielded inconsistent results when attempting to predict or explain behavior of people diagnosed with heart disease. The review found somewhat more support for the theory of reasoned action and the theory of planned behavior, largely because both these theories include the concept of intention, which is a strong factor in predicting health-related behaviors. The review also included 14 studies on self-efficacy and concluded that efficacy expectations can be important in a person's decision to initiate health-related behaviors, but its role in maintaining change is much less clear.

Why are these theories somewhat less than adequate in explaining and predicting health-related behaviors? Several reasons exist. First, health-seeking behavior is determined by factors other than an individual's beliefs or perceptions. Rosenstock (1990) pointed out that interpersonal processes, institutional factors, community factors, and public policy (including law) all affect health-seeking behaviors. Rosenstock further commented that some health-related behaviors, such as cigarette smoking and dental care, can develop into habits that become so automatic that they are largely beyond the personal decision-making process. In addition, other health-producing behaviors, such as dietary changes, may be undertaken for the sake of personal appearance rather than health.

Another reason for the failure of theories to better predict health-seeking behaviors is that they must rely on consistent and accurate instruments to assess their various components, and such measures have not yet been developed. The health belief model, for example, might more accurately predict health-seeking behavior if valid measurements existed for each of its components. If a person feels susceptible to a disease, perceives his or her symptoms to be severe, believes that treatment will be effective, and sees few barriers, then logically, that person should seek health care. But each of these four factors is difficult to reliably and validly assess.

Also, a model may have some value for predicting health-seeking behaviors related to one disorder but not to another. Similarly, a theory may relate to health-seeking behavior but not to prevention behavior or to adherence to medical advice. No current theory is comprehensive enough to encompass all these areas. Also, the theories seldom consider that many people, such as children and some elderly persons, are often sent to health care professionals by someone else and have only limited choice in seeking care.

Finally, most of the models postulate some type of barrier or obstacle to seeking health care, and an almost unlimited number of barriers are possible. Often these barriers are beyond the life experience of researchers. For example, barriers for affluent European Americans may be quite different from those of poor Hispanic Americans or African Americans; thus, the health belief model and the theory of reasoned action may not apply equally to all ethnic groups (Poss, 2001). Models for health-seeking behavior tend to emphasize the importance of direct and personal control of behavioral choices. Little allowance is made for such barriers as racism and poverty.

In Summary

If and how people go about seeking medical attention when they feel unwell depends on several factors, many of which are included in one or more of the theories of health-seeking behaviors. Some of these determinants are (1) the characteristics of the symptoms being experienced, (2) the cost of seeking help, (3) the perceived severity of the disease, (4) a person's intention to act, (5) a person's stage of readiness for change, and (6) multiple social and demographic factors.

People adopt health-related behaviors in order to stay healthy and to combat disease. Several theoretical models have been formulated in an effort to explain and predict health behaviors, and most of these theories have some value in predicting and explaining health-related behavior. However, all of them have some limitations, especially in their ability to predict the health-related behaviors of people who lack the financial resources necessary to pursue proper medical attention.

Current theories drawing the most interest among researchers include the health belief model, the theory of reasoned action, the theory of planned behavior, self-efficacy theory, the precaution adoption process model, and the transtheoretical model. The health belief model includes the concepts of perceived severity of the disease, personal susceptibility, and perceived benefits of and barriers to health-enhancing behaviors. Research has shown that the health belief model has only limited success in predicting health-related behaviors.

The theory of reasoned action and the theory of planned behavior both include attitudes, subjective norms, and intention in an effort to predict and explain behavior. Moreover, the theory of planned behavior adds the person's perceived behavioral control. Research has found that the concepts of intention and perceived behavioral control are powerful predictors of health-seeking behaviors. Weinstein's precaution adoption process model assumes that when people are faced with adopting health-protective behaviors, they go through seven possible stages of belief about their personal susceptibility. Among these stages is the necessity of overcoming their optimistic bias; that is, their belief that although certain behaviors are dangerous, the danger pertains to other people and not to them. A limitation of each of these models is their inability to accurately measure myriad social, ethnic, and demographic factors that also affect people's health-seeking behavior. The balance of this chapter discusses issues involved in seeking medical attention, the problems of being in the hospital, and the preparations necessary to cope with stressful medical procedures.

Seeking Medical Attention

How do people know when to seek medical attention? How do they know whether they are ill or not? When Jeff injured his hand, he experienced pain that persisted for hours, yet he tried several alternatives before he sought medical attention. Those alternatives included home care and consulting nonexperts about his injury. Was Jeff unusually reluctant to seek medical care or was his behavior typical? Deciding when formal medical care is necessary is a difficult problem, compounded by personal, social, and economic factors.

We discuss these issues later, but first we define three terms: health, illness, and disease. Although the meaning of these concepts may seem obvious, their definitions have been elusive. Is health the absence of illness, or is it the attainment of some positive state? In the first chapter, we saw that the World Health Organization (WHO) defined health as positive physical, mental, and social well-being, and not merely as the absence of disease or infirmity. Unfortunately, this definition has little practical value for people trying to make decisions about their state of health or illness. Another difficulty for many people is the difference between illness and disease. These terms are often used interchangeably, but most health scientists make a distinction between illness and disease. Disease refers to the process of physical damage within the body and can exist even in the absence of a label or diagnosis. Illness, on the other hand, refers to the experience of being sick and having been diagnosed as being sick. People can have a disease and not be ill. For example, people with undiagnosed hypertension, HIV infection, or cancer all have a disease, but they may appear quite healthy and be completely unaware of their disease. Although illness and disease are separate conditions, they often overlap, for example, when a person feels ill and has been officially diagnosed.

People frequently experience physical symptoms, but these symptoms may or may not indicate a disease. Symptoms such as a headache, a painful shoulder, sniffles, and sneezing would probably not prompt a person to seek medical care, but an intense and persistent stomach pain probably would. At what point should a person decide to seek health care? Errors in both directions are possible. People who decide to go to the doctor when they are not really sick feel foolish, must pay the bill for an office visit, and lose credibility with people who know about the error, including the physician. If they choose not to seek health care, they may get better, but they may also get worse because they have tried to ignore their symptoms, which may make treatment more difficult and seriously endanger their health or increase their risk of death. A prudent action would seem to be to chance the unnecessary visit, but people are often reluctant to go to the doctor.

In the United States and other Western countries, people are not "officially" ill until they are diagnosed by a physician, making physicians the gatekeepers to further health care. They not only *determine* disease by their diagnoses but also *sanction* it by giving a diagnosis. Hence, the person with symptoms is not the one who officially determines his or her health status. Jeff's case illustrates this process. The imaging center would not provide him with an X ray of his hand without a physician's referral—the gate to medical care was closed without a physician's permission to receive these services.

Dealing with symptoms occurs in two stages, which Stanislav Kasl and Sidney Cobb (1966a, 1966b) called illness behavior and sick role behavior. **Illness behavior** consists of the activities undertaken by people who experience symptoms but who have not yet received a diagnosis. That is, illness behavior occurs *before* diagnosis. These activities are oriented toward determining one's state of health and discovering suitable remedies. Jeff was engaging in illness behavior when he sought the opinion of his colleagues, when he went to the imaging center, and when he called his internist for a referral. All these actions took place before his diagnosis and were oriented toward receiving a diagnosis. In contrast, **sick role behavior** is the term applied to the behavior of people after a diagnosis, either from a health care provider or a self-diagnosis. The activities of sick role behavior are oriented toward getting well. Jeff was exhibiting sick role behavior when he got his broken hand put in a cast, kept his appointments to have his hand checked, stopped playing basketball for 6 weeks, and took care not to reinjure his hand. All these activities occurred after diagnosis and were oriented toward getting well. A *diagnosis,* then, is the event that separates illness behavior from sick role behavior.

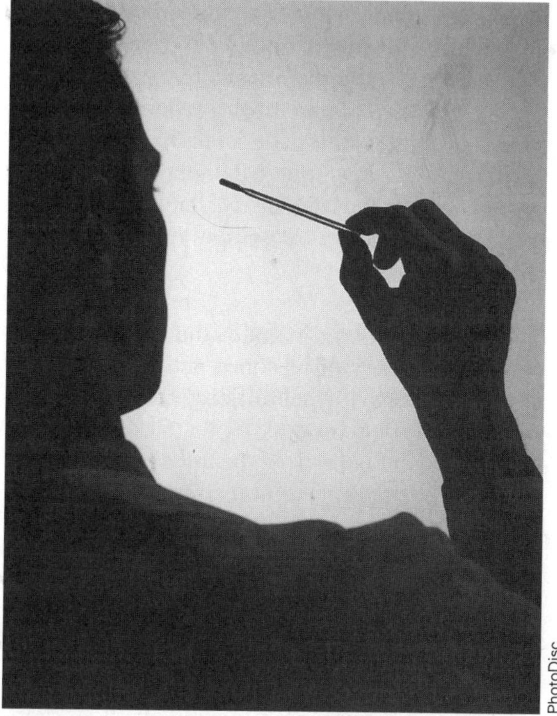
PhotoDisc

Illness behavior is directed toward determining health status.

Illness Behavior

Illness behavior takes place before one is officially diagnosed. It is directed toward determining health status in the presence of symptoms. People routinely experience symptoms that may signal disease. Symptoms are a critical element in seeking medical care, but the presence of symptoms is not sufficient to prompt a visit to the doctor. Given similar symptoms, some people readily seek help, others are reluctant, and still others do not seek help. What determines people's decision to seek professional care? At least six factors may shape their response to symptoms: (1) personal factors, (2) gender, (3) age, (4) socioeconomic and cultural factors, (5) characteristics of the symptoms, and (6) conceptualization of disease.

Personal Factors Personal factors include people's way of viewing their own body, their level of stress, and their personality traits. For example, people view some body parts, such as the anus, as stigmatized and other body parts, such as the genitalia, as private (Klonoff & Landrine, 1993). These perceptions lead the college students in this study to be reluctant to seek medical care for these two body parts. In addition, they were more likely to seek help for body parts perceived as important and vulnerable, such as the heart and blood.

Stress is another personal factor in people's readiness to seek care. People who experience a great deal of stress are more likely to seek health care than those under less stress, even with equal symptoms. Those who experience concurrent and prolonged stress are more likely to seek care when the symptoms are ambiguous (Cameron, Leventhal, & Leventhal, 1995).

Ironically, complaining about or being perceived as being under high stress makes it less likely that people will be considered to have a disease. Symptoms that vary along with stress tend to be discounted as not real (Leventhal & Diefenbach, 1991). This discounting occurs selectively, with women under high stress judged as less likely to have a physical disease than men in the same circumstances (Martin & Lemos, 2002). This tendency to discount symptoms may be very important for both women who experience symptoms and for the health care providers who hear their reports.

Personality traits may also contribute to illness behavior. Sheldon Cohen and his colleagues (Feldman, Cohen, Gwaltney, Doyle, & Skoner, 1999) inoculated a group of healthy volunteers with a common cold virus to see if participants with different personality traits would report symptoms differently. Participants who scored high on neuroticism, that is, those with strong emotional reactions, generally had high self-reports of illness whether or not objective evidence confirmed their reports. These people also reported more symptoms than other participants, suggesting that people with strong emotional reactions are more likely to complain of an illness.

Gender Differences In addition to personal factors, gender plays a role in the decision to seek treatment, with women more likely than men to use health care. The reasons for this difference are somewhat complex. Women tend to be more sensitive to their internal body signals than men, and this sensitivity makes women more likely to perceive and thus to report symptoms, even if they are not sicker than men. When asked about their symptoms, men tended to report only life-threatening situations, such as heart disease (Benyamini, Leventhal, & Leventhal, 2000). In contrast, women, reported not only these symptoms but also non-life-threatening symptoms, such as joint disease. Given the same level of symptoms, the female gender role allows women to seek many sorts of assistance whereas the male gender role teaches men to act strong and to deny pain and discomfort unless their disease is life threatening.

In addition, men's social role permits them to take more risks, and failure to seek health care is among these risks. Men are more likely to need health care because they have greater risks from alcohol consumption and job hazards, but women are at greater risk through physical inactivity, unemployment, and stress. When all risk factors are controlled, the illness gap between men and women may be quite narrow (Lahelma, Arber, Martikainen, & Silventoinen, 2001).

Age Age is yet another factor that influences people's willingness to seek medical care. Young and middle-aged adults show the greatest reluctance to see a health professional, probably because they feel more indestructible. Also, children are more willing to seek help than adolescents, especially male adolescents (Garland & Zigler, 1994).

As people age, they must make distinctions between symptoms of aging and those of disease, discriminating between what is normal and symptoms that signal problems. This distinction is not always easy, but people tend to interpret problems with a gradual onset and mild symptoms as resulting from age, compared to those with sudden onset and severe symptoms. People who are able to attribute their symptoms to age tend to delay in seeking medical care, but older adults are not as strongly influenced by this tendency as the middle aged. Although older and middle-aged people do not differ in type of complaint or ease of access to health care, older people are quicker to seek medical care for symptoms that they cannot identify. This difference may reflect a lack of tolerance for uncertainty in older adults and a desire to deny or minimize the severity of illness in middle-aged adults (Leventhal & Diefenbach, 1991).

Socioeconomic and Cultural Factors Socioeconomic and cultural factors also relate to people's frequency of seeking medical care. People in higher socioeconomic groups experience fewer symptoms and report a higher level of health than people at lower socioeconomic levels (Pennebaker, 1982). Yet, when higher income people are sick, they are more likely to seek health care. Nevertheless, poor people are overrepresented among the hospitalized, an indication that they are much more likely than middle- and upper-class people to become seriously ill. In addition, people in lower socioeconomic groups tend to wait longer before seeking health care, thus making treatment more difficult and hospitalization more likely. The poor also have less access to medical care, have to travel longer to reach health care facilities, and must wait longer once they arrive at those facilities.

Ethnic background is another factor in seeking health care, with European Americans being more likely than other groups to report a visit to a physician. Part of the National Health and Nutrition Examination Survey (Harris, 2001) examined some of the reasons behind these ethnic differences, comparing European Americans, African Americans, and Mexican Americans with Type 2 diabetes on access to and use of health care facilities. Ethnic differences appeared in health insurance coverage as well as common risk factors for diabetes and heart disease.

Symptom Characteristics Symptom characteristics also influence when and how people look for help. Symptoms themselves do not inevitably lead people to seek care, but certain characteristics are important in their response to symptoms. David Mechanic (1978) listed four characteristics of the symptoms that determine one's response to disease.

First is the *visibility of the symptom*—that is, how readily apparent the symptom is to the person and to others. A study on intentions to adopt osteoporosis prevention (Klohn & Rogers, 1991) confirmed the importance of the visibility of symptoms. Young women who received messages about osteoporosis as a disfiguring condition were significantly more likely to say that they intended to adopt precautions against osteoporosis than young women who were not alerted to the disfiguring aspects of osteoporosis.

Mechanic's second symptom characteristic was *perceived severity of the symptom*. He contended that symptoms seen as severe would be more likely to prompt action than less severe symptoms. In part, Jeff did not seek immediate medical care because his hand did not appear to be broken, nor was it discolored until the second day. The perceived severity of the symptom highlights the importance of personal perception and distinguishes between the perceived severity of a symptom and the judgment of severity by medical authorities. Indeed, patients and physicians differ in their perceptions of the severity of a wide variety of symptoms (Peay & Peay, 1998). Symptoms perceived as more serious produced greater concern and a stronger belief that treatment was urgently needed. Therefore, perceived severity of symptoms rather than the presence of symptoms is critical in the decision to seek care.

The third symptom characteristic mentioned by Mechanic was the *extent to which the symptom interferes with a person's life,* and some evidence (Suchman, 1965) indicates that the degree of incapacitation affected the person's action in seeking care. That is, the more incapacitated the person is, the more likely he or she is to seek medical care. On the third day after his injury, Jeff's broken hand began to seriously interfere with daily activities, a condition that motivated him to seek medical attention

Mechanic's fourth hypothesized determinant of illness behavior is the *frequency and persistence of the symptoms.* Conditions that people view as requiring care tend to be those that are both severe and continuous, whereas intermittent symptoms are less likely to generate illness behavior (Suchman, 1965). Severe symptoms prompt people to seek help, but even mild symptoms can motivate people to seek help if those symptoms persist. When ice packs could not reduce the swelling of his hand and when the pain persisted, Jeff decided to take action.

In Mechanic's description and subsequent research, symptom characteristics alone are not sufficient to prompt illness behavior. However, if symptoms persist or are perceived as severe, people are more likely to evaluate them as indicating a need for care. Thus, people are prompted to seek care on the basis of their interpretation of their symptoms, which relates to each person's view of illness.

Conceptualization of Disease Despite a vast amount of knowledge in the fields of physiology and medicine, most people are largely ignorant of how their bodies work and how diseases develop. When people gain information, they integrate it into their existing knowledge structure. If the new information seems incompatible with what they already "know," they may modify this new information to make it fit their preexisting knowledge rather than changing their knowledge to conform to the new information. This process may, of course, lead to personal conceptualizations of disease that vary substantially from the medical explanation. Both children (Veldtman et al., 2001) and college students (Nemeroff, 1995) showed inaccurate and incomplete conceptualizations of diseases in describing diseases they had and how they became ill.

Howard Leventhal and his colleagues (Benyamini, Leventhal, & Leventhal, 1997, 2000; Leventhal, Leventhal, & Cameron, 2001) have explored how people conceptualize various diseases. They have studied five components in the conceptualization of disease: (1) identity of the disease, (2) time line (the time course of both disease and treatment), (3) cause of the disease, (4) consequences of the disease, and (5) controllability of the disease. Further research (Lau, 1997; Veldtman et al., 2001) has confirmed the factors identified by Leventhal and his colleagues in samples of healthy adults as well as adults with acute and chronic diseases.

The *identity of the disease,* the first component identified by Leventhal and his associates, is very important to illness behavior. A person who has identified his symptoms as a "heart attack" should react quite differently from one who labels the same symptoms as "heartburn." The presence of symptoms is not sufficient to initiate help seeking, but the labeling that occurs in conjunction with symptoms may be critical in a person's either seeking help or ignoring symptoms.

Labels provide a framework within which symptoms can be interpreted. People experience less emotional arousal when they find a label that indicates a minor problem (heartburn rather than heart attack). Initially, they will probably adopt the least serious label that fits their symptoms. For example, Jeff initially interpreted his broken hand as a bruise. To a large extent, a label carries with it some prediction about the time course of the disease, so if the time course does not correspond to the expectation implicit in the label, the person has to relabel the symptoms. When Jeff's hand failed to respond to the ice packs and the pain continued, he began to doubt the label he had applied. His friends told him he was foolish to ignore the swelling and pain out of a belief that these symptoms would disappear. However, the tendency to interpret symptoms as indicating minor rather than major problems is the source of many optimistic self-diagnoses, and Jeff's was no exception.

The second component in conceptualizing an illness is the *time line.* Even though the time course of a disease is usually implicit within the diagnosis, people's understanding of the time involved is not necessarily accurate. People with hypertension, a chronic disease, tended to conceptualize their disease as acute (Meyer, Leventhal, & Gutman, 1985); that is, these patients saw their disease as corresponding to the pattern of most temporary diseases, with the onset of symptoms followed by treatment, a remission of symptoms, and then a cure. This belief was frequent among patients who had been recently diagnosed as hypertensive; 40% of those patients expressed the belief that they would be cured. It was much less common among those who had stayed in treatment for at least 3 months; only 12% of these patients holding an acute concept of their disease.

The third component of the personal view of illness is the *determination of cause.* For the most part, determining causality is more a facet of the sick role than of illness behavior because it usually occurs after a diagnosis has been made. But the attribution of causality for symptoms is an important factor in illness behavior. For example, if a person can attribute the pain in his hand to a blow received on the day before, he will not have to consider the possibility of bone cancer as the cause of the pain.

Attribution of causality, however, is often faulty. People may attribute a cold to "germs" or to the weather, and they may see cancer as caused by microwave ovens or by the will of God. The belief that God's will and sin play a role in disease is not unusual (Klonoff & Landrine, 1994), and these conceptualizations have important implications for illness behavior. People are less likely to seek professional treatment for conditions they consider as having emotional or spiritual causes. Among a group of adults with coronary artery disease, older patients were more likely than younger ones to believe that age rather than smoking or high cholesterol was the cause of their disease (Gump et al., 2001). These beliefs may affect how these patients care for themselves and manage their cardiovascular disease. Therefore, people's conceptualizations of disease causality can influence their behavior.

The *consequences of a disease* are the fourth component in Leventhal's description of illness conceptualizations. Again, the consequences of a disease are implied by the diagnosis. However, an incorrect understanding of the consequences can have a profound effect on illness behavior. Many people view a diagnosis of cancer as a death sentence. Some neglect health care because they believe themselves to be in a hopeless situation. Women who find a lump in their breast sometimes delay making an appointment with a doctor (Champion & Miller, 1997), not because they fail to recognize this symptom of cancer, but because they fear the possible consequences—surgery and possibly the loss of a breast, chemotherapy, radiation, or some combination of these consequences.

The *controllability* of a disease relates to people's perception of the responsiveness of the condition to treatment. People who believe that their behaviors will not change the course of a disease are less likely to seek treatment than those who believe that prompt treatment will be effective. In addition, the perception that a person can control the outcome of a disease will make the person less likely to seek care from a professional than a person who believes that expert care is necessary.

The Sick Role

Kasl and Cobb (1966b) defined sick role behavior as the activities engaged in by those who believe themselves ill, for the purpose of getting well. In other words, sick role behavior occurs *after* a person has been diagnosed. Alexander Segall (1997) modified this concept, proposing that the sick role concept includes three rights or privileges and three duties or responsibilities. The privileges are (1) the right to make decisions concerning health-related issues, (2) the right to be exempt from normal duties, and (3) the right to become dependent on others for assistance. The three responsibilities are (1) the duty to maintain health as well as get well, (2) the duty to perform routine health care management and, (3) the duty to use a range of health care resources.

Segall's formulation of rights and duties is meant to be an ideal—not a realistic conception of sick role behavior in the United States. The first right—to make decisions concerning health-related issues—does not extend to children and to many people living in poverty (Bailis, Segall, Mahon, Chipperfield, & Dunn (2001).

The second feature of the sick role is the exemption of the sick person from normal duties. Sick people are usually not expected to go to work, school, or meetings; to cook, clean house, or care for children; to do homework or mow the lawn. However, meeting these expectations is not always possible. Many sick people do not stay home or go to the hospital, but rather they continue to go to work. Similarly, the third privilege—to be dependent on others—is more of an ideal than a reflection of reality. For example, sick mothers often must continue to be responsible for their children.

Each of Segall's three duties of sick people can be grouped under the single obligation to do whatever is necessary to get well. However, the goal of getting well applies more to acute than to chronic diseases. People with chronic diseases will never be completely well. This situation presents a conflict for many people with a chronic disease, who have difficulty accepting their condition as one of continuing disability and instead believe that their disease is a temporary state.

In Summary

No easy distinction exists between health and illness. The World Health Organization sees health as more than the absence of disease; rather health is the attainment of positive physical, mental, and social well-being. Curiously, the distinction between disease and illness is clearer. Disease refers to the process of physical damage within the body, whether or not the person is aware of this damage. Illness, on the other hand, refers to the experience of being sick; people can feel sick but have no identifiable disease.

At least six factors determine how people respond to illness symptoms: (1) personal factors, such as personality traits and the way people look upon their own body; (2) gender, with women being more likely than men to seek professional care; (3) age, with older people attributing many ailments to their age; (4) socioeconomic and cultural factors; people who cannot afford medical care are more likely than affluent people to become ill, but they are less likely to seek health care; (5) characteristics of the symptoms—symptoms that interfere with daily activities and that are visible, severe, and frequent are most likely to prompt medical attention; and (6) people's conceptualization of disease.

People tend to incorporate five components into their concept of disease: (1) the identity of the disease, (2) the time line of the disease, (3) the cause of the disease, (4) the consequences of the disease, and (5) controllability of the disease. If a disease has been officially identified or diagnosed, then its time course and its consequences are implicit. However, people who know the name of their disease do not always have an accurate concept of its time course and consequence and may wrongly see a chronic disease as having a short time course. People want to know the cause of their illness and understand how it can be controlled.

Once people's symptoms are diagnosed and they believe themselves to be ill, they engage in sick role behavior in order to get well. People who are sick should be relieved from normal responsibilities and should have the obligation of trying to get well. However, these rights and duties are often impossible to fulfill.

Receiving Health Care

People have a wide experience of receiving health care, from the time they are children, when they get bandages from caregivers and injections from pediatricians, to the time they are adults, when they are faced with a wide variety of health problems as well as choices of locations for and professionals who provide health care services. People may make those choices based on their personal preferences, but the cost of health care prevents many people from having access to all possibilities.

Limited Access to Health Care

Access to health care is more restricted in the United States than in other industrialized countries (Weitz, 2001). Many countries developed national health insurance or other plans for coverage for all citizens, but the United States has resisted this strategy. Hospitalization and other complex medical treatments are so expensive that most people cannot afford these services. This situation led to the development of insurance, and people may purchase health insurance as individuals or as members of groups that offer coverage to all members. Individual insurance tends to be expensive, especially for people with health problems, but these individuals may be able to get insurance as part of a workplace group. Thus, employment is an important factor in access to health care in the United States. People who are unemployed or whose jobs do not offer the benefit of health insurance are often uninsured.

The problem of providing health care for those who cannot afford to pay for these services was a concern throughout the 20th century (Weitz, 2001). As a response to these concerns, the U.S. Congress created two programs in 1965 to provide health care: Medicare and Medicaid. Medicare pays hospital expenses for most Americans over the age of 65. This program also offers insurance that those who participate may purchase for a monthly fee, but many medical expenses are not covered, such as prescription drugs. This situation leaves those people who are part of this program with substantial expenses that they must pay. In addition, the future funding for this program is uncertain, and the expense is rising while the benefits are decreasing. Medicare provides care to people based on their age, and Medicaid provides health care based on low income and physical problems, such as disability or pregnancy. These restrictions make many poor people ineligible; only about 40% of poor people receive Medicaid (Campbell, 1999). Therefore, many people in the United States have no insurance or have insurance that fails to pay for many of their health care expenses.

People without insurance face barriers in obtaining health care. These people are less likely to have a regular physician, more likely to have a chronic health problem, and less willing to seek medical care because of the cost (Washington, 2001). This reluctance has consequences for the management of their diseases; people with chronic diseases and without health insurance have poorly controlled conditions, more health crises, difficulty in obtaining medications, and higher risk of mortality than people with insurance (Becker, 2001). Therefore, health insurance coverage is an important issue in the access to medical care and in choosing a practitioner.

Choosing a Practitioner

As part of their attempts to get well, sick people usually consult a health care practitioner. Beginning during the 19th century, physicians became the dominant health care providers (Weitz, 2001). Most middle-class people in industrialized nations seek the services of a physician. Toward the end of the 20th century, however, medical dominance began to decline and other types of health care providers became more prominent. For example, midwives, nurses, physical therapists, psychologists, osteopaths, chiropractors, dentists, nutritionists, and herbal healers all provide various types of health care.

Some of these sources of health care are considered "alternative" because they provide alternatives to traditional medicine. Almost a third of U.S. residents seek some form of alternative health care (Cowley, King, Hager, & Rosenberg, 1995). Some people who consult practitioners such as herbal healers do so because these healers are part of a cultural tradition, such as *cuaranderos* in Latin American culture. However, the recent growth of alternative medicine has come mainly from well-educated people who are dissatisfied with traditional medical care and who hold attitudes that are compatible with the alternative care they seek (Austin, 1998). Well-educated people are disproportionately represented because they are more able to pay for this care, which is less likely to be covered by insurance than traditional care.

People without health insurance are less likely to have a regular health care provider than those with insurance (Washington, 2001). Their experience of receiving health care may consist of going to a hospital emergency room for care, even for chronic conditions. This strategy may result in these people receiving care only after their condition meets the definition of emergency. Thus, these patients are sicker than they might have been if they had easier access to care. In addition, seeking care from emergency rooms overburdens these facilities, decreasing their ability to provide care to those with acute conditions.

The health care system is changing and so are attitudes about receiving health care. Access to health care has become increasingly restricted, but attitudes concerning health care have become more consumer oriented. Younger people are particularly more likely to view patients as consumers of health care who, like any consumers, have choices in their selection of services and service providers (DiMatteo, 1997). This attitude is a sharp contrast with the trend toward restricting access to health care and limiting treatment options. This combination seems to be a guarantee for dissatisfaction, and many people believe that they are not receiving good quality health care (Vastag, 2001). Much of that dissatisfaction centers around health maintenance organizations (HMOs) and managed care.

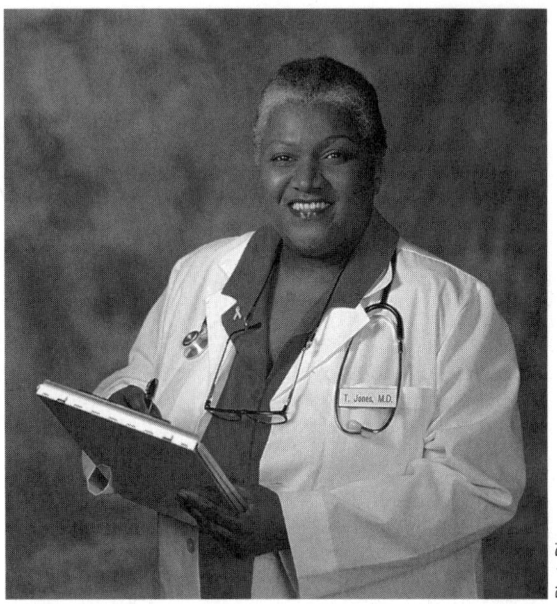

PhotoDisc

Patients are most pleased with health care providers who are friendly and willing to discuss health problems.

The Rise of Managed Health Care

Health maintenance organizations (HMOs) originated with the concept that prevention is preferable to treatment. Kaiser Permaente and the Group Health Cooperative of Puget Sound were organized to provide affordable care oriented toward keeping people healthy (Weitz, 2001). HMOs hire health care workers, including physicians, and pay them salaries for their services.

This arrangement differs from the fee-for-service payments that most physicians in private practice receive. Physicians in HMOs cannot boost their salaries by performing more procedures or seeing more patients. Thus, HMOs came to be seen as a way to contain rising health care costs. They have spread from a limited number to institutions that provide health care for over 80 million U.S. residents (Paul & Clarke, 2001).

The hope that HMOs could help contain escalating medical care costs led to changes in their operations. Rather than allowing HMO members to choose their services, HMOs began to limit services. That is, HMOs began to manage the amount of health care available to members. A typical arrangement includes a gatekeeper, a primary care physician who is often a general practitioner or family care specialist. Under this arrangement, patients must see a primary care physician when they visit the HMO, and this provider decides if the patient may see specialists or receive additional care. HMOs may pressure their primary care physicians to limit referrals and additional treatment as ways to cut costs (sometimes giving physicians bonuses for limiting these options). This strategy denies access to health care and has led to patient dissatisfaction and loss of members for HMOs (Paul & Clarke, 2001).

The trend toward managed care and limiting access to health care as ways to control costs also have affected insurance plan members. Rather than seeking health care from a practitioner of the person's choice, many insurance plans now have lists of preferred or exclusive providers whom members may consult (Weitz, 2001). Members may choose practitioners who are not on the list, but the financial penalty for this choice is high. Practitioners who are on such lists have agreements with the insurance companies to provide health care at lower cost.

Managed care has limited the amount and type of care that individuals receive and has restricted their choice of health care professionals. This situation may prevent people form creating ongoing relationships with health care providers and severely limits the option to seek any but traditional types of health care.

For physicians who provide health care, the practice of medicine has changed. The era of the solo practitioner is coming to an end; most physicians now practice within a multispecialty group of other health care providers or are employed by HMOs. These physicians have less autonomy to make treatment decisions and feel pressure to cut costs, possibly at their patients' health expense. The traditional authoritarian role of various health care providers is changing, with physicians' authority and power diminishing.

Therefore, health care has become less personal, more difficult to obtain, and more technology oriented. These factors have an impact on all facets of receiving health care, but depersonalization and technology are important factors for the experience of being in the hospital.

Being in the Hospital

Over the past 25 years, hospitals and the experience of being in the hospital have both changed. First, many types of surgery and tests that were formerly handled through hospitalization are now performed on an outpatient basis; second, hospital stays have become shorter; third, an expanding array of technology is available for diagnosis and treatment; and fourth, most patients now feel free to voice their concerns to their physician (Bell, Kravitz, Thom, Krupat, & Azari, 2001). As a result of these changes, people who are not severely ill are not likely to be hospitalized. Therefore, people who are admitted to a hospital are more severely ill than those admitted 30 years ago.

Ironically, managed care directives have resulted in shorter hospital stays in the interest of controlling health care costs (but not always in the interest of the patient). Technological medicine has become more prominent in patient care, and personal treatment by the hospital staff has become less so. These factors can combine to make hospitalization a stressful experience (Weitz, 2001). In addition, understaffing

WOULD YOU BELIEVE

Medical Care Can Be Dangerous

Would you believe that receiving medical care, especially in a hospital, can be fatal? Recent reports have painted an alarming picture of the dangers of receiving health care. In 1999, a study from the Institute of Medicine made headlines with its findings that at least 44,000, and perhaps as many as 98,000 people die in U.S. hospitals every year as a result of medical errors (Kohn, Corrigan, & Donaldson. 1999). Why such a large discrepancy in these estimates? Perhaps it was because the 44,000 figure was based on a study in Utah and Colorado (Thomas et al., 1999), whereas the 98,000 estimate was based on the earlier Harvard Medical Practice Study I (Brennan et al., 1991).

These figures created both sensational headlines and immediate controversy. *The New York Times* ("Preventing Fatal Medical Errors," 1999) compared these numbers with fatalities from the Vietnam War, stating that more Americans are killed in U.S. hospitals every 6 months than during the entire war in Vietnam, and the *Washington Post* (Weiss, 1999) calculated that medical errors are the fifth leading cause of death in the United States.

The purpose of the Harvard Medical Practice Study I (Brennan et al., 1991) was not to blame the medical profession but to discover the extent of medical errors that might lead to law suits for malpractice and the huge monetary claims often awarded to patients. This study was limited to New York State, but it provided the data for the Institute of Medicine's 98,000 estimate of deaths from medical errors, most of which were from mistakes associated with surgery.

Unfortunately, medical errors are not the only cause of unnecessary deaths of patients in U.S. hospitals. Medication, too, can kill. A meta-analysis of studies on adverse drug reactions (Lazarou, Pomeranz, & Corey, 1998) found that, even when prescribed and taken properly, prescription drugs account for between 76,000 and 137,000 deaths each year. This analysis included both patients admitted to a hospital for an adverse drug reaction and those already in the hospital who suffered a fatal drug reaction. This meta-analysis also estimated the total number of toxic drug reactions among hospitalized patients at more than 2 million. As with the reports on medical errors, these results created interest in the popular media. *Newsweek* carried an article on the report (Kalb, 1998) and estimated that death from adverse drug reactions is the fourth leading cause of death in the United States, exceeded only by cardiovascular disease, cancer, and stroke.

In summary, a conservative estimate of deaths from medical errors plus drug reactions would be about 120,000 (44,000 + 76,000), whereas the higher estimates (98,000 + 137,000) would suggest that 235,000 people die unnecessarily every year in the United States. Or stated another way, every 3 years medical errors may kill the equivalent of the entire population of the city of San Francisco.

---

and the challenges of monitoring complex technology and medication regimens have created an alarming number of medical mistakes. (See Would You Believe . . . ? box, "Medical Care Can Be Dangerous.")

The Hospital Patient Role Part of the sick role is to be a patient, and being a patient means conforming to the rules of the health care institution and complying with medical advice. When a person enters the hospital as a patient, that person becomes part of a complex institution and assumes a role within that institution. That role includes some difficult aspects: being treated as a "nonperson," tolerating lack of information, and losing control of daily activities.

Being referred to as "the multiple fracture in Room 458" may be both startling and annoying, but such a reference is not uncommon. When people are hospitalized, all but their illness becomes invisible, and their status is reduced to that of a "nonperson." Not only are patients' identities ignored but their comments and questions may also be overlooked. The hospital procedure focuses on the technical aspects of medical procedures, but it usually ignores patients' emotional needs and

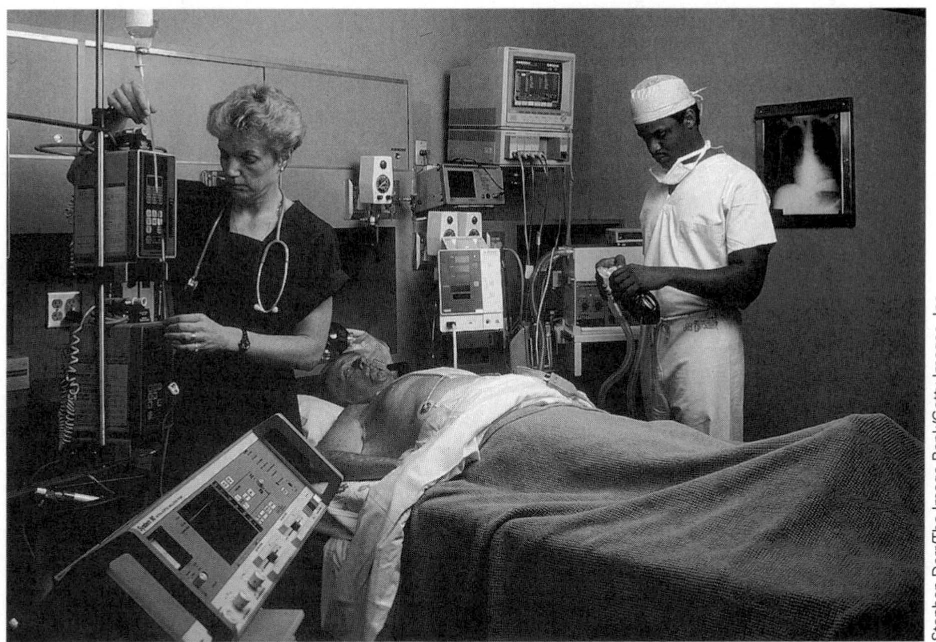
Stephen Derr/The Image Bank/Getty Images, Inc.

Hospitalized patients lack control of their lives and information about their conditions, resulting in increased distress.

leaves them less satisfied with their treatment than patients who are treated as persons and informed about their condition (Yarnold, Michelson, Thompson, & Adams, 1998).

The lack of information that patients experience comes from hospital routine rather than from an attempt to keep information from patients. The philosophy that physicians should decide how much patients ought to know has faded, and most physicians believe that patients should be fully informed about their conditions. However, an open exchange of information between patient and practitioner is difficult to achieve in the hospital; physicians spend only a brief amount of time in the hospital talking to patients. In addition, information may be unavailable because patients are undergoing diagnostic tests. The hospital staff may not explain the purpose or results of diagnostic testing, leaving the patient without information and filled with anxiety.

Hospitalized patients are expected to conform submissively to the rules of the hospital and the orders of their doctor, thus relinquishing much control over their lives. This loss of control can be very stressful. Henry Bennett and Elizabeth Disbrow (1993) suggested that research findings on loss of control can readily be applied to patients in hospital settings. For example, when exposed to uncontrollable, unpleasant stimulation, people experience more discomfort than they do when the situation is equally unpleasant but under their control. People tend to manifest heightened physiological responses and to react on a physical level to uncontrollable stimulation more strongly than they do when they can exert some control over the condition. Lack of control can decrease people's capacity to concentrate and can increase their tendency to report physical symptoms.

For the efficiency of the organization, uniform treatment and conformity to hospital routine are desirable, even though they deprive patients of information and control. Hospitals have no insidious plot to deprive patients of their freedom, but that is the result when hospitals impose their routine

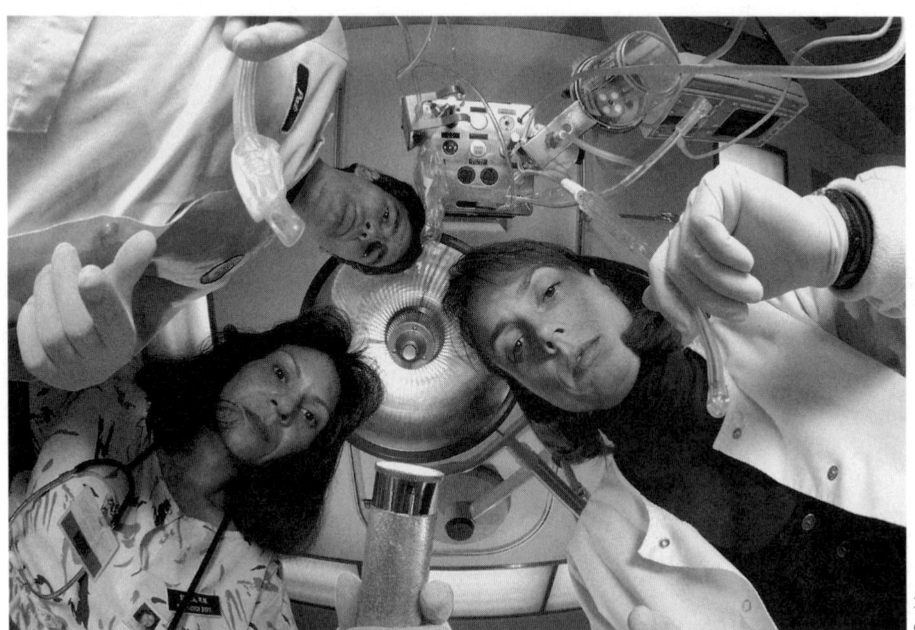
Corbis

Preparation for surgery can ease the stress associated with such procedures.

on patients. Restoring control to patients in any significant way would further complicate an already complex organization, but the restoration of small types of control may be effective. For example, many hospitals allow patients some choice of foods and provide TV remote controls to give patients the power to select a program to watch (or not watch). These aspects of control are small but possibly important (Langer & Rodin, 1976), as we discuss in Chapter 8. More important is the control that hospitalized patients have using patient-controlled systems of pain medication. Such systems allow patients to control the delivery of their intravenous pain medication, and these systems usually decrease medication use and increase patients' satisfaction (Siwek, 1997).

Children and Hospitalization Hospitalization is a common experience for children as well as for adults. Few children negotiate childhood without some injury, disease, or condition that requires hospitalization, and the commonalties of the hospitalization experience are sources of stress and anxiety—separation from parents, an unfamiliar environment, diagnostic tests, administration of anesthesia, surgery, and postoperative pain (Blount, Smith, & Frank, 1999). Since the middle of the 20th century, health care professionals have known and attended to the special problems of children in hospitals.

Training children to cope with their fear of treatment presents special problems to health psychologists. Pediatric hospitals often offer some type of preparation program for children (Blount et al., 1999). Group tours and discussions are the most common type of preparation, but the effectiveness of such interventions is questionable. Providing children and parents with information about hospital procedure and equipment is a more effective way to decrease anxiety.

Slide presentations or interactive computer programs have both demonstrated effectiveness in improving knowledge about hospitals (Nelson & Allen, 1999). Modeling can be even more effective, especially in allowing children to see another child who successfully copes with a procedure similar to the one that they are facing.

For example, pediatric patients facing first-time elective surgery experienced less emotional arousal after seeing a videotape about surgery (Pinto & Hollandsworth, 1989). In addition, children who viewed the video with their parents seemed to benefit more than children who saw the video alone, and the video also helped the parents control their anxiety. The results of this study indicate an advantage for both the videotape presentation and the presence of parents during psychological preparation for medical procedures.

Other research indicates that parents are able to help their children cope with hospitalization and painful medical procedures, but some parental reactions can make the situation worse (Manne et al., 1992). The time-honored parental technique of persistently reassuring a child facing medical treatment is not only ineffective but also tends to increase the child's feelings of distress (Bush, Melamed, Sheras, & Greenbaum, 1986). Training parents to be less anxious and to help their children cope may decrease the anxiety for both (Streisand, Rodrigue, Houck, Graham-Pole, & Berlant, 2000) and also aid in children's recovery (Melnyk & Feinstein, 2001).

Susan Jay and her colleagues (Jay, Elliott, Woody, & Siegel, 1991) devised a cognitive behavioral intervention for reducing children's distress that combines filmed modeling with relaxation training, distraction, and instruction on self-talk techniques. This program has been successful with children who were receiving painful treatments for leukemia. Indeed, this intervention was more successful than no treatment in lowering distress, pain ratings, and pulse rates, and it was also more successful than a drug treatment that included Valium. Thus, even though drugs are often considered an easier way to promote relaxation during stressful medical procedures, this research demonstrated the effectiveness of behavioral techniques.

Cost, not effectiveness, is the main problem with intervention strategies to reduce children's distress resulting from hospitalization or specific medical procedures. The trend is toward cost cutting, and all interventions add to medical care costs. Some of these interventions may be cost effective if they reduce the need for additional care or decrease other expenses. However, patient satisfaction is only one (and not always the primary) concern in determining care.

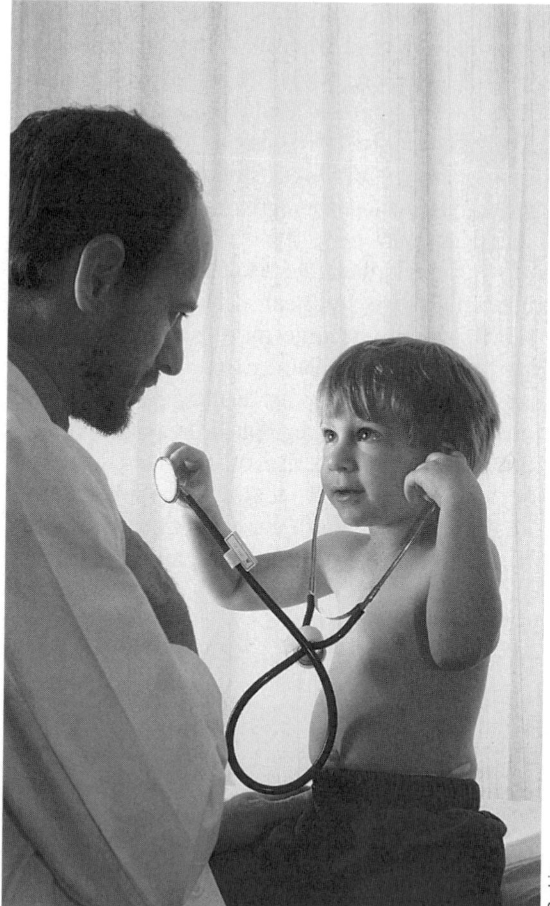
Corbis

Allowing children to become comfortable with medical apparatus can ease distress.

In Summary

The expense of health care has led to restricted access for most U.S. residents. Those people who have health insurance receive better care and have more choices about their health care than people without insurance. Concerns about health care costs led to the creation of two U.S. government-sponsored programs—Medicare, which pays for hospitalization for those over age 65, and Medicaid, which pays for care for poor people who are aged, blind, disabled, pregnant, or the parent of a dependent child.

Sick people usually seek care; physicians are traditional sources of health care, but alternative health care has become more popular over the past two decades. Again, people without health insurance often have disadvantages and limitations in securing a regular health care practitioner. However, the rise of managed care has affected the health care that most people receive. The drive to cut health care costs has prompted the proliferation of health maintenance organizations and preferred or exclusive provider networks, sometimes at the expense of patient care. Satisfaction with health care has declined.

Hospitalized patients often experience added stress as a result of being in the hospital. They are typically regarded as "nonpersons," receive inadequate information concerning their illness, and experience some loss of control over their lives. They are expected to conform to hospital routine and to comply with frequent requests of the hospital staff. Hospitalized children and their parents experience special problems and often receive special training to help them deal with hospitalization. Several types of interventions, including modeling, providing information and support, and cognitive behavioral programs, are effective in helping children and their parents cope with this difficult situation.

Answers

This chapter addressed three basic questions:

1. **Why do people adopt health-related behaviors?** Most people value good health and wish to avoid disease, but many fail to seek health care when necessary. Several theories attempt to explain health-related behavior. The health belief model was developed specifically to predict and explain health-related behaviors and includes the concepts of perceived severity of the disease, personal susceptibility, and perceived benefits and barriers of health-enhancing behaviors. Although recent research has demonstrated some utility for the original health belief model, other studies have introduced new concepts and have had only limited success in predicting health-seeking behavior.

   The theory of reasoned action and the theory of planned behavior are general behavior theories that have also been applied to health-related situations. Both theories include attitudes, subjective norms, and intention; in addition, the theory of planned behavior includes the person's perceived behavioral control. These two theories have not yet produced the volume of research generated by the health belief model, but some research suggests that the concepts of intention and perceived behavioral control add to the predictive ability of theories of reasoned action and planned behavior.

   Weinstein's precaution adoption process model assumes that when people are faced with adopting health protective behaviors, they go through seven possible stages of belief about their personal susceptibility. Built into one stage is optimistic bias, a topic that has been heavily researched. However, most research on the total precaution adoption model has been limited to Weinstein and his colleagues. A limitation of each of these models is their inability to accurately assess various social, ethnic, and other demographic factors that also affect people's health-seeking behavior.

2. **What factors are related to seeking medical attention?**
How people determine their health status when they do not feel well depends not only on social, ethnic, and demographic factors but also on the characteristics of their symptoms and their concept of illness. In deciding whether they are ill, people consider at least four characteristics of their symptoms: (1) the obvious visibility of the symptoms, (2) the perceived severity of the illness, (3) the degree to which the symptoms interfere with their lives, and (4) the frequency and persistence of the symptoms.
Once people are diagnosed as sick, they adopt the sick role that involves relief from normal social and occupational responsibilities and the duty to try to get better.
3. **What problems do people encounter in receiving medical care?**
People encounter problems in paying for medical care, and those without insurance often have limited access to health care. The U.S. government's creation of Medicare and Medicaid has helped people over 65 and some poor people with access to health care, but many people have problems in finding a regular practitioner and receiving optimal health care.
The escalating cost of medical care has changed receiving care. The system of private practitioners who provide care to individuals has become a system of managed care in which health care is restricted by gatekeepers in health maintenance organizations or by preferred providers specified by insurance companies.
Although hospital stays are shorter than 25 years ago, being in the hospital is a difficult experience for both adults and children. As a hospital patient, people must conform to hospital procedure and policy, which includes being treated as a "nonperson," tolerating lack of information, and losing control of daily activities. Children who are hospitalized are placed in an unfamiliar environment and may be separated from parents and undergo surgery or other painful medical procedures. Interventions that help children and parents manage this stressful experience may ease the distress, but cost is also a factor in providing these services.

Suggested Readings

Leventhal, H., Leventhal. E. A., & Cameron, L. (2001). Representations, procedures, and affect in illness self-regulation: A perceptual-cognitive model. In A. Baum, T. A. Revenson, & J. E. Singer (Eds.), *Handbook of health psychology* (pp. 19–47). Mahwah, NJ: Erlbaum. This article presents the self-regulation model, one of the models that explains how people conceptualize illness, along with the personal and social context of these cognitions. In contrasting the self-regulation model with other theories of health-related behaviors, the article provides a review of all these theories.

Strecher, V. J., & Rosenstock, I. M. (1997). The health belief model. In A. Baum, S. Newman, J. Weinman, R. West, & C. McManus (Eds.), *Cambridge handbook of psychology, health and medicine* (pp. 113–117). Cambridge, United Kingdom: Cambridge University Press. This short article discusses the health belief model and reviews research that the model has generated.

Weitz, R. (2001). *The sociology of health, illness, and health care: A critical approach.* (2nd ed.) Belmont, CA: Wadsworth. Weitz critically reviews the health care situation in the United States in this medical sociology book. Chapters 10, 11, and 12 provide a description of health care settings and professions, including many alternatives to traditional health care.

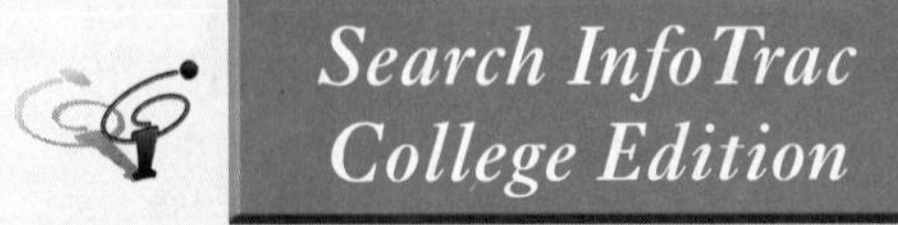

Search these terms to learn more about topics in this chapter:

- Health belief model
- Self-efficacy and health behavior
- Theory of planned behavior and health
- Illness behavior
- Sick role
- Gender and medical care
- Culture and medical care
- Managed care and patient satisfaction
- Health insurance and access to health care
- Medical errors and statistics
- Children and hospitalization and coping

4

Adhering to Medical Advice

The Story of Paul

CHAPTER OUTLINE

Theories That Apply to Adherence

Problems of Adherence

What Factors Predict Adherence?

Improving Adherence

QUESTIONS

This chapter focuses on four basic questions:

1. What theoretical models have been used to explain adherence?
2. What is adherence, how can it be measured, and how frequently does it occur?
3. What factors predict adherence?
4. How can adherence be improved?

The Story of Paul

Two years ago, Paul, a 47-year-old European American, suffered a heart attack (myocardial infarction), and since that time he has been under treatment for coronary heart disease. Paul returned to his job as a college professor soon after his release from the hospital. After his heart attack, Paul visited his physician on a regular basis and never missed a scheduled appointment. In addition, he strictly followed his doctor's orders concerning his prescribed medication. Despite these dutiful deeds, Paul was not a compliant patient. He continued to smoke a pack and a half of cigarettes a day, remained 60 to 70 pounds overweight, and refused to follow a regular exercise regimen. Paul knew that smoking, being overweight, and leading a sedentary lifestyle were associated with increased risk of a second heart attack, yet he continued to engage in these unhealthy behaviors. Why?

No completely satisfactory answer to this question is possible. However, some additional information may be illuminating. First, Paul had been smoking for 30 years and had never seriously tried to quit. Second, he had had a weight problem since he was about 25 and had tried several diets in years past, but none had been successful. Third, Paul had not exercised regularly since he played football in high school and college. For Paul, therefore, failure to comply with known healthy behaviors was simply a matter of continuing his longstanding lifestyle. There was a fourth factor involved in his nonadherence His physician was himself a model for unhealthy behaviors. He smoked heavily, was considerably overweight, and did not exercise regularly. Moreover, he had never made clear to Paul what he should do to lower his risk of future coronary problem. Paul, who was divorced and lived alone, had little support or encouragement from family or physician to change his lifestyle.

Paul had gone to considerable effort and expense to seek medical care only to undermine his own progress by neglecting to follow recommended medical regimens. What theoretical models explain Paul's self-defeating, nonadherent behavior? What is adherence and how can it be measured and predicted? Is nonadherence a matter of situational factors, such as money, convenience, and time, or do certain personality characteristics relate to adherence? How can adherence be improved? This chapter addresses each of these questions.

Theories That Apply to Adherence

Why do some people comply with medical advice whereas others fail to comply? Several theoretical models that apply to behavior in general have also been applied to the problem of adherence and nonadherence. These models include the behavioral model, the self-efficacy theory, the theories of reasoned action and planned behavior, and the transtheoretical model.

Behavioral Theory

The *behavioral model* of adherence is based on the principles of operant conditioning proposed by B. F. Skinner (1953). The key to operant conditioning is the immediate *reinforcement* of any response that moves the organism (person) toward the target behavior—in this case better adherence to medical recommendations. Reinforcement, which strengthens the behavior it follows, can be either positive or negative. With **positive reinforcement,** a positively valued stimulus is added to the situation, thus strengthening that behavior and increasing the probability that it will recur. An example of positive reinforcement of adherent behavior would be a monetary payment contingent on a patient's keeping a doctor's appointment. With **negative reinforcement,** behavior is strengthened by the removal of an unpleasant or negatively valued stimulus. An example of negative reinforcement would be going to a clinic to receive a powerful pain medication, thus increasing the probability that that behavior will be repeated in future similar situations.

Punishment may also change behavior, but psychologists seldom use it to lessen noncompli-

CHECK YOUR HEALTH RISKS

Check the items that apply to you.

- ☐ 1. I usually stop taking prescription medicine whenever I begin to feel better, even though some of the medication is still left.
- ☐ 2. If my prescription medicine doesn't seem to be working, I will continue taking it.
- ☐ 3. I believe that faith will cure disease and heal injuries much more certainly than modern medicine.
- ☐ 4. I won't have a prescription filled if it costs too much.
- ☐ 5. I see my dentist twice a year whether or not I have a problem.
- ☐ 6. Often when I don't feel well, I take medication left over from a previous illness, or I borrow someone else's medication.
- ☐ 7. I am a woman who doesn't worry about breast cancer because I don't have any symptoms.
- ☐ 8. I am a man who doesn't worry about testicular cancer because I don't have any symptoms.
- ☐ 9. I take all my prescribed medication whether or not they seem to be working.
- ☐ 10. I find prescription labels difficult or confusing to read.
- ☐ 11. People have advised me to stop smoking, but I have never been able to quit.
- ☐ 12. I frequently forget to take my medication.
- ☐ 13. I will take all my prescribed medication even if it makes me feel worse.
- ☐ 14. The last time I was sick, the doctor gave me advice that I didn't completely understand, but I was too embarrassed to say so.

Questions 2, 5, 9, and 13 represent good adherence habits, but each of the other items represents a health risk from failure to follow medical advice. Although it may be nearly impossible to adhere to all good health recommendations (such as not smoking, eating a healthy diet, exercising, and having regular dental and medical checkups), you can improve your health by adhering to sound medical advice. As you read this chapter, you will learn more about the health benefits of adherence.

ant behaviors. Whereas positive and negative reinforcers strengthen behavior, the effects of punishment are limited and difficult to predict. At best, punishment will merely inhibit or suppress a behavior. At worst, it conditions strong negative feelings toward any persons or environmental conditions associated with it. Punishment, including threats of harm, is seldom useful in improving a person's adherence with medical advice.

Advocates of the behavioral model use cues, rewards, and contracts to reinforce compliant behaviors. Cues include written reminders of appointments, telephone calls from the practitioner's office, and a variety of self-reminders. Rewards can be extrinsic (money and compliments) or intrinsic (feeling healthier). Contracts can be verbal, but they are more often written agreements between practitioner and patient. Most adherence models recognize the importance of incentives in improving adherence.

Some research (Wysocki et al., 1997) shows that behavioral strategies are superior to support groups in reducing friction in families with adolescent diabetics—a serious problem in many households where an insulin-dependent adolescent resists complying with an unpleasant lifestyle.

Self-Efficacy Theory

Albert Bandura (1986, 1997, 2001) has proposed a social cognitive theory that assumes that humans have the capacity to exercise some control over their lives. This control, however, is not absolute; people have limited power to use their

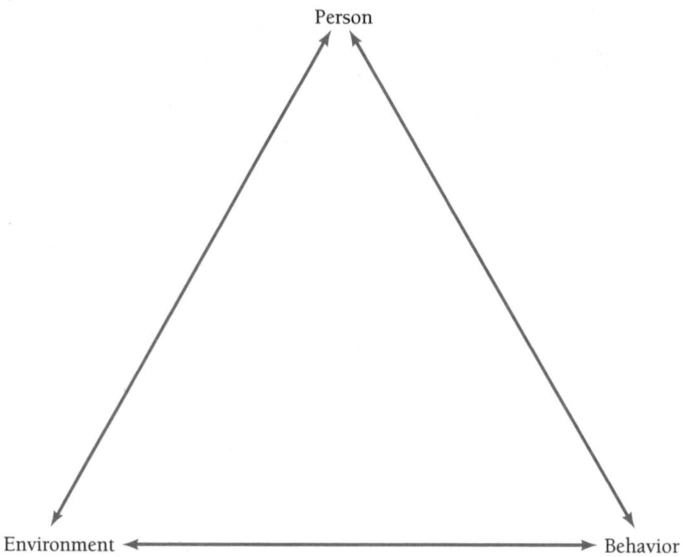

Figure 4.1 Bandura's concept of reciprocal determinism. Human functioning is a product of the interaction of behavior, environment, and person variables, especially self-efficacy and other cognitive processes.

Source: From "The self system in reciprocal determinism," by A. Bandura, 1978, American Psychologist, *33, p. 345. Adapted by permission of Albert Bandura.*

cognitive processes for self-regulation. Bandura suggests that human action results from an interaction of behavior, environment, and person factors, especially cognition. Bandura (1986, 2001) referred to this interactive triadic model as **reciprocal determinism.** The concept of reciprocal determinism can be illustrated by a triangle, with behavior, environment, and person factions occupying the three corners of the triangle and each having some influence on each of the other two factors (see Figure 4.1). An important component of the person factor is **self-efficacy,** defined by Bandura (2001) as "people's beliefs in their capability to exercise some measure of control over their own functioning and over environmental events" (p. 10).

Self-efficacy is a specific rather than a global concept and refers to people's beliefs that they can perform those behaviors that will produce desired outcomes in any *particular* situation. Bandura (1986) suggested that self-efficacy can be acquired, enhanced, or decreased through one of four sources: (1) performance, or enacting a behavior; (2) vicarious experience, or seeing another person with similar skills perform a behavior; (3) verbal persuasion, or listening to the encouraging words of a trusted person; and (4) physiological arousal states such as feelings of anxiety, which ordinarily *decrease* self-efficacy. Bandura believes that the combination of self-efficacy and outcome expectations plays an important role in predicting behavior.

According to self-efficacy theory, people's beliefs concerning their ability to initiate difficult behaviors (such as an exercise program) predict their accomplishment of those behaviors. Self-efficacy is a situation-specific concept that refers to people's confidence that they can perform necessary behaviors to produce desired outcomes in any particular situation.

Self-efficacy theory has been used to predict adherence to a variety of health recommendations, including two of the most difficult health-related behaviors—smoking cessation and adherence to a diabetic diet. For example, one study on self-efficacy and smoking relapse (Shiffman, et al., 2000) found that daily fluctuations in self-efficacy closely tracked daily lapses in smoking. That is, after an initial lapse, smokers with high self-efficacy tended to remain abstinent, whereas those with waning self-efficacy were likely to relapse.

Self-efficacy also predicts adherence to a proper diet among diabetic patients. One team of researchers (Senécal, Nouwen, & White, 2000) studied the dietary self-care of adults diagnosed with either Type 1 or Type 2 diabetes and found that self-efficacy correlated with adherence to a recommended diet. These researchers suggested that health care professionals should focus on increasing self-efficacy for adherence to a prescribed diet as a means of improving dietary self-care.

Theories of Reasoned Action and Planned Behavior

The *theory of reasoned action* (Ajzen & Fishbein, 1980; Fishbein & Ajzen, 1975) and the *theory of planned behavior* (Ajzen, 1991) both assume that the immediate determiner of behavior is people's *intention* to perform that behavior. The theory of reasoned action suggests that behavioral intentions, in turn, are (1) a function of people's *attitudes* toward the behavior, which are determined by their beliefs that the behavior will lead to positively or negatively valued outcomes, and (2) their *subjective norm,* which is shaped by their perception of the value that significant others place on that behavior and by their *motivation* to comply with those norms (see Chapter 3, Figure 3.1). The theory of planned behavior includes an additional determinant of intentions to act, namely, people's perception of how much *control* they have over their behavior (see Chapter 3, Figure 3.2). Both theories have been used to predict adherence to a number of health-related behaviors.

A meta-analysis of studies on the usefulness of the theory of reasoned action and the theory of planned behavior (Hausenblas, Carron, & Mack, 1997) found that both theories had value in predicting who will adhere to an exercise program and who will not. More specifically, the analysis revealed a strong connection between attitude toward exercising and intention to exercise and a strong link between intention and exercise behavior. However, the relationship between subjective norms and intention was only moderate. Other researchers (Orbell et al., 2001; Sheeran, Conner, & Norman, 2001) found similar results when they applied the variables of these two theories to adherence to two health-related behaviors, namely use of illicit substance and attendance at health-screening programs. Results from each of these studies suggested that the theory of reasoned action and the theory of planned behavior have at least some value in predicting adherence to healthy behaviors.

Why are these two common-sense theories only moderately successful at predicting adherence to health-related behaviors? Perhaps their predictive value is limited by people's past experience in adhering or not adhering to healthy behaviors. That is, people's past experience may be a better predictor of future behavior than either the theory of reasoned action or the theory of planned behavior. Some evidence supports this notion. For example, one study (Sutton, McVey, & Glanz, 1999) showed only weak evidence that these two theories were related to young people's use of condoms and that neither theory could overcome the effects of past behaviors as a predictor of condom use. Thus, past adherence seems to predicts future adherence more effectively than either the theory of reasoned action or the theory of planned behavior.

The Transtheoretical Model

Another theory that attempts to explain and predict adherence behavior is called the *transtheoretical model* because it cuts across and borrows from other theoretical models. The transtheoretical model, developed by James Prochaska, Carrlo DiClemente, and John Norcross (1992, 1994), assumes that people progress as

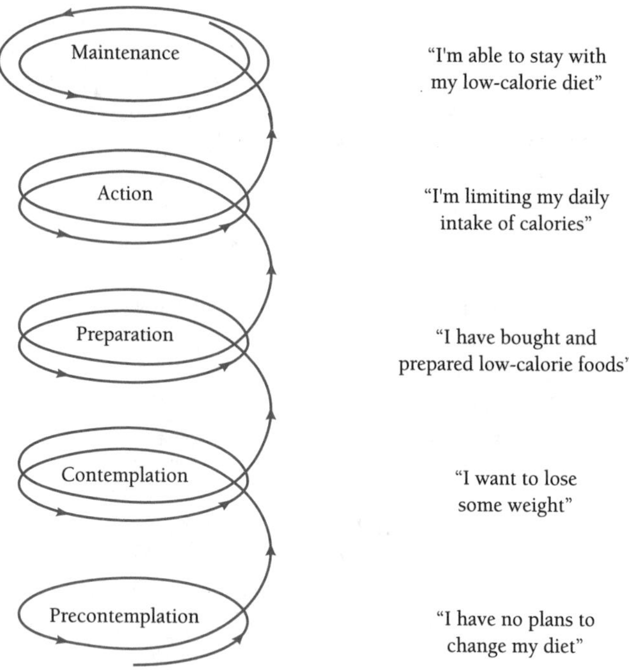

Figure 4.2 The transtheoretical model and stages of changing from a high-calorie diet to a low-calorie diet

well as regress through five spiraling stages in making changes in behavior. These stages are precontemplation, contemplation, preparation, action, and maintenance. An overweight person's progression through these five stages of change in adopting a low-calorie diet is illustrated in Figure 4.2.

During the *precontemplation stage,* the person has no intention of changing to a low-calorie diet. In the *contemplation stage,* the person is aware of the problem, has thoughts about adopting a new diet, but has not yet made an effort to change. The *preparation stage* includes both thoughts (such as intending to adopt a diet within the next month) and action (such as purchasing low-calorie food). During the *action stage,* the person makes overt changes in behavior, such as adhering to a low-calorie diet. In the *maintenance stage,* the person tries to sustain the changes previously made and to resist temptation to relapse.

Prochaska et al. maintained that a person moves from one stage to another in a spiral rather than a linear fashion. Relapses spiral people back into a previous stage, or perhaps all the way back to the contemplation or precontemplation stages. From that point, the person may progress several times through the stages until finally completing behavioral change. Thus, relapses are to be expected and can serve as learning experiences that help a person recycle upward through the stages.

Prochaska et al. suggested that people in each of these stages need different types of assistance in making changes. For example, attempts to change people in the precontemplation stage will be unsuccessful because these people do not believe they have a problem. On the other hand, people in the preparation stage do not need to be convinced to change their behavior; they need specific suggestions about how to change. People in the maintenance stage need help or information oriented toward preserving their changes.

Research tends to support these assumptions. For example, a study on people with one or more risk factors for heart attack (Steptoe, Kerry, Rink, & Hilton, 2001) used behavioral counseling to move people from lower level stages to action and maintenance stages. Similarly, a study on exercise (Rosen, 2000a) found that messages tailored toward the value of physical activity were sufficient to move previously sedentary college students to adopt an exercise program.

Does the transtheoretical model apply equally to different problem behaviors? A meta-analysis of 47 studies (Rosen, 2000b) attempted to answer this question by looking at the model across several health-related issues, including smoking, substance abuse, exercise, diet, and psychotherapy. The results showed that the transtheoretical model works better with some behaviors than with others. For example, with techniques to stop smoking, cognitive processes were more frequently used in deciding to quit, whereas behavioral techniques were more effective during abstinence. Similar variations occurred with the other health-related areas. Craig Rosen (2000b) summed up these findings saying that people who look to the transtheoretical model for "a one-size-fits-all blueprint for interventions are likely to be disappointed" (p. 602).

In Summary

Several theoretical models attempt to predict and explain compliant and noncompliant behavior. The behavioral model uses contingency contracts and reinforcement for compliant behaviors. Bandura's self-efficacy theory emphasizes people's beliefs about illness and their limited ability to control their own health. Ajzen and Fishbein's theory of reasoned action assumes that intentions, attitudes, subjective norms, and motivation predict adherence; and Ajzen's theory of planned behavior adds people's subjective belief that they can control their adherence to health-related behaviors. Prochaska's transtheoretical model assumes that people spiral through five stages in making changes in behavior—precontemplation, contemplation, preparation, action, and maintenance. Relapse should be expected, but after relapse, people can again move forward through the various stages.

Research on the effectiveness of these models suggests that people's belief that they can perform healthy behaviors (self-efficacy) combined with their intention to enact these behaviors contribute to a better understanding of reasons for adherence and nonadherence. However, more research is needed to establish the usefulness of these models to explain and predict adherent and nonadherent behaviors.

Problems of Adherence

For medical advice to benefit the health of patients, two contingencies must be met. First, the advice must be accurate. Second, patients must follow this good advice. Both conditions are essential. Ill-founded advice that patients strictly follow may introduce new health problems that lead to disastrous outcomes for the compliant patient. On the other hand, excellent advice is essentially worthless if patients do not follow it. In this section we look at three questions regarding adherence: What is adherence? How is adherence measured? How frequent is adherence?

Definition of Adherence

Traditionally, people in the medical profession have used the term **compliance** to refer to patient behaviors that conform to physicians' orders. But because the term compliance connotes reluctant obedience, many health psychologists and some physicians advocate the use of other words, especially *adherence.* However, the terms *cooperation, obedience,* and *collaboration* have also been suggested as substitutes for compliance. Perhaps the most accurate term to describe the ideal relationship between physician and patient would be *cooperation,* a word that implies a relationship in which both the health care provider and the consumer are actively involved in the restoration and/or the maintenance of the patient's health. However, because cooperation is neither a common practice nor an accepted label for this relationship, the terms *compliance* and *adherence* are still the most frequently used words, and we employ these two words interchangeably.

What does it mean to be adherent? We define **adherence** as a person's ability and willingness to follow recommended health practices, but R. Brian Haynes (1979) has suggested a broader definition of the term. Haynes defined adherence as "the extent to which a person's behavior (in terms of taking medications, following diets, or executing lifestyle changes) coincides with medical or health advice" (pp. 1–2). This definition expands the concept of compliance beyond merely taking medications to include maintaining healthy lifestyle practices, such as eating properly, getting sufficient exercise, avoiding undue stress, abstaining from smoking cigarettes, and not abusing alcohol. In addition, adherence includes making and keeping periodic medical and dental appointments, using seatbelts, and engaging in other behaviors that coincide with the best health advice available. Moreover, adherence is a complex concept, with people being compliant in one situation and noncompliant in another (Johnson, 1993).

Assessment of Adherence

The assessment of adherence raises at least two questions. First, how do researchers know the percentage of patients who fail to comply with practitioners' recommendations? Second, how can nonadherent behaviors be identified? The answer to the first question is that compliance rates are not known with certainty, and that any reported percentage is usually only an estimate.

Second, at least six basic means of measuring patient compliance are available: (1) ask the clinician, (2) ask the patient, (3) ask other people, (4) count pills, (5) examine biochemical evidence, and (6) use a combination of these procedures. The first of these methods, asking the clinician, is usually the poorest choice. Physicians generally overestimate their patients' compliance rates, and even when their guesses are not overly optimistic, they are usually wrong. In general, the accuracy of the estimates made by physicians and other health care practitioners is only slightly better than chance (Blackwell, 1997).

Asking patients themselves is a more valid procedure, but it is fraught with many difficulties. Self-reports are inaccurate for at least two reasons: First, patients may lie to avoid the disapproval of their health care provider; second, they may simply not know their own rate of compliance. Patients not only underreport poor adherence, but they also overreport good compliance. In addition, some patients take more medication than recommended, whereas others take less. Thus, self-report measures have questionable validity and should be supplemented by other assessment techniques.

One other technique is to ask hospital personnel and family members to monitor the patient, but this procedure also has at least two inherent problems. First, constant observation may be physically impossible, especially with regard to such regimens as diet and alcohol consumption. Second, persistent monitoring creates an artificial situation and frequently results in higher rates of compliance than would otherwise occur. This outcome, of course, is desirable, but as a means of assessing compliance, it contains a built-in error that makes observation by others inaccurate.

A fourth method of assessing compliance is to count pills. This procedure may seem ideal because very few errors would be made in counting the number of pills absent from a bottle or a drug dispenser. Unfortunately, this method also may be inaccurate. Even if the required number of pills are gone, the patient may not have been compliant. Once again, there are at least two possible problems with pill counts. First, the patient, for a wide variety of reasons, may have simply discarded some of the medication. Second, the patient may have taken all the pills, but in a manner other than the prescribed one.

Several investigators have developed automated devices that facilitate pill counting and determine whether patients take their medication at the prescribed time. One group of investigators (Cramer, Mattson, Prevey, Scheyer, & Ouellette, 1989) reported on a novel assessment technique in which a microprocessor in the pill cap recorded every bottle opening and closing and yielded information concerning the time of day that the bottle was opened. These researchers assumed that each bottle opening equaled one dose of medication. The procedure did not detect the number of pills removed with each opening, and although this procedure represents an improvement over the pill-counting technique, it too cannot ascertain that patients are taking medication according to their doctor's recommendations.

Examination of biochemical evidence is a fifth method of measuring compliance. This procedure looks at the outcome of compliant behavior to find some biochemical evidence, such as analysis of blood or urine samples, to determine whether the patient has behaved in a compliant fashion. Some research (Liu et al., 2001) used biochemical evidence in HIV patients and found that a combination of adherence measures was related to a decrease in the virus that may lead to AIDS. However, problems can arise with the use of biochemical evidence as a means of assessing compliance. First, some drugs are not easily detected in blood or urine samples. Second, individual differences in absorption and metabolism of drugs can lead to wide variations among people who are equally compliant. Third, biochemical checks must be carried out frequently and regularly to assess compliance rates accurately.

Finally, clinicians can use a combination of these methods of assessing compliance. One study (Liu et al., 2001) interviewed patients about their level of adherence, counted pills, and used an electronic pill bottle as well as a combination of all of these three methods to measure compliance among HIV patients. As with most studies on adherence, this one found that compliance decreased over time, but it also found that each of the three methods (pill count, ask the patients, and electronic pill bottle) were independently related to improved health. However, a combination of the three methods showed the strongest relationship with biological evidence. A weakness of this approach to measuring adherence is its cost.

Frequency of Nonadherence

How pervasive is the problem of nonadherence? The answer to this question depends in part on how nonadherence is defined, the nature of the illness under consideration, the demographic features of the population, and the methods used to assess compliance. In general, the rate of noncompliance with medical or health advice is approximately 50% (Haynes, McKibbon, & Kanani, 1996). Robin DiMatteo (1994) reported that at least 38% of patients do not follow short-term treatment plans, and more than 45% fail to adhere to recommendations for long-term treatment. Moreover, as many as three fourths of all people are unwilling or unable to stick to recommended healthy lifestyles, such as eating a low-fat diet, avoiding cigarette smoking, or exercising regularly.

In the late 1970s, David Sackett and John C. Snow (1979) reviewed more than 500 studies that dealt with the frequency of compliance and noncompliance and found that about 75% of the patients kept their scheduled appointments when they had initiated them, but only about 50% kept appointments that had been scheduled by the health care professional. As expected, compliance rates were higher when treatment was to cure a disease than when it was to prevent a disease. However, when medication must be taken over a long period, compliance is around 50% for either prevention or cure. Sackett and Snow also found that compliance rates for dietary regimens ranged from 30% to 70%, again with a mean of about 50%.

Unfortunately, little evidence exists that compliance rates have risen since this early review. Indeed, compliance rates have remained quite constant, with about half of all patients failing to comply with recommended medical programs (Dishman & Buckworth, 1997).

In Summary

Adherence is the extent to which a person is able and willing to follow medical and health advice. In order for people to profit from adherence, the advice must first be valid, and second, patients must follow that advice. Inability or unwillingness to adhere to health-related behaviors increases people's chances of developing serious health problems or even death.

At least six basic ways of measuring patient adherence have been suggested: (1) ask the physician, (2) ask the patient, (3) ask other people, (4) count pills, (5) examine biochemical evidence, (6) use a combination of these procedures. No one of these procedures is both reliable and valid. However, with the exception of clinician judgment, most have some limited validity and usefulness. Therefore, when accuracy is crucial, it seems appropriate to use two or more of these basic measures for assessing patient compliance, a procedure that yields greater accuracy than reliance on a single assessment technique.

Assessing the frequency of nonadherence is complicated by the different definitions of the term, the nature of the illness, the population being studied, and the methods used to assess compliance. In general terms, however, the rate of nonadherence has remained around 50% for the past 2 or 3 decades.

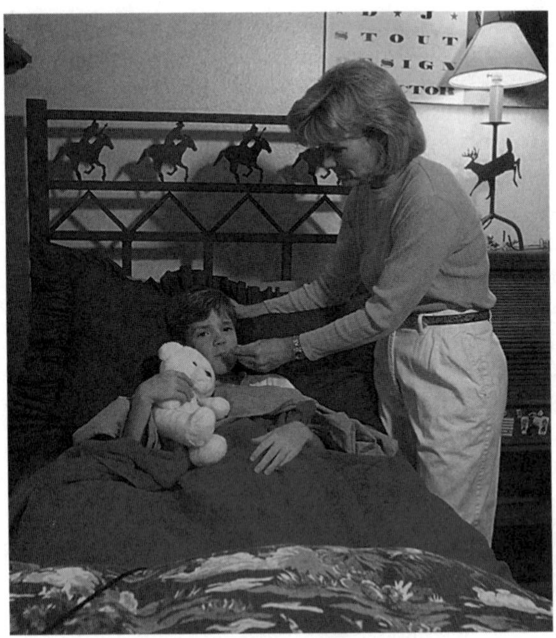
Corbis

Parents follow medical advice for their sick children at a similar rate as for themselves—about 50%

What Factors Predict Adherence?

What factors determine who will be compliant and who will be not? If we assume that people always act in their own best interests, we may be at a loss to explain the factors that do and do not relate to adherence. For example, it may seem intuitively obvious that the amount of money invested in the treatment procedure would predict compliance. Intuition, however, does not always agree with scientific evidence. What are the factors that do or do not predict compliance? Possible predictors can be divided into five groups: severity of the disease; treatment characteristics, including side effects and complexity of the treatment; personal characteristics, such as age, gender, personal beliefs, and so on; cultural norms; and characteristics of the relationship between the health care provider and the patient, including verbal communication and the personal characteristics of the health care practitioner.

Severity of the Disease

Common wisdom might suggest that people with severe, potentially crippling or life-threatening illnesses will be highly motivated to adhere to regimens that protect them against such major catastrophes. Interestingly, little evidence exists to support this logical hypothesis. In general, people with a serious disease are no more likely than people with a mild illness to seek medical treatment or to comply with medical advice. Indeed, people sometimes seek health care not because they have a serious medical problem but because someone might casually mention that they looked bad. For example, Robin DiMatteo and Dante DiNicola (1982) reported a woman who had been hit by a baseball bat and had suffered some loss of vision in her left eye. The loss of vision, however, did not prompt her to go to a doctor. She sought treatment only after a friend casually commented that her eyelid drooped!

Indeed, studies on the relationship between adherence and severity of a disease reveal no consistent evidence that people are more likely to comply with treatment regimens for a serious illness than they are when the disorder is minor. One study (Catz, Kelly, Bogart, Genosch, & McAuliffe, 2000) found that nearly one third of patients diagnosed with HIV (an extremely severe disease) failed to take their medication within the 5 days prior to the study.

Although severity of the disease is a poor predictor of adherence, *pain* associated with the illness does seem to increase people's level of adherence (Becker, 1979). When people suffer great pain, they have strong motivation to comply with any treatment that might cure their illness or reduce their discomfort.

In summary, results of research on adherence and the severity of a disease suggest two general conclusions. First, little direct relationship exists between the severity of a disease and a patient's probability of complying with recommended medical regimens. Second, if patients have experienced pain from a disorder, they are more likely to comply with their physician's recommendations. Pain by itself, of course, is not a true indicator of the severity of an illness, but it may be one of several factors that help convince patients to cooperate in protecting their own health.

Treatment Characteristics

A second set of predictors of adherence includes the side effects of the medication and the complexity of the treatment.

Side Effects of the Medication A second illness characteristic that might relate to adherence is the potential unpleasantness of the medication's side effects. Early research (Masur, 1981) found little evidence to suggest that unpleasant side effects are a major reason for discontinuing a drug or dropping out of a treatment program. Recent research with the complex regimen of drugs for HIV (Catz et al., 2000) indicated that patients who experience severe side effects are less likely to take their medications than those with less severe side effects.

Complexity of the Treatment Are people less likely to comply as the treatment procedures become increasingly more complex? In general, the greater the variety of medications a person must take, the greater is the likelihood that people will not take pills in the prescribed manner. For example, one study (Cramer et al., 1989) found that as the number of pills per day increased from one to three, the rate of compliance decreased from 88% to 77%—a small but significant decline. However, patients who were prescribed four doses per day achieved only a 39% compliance rate. These data indicate that compliance drops dramatically when pills are to be taken more than three times a day.

The reason seems obvious. For most people, a day has one, two, or three prominent periods, and medicine can be cued to each. For example, pills prescribed once a day can be taken early in the morning; those prescribed twice a day can be cued to early morning and late night; and those prescribed three times a day can be taken after each meal. Adherence to any of these three schedules is quite high. Schedules calling for medication to be taken four or more times a day create an unnatural division of the day for most people, resulting in low compliance rates.

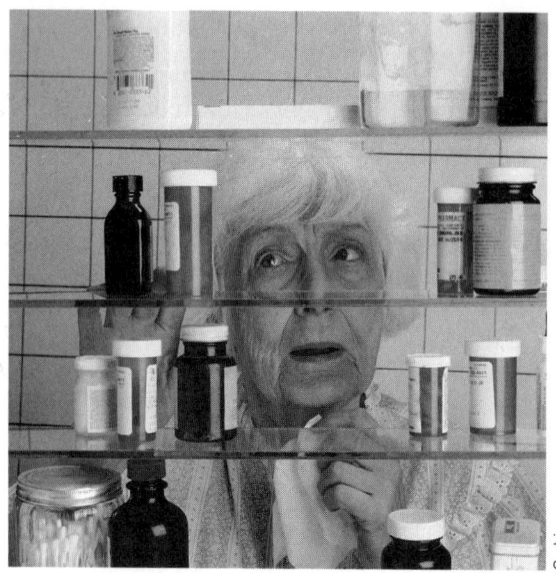
Corbis

More complex treatments tend to lower compliance rates.

In summary, the more complex the treatment, the lower the rate of compliance. After looking at the evidence, Philip Ley, who has studied adherence for more than 30 years, concluded that "the simpler the treatment schedule, and the shorter its duration, the greater is compliance" (Ley, 1997, p. 282).

Personal Factors

Researchers have investigated such factors as age, gender, social support, emotional support, personality patterns, emotional factors, and personal beliefs about health to determine their association with adherence.

Age The relationship between adherence and age is complicated by several factors. Depending on the specific illness, the time frame, and the adherence regimen, studies show that compliance can either increase or decrease with age. For example, a study of adherence to an exercise program for 26- to 68-year-old adults with high cholesterol initially revealed a positive correlation between age and adherence (Lynch et al., 1992). This might suggest that as people get older they become more concerned with their health and are more likely to comply with an exercise program designed to reduce cholesterol. However, as the program continued beyond 4 months, age was not significantly related to adherence, a finding that prompted the authors to suggest that older participants may have suffered some minor physical discomfort that interfered with exercise.

A later study (Thomas et al., 1995) added a further complication to this issue by finding a curvilinear relationship between age and compliance with colorectal cancer screening. In this large-scale, longitudinal study of both men and women, the best compliers were around 70 years old; the worst were below 55 or over 80. Perhaps after age 80 people simply do not regard screening for colorectal cancer to be important. Some evidence (Monane et al., 1996; Sherbourne, Hays, Ordway, DiMatteo, & Kravitz, 1992) suggests that, among adults, adherence to regimens for diabetes, hypertension, and heart disease tends to increase as people get older. However, with young diabetic patients, age may be inversely related to compliance. One study of 10- to 19-year-old diabetics reported that as the patients' age increased, their compliance with their exercise program and insulin self-injection decreased (Bond, Aiken, & Somerville, 1992). Another study (Olsen & Sutton, 1998) found that as young adolescent diabetics grow into late adolescence, they feel more isolated from their family and tend to show greater noncompliance with an inconvenient health-protective regimen.

Gender With regard to gender, researchers have found few differences between the overall adherence rates of women and men but some differences in following specific recommendations. In general, men and women are about equal in adhering to taking medication for high blood pressure (Monane et al., 1996) and in dropping out or staying with an exercise program when the exercise is conducted in a class (Oman & King, 2000). However, when the exercise was performed at home, women report higher compliance rates than men. Also, women seem to be better at adhering to healthy diets with lots of vegetables (Laforge, Greene, & Prochaska, 1994) and at taking medication for a mental disorder (Sellwood & Tarrier, 1994).

Social Support **Social support** is a broad concept that refers to both tangible and intangible help a person receives from family members and from friends. The introduction to this chapter presented the case of Paul, the heart attack patient who experienced very limited social support. He was divorced, lived alone, and enjoyed no close personal relationships. Although Paul faithfully adhered to his physician's prescriptions concerning medication, he was less compliant with regard to good health practices. His story suggests an association between compliance and the support a patient receives from family and friends.

One of the strongest predictors of adherence is the level of social support one receives from friends and family, but even this factor is not invariably related to compliance. In general, people who are isolated from others are likely to be noncompliant; those whose lives are filled with close interpersonal relationships are more likely to follow medical advice. For example, compliance by hemodialysis patients increases when family members are neither emotionally distant nor emotionally overinvolved and when they have some understanding of the emotional effects of the illness (Sherwood, 1983).

Social support also increases rates of adherence to appointment in chronically ill patients. In an experimental design (Tanner & Feldman, 1997), low-income patients with no symptoms of their chronic illness were divided into four groups: (1) a control group that received only an exit interview; (2) an experimental group that received the interview plus social support counseling of the patient's significant other; (3) an experimental group that received the interview and counseling plus a postcard reminder; and (4) an experimental group that received the interview, counseling, and postcard plus a telephone call. Results revealed that social support counseling of the significant other led to significantly better adherence to appointment keeping than the interview and was at least as effective alone as it was when combined with the postcard and the telephone call.

Support of family and friends also increases compliance among heart patients. For example, strong social support is positively related to the likelihood that hypertensive patients will adhere to medical advice, including keeping appointments with the doctor (Stanton, 1987). Also, men with high cholesterol whose wives are highly supportive are more likely to adhere to their diet than men whose wives offer little support (Bovbjerg et al., 1995).

Emotional Support Some evidence suggests that *quality* rather than *quantity* of social support predicts diabetics' adherence to complex medical recommendations. The number of friends may be unrelated to a patient's compliance, but quality of interpersonal relations is a significant predictor of adherence (Sherbourne et al., 1992). Similarly, emotional support may be a better predictor of compliance than marriage. One study (Kulik & Mahler, 1993) found that, although married men who had undergone artery bypass surgery were more likely than unmarried men to have followed their doctor's advice, the key to adherence was the level of emotional support they received from their wives rather than marriage itself.

Personality Patterns Are people with certain personality patterns more likely than others to be noncompliant? If personality can predict noncompliance, then the same people should be noncompliant in a variety of situations. However, little evidence exists that would support this conclusion. On the contrary, some indications exist that noncompliance is specific to the situation (Lutz, Silbret, & Olshan, 1983) and that adherence to one treatment program is independent of adherence to others (Orme & Binik, 1989). Thus, the evidence suggests that noncompliance is not a global personality trait but is specific to a given situation.

Nevertheless, some researchers have identified two personality patterns—obsessive-compulsive disorders and cynical hostility—as possible predictors of compliance or noncompliance. **Obsessions** are persistent and pathological thoughts that often lead to compulsive behavior, whereas **compulsions** are pathological repetitions of behaviors.

Intuitively, it would seem that obsessive-compulsive individuals should be more compliant than other people, and some evidence supports this hypothesis. Using the Symptoms Checklist-90-R, Jon Kabat-Zinn and Ann Chapman-Waldrop (1988) found that scores on the obsessive-compulsive scale predicted which patients would adhere to an 8-week stress-reduction regimen and which ones would not. Obsessive-compulsive people, as one might guess, were more likely to complete the program.

The second personality pattern that may be related to nonadherence is **cynical hostility,** or feelings of resentment and distrust of other people. One group of researchers (Christensen, Wiebbe, & Lawton, 1997) used the Cook-Medley Hostility (Ho) Scale to measure cynical hostility in hemodialysis patients. They found that high hostility scores were associated with poor dietary and medication adherence. People who score high on the Cook-Medley Hostility Scale are generally suspicious, mistrustful, and resentful of others and have frequent outbursts of anger, which may predispose them to reject or disregard the advice that health care professionals provide. (We discuss the Cook-Medley Hostility Scale and its relation to cardiovascular disease in Chapter 9.). In summary, although the noncompliant personality seems to be a myth, some evidence exists that obsessive-compulsiveness is positively related to good compliance, whereas cynical hostility is positively related to poor adherence.

Emotional Factors Can such emotional factors as stress and anxiety predict adherence? Some evidence suggests a positive answer to this question. A study (Oman & King, 2000) that investigated the effects of stressful life events on subsequent exercise adherence found that people who experience several stressful experiences are likely to drop out of an exercise program. This research defined stress by items on the Holmes and Rahe (1967) Social Readjustment Rating Scale (SRRS). The SRRS is a list of more than 40 potential stressful life events such as death of a spouse, divorce, fired at work, death of a close friend, change in residence, and new home mortgage. The results of the exercise adherence study showed that people who experienced three or four of these stressful life events during the previous 6 months were much more likely to drop out of an exercise program than were people who reported zero to one life event. This relationship emerged regardless of the intensity of the exercise or whether the exercise was conducted at home or in an exercise class.

A second emotional factor is anxiety. Can a high level of anxiety reduce adherence rates? The evidence on this question was not clear, so Kate Brain and her associates (Brain, Norman, Gray, & Mansel, 1999) attempted to clarify previous, conflicting studies concerning the relationship between anxiety and breast self-examination. When they divided anxiety into generalized anxiety and cancer-specific anxiety, Brain et al. found that high general anxiety may lead to excessive self-examination and that cancer-specific anxiety can motivate women to adhere to a periodic breast self-examination program. That is, the higher a woman's general anxiety, the more likely she is to be hypervigilant, whereas the higher her cancer anxiety, the more likely she is to routinely examine her breasts.

Personal Beliefs Some evidence suggests that patients' personal beliefs are related to compliance. We have seen that perceived self-efficacy and the theory of reasoned action have some ability both to predict and to explain adherence and nonadherence. In general, when patients believe that adherence to treatment recommendations will result in health benefits, they are likely to comply with those recommendations. During the past 25 years, some evidence has accrued suggesting that health beliefs might be a promising alternative to traditional personality traits in explaining adherence.

Martha Brownlee-Duffeck and her colleagues (Brownlee-Duffeck et al. (1987) examined health beliefs and their effects on adherence to diabetic treatment regimens for both adults and adolescents. For adults, the belief that compliance will benefit one's health predicted adherence. For adolescents, however, the perceived health benefits of compliance were not important. Young diabetic patients have notoriously low levels of compliance, and this study suggested that even when they see the long-range value of following treatment recommendations, they are not very likely to comply.

Some people cope with illness by denying personal vulnerability or by avoiding personal responsibility for taking actions that might restore health. These people use **avoidance coping** strategies to reduce the stress of being sick. They may smoke more, overeat, abuse alcohol or other drugs, or simply hope for a miracle. Such strategies are often effective for a short time, but in the long run they are usually hazardous to health. People who use avoidance coping are less likely than others to adhere to their doctor's advice, perhaps because they either deny the efficacy of such advice or because they reject responsibility for their own health care (Sherbourne et al., 1992).

On the other hand, people who believe they are personally responsible for their own health are more likely to adhere to medical advice. For example, one study (Helby, Gafarian, & McCann, 1989) found that those diabetic patients who assumed responsibility for their health care were more likely than others to adhere to their treatment program. Similarly, hypertensive patients are more likely to adhere to their medical regimens when they believe that they exercise some personal control over both their blood pressure and their health (Stanton, 1987). In summary, people who believe they have little control over their own health tend to be noncompliant, whereas those patients who believe that their own actions will bring about a health benefit are more likely to adhere to medical advice.

Cultural Norms Cultural beliefs and norms have a powerful effect not only on rates of compliance but even what constitutes compliance. For example, if one's family or tribal traditions include strong beliefs in the efficacy of tribal healers, it seems reasonable that the individual's compliance with modern medical recommendations might be low. A study of diabetic and hypertensive patients in Zimbabwe (Zyazema, 1984) found a large number of people who were not adhering to their recommended therapies. As might be expected, many of these patients still believed in traditional healers, and they had little faith in modern medical procedures. Another study (Ruiz & Ruiz, 1983) reported that Latino patients were more likely to comply with medical advice when their physicians demonstrated some understanding of Hispanic cultural norms and practices.

Physicians are influenced by their patients' ethnic background and socioeconomic status, and this influence relates to patient compliance. Physicians tend to have stereotypical and negative attitudes toward African American and low- and middle-income patients (van Ryn & Burke, 2000). Moreover, these physicians had pessimistic beliefs about African American and low-income patients to adhere to medical advice. These findings have important implications for physicians and other health care providers whose clientele consists largely of people from different cultural backgrounds.

Practitioner-Patient Interaction

In addition to looking at disease characteristics and personal factors, researchers have studied the patient-practitioner interaction and its relationship to adherence and nonadherence. Patients who dislike their physicians or who have trouble talking openly with them are more likely than other patients to be nonadherent (Ciechanowski, Katon, Russo, & Walker (2001).

Practitioner-patient interaction includes the verbal communication, the practitioner's personal characteristics, the amount of time between referral and treatment, and the length of time patients must spend in the practitioner's waiting room.

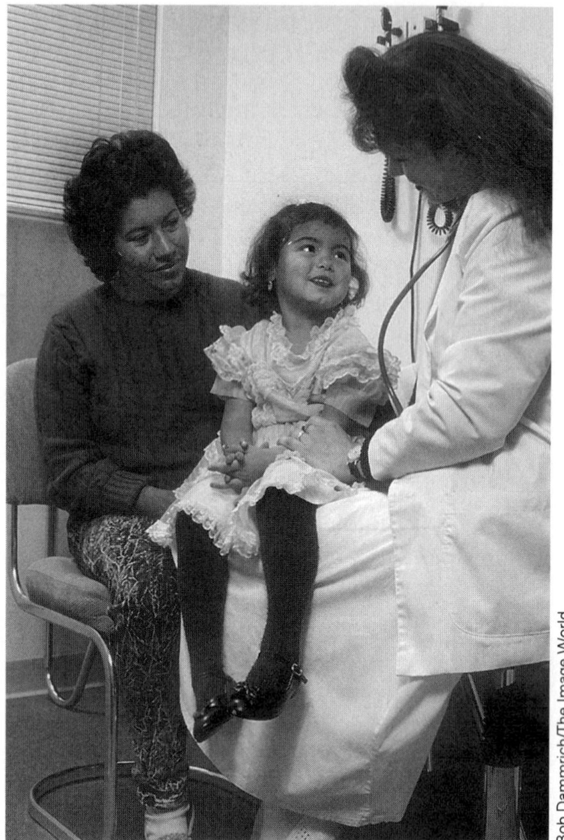

Bob Daemmrich/The Image World

Patient compliance is high when practitioners convey information about the condition and reasons for treatment.

Verbal Communication Perhaps the most crucial factor in patient noncompliance is poor verbal communication between the practitioner and the patient. Again, Paul's case illustrates this point. Because Paul recalled only vague and general information regarding diet and smoking, either his physician was remiss in detailing the precise healthful practices that Paul was to follow, or Paul was less than receptive to the information—or perhaps both.

The miscommunication can start when physicians ask patients to report on their symptoms and fail to listen to patients' concerns. What constitutes a concern for the patient may not be essential to the diagnostic process, and practitioners may seem unconcerned when they are, in fact, trying to elicit information relevant to making a diagnosis. However, patients may misinterpret the physician's focus as a lack of personal concern or as overlooking what patients consider important symptoms. After practitioners have made a diagnosis, they typically tell patients about that diagnosis. If the diagnosis is minor, patients are relieved and not highly motivated to adhere to (or even listen to) any instructions that may follow. If the verdict is serious, patients are likely to become highly anxious, and this anxiety may then interfere with their concentration on subsequent medical advice.

For a variety of reasons, physicians and patients frequently do not speak the same language. First, physicians operate in familiar territory. They know the subject matter, are comfortable with the physical surroundings, and are ordinarily calm and relaxed with procedures that have become routine to them. Patients, in contrast, may be unfamiliar with medical terminology; distracted by the strange environs; and distressed by anxiety, fear, or pain (Charlee, Goldsmith, Chambers, & Haynes, 1996). Differences in native language, educational level, ethnic background, or social class may also contribute to problems in communication (van Ryn & Burke, 2000). As a result, patients either fail to remember or misunderstand much of the information their doctors give them.

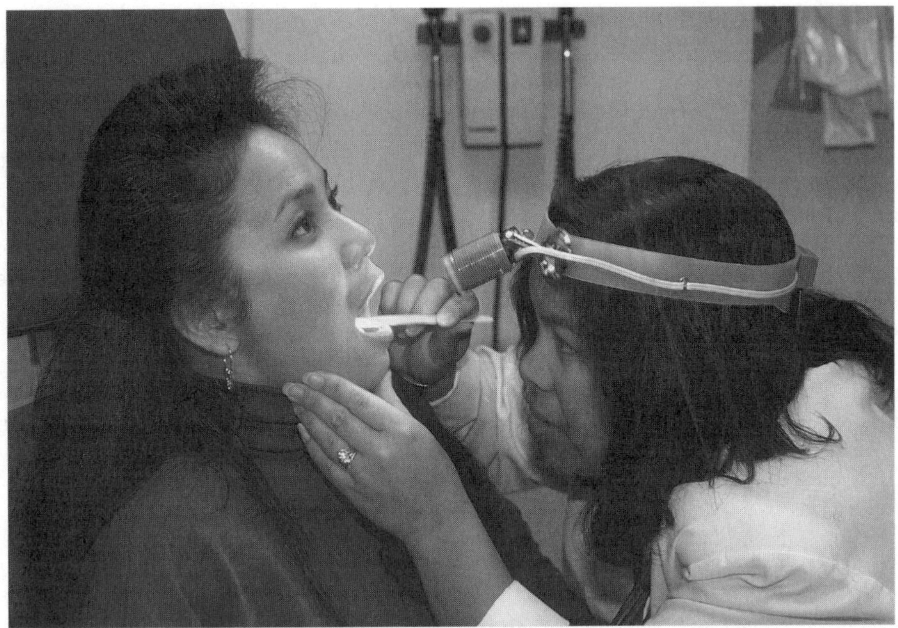

Female physicians encourage patient interaction, which can boost compliance rates.

How often do physicians offer patients health-promotion advice during office visits? One study (Russell & Roter, 1993) found that doctors provided information or made suggestions about changes in patients' lifestyle and health behaviors in only about half the visits. The most frequent suggestions were about diet and weight control, but physicians also mentioned exercise, stress, smoking, and alcohol. Unfortunately, physicians tended not to use the most effective behavioral strategies for getting their patients to adopt the suggested changes, leading to the conclusion that physicians miss important opportunities to urge their patients to change unhealthy behaviors.

The Practitioner's Personal Characteristics A second aspect of the practitioner-patient interaction is the perceived personal characteristics of the physician. As might be expected, patients' compliance improves as confidence in their physician's technical ability increases (Gilbar, 1989). In addition, several physician personality variables—as perceived by the patient—are related to compliance. DiNicola and DiMatteo (1984) reported that people were more likely to follow the advice of doctors they saw as warm, caring, friendly, and interested in the welfare of patients. When physicians display a good bedside manner, such as making eye contact, smiling, leaning forward, and even joking and laughing, patient compliance improves.

The physicians' gender also may play a role in the exchange of information between doctor and patient. A study of both female and male physicians during patient visits (Hall, Irish, Roter, Ehrlich, & Miller, 1994) found that female physicians made more partnership statements, made more positive statements, and asked more questions than did male physicians. In addition, patients talked to female physicians more than to male physicians, and the gender of both physician and patient contributed to the communication pattern during the visit.

WOULD YOU BELIEVE

Nonadherence to a Placebo Is Risky

Would you believe that people who are nonadherent to a placebo have much higher death rates than people who conscientiously take a placebo drug?

In Chapter 2, we discussed the potentially powerful effects of a placebo—an inactive substance that may cause participants in an experiment to improve or change behavior due to their belief in the placebo's effectiveness. We saw that the placebo effect applies to all types of treatment, including depression, pain, and even surgery. That is, people who had sham knee surgery benefited as much as those who had actual surgery (Moseley et al., 2002). Do the effects of the placebo extend to nonadherence of prescribed medications? Is poor adherence to a placebo more risky than poor adherence to medication?

Two studies from the National Heart, Lung, and Blood Institute's Beta-Blocker Heart Attack Trial (Gallagher, Viscoli, & Horwitz, 1993; Horwitz et al., 1990) indicated that, as expected, heart patients who took their prescribed medication were less likely to have died from all causes than those patients who did not. Both women and men who were poor adherers were about two and a half times more likely to have died than heart patients who were good adherers. Interestingly, the poor adherers in both studies had a greater risk of death whether they were in the medication group or in the placebo group. Women who were poor adherers to the placebo were 2.8 times more likely to have died than women in the placebo group who were good adherers. Noncompliant men in the placebo group were 2.5 times as likely to have died than compliant men in the placebo group.

These findings suggest that noncompliance itself may contribute to all-cause mortality. Perhaps noncompliant people are not conscientious and have little regard for their own health. These two studies suggest that either the power of the placebo is much stronger than earlier studies indicated or that some heart patients do not protect themselves well from a variety of potentially fatal conditions.

The studies indicate that adherence to heart medication can be effective in reducing death rate, but it is no more effective than adherence to a placebo. Moreover, nonadherence can be dangerous—whether the medication is genuine or a placebo. The bottom line is this: People who are part of drug study should take their medication as prescribed and not be concerned whether they may be taking a placebo.

In Summary

Several conditions predict nonadherence: (1) patients' perception of the severity of their disease; (2) side effects of the medication; (3) long and complicated treatment regimens; (4) personal factors, such as old age, male gender, lack of social support, and lack of emotional support; (5) personality patterns such as cynical hostility; (6) stressful life events and anxiety; (7) patient's beliefs that their own behavior cannot benefit their health; (8) patients' cultural beliefs that modern medicine is ineffective; (9) inaccurate patient-practitioner communication, including poor verbal communication and an unfriendly, incompetent, or authoritarian physician. Table 4.1 summarizes the research on what factors predict adherence.

Improving Adherence

We have surveyed several issues related to adherence, including examinations of theoretical models that might explain or predict compliance, techniques of measuring compliance, the frequency of compliance, and factors that do or do

TABLE 4.1 *Predictors of Patient Adherence*

	Findings	Studies
I. Disease Characteristics		
A. Severity of illness		
HIV	No relationship	Catz et al., 2000
Blindness	No relationship	Vincent, 1971
If illness interferes with daily activities or appearance	Increases compliance	DiMatteo & DiNicola, 1982
Pain with the illness	Increases compliance	Becker, 1979
B. Side effects of medication		
Unpleasant HIV drugs	Decreases compliance	Catz et al., 2000
C. Complex treatment procedures		
Number of doses over three	Decreases compliance	Cramer et al., 1989
II. Personal Factors		
A. Increasing Age		
Adults		
Exercise up to 4 months	Increases compliance	Lynch et al., 1992
Exercise after 4 months	No relationship	Lynch et al., 1992
Cancer screening	Curvilinear relationship	Thomas et al., 1995
Hypertension medication	Increases compliance	Monane et al., 1996
Diabetes medication	Increases compliance	Sherbourne et al., 1992
Heart disease medication	Increases compliance	Sherbourne et al., 1992
Adolescents		
Diabetes	Decreases compliance	Bond et al., 1992
Diabetes	Decreases compliance	Olsen & Sutton, 1998
B. Gender		
Exercise program	No difference for class-based exercise	Oman & King, 2000
	Women report greater adherence for home exercise	Oman & King, 2000
Hypertensive medication	Men and women equal	Monane et al., 1996
Eating a healthy diet	Women more compliant	Laforge et al., 1994
Mental disorder medication	Women more compliant	Sellwood & Tarrier, 1994
C. Social support		
Wives support of husbands' diet	Increases compliance	Bovbjerg et al., 1995
Hemodialysis regimen	Increases compliance	Sherwood, 1983
Appointment keeping	Increases compliance	Tanner & Feldman, 1997
D. Emotional support		
Diabetes medication	Increases compliance	Sherbourne et al., 1992
Heart regimen	Emotional support better predictor than marriage	Kulik & Mahler, 1993
E. Personality factors		
Obsessive-compulsive	Increases compliance	Kabat-Zinn & Chapman-Waldrop, 1988
Cynical hostility	Decreases compliance	Christensen et al., 1997
F. Emotional factors		
Stressful life events	Decrease compliance	Oman & King, 2000
Anxiety	Decreases compliance	Brain et al., 1999

continued

TABLE 4.1 *Predictors of Patient Adherence—continued*

	Findings	Studies
II. Personal Factors—*continued*		
F. Personal beliefs		
Avoidance coping	Decreases compliance	Sherbourne et al., 1992
Personal control	Increases compliance	Helby et al., 1989; Stanton, 1987
III. Cultural Norms		
A. Diabetic and hypertensive patients in Zimbabwe		
Belief in traditional healers	Decreases compliance	Zyazema, 1984
B. Latino patients		
Physician's knowledge of Hispanic culture	Increases compliance	Ruiz & Ruiz, 1983
C. Physician's stereotype		
of African Americans	Decreases compliance	van Ryn & Burke, 2000
of low-income patients	Decreases compliance	van Ryn & Burke, 2000
IV. Practitioner-Patient Interaction		
A. Verbal communication		
Patients' confidence in physician's competence	Increases compliance	Gilbar, 1989
Physician disinterest	Decreases compliance	Russell & Roter, 1993
B. Practitioner's personal qualities		
Friendliness	Increases compliance	DiNicola & DiMatteo, 1984
Being a woman	Female doctors provide more information	Hall et al., 1994

not relate to compliance. This information, along with knowledge of why some people are nonadherent, can help answer the basic question of this chapter: How can adherence be improved?

Why Are Some People Nonadherent?

After his heart attack, Paul's physician told him, "Well, I guess we're going to have to get you off those damned weeds." This statement may have been meant as a requirement to quit smoking, but Paul interpreted it as a mere comment. Unfortunately, many patients leave the doctor's office still unclear about their instructions and with no specific plan for carrying out their medical regimen. Vagueness of physician advice is one of the communication problems between patient and physician, but it is only one of several reasons people fail to follow medical advice.

One reason for high rates of nonadherence is that the current definition of adherence demands certain difficult lifestyle changes. At the beginning of the 20th century, when the leading causes of death and disease were infectious diseases, compliance was simpler. Patients were compliant when they followed the doctor's advice with regard to medication, rest, diet, and so on. With health restored, patients could return to their former way of living. Adherence is no longer a matter of taking the proper pills and following short-term advice. The three leading causes of death in the United States—cardiovascular disease, cancer, and chronic obstructive lung disease—are all affected by unhealthy lifestyles. Thus compliance, broadly defined, currently includes adherence to healthy and safe behaviors as part of an ongoing lifestyle. To be compliant, people must now avoid cigarette smoking, use alcohol wisely or not at all, eat properly, and exercise regularly. In addition, of course, they must also make and keep medical and dental appointments, listen with understanding to the advice of health care providers, and finally, follow that advice. These requirements present a complex array of requirements that are difficult to fulfill.

The second category of reasons for nonadherence includes all those problems inherent in hearing and heeding physicians' advice. Patients may reject the prescribed regimen as being too difficult, time consuming, or expensive; or they may reject the practitioner as being incompetent, arrogant, or unfriendly. Also, many patients stop taking their medication when their symptoms disappear. Paradoxically, others stop because they begin to feel worse, leading them to believe that the medication is useless. Still others, in squirrel-like fashion, save a few pills for the next time they get sick. Responsibility for adherence rests with both the patient and the health care professional, and both contribute to patients' noncompliant behavior. Many patients do not understand their physician's criteria for specific adherence (Orme & Binik, 1989), and others stop taking their medication because adherence is simply too much trouble or it does not fit into the routine of their daily lives (Hunt, Jordan, Irwin, & Browner, 1989). Still other patients may make irrational choices about adherence because they have an **optimistic bias;** that is, a belief that they will be spared the same negative consequences of nonadherence that afflict other people (Brock & Wartman, 1990). Another suggestion is that some patients fail to follow medical advice because they hope for a miracle (Sherbourne et al., 1992). Other patients may be noncompliant because prescription labels are too difficult to read. For example, one study (Mustard & Harris, 1989) found that fewer than half of college students were able to correctly understand prescription labels that had been randomly selected from a pharmacist's records. Table 4.2 summarizes some of the reasons patients give for not complying with medical advice.

TABLE 4.2 *Reasons Given by Patients for Not Complying with Medical Advice*

"It's too much trouble."
"I won't get sick. God will save me."
"I just didn't get the prescription filled."
"The medication was too expensive."
"The medication didn't work very well. I was still sick, so I stopped taking it."
"The medication worked after only one week, so I stopped taking it."
"I have too many pills to take."
"I forgot."
"I want to remain sick."
"I don't want to become addicted to pills."
"If one pill is good, then two pills should be twice as good."
"I saved some pills for the next time I get sick."
"I gave some of my pills to my husband so he won't get sick."
"They're trying to poison me."
"This doctor doesn't know as much as my other doctor."
"The medication makes me sick."
"The medication tastes bad."
"Taking medication is just another bad habit."
"I was hoping for a miracle."
"I don't see any reason to take something to prevent illness."
"My doctor prescribes too many pills. I don't need all of them."
"I don't like my doctor. He thinks he knows everything."
"I didn't understand my doctor's instructions and was too embarrassed to ask her to repeat them."
"I don't like the taste of nicotine chewing gum."
"I won' t get very sick anyway, so I don't need to take anything."
"I didn't understand the directions on the label."

How Can Adherence Be Improved?

Knowing these reasons for nonadherence may help health care providers to improve patient compliance. Methods for improving compliance can be divided into educational and behavioral strategies. Educational procedures are those that impart information, sometimes in an emotion-arousing manner designed to frighten the noncompliant patient into becoming compliant. Included with educational strategies are such procedures as health education messages, individual patient counseling with various professional health care providers, programmed instruction, lectures, demonstrations, and individual counseling accompanied by written instructions. Haynes (1976) reported that strategies that relied on education and threats of disastrous consequences for nonadherence were only marginally effective in bringing about a meaningful change in patients' behaviors.

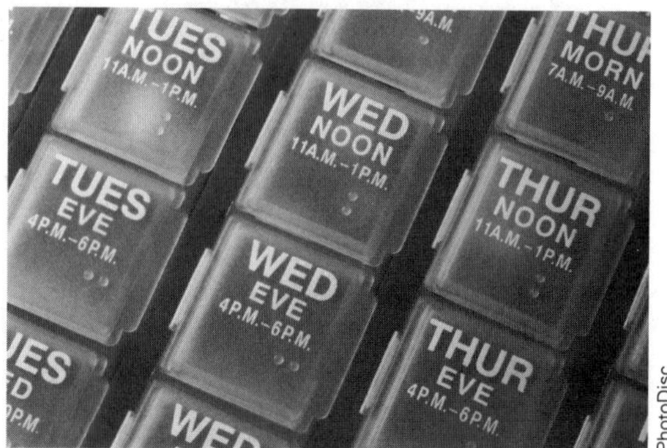

Finding ways to fit medication into patients' schedules can improve adherence rates.

Behavioral strategies, on the other hand, focus more directly on changing the person's behaviors involved in compliance. They include a wide variety of techniques, such as reducing economic barriers to compliance, using reward to reinforce compliance, notifying patients of upcoming appointments, simplifying medical schedules, making home visits, and persistently monitoring and rewarding the patients' compliant behaviors. Behavioral techniques have been found to be more effective than educational strategies in improving patient compliance. Educational methods may increase patients' knowledge, but behavioral approaches aimed at increasing patient involvement and encouraging an active, ongoing relationship between patient and practitioner offer a more effective approach to enhancing adherence (Haynes, 1976). People, it seems, do not misbehave because they do not know better, but because proper behavior, for a variety of reasons, is less appealing.

A review of the literature on interventions to improve compliance and keep appointments (Macharia, Leon, Rowe, Stephenson, & Haynes, 1992) found that, once again, education was not an effective means of improving adherence. The ineffectiveness of educational and instructional procedures has instigated a growing interest in various behavioral and cognitive strategies for improving patient compliance. These interventions include self-monitoring, home visits, cues and rewards, and peer group discussions. One group of researchers (Haynes, Wang, & da Mota Gomes, 1987) found that cues and rewards seem to be the most consistently effective means of improving compliance. Cues include using one's toothbrush or a completed meal as a signal to take one's medication. Rewards might include small sums of money given by the health care provider or self-reinforcement, such as seeing a movie or treating oneself to a nice meal. Both cues and rewards have been shown to increase the chances that patients will take their prescribed medication.

Robin DiMatteo and Dante DiNicola (1982) recommended four behavioral strategies for improving adherence. First, various *prompts* can be used to remind patients to initiate health-enhancing behaviors. These prompts may be cued by regular events in the patient's life, such as taking medication before each meal, or they may take the form of telephone calls from a clinic to remind the person to keep an appointment or to refill a prescription. A second behavioral strategy, *tailoring the regimen,* involves fitting the treatment to habits and routines in the patient's daily life. Third, these authors suggested a *graduated regimen implementation* that reinforces successive approximations to the desired behavior. Such shaping procedures should be effective with exercise and diet, but of course they are not appropriate to the taking of medica-

BECOMING HEALTHIER

You can improve your health by following sound health-related advice. Here are some things you can do to make adherence pay off.

1. Adopt an overall healthy lifestyle—one that includes not smoking, using alcohol in moderation or not at all, eating a diet high in fiber and low in saturated fats, getting an optimum amount of regular physical activity, and incorporating safety into your life. Procedures for adopting each of these health habits are discussed in *Becoming Healthier* boxes, Chapters 12 to 16.
2. Establish a relationship with your physician that is one of cooperation and not servile obedience. You and your doctor are the two most important people involved in your health, and the two of you should cooperate in designing your health practices.
3. Another important person interested in your health is your spouse, parent, friend, or sibling. Enlist the support of a significant person or persons in your life. Research shows that high levels of social support improve one's rate of adherence.
4. Before visiting a health care provider, jot down some questions you would like to have answered; ask the questions, and write down the answers during the visit. If you receive a prescription, ask the doctor about possible side effects—you don't want an unanticipated unpleasant side effect to be an excuse to stop taking the medication. Also, be sure you know how long you must take the medication—some chronic diseases require a lifetime of treatment.
5. If you feel that your physician gives you complex medical information that you don't comprehend, ask for clarification in a language that you can understand.
6. Remember that some recommendations (such as beginning a regular exercise program) should be adopted gradually. (If you do too much the first day, you won't feel like exercising again the next day.)
7. Find a doctor who understands and appreciates your cultural beliefs, ethnic background, language, and religious beliefs.
8. Reward yourself for following your good health practices. If you faithfully followed your diet for a day or week, do something nice for yourself.

tions. The final behavioral strategy listed by DiMatteo and DiNicola was a *contingency contract,* an agreement (usually written) between patients and the health care professionals that provides for some kind of reward to patients contingent on their achieving compliance. The ultimate goal of each of these approaches is self-regulation. However, before reaching this goal, patients often need help from others. This outside help, whether from family members or from professionals, ordinarily is given extensively at first and then is gradually withdrawn as patients begin to acquire more control over their health-related behaviors.

Cognitive-behavioral interventions attempt to enhance patients' social support and to increase their self-efficacy for adherence to healthy behaviors. These strategies include training patients to monitor their health-related behaviors, to evaluate those behaviors against a predetermined criterion, and to use positive self-reinforcement for any progress toward meeting the criterion. Several studies have demonstrated the effectiveness of cognitive-behavioral methods in improving patient compliance with a variety of health and medical regimens, including exercise (McAuley, 1993), lithium treatment for bipolar disorders (Cochran, 1984), and weight control for hemodialysis patients (Hegel, Ayllon, Thiel, & Oulton, 1992).

In addition to these behavioral and cognitive-behavioral strategies, several novel but simple interventions have shown promising results. Obtaining a *verbal commitment* from mothers increased their adherence to the recommended medical regimen for their children (Kulik & Carlino, 1987). Also, the simple process of a *service fee* for missed appointments was effective in decreasing missed appointments at a college health center (Wesch, Lutzker, Frisch, & Dillon, 1987). *Hypnosis* can be effective in initiating and maintaining dental flossing by college students, increasing the rate from 15% to 67% of students who flossed daily (Kelly, McKinty, & Carr, 1988). Hypnosis can also improve compliance in adolescent diabetics who previously showed poor control of their blood glucose (Ratner, Gross, Casas, & Castells, 1990). Finally, an instructional audiotape helped undergraduate women improve their proficiency at breast self-examination (Jones et al., 1993). Although these studies generally used few participants and lacked rigorous controls, they point to potentially promising means of improving patient adherence.

Haynes et al. (1987) proposed several other means of improving adherence to medical recommendations. For all treatment regimens, they suggested that the prescription should be as simple as possible and that patients should receive clearly written instructions on the exact behaviors to follow. For long-term treatments, these authors recommended reminders, rewards, and social support. More specifically, they suggested that health care providers can increase compliance by (1) calling patients who miss an appointment, (2) providing medication that fits easily into a patient's daily schedule, (3) reinforcing the importance of adherence at each visit, (4) tailoring the number of visits to fit the patient's level of compliance, (5) verbally rewarding the patient's efforts to comply, (6) decreasing the frequency of visits as a reward for good adherence, and (7) involving the patient's spouse or other partner.

Despite these suggestions, a review of research on adherence (Haynes et al., 1996) concluded that little evidence existed that adherence can be improved and also that complex and labor-intensive interventions are "not very effective despite the amount of effort and resources they consumed" (p. 386).

In Summary

To improve adherence, many health care professionals first look for reasons why people are nonadherent. These reasons include the difficulty of altering lifestyles of long duration, incomplete practitioner-patient communication, and erroneous beliefs as to what advice they should follow. Effective programs to improve compliance rates frequently include clearly written instructions, simple prescriptions, follow-up calls for missed appointments, prescriptions tailored to the patient's daily schedule, rewards for compliant behavior, cues to signal the time for taking medication, and involvement of the patient's spouse or support network.

Answers

This chapter addressed four basic questions:

1. What theoretical models have been used to explain adherence?

Several theoretical models attempt to predict and explain compliant and noncompliant behavior. These include the behavioral model, which relies on contingency contracts and reinforcement for compliant behaviors; the self-efficacy model, which holds that people's beliefs that they can perform certain behaviors strongly predict what behaviors they will enact; the theories of reasoned action and planned behavior, both of which assume that intentions, attitudes, subjective norms, and motivation predict adherence; and the transtheoretical model, which assumes that people progress in spiral fashion through five stages in making changes in behavior—precontemplation, contemplation, preparation, action, and maintenance. Each of these models has some use in predicting and explaining compliance and noncompliance.

2. **What is adherence, how can it be measured, and how frequently does it occur?**
Adherence is the extent to which a person's behavior coincides with appropriate medical and health advice. For people to profit from medical advice, that advice first must be accurate and second, patients must follow that advice. When people do not adhere to sound health behaviors, they may risk developing serious health problems or even death. When participants in a health intervention study fail to comply, the results of the study may be seriously contaminated.

There are at least six basic ways of measuring patient adherence: (1) ask the physician, (2) ask the patient, (3) ask other people, (4) count pills, (5) examine biochemical evidence, (6) use a combination of these procedures. Of these, physician judgment is the least valid, but each of the others also has serious flaws.

Assessing the frequency of nonadherence is complicated by the different definitions of the term, the nature of the illness, the population being studied, and the methods used to assess compliance. In general terms, however, the rate of nonadherence has remained around 50% for the past 2 or 3 decades.

3. **What factors predict adherence?**
Researchers have found little evidence that the severity of a disease is an accurate predictor of adherence. Unpleasant or painful side effects of medication tend to lower adherence. Personal dispositions are mostly unrelated to compliant behavior, but people with an obsessive-compulsive pattern of relating to the world are more likely to comply, whereas cynically hostile people are less likely to comply.

Researchers have found some evidence for each of the following predictors to lead to increased levels of nonadherence: (1) long and complicated treatment regimens; (2) lack of emotional and social support for adherence; (3) increasing age of adolescent diabetics, (4) male gender for exercising at home, maintaining a healthy diet, or taking medication as scheduled; (5) high levels of stress and anxiety (6) avoidance coping, (7) lack of personal control, (8) patients' cultural beliefs that modern medicine is ineffective; (9) patients' lack of confidence in their doctor's competence; (10) poor patient-practitioner communication; and (11) unfriendly or authoritarian physicians.

4. **How can adherence be improved?**
Knowing reasons for nonadherence may help health care professionals detect methods of improving compliance, and they have suggested a variety of behavioral strategies to enhance adherence. Effective programs frequently include clearly written instructions, simple prescriptions, follow-up calls for missed appointments, prescriptions tailored to the patient's daily schedule, rewards for compliant behavior, cues to signal the time for taking medication, and involvement of the patient's spouse or support network.

Suggested Readings

Blackwell, B. (1997). From compliance to alliance: A quarter century of research. In B. Blackwell (Ed.), *Treatment compliance and the therapeutic alliance* (pp. 1–15). Amsterdam: Harwood Academic Publishers. This concise overview of compliance addresses many of the basic issues in the field, including the meaning of compliance, its effectiveness, how it can be measured, and how it can be improved.

Haynes, R. B., McKibbon, K. A., & Kanani, R. (1996). Systematic review of randomized trials of interventions to assist patients to follow prescriptions for medications. *Lancet, 348,* 383–386.R. Brian Haynes, K. Ann McKibbon, and Ronak Kanani review various techniques of improving adherence and conclude that most of these attempts are only marginally effective. Taking all techniques into consideration, the reviewers conclude that only about half of all medical and health advice is correctly followed.

Prochaska, J. O., Norcross, J. C., & DiClemente, C. C. (1994). *Changing for good.* New York: Avon Books.In this popular, easy-to-read book, the authors of the transtheoretical model offer many practical pointers for changing unhealthy behaviors. The book offers readers suggestions for recognizing their readiness to change and advice on how to accomplish change.

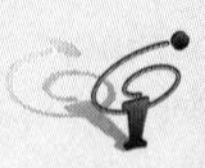

Search InfoTrac College Edition

Search these terms to learn more about topics in this chapter:

Self-efficacy and adherence

Reinforcement and compliance

Transtheoretical and compliance

Stages of change and compliance

Compliance and HIV

Social support and adherence

Improving compliance

Improving adherence

5

Defining and Measuring Stress

The Story of René

CHAPTER OUTLINE

The Nervous System and the Physiology of Stress

Theories of Stress

Sources of Stress

Measurement of Stress

QUESTIONS

This chapter focuses on four basic questions:

1. What is the physiology of stress?
2. What theories explain stress?
3. What sources produce stress?
4. How has stress been measured?

The Story of René

At age 25, René feels that her life is almost more stressful than she can manage. An African American college sophomore majoring in health a… ance, René's busy life leaves little room … self or for fostering new friendships.

A single mother of two children, R… ries a full academic load while working … child care center. At work, she looks aft… young children, including her own 1-ye… ever, the most stressful part of her life i… watching her 7-year-old son Michael, w… nosed as having attention-deficit/hyper… (ADHD). Michael's hyperactivity dem… ual vigilance by René.

Three years ago, René's father died … thinks of him every day. Her mother, w… town as René, works two jobs and is not…

daughter care for the two children. Thus, the only break René has from her two needy … is the time she spends … l. After attending … during the evening, she … consequence, her … like them to be, and be… …nts yet another source … uggling with school… students who seem to … ppear to be making … Later, we return to the … sors and to see how she …

…s is and how it can be … question of whether … and even death. Chap… people cope with stress, … bases for stress.

The Nervous System and the Physiology of Stress

The basic function of the nervous system is to integrate all the body's systems. Small, simple organisms do not need (nor do they have) nervous systems. In larger and more complex organisms, nervous systems provide internal communication and relay information to and from the environment.

The human nervous system contains billions of individual cells called **neurons.** The action of neurons is electrochemical. Within each neuron, electrically charged ions hold the potential for an electrical discharge. This discharge, a minute electrical current, travels the length of the neuron. The electrical charge leads to the release of chemicals called **neurotransmitters** that are manufactured within each neuron and stored in vesicles at the ends of the neurons. The released neurotransmitters diffuse across the **synaptic cleft,** the space between neurons.

A number of different neurotransmitters have been identified; more remain unidentified. Of those that are understood, the chemical action is quite complex. Some neurotransmitters produce an excitatory action, which promotes the development of the neurons' electrical potential. Other neurotransmitters inhibit transmission, making neurons more difficult to activate. When a neuron is stimulated and releases its transmitter chemical, the excitatory and inhibitory messages have a cumulative effect. The next neuron's threshold must be exceeded for it to be activated. If the threshold is reached, then the next neuron "fires." If the threshold is not reached, then the next neuron will not be activated.

Neurons do not form an end-to-end chain; rather, they are more like a net, with each neuron having as many as several hundred synaptic connections to other neurons. One neuron may form multiple connections with another neuron and, in addition, it may synapse with several other neurons. The many avenues for communication among neurons, excitatory and inhibitory effects, and

CHECK YOUR HEALTH RISKS

Undergraduate Stress Questionnaire

Has this stressful event happened to you at any time during the last two weeks? If it has, please check the space next to it. If it has not, then please leave it blank.

- ☐ Lack of money
- ☐ Someone broke a promise
- ☐ Death (family member or friend)
- ☐ Dealt with incompetence at the Registrar's office
- ☐ Can't concentrate
- ☐ Had a lot of tests
- ☐ Thought about unfinished work
- ☐ Someone did a "pet peeve" of yours
- ☐ It's finals week
- ☐ Living with boy-/girlfriend
- ☐ No sleep
- ☐ Applying to graduate school
- ☐ Felt need for transportation
- ☐ Sick, injury
- ☐ Bad haircut today
- ☐ Victim of a crime
- ☐ Had a class presentation
- ☐ Job requirements changed
- ☐ Applying for a job
- ☐ Assignments in all classes due the same day
- ☐ Fought with boy-/girlfriend
- ☐ No time to eat
- ☐ You have a hard upcoming week
- ☐ Felt some peer pressure
- ☐ Lots of deadlines to meet
- ☐ Went into test unprepared
- ☐ Working while in school
- ☐ Arguments, conflict of values with friends
- ☐ You have a hangover
- ☐ Problems with your computer
- ☐ Lost something (especially wallet)
- ☐ Death of a pet
- ☐ Bothered by having no social support of family
- ☐ Performed poorly at a task
- ☐ Did worse than expected on test
- ☐ Problem getting home from bar when drunk
- ☐ Used a fake ID
- ☐ Had an interview
- ☐ Had projects, research papers due
- ☐ Did badly on a test
- ☐ Can't finish everything you needed to do
- ☐ Heard bad news
- ☐ No sex for a while
- ☐ Someone cut ahead of you in line
- ☐ Had confrontation with an authority figure
- ☐ Maintaining a long-distance boy-/girlfriend
- ☐ Crammed for a test
- ☐ Parents getting divorce
- ☐ Dependent on other people
- ☐ Feel unorganized
- ☐ Breaking up with boy-/girlfriend
- ☐ Trying to decide on major
- ☐ Feel isolated
- ☐ Having roommate conflicts
- ☐ Checkbook didn't balance
- ☐ Visit from a relative and entertaining them
- ☐ Decision to have sex on your mind
- ☐ Car/bike broke down, flat tire, etc.
- ☐ Parents controlling with money
- ☐ Couldn't find a parking space
- ☐ Noise disturbed you while trying to study
- ☐ Someone borrowed something without permission
- ☐ Had to ask for money
- ☐ Got a traffic ticket
- ☐ Talked with a professor
- ☐ Change of environment (new doctor, dentist, etc.)
- ☐ Exposed to upsetting TV show, book, or movie
- ☐ Got to class late
- ☐ Erratic schedule
- ☐ Found out boy-/girlfriend cheated on you
- ☐ Can't understand your professor
- ☐ Trying to get into your major or college
- ☐ Missed your period and waiting
- ☐ Coping with addictions
- ☐ Registration for classes
- ☐ Stayed up late writing a paper
- ☐ Property stolen
- ☐ Someone you expected to call did not
- ☐ Holiday
- ☐ Sat through a boring class
- ☐ Favorite sporting team lost
- ☐ Thoughts about future

Add the number of check marks. Student with higher scores are more likely to need health care (as measured by going to the student health center or infirmary) than students with lower scores.

Source: "Measuring life event stress in the lives of college students: The Undergraduates Stress Questionnaire (USQ)," by C. S. Crandall, J. J. Preisler, & J. Aussprung, 1992, *Journal of Behavioral Medicine,* vol. 15, pp. 627–662. Reprinted by permission of Chris Crandall and Kluwer Academic.

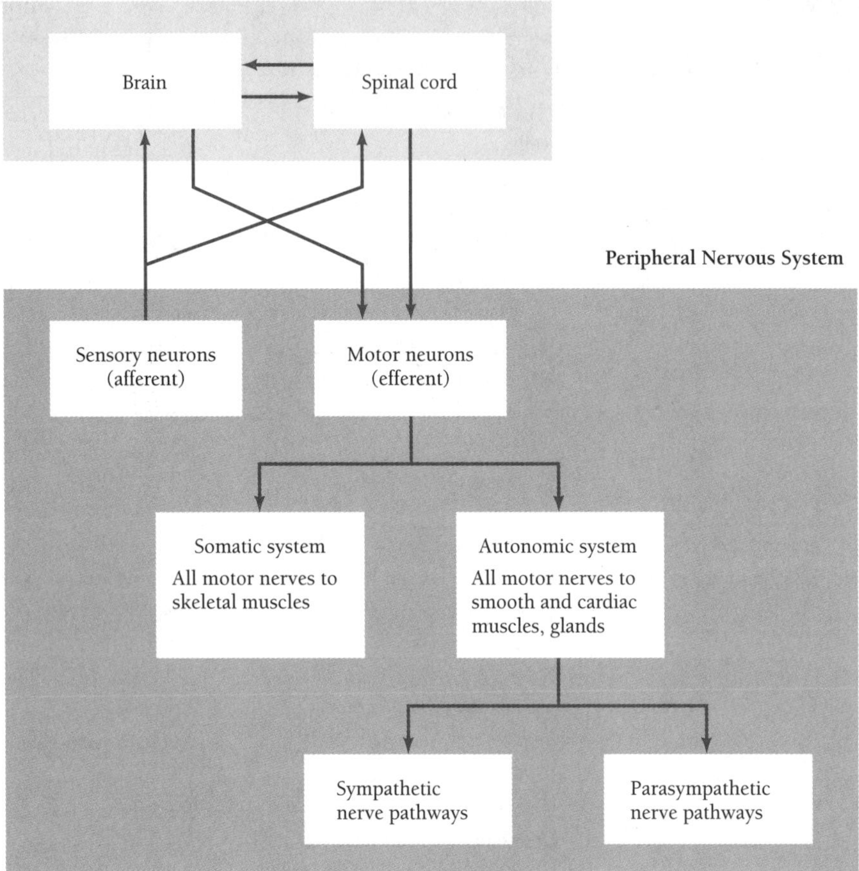

Figure 5.1 Divisions of the human nervous system.

billions of neurons in each person's nervous system ensure great complexity in neural transmission.

The billions of neurons fall into three types. **Afferent neurons** (sensory neurons) relay information from the sense organs toward the brain. The action of **efferent neurons** (motor neurons) results in movement of muscles or stimulation of organs or glands. **Interneurons** connect sensory neurons to motor neurons.

The nervous system is organized hierarchically, with major divisions and subdivisions. The two major divisions of the nervous system are the **central nervous system (CNS)** and the **peripheral nervous system (PNS).** The CNS is composed of the brain and the spinal cord, and the PNS consists of all other neurons. The divisions and subdivisions of the nervous system are illustrated in Figure 5.1.

The next section describes the nervous system from the bottom of its organizational hierarchy to the top—that is, beginning with the PNS and ending with the brain. This approach traces the path of information from the periphery of the nervous system to the brain.

The Peripheral Nervous System

The peripheral nervous system, that part of the nervous system lying outside the brain and spinal cord, is divided into two parts: the **somatic nerv-**

ous system and the **autonomic nervous system (ANS).** The somatic nervous system has both sensory and motor components, primarily serving the skin and the voluntary muscles. The autonomic nervous system primarily serves internal organs.

The Somatic Nervous System The somatic division of the peripheral nervous system serves muscles and skin. Sensory impulses begin with stimulation of the skin and muscles, and these neural impulses travel toward the spinal cord by way of sensory nerves in the somatic nervous system. Motor messages that originate in the brain travel down the spinal cord, are relayed to muscles, and initiate muscle movement. The motor nerves that activate muscles are part of the somatic nervous system.

Sensory and motor impulses in the head and neck region do not travel through the spinal cord. Instead, 12 pairs of cranial nerves enter and exit directly from the lower part of the brain. The cranial nerves are also part of the somatic nervous system. They function like the sensory and motor neurons that run through the spinal cord.

The Autonomic Nervous System The term *autonomic* means "self-governing." It has been applied to this division of the peripheral nervous system because, traditionally, the autonomic nervous system has been considered outside the realm of conscious or voluntary control. Although the functions of the ANS do not require conscious thought, we now know it is possible for people to learn to exert conscious control over many ANS functions. Neal Miller's (1969) famous experiments with biofeedback demonstrated that rats could learn to accelerate or decelerate their heart rate, a function under autonomic control. Many types of biofeedback have been developed, and several have clinical applications in health psychology (as Chapter 8 explains). Learning to control autonomic functions requires both effort and training, but some control of the ANS is within the realm of human capability.

The ANS allows for a variety of responses through its two divisions: the **sympathetic nervous system** and the **parasympathetic nervous system.** These two subdivisions differ anatomically as well as functionally. They, along with their target organs, appear in Figure 5.2.

The sympathetic division of the ANS mobilizes the body's resources in emergency, stressful, and emotional situations. The reactions include an increase in the rate and strength of cardiac contraction, constriction of blood vessels in the skin, a decrease of gastrointestinal activity, an increase in respiration, stimulation of the sweat glands, and dilation of the pupils in the eyes.

The parasympathetic division of the ANS, on the other hand, promotes relaxation and functions under normal, nonstressful conditions. The parasympathetic and sympathetic nervous systems serve the same target organs, but they tend to function reciprocally, with the activation of one increasing as the other decreases. For example, the activation of the sympathetic division reduces the secretion of saliva, producing the sensation of a dry mouth, whereas activation of the parasympathetic division promotes secretion of saliva.

Neurons in the ANS are activated by neurotransmitters, principally by **acetylcholine** and **norepinephrine.** These neurotransmitters have complex effects; each has different effects in different organ systems because the organs contain different neurochemical receptors. In addition, the balance of these two main neurotransmitters, as well as their absolute quantity, is important. Therefore, even though there are only two major ANS neurotransmitters, they produce a wide variety of responses.

Whether sympathetic or parasympathetic activation is appropriate depends on the situation. Maintaining the appropriate level of activation is referred to as **allostasis,** the concept that different circumstances requires different levels of physiological activation. Activation of the sympathetic nervous system is the body's attempt to meet the needs of the situation during emergencies and so is the activation of the parasympathetic nervous

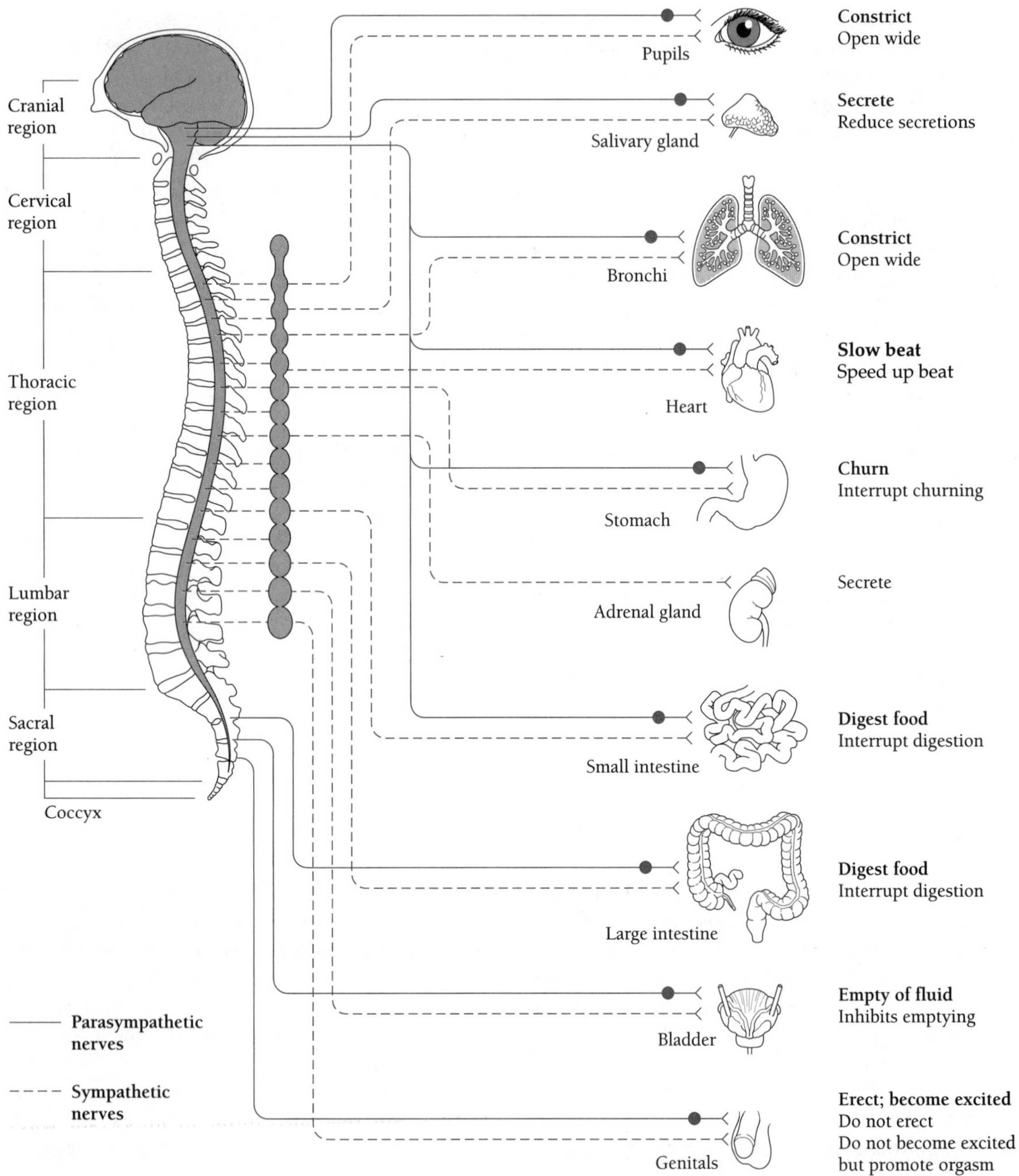

Figure 5.2 Autonomic nervous system and target organs.

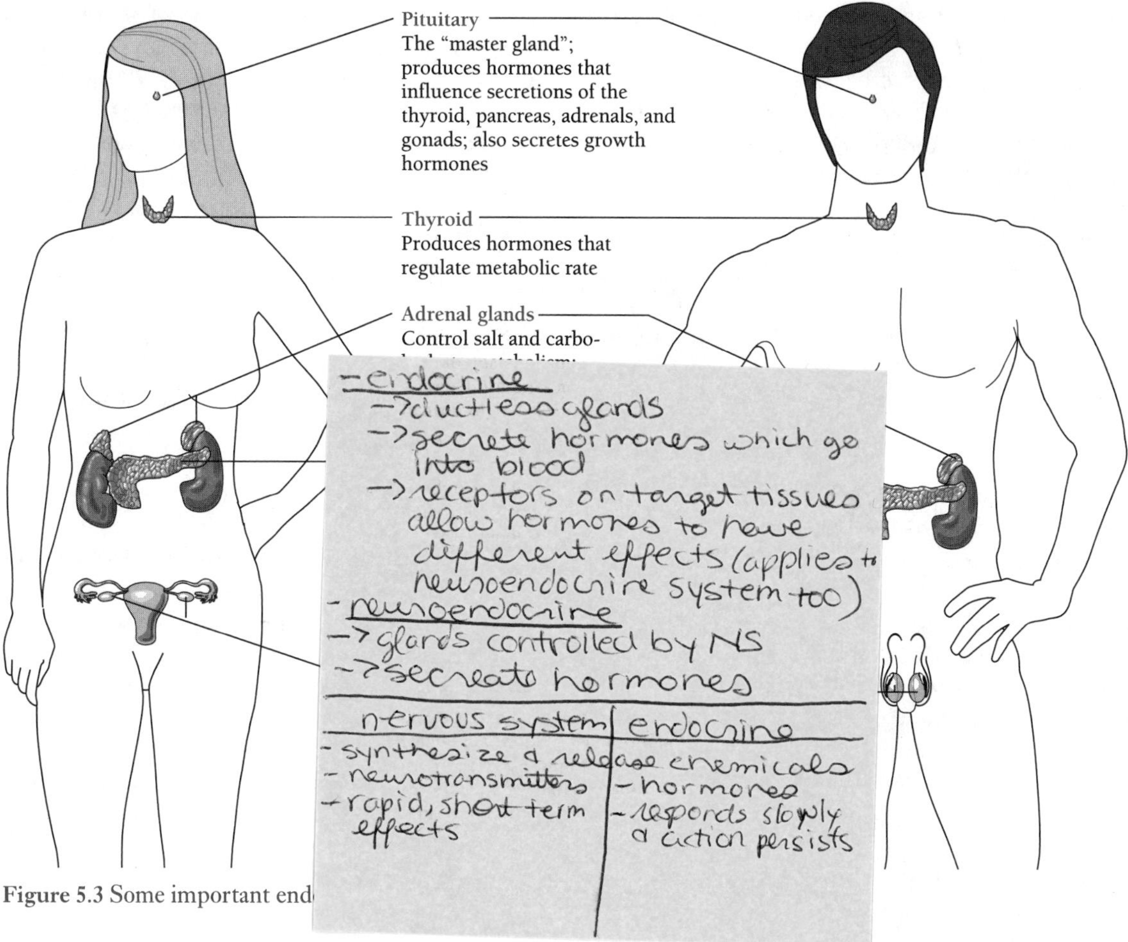

Figure 5.3 Some important end

system during normal circumstances. At its optimum in maintaining allostasis, the autonomic nervous system adapts smoothly, rapidly mobilizing resources by sympathetic activation and adjusting to normal demands by parasympathetic activation.

The Neuroendocrine System

The **endocrine system** consists of ductless glands distributed throughout the body (see Figure 5.3). The **neuroendocrine system** consists of those endocrine glands that are controlled by the nervous system. Glands of the endocrine and neuroendocrine systems secrete chemicals known as **hormones,** which move into the bloodstream to be carried to different parts of the body. Specialized receptors on target tissues or organs allow hormones to have specific effects, even though the hormones circulate throughout the body. At the target, hormones may have a direct effect, or they may cause the secretion of another hormone.

The endocrine and nervous systems can work closely together because they have several similarities, but they also differ in important ways. Both systems share, synthesize, and release chemicals. In the nervous system these chemicals are called neurotransmitters. In the endocrine system they are called hormones. The activation of neurons is usually rapid and the effect is short term; the endocrine system responds more slowly, and its action persists longer. In the nervous system, neurotransmitters are released by stimulation of neural impulses, flow across the synaptic cleft, and are immediately either reabsorbed or inactivated. In the endocrine system, hormones are synthesized by the endocrine cells, are released into the blood, reach their targets in minutes or even hours, and have prolonged effects. The endocrine and nervous systems both have communication and control functions, and both work toward integrated, adaptive behaviors. The two systems are related in function and interact in neuroendocrine responses.

The Pituitary Gland Located within the brain, the **pituitary gland** is an excellent example of the intricate relationship between the nervous and endocrine systems. The pituitary is connected to the hypothalamus, a structure in the forebrain. These two structures work together to regulate and produce hormones. The pituitary has been referred to as the "master gland" because it produces a number of hormones that affect other glands and prompts the production of other hormones.

Of the seven hormones produced by the anterior portion of the pituitary gland, **adrenocorticotropic hormone (ACTH)** plays an essential role in the stress response. When stimulated by the hypothalamus, the pituitary releases ACTH, which in turn acts on the **adrenal glands.**

The Adrenal Glands The adrenal glands are endocrine glands located on top of each kidney. Each gland is composed of an outer covering, the **adrenal cortex,** and an inner part, the **adrenal medulla.** Both secrete hormones that are important in the response to stress. The **adrenocortical response** occurs when ACTH from the pituitary stimulates the adrenal cortex to release **glucocorticoids,** one type of hormone. **Cortisol** is the most important of these hormones and is capable of affecting every major organ in the body (Lovallo, 1997). This hormone is so closely associated with stress that the level of cortisol circulating in the blood can be used as an index of stress.

The **adrenomedullary response** occurs when the sympathetic nervous system activates the adrenal medulla. This action prompts secretion of **catecholamines,** a class of chemicals containing epinephrine and norepinephrine. **Epinephrine** (sometimes referred to as adrenaline) is produced exclusively by the adrenal medulla and accounts for about 80% of the hormone production of the adrenal glands. **Norepinephrine** is not only a hormone; it is also a neurotransmitter produced in many places in the body besides the adrenal medulla. Neurotransmitters work at the synapse, whereas hormones circulate through the blood. Norepinephrine has both actions and is produced at many places in the body, not exclusively in the adrenal medulla.

Epinephrine, on the other hand, is produced exclusively in the adrenal medulla. It is so closely and uniquely associated with the adrenomedullary stress response that it is sometimes used as an index of stress. The amount of epinephrine secreted can be determined by assaying a person's urine, thus measuring stress by tapping into the physiology of the stress response. Such an index can be helpful because it does not rely on personal perceptions of stress and its use as a measure of stress can give an alternative perspective. Like other hormones, epinephrine and norepinephrine circulate through the blood stream, and their action is both slower and more prolonged than the action of neurotransmitters.

Physiology of the Stress Response

The physiological reactions to stress begin with the perception of stress. That perception results in activation of the sympathetic division of the autonomic nervous system, which mobilizes the body's resources to react in emotional, stressful, and emergency situations. Walter Cannon (1932) termed this configuration of responses the "fight-or-flight" reaction because this array of responses prepares the body for either option. Sympathetic activation prepares the body for intense motor activity, the sort necessary for attack, defense, or escape. This mobilization occurs through two routes and affects all parts of the body.

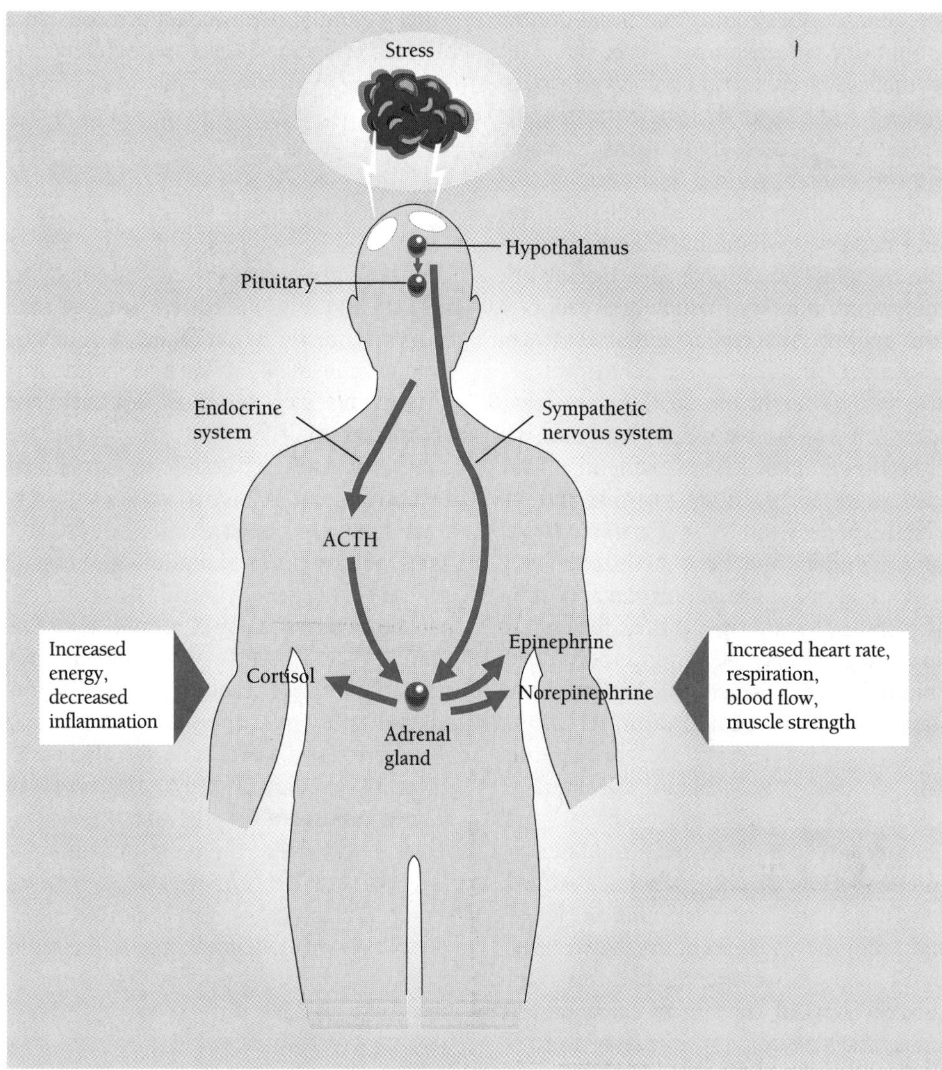

Figure 5.4 Physiological effects of stress.

One route is through direct activation of the sympathetic division of the ANS, which activates the adrenal medulla to secrete epinephrine and norepinephrine. These effects occur throughout the body, affecting the cardiovascular, digestive, and respiratory systems. The other route of action begins with the anterior pituitary (the part of the pituitary gland at the base of the brain), which secretes adrenocorticotropic hormone (ACTH). This hormone stimulates the adrenal cortex to secrete glucocorticoids, including cortisol. Its secretion mobilizes the body's energy resources, raising the level of blood sugar to provide energy for the cells. Cortisol also has an anti-inflammatory effect, giving the body a natural defense against swelling from injuries that might be sustained during a fight or a flight. Figure 5.4 shows these two routes of activation.

Shelly Taylor and her colleagues (2000) raised objections to the traditional conceptualization of the stress response, questioning the basic notion that it is a fight-or-flight response. These theorists contended that research and theory on stress responses have been biased by concentrating on men, for whom fight-or-flight is a more valid model than for women. Although they acknowledged that men's and women's nervous system responses to stress are virtually identical, they argued that women exhibit neuroendocrine responses to stress that differ from men's reactions and that these differences lay the biological foundation for gender differences in behavioral responses to stress. They proposed that the stress response in women is better characterized as "tend-and-befriend" than "fight-or-flight." That is, women tend to respond to stressful situations by nurturing responses and by seeking and giving social support rather than by either fighting or fleeing. Taylor and her colleagues argued that this pattern of responses arose in women during human evolutionary history and is more consistent with the biological and behavioral evidence than the fight-or-flight conceptualization of stress responses.

In Summary

The physiology of the stress response is extremely complex. When a person perceives stress, the sympathetic division of the autonomic nervous system rouses the person from a resting state in two ways: by stimulating the sympathetic nervous system and by producing hormones. The ANS activation is rapid, as is all neural transmission, whereas the action of the neuroendocrine system is slower. The pituitary releases ACTH, which in turn affects the adrenal cortex. Glucocorticoid release prepares the body to resist the stress and even to cope with injury by the release of cortisol. Together the two systems form the physiological basis for the stress response as well as the potential for illness.

An understanding of the physiology of stress does not completely clarify the meaning of stress. Thus, several models have been constructed in an attempt to better define and explain stress.

Theories of Stress

Despite a great deal of scientific research on the subject and the widespread use of the term in everyday conversation, *stress* has no simple definition. Indeed, it has been defined in three different ways: as a stimulus, as a response, and as an interaction. When some people talk about stress, they are referring to an environmental *stimulus,* as in "I have a high-stress job." Others consider stress a physical *response,* as in "My heart races when I feel a lot of stress." Still others consider stress to result from the *interaction* between environmental stimuli and the person, as in "I feel stressed when I have to make financial decisions at work, but other types of decisions do not stress me."

These three views of stress also appear in the different theories of stress. The view of stress as an external event was the first approach taken by stress researchers, the most prominent of whom was Hans Selye. During the course of his research, Selye changed to a more response-based view of stress, concentrating on the biological aspects of the stress response. The most influential view of stress among psychologists has been the interactionist approach, proposed by Richard Lazarus. The next two sections discuss the views of Selye and Lazarus.

Selye's View

Beginning in the 1930s and continuing until his death in 1982, Hans Selye (1956, 1976, 1982) researched and popularized the concept of stress, making a strong case for its relationship to physical illness and bringing the importance of stress to the attention of the public. Although he did not originate the concept of stress, he researched the effects of stress on physiological responses and tried to connect these reactions to the development of illness.

Over the course of his career, Selye first considered stress to be a stimulus and later saw it as a response. His original position was that stress was a stimulus, concentrating on the environmental conditions that produced stress. In the 1950s, Selye started to use the term *stress* to refer to a response that the organism makes. To distinguish the two, Selye started using the terms *stressor* to refer to the stimulus and *stress* to mean the response.

Selye's contributions to stress research included a concept of stress and a model for how the body defends itself in stressful situations. Selye conceptualized stress as a nonspecific response, repeatedly insisting that stress is a general physical response caused by any of a number of environmental stressors. He believed that a wide variety of different situations could prompt the stress response, but that response would always be the same.

The General Adaptation Syndrome The body's generalized attempt to defend itself against noxious agents became known as the **general adaptation syndrome (GAS).** This syndrome is divided into three stages, the first of which is the **alarm reaction.** During alarm, the body's defenses against a stressor are mobilized through activation of the sympathetic nervous system. This division activates body systems to maximize strength and prepares them for the fight-or-flight response. Adrenaline (epinephrine) is released, heart rate and blood pressure increase, respiration becomes faster, blood is diverted away from the internal organs toward the skeletal muscles, sweat glands are activated, and the gastrointestinal system decreases its activity. As a short-term response to an emergency situation, these physical reactions are adaptive, but many modern stress situations involve prolonged exposure to stress but do not require physical action.

Selye called the second phase of the GAS the **resistance stage.** In this stage the organism adapts to the stressor. How long this stage lasts depends on the severity of the stressor and the adaptive capacity of the organism. If the organism can adapt, the resistance stage will continue for a long time. During this stage, the person gives the outward appearance of normality, but physiologically the body's internal functioning is not normal. Continuing stress will cause continued neurological and hormonal changes. Selye believed that these demands take a toll, setting the stage for what he described as *diseases of adaptation,* those diseases related to continued, persistent stress. Figure 5.5 illustrates these stages and the point in the process at which diseases develop.

Among the diseases Selye considered to be the result of prolonged resistance to stress are peptic ulcers and ulcerative colitis, hypertension and cardiovascular disease, hyperthyroidism, and bronchial asthma. In addition, Selye hypothesized that resistance to stress would cause changes in the immune system, making infection more likely.

The capacity to resist stress is finite, and the final stage of the GAS is the **exhaustion stage.** At the end, the organism's ability to resist is depleted, and a breakdown results. This stage is characterized by activation of the parasympathetic division of the autonomic nervous system. Under normal circumstances, parasympathetic activation keeps the body functioning in a balanced state. In the exhaustion stage, however, parasympathetic functioning is at an abnormally low level, causing a person to become exhausted. Selye believed that exhaustion frequently results in depression and sometimes even death.

Evaluation of Selye's View Selye's early concept of stress as a stimulus as well as his later concentration on the physical aspects of stress have both been influential in researching and measuring stress. The stimulus-based view of stress prompted researchers to investigate the various environmental conditions that lead people to experience stress and also led to the construction of stress inventories. Such inventories ask people to check or list the events they have

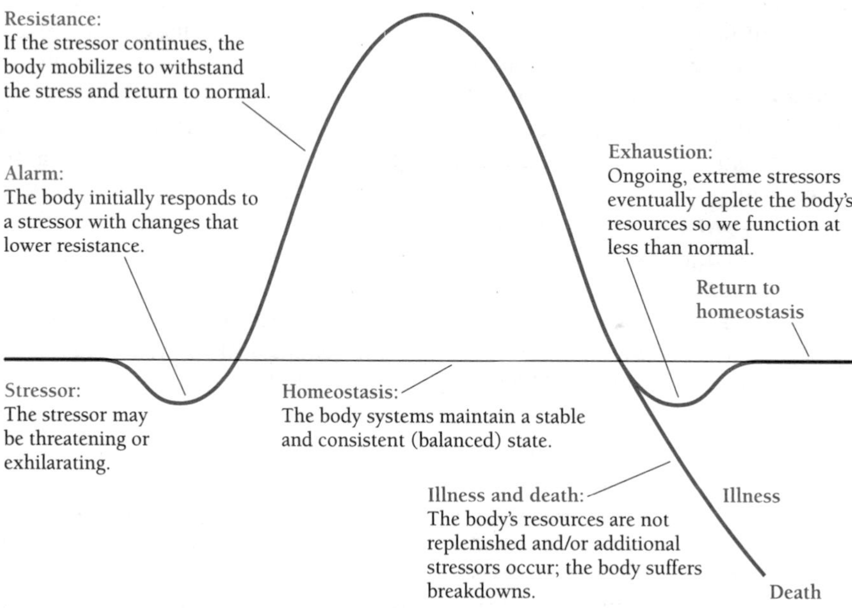

Figure 5.5 The three stages of Selye's General Adaptation Syndrome and their consequences.

Source: An Invitation to Health *(7th ed. p. 40) by D. Hales, 1997, Belmont, CA: Brooks/Cole. Copyright 1997 by Brooks/Cole Publishing Company. Reprinted by permission.*

experienced in the recent past and measure the amount of stress by totaling these events. We consider both the environmental sources of stress and the life event approach to measuring stress later in this chapter.

In considering stress as a set of physical responses, Selye largely ignored psychological factors, including the emotional component and the individual interpretation of stressful events. John Mason (1971, 1975) criticized Selye for ignoring the element of emotion in stress and hypothesized that the consistency in the stress response is due to this underlying element of emotion.

Selye emphasized the physiology of stress and conducted most of his research on nonhuman animals. By downplaying the differences between humans and other animals, he neglected the factors that are unique to humans, such as perception and interpretation of stressful experiences. Selye's view has had a great influence on the popular conception of stress, but an alternative model formulated by psychologist Richard Lazarus has had a greater impact among psychologists.

Lazarus's View

In Lazarus's view, the interpretation of stressful events is more important than the events themselves. Neither the environmental event nor the person's response defines stress, but rather the individual's *perception* of the psychological situation is the critical factor. This perception includes potential harms, threats, and challenges as well as the individual's perceived ability to cope with them.

Psychological Factors Lazarus's emphasis on interpretation and perception differs from that of Selye. Also, Lazarus worked largely with humans rather than nonhuman animals. The ability of people to think about and evaluate future events makes them vulnerable in ways that other animals are not. Humans encounter stresses because they have high-level cognitive abilities that other animals lack.

According to Lazarus (1984, 1993), the effect that stress has on a person is based more on that person's feelings of threat, vulnerability, and ability to cope than on the stressful event itself. For example, losing a job may be extremely stressful for someone who has no money saved or who believes that finding another job would be very difficult. Prior to her job at the child care center, René worked at a clerk in a large department store, but she was fired from that job because of difficulties with her assistant manager. Although being fired at work might be stressful for many single parents, René felt little additional stress from that experience: she had confidence that she could easily find a new job, which she did. In Lazarus's view, a life event is not what produces stress; rather, it is one's view of the situation that causes an event to become stressful.

Lazarus and Susan Folkman defined psychological stress as a "*particular relationship between the person and the environment that is appraised by the person as taxing or exceeding his or her resources and endangering his or her well-being*" (1984, p. 19). You should note several important points in this definition. First, Lazarus and Folkman's theory takes an interactional or *transactional* position, holding that stress refers to a relationship between person and environment. Second, this theory holds that the key to that transaction is the person's appraisal of the psychological situation. Third, the situation must be seen as threatening, challenging, or harmful.

Appraisal Lazarus and Folkman (1984) recognized that people use three kinds of appraisal to assess situations: primary appraisal, secondary appraisal, and reappraisal. **Primary appraisal** is not necessarily first in importance, but it is first in time. When a person first encounters an event, such as an offer of a job promotion, the person appraises it in terms of its effect on his or her well-being. The person may view the event as irrelevant, benign–positive, or stressful. It is unlikely that an offer of a job promotion would be seen as irrelevant, but many environmental events, such as a snowstorm in another state, have no implications for a person's well-being. A benign–positive appraisal means that the event is seen as having good implications. A stressful appraisal can mean that the event is seen as harmful, threatening, or challenging. Each of these three—harm, threat, and challenge—is likely to generate an emotion. Lazarus (1993) defined *harm* as the psychological damage that has already been done, such as an illness or injury; *threat* as the anticipation of harm; and *challenge* as a person's confidence in overcoming difficult demands. An appraisal of harm may produce anger, disgust, disappointment, or sadness; an appraisal of threat is likely to generate worry, anxiety, or fear; an appraisal of challenge may be followed by excitement or anticipation. It is important to remember that these emotions do not produce stress; instead, they are generated by the individual's appraisal of an event.

After a person's initial appraisal of an event, that person forms an impression of his or her ability to control or cope with harm, threat, or challenge, an impression called **secondary appraisal.** A person asks three questions in making secondary appraisals. The first is "What options are available to me?" The second is "What is the likelihood that I can successfully apply the necessary strategies to reduce this stress?" The third is "Will this procedure work, that is, will it alleviate my stress?"

As an example, let's look at our case study René after she had lost her job in a department store and felt the stress of earning a living for herself and her two children. René's secondary appraisal would begin with an assessment of the choices open to her, including moving in with her mother. However, René quickly dismissed that option because she believed that she and her mother would resort to their previous mode of relating, namely constantly quarreling. Answers to René's second question included her confidence that she could secure another job, one that would allow her to continue pursuing a college degree and to spend some time with her children. Answers to the third question included her belief that juggling three roles (college student, child care worker, and single parent) might be more than she could handle. In René's situation, the first two questions did not leave her with overwhelming feelings of stress, but the third question led to doubt and uncertainty. When people believe they can do something that will make a difference—when they believe they can successfully cope with a situation—stress is reduced, but René did not have that confidence.

The third type of appraisal is **reappraisal.** Appraisals change constantly as new information becomes available. René lost much of her confidence that she could handle three roles when her mother took a second job and was thus not able to help René with the children. René experienced even more stress when she learned that her schoolwork was more difficult than she had expected. This new information may lead René to reappraise the confidence she initially had that she could effectively cope with her multiple roles. Reappraisal does not always result in more stress; sometimes it decreases stress. During the first week of her sophomore year, René learned that she had access to the swimming pool, weight room, and the indoor track, and she also learned that physical exercise was one way to cope with stress.

Vulnerability Stress is most likely to be aroused when people are vulnerable, when they lack resources in a situation of some personal importance. These resources may be either physical or social, but their importance is determined by psychological factors, such as perception and evaluation of the situation. An arthritic knee, for example, would produce physical vulnerability in a professional athlete but would be a minor inconvenience to the professional life of someone who works behind a desk.

Lazarus and Folkman (1984) insisted that physical or social deficits alone are not sufficient to produce vulnerability. What matters is whether one considers the situation personally important. Vulnerability differs from threat in that it represents only the *potential* for threat. Threat exists when one perceives that self-esteem is in jeopardy; vulnerability exists when the lack of resources creates a potentially threatening or harmful situation.

Coping An important ingredient in Lazarus's theory of stress is the ability or inability to cope with a stressful situation. Lazarus and Folkman defined coping as *"constantly changing cognitive and behavioral efforts to manage specific external and/or internal demands that are appraised as taxing or exceeding the resources of the person"* (1984, p. 141). This definition spells out several important features of coping. First, coping is a process, constantly changing as one's efforts are evaluated as more or less successful. Second, coping is not automatic; it is a learned pattern of responding to stressful situations. A response that is automatic (such as closing one's eyes to block out intense light) or that becomes automatic through experience (such as shifting one's weight while riding a bicycle) would not be considered coping. Third, coping requires effort. A person need not be completely aware of his or her coping response, and the outcome may or may not be successful, but effort must have been expended. Fourth, coping is an effort to *manage* the situation; control and mastery are not necessary. For example, most of us make an effort to manage our physical environment by striving for a comfortable air temperature. Thus, we cope with our environment even though complete mastery of the climate is impossible.

How well people are able to cope depends on several factors. Lazarus and Folkman (1984) listed *health and energy* as one important coping resource. Healthy, robust individuals are better able to manage external and internal demands than are frail, sick, tired people. A second resource is a *positive belief*—the ability to cope with stress is enhanced when people believe they can successfully bring about desired consequences. This ability is related to the third resource: *problem-solving skills.* Knowledge of anatomy and physiology, for example, can be an important source of coping when receiving information about one's own health from a physician who is speaking in technical terms. A fourth coping resource is *social skills.* Confidence in one's ability to get other people to cooperate can be an important source of stress management. Closely allied to this resource is *social support,* or the feeling of being accepted, loved, or prized by others. (Chapter 8 presents information on the importance of social support in coping.) Finally, Lazarus and Folkman list *material resources* as an important means of coping. Having the money to get one's car repaired decreases the stress of having a transmission problem.

In Lazarus's transactional view, of course, material and social resources by themselves are not as important as one's personal belief about these resources. Perceiving that you can manage or alter a stressful environmental situation and feeling confident that you can regulate your own emotional distress are the two main ways to cope with stress. The ways people cope with stressful life events, including daily annoyances, play a leading role in stress-related illnesses.

In Summary

Two leading theories of stress are those of Hans Selye and Richard Lazarus. Selye, the first researcher to look closely at stress, first saw stress as a stimulus, but he later viewed it a response. Whenever animals (including humans) encounter a threatening stimulus, they mobilize themselves in a generalized attempt to adapt to that stimulus, and this mobilization is called the general adaptation syndrome (GAS). The GAS has three stages—alarm, resistance, and exhaustion—and the potential for trauma or illness exists at all three stages.

In contrast, Lazarus held a cognitively oriented, transactional view of stress and coping. Stressful encounters are dynamic and complex, constantly changing and unfolding, so that the outcomes of one stressful event alter the subsequent appraisal of new events. Individual differences in coping strategies and in the appraisal of stressful events are crucial to a person's experience of stress; therefore, the likelihood of developing any stress-related disorder also varies with individuals. The relationship between stressful events and subsequent health is complex, according to Lazarus, and any attempt to measure stress and a person's attempts to cope with it must also be complex.

Sources of Stress

Searching for sources of stress in the environment is consistent with the conceptualization of stress as a stimulus (Kasl, 1996). This view leads researchers to investigate factors that produce stress, to quantify those sources of stress, and to relate them to health outcomes. One way to consider such sources of stress is to look for its sources from family relationships, workplace demands, balancing multiple roles, and community conditions.

Family Relationships

Family relationships are a potential source of stress, but they can also buffer against stress. That is, problems in family relationships can create stress, but these relationships also have the potential to protect against stress. In René's case, her relationship with her mother is a significant source of stress, but in her view, keeping up with a hyperactive 7-year-old child is her major cause of stress.

Philip Blumstein and Pepper Schwartz's (1983) classic survey of couples showed that work, money, and sex were all potential sources of stress for married as well as cohabiting and gay

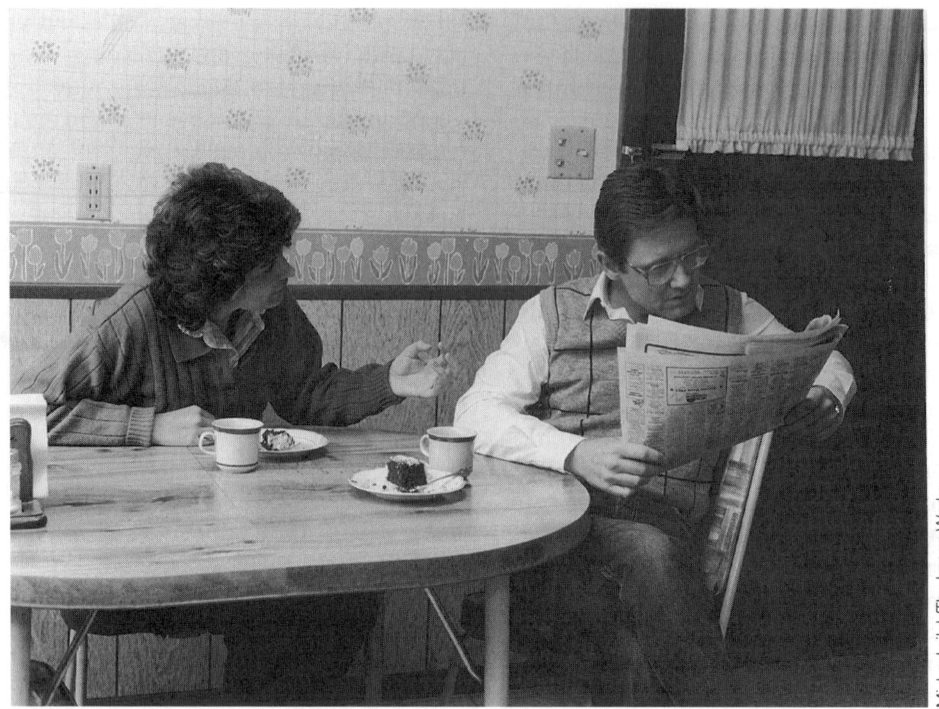

Michael siluk/The Image Works

Personal relationships can be a source of stress, and physical stress reactions are related to marital instability.

and lesbian couples. Differing attitudes in any of these areas may lead to conflict, which can result in couples' failing to support each other. Partners perceive a lack of support as stressful (Dehle, Larsen, & Landers, 2001).

Research on couples has indicated that those whose interactions provoked the physiological responses associated with stress tended to have marriages that dissolved (Gottman, 1998). Thus, stress responses were a good predictor of marital stability. Research measuring neuroendocrine measures of stress showed that hostile marital interaction raised these indices in both recently married (Kiecolt-Glaser et al., 1996) and long-married (Kiecolt-Glaser et al., 1997) couples. Of course, partner violence increases stress and decreases the quality of the relationship (Testa & Leonard, 2001). These studies show that conflict produces stress in marital relationships.

Children change the family and add the role of parent to that of partner. Beginning during pregnancy, the complexities of parenthood provide many situations that require adaptation (Pancer, Pratt, Hunsberger, & Gallant, 2000). For both women and men, having young children at home increases their level of stress, and many children create more stress than fewer children, especially for women (Moen & Yu, 2000). However, for couples who want children, infertility is a serious source of stress, and treatments for infertility add emotional and financial burdens (Domar et al., 2000).

Violence is an extreme case of conflict within the family. Domestic violence can occur between partners or in the form of child maltreatment. Although violence may be a reaction to stress, the threat of violence within the family is a source of stress for the targets. For children and adults, family violence is a serious source of stress that can end marriages (Testa & Leonard, 2001) and produce long-lasting emotional as well as physical damage (Golding, 1999).

Although family relationships can be stressful, dissolving these relationships is even more so; ending a relationship with a partner or with a child is stressful for all involved. Individual reactions to divorce vary a great deal, with some people experiencing permanent distress and others benefiting from the divorce (Amato, 2000). Factors that decrease stress for divorcing partners include having an adequate income and other relationships (Wang & Amato, 2000). For children, arguments between parents are stressful, and when divorce occurs, it is a major disruption to their lives (Ellis, 2000). Custody battles increase the stress for children. Remarriage and the establishment of relationships with stepparents and their children present more possibilities for stress. Therefore, no type of family relationship is without the possibility for stress, but relationships with family members also provide the support that people need to help them cope with other sources of stress.

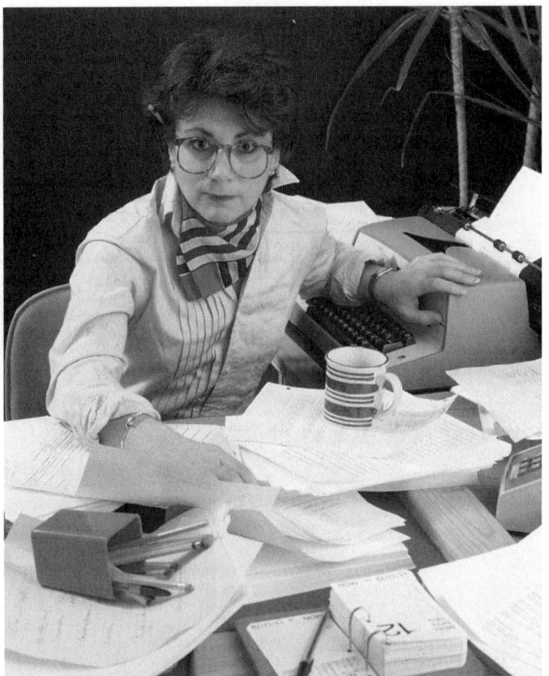
Corbis

High job demands can produce stress, especially when combined with low levels of control.

Workplace Demands

Do business executives who must make many decisions every day suffer more from a higher level of stress than do their employees who merely carry out those decisions? Most executives have jobs in which the demands are high but so is their level of control, and research indicates that lack of control is more stressful than the burden of decision making. Lower level occupations are actually more stressful than executive jobs (Wamala, Mittleman, Horsten, Schenck-Gustafsson, & Orth-Gomér, 2000). Using stress-related illnesses as a criterion, the jobs of construction worker, secretary, laboratory technician, waiter or waitress, machine operator, farm worker, and painter were among the most stressful. These jobs have factors in common: all share a high level of demand combined with a low level of control, status, and compensation. Middle-level managers such as foreman or supervisor also have highly stressful jobs. They must meet demands from two directions: their bosses and their workers. Thus, they have more than their share of stress (and stress-related illnesses).

At least two models have been constructed to explain and predict workplace demands. Robert Karasek and Tores Theorell (1990) proposed a model in which a combination of high job demands and low decision latitude interact to create stress for workers. The second model, developed by Jeffery Johnson and Ellen Hall (1988), suggests that high job-related social support would serve as a buffer to high demands and low control. A subsequent review of the research (van der Doef & Maes, 1999) found significant support for the high-demand/low-control hypothesis but less consistent evidence for the buffering effects of job-related social support.

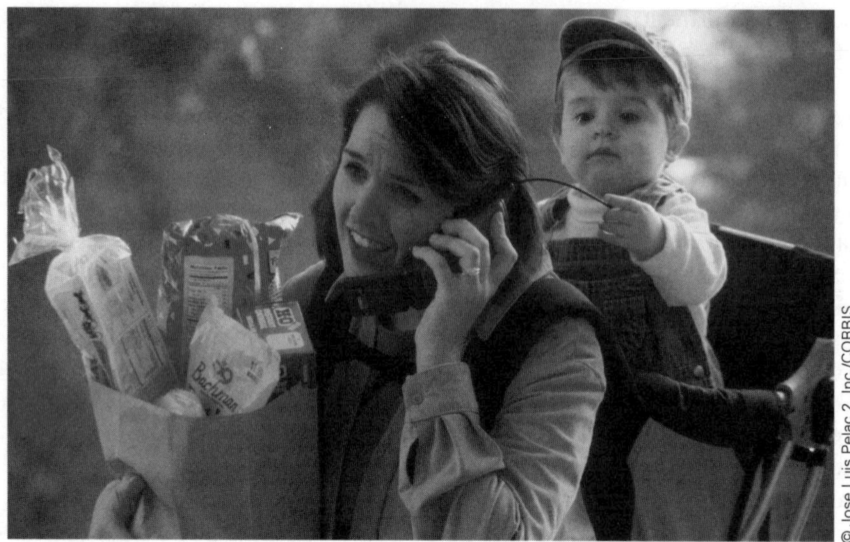

© Jose Luis Pelac 2, Inc./CORBIS

Multiple roles can be a source of stress.

Additional research (Cheng, Kawachi, Coakley, Schwartz, & Colditz, 2000; Dollard, Winefield, Winefield, & de Jonge, 2000) has supported the high-demand/low-decision hypothesis, and other research (Vermeulen & Mustard, 2000) has reported that lack of job-related social support also adds to workers' stress. This combination of high demands, low control, and lack of support relates to poor health and increased risk for heart disease (Sacker, Bartley, Frith, Fitzpatrick, & Marmot, 2001).

High demands and low control also combine with other workplace conditions to increase on-the-job stress. A situation such as working in a noisy environment is not sufficient to produce stress, but when combined with other workplace factors such as rotating shift work (Cottington & House, 1987) or high job complexity (Melamed, Fried, & Froom, 2001), signs of stress appear, such as increased blood pressure and stress hormone production. In addition, shift work can lead to a variety of physical complaints, including sleep and gastrointestinal problems, and rotating shifts can interfere with family life (Taylor, Briner, & Folkard, 1997). Workers identified night and overtime schedules, ongoing stress on the job, and high job pressure as factors that have negative influences on their health (Ettner & Grzywacz, 2001). Therefore, several job-related factors create workplace stress.

Multiple Roles

Within families people may occupy different roles, such as spouse and parent. Employment adds another role, and the conflict between the demands of family and work present additional possibilities for stress. These multiple roles are increasingly common—half of all workers are married to someone who is also employed (Moen & Yu, 2000). Problems may arise from work stress spilling over into the family or from family conflicts intruding into the workplace (Fu & Shaffer, 2001).

The differences in men's and women's roles and expectations within the family mean that family and work conflicts influence women and men in different ways. Women often encounter stress because of the increased burden of doing the work associated with their multiple roles as employee, wife, and mother (Moen & Yu, 2000).

Although changes in gender roles have resulted in a more equitable distribution of household work, that equity disappears when the family includes children (Lundberg, 1998). Women carry out the great majority of child care responsibilities; for women with full-time employment, household and child care responsibilities makes their work load larger than men's. Thus, women who have employment and child care obligations experience more stress than women without children (Luecken et al., 1997). In a variety of ethnic groups, conflict over household work is both common and a source of stress (Bird, 1999; Stohs, 2000). Some intriguing research (Gottman, 1991) suggested that men who perform household work experience better physical health than those who do not, and other research (Bird, 1999) indicated that women are doing too much and men too little household work for maximum health benefits.

The positive or negative effects of work and family roles depend on the resources people have available (E. Taylor et al., 1997). Both men and women are affected by partner and family support, but women's health is more strongly affected by these sources of stress (Walen & Lachman, 2000). Therefore, filling multiple obligations is not necessarily stressful for women, but low control and poor support for multiple roles can produce stress.

Community Conditions

Many people associate environmental sources of stress with urban life. They think of noise, pollution, crowding, fear of crime, and personal alienation as being associated with city living. Although they are frequently more concentrated in urban settings, rural life can also be noisy, polluted, hot, cold, humid, or even crowded, with many people living in a one- or two-room dwelling. And although air and water pollution usually originate in urban or industrial settings, they may then disperse to other parts of the world. Therefore, environmental sources of stress are not limited to urban settings, but the crowding, noise, pollution, fear of crime, and personal alienation combine to produce what Eric Graig (1993) termed **urban press.** The results from one study (Christenfeld, Glynn, Phillips, & Shrira, 1999) suggested that the combined sources of stress affecting residents of New York City are factors in that city's higher heart attack death rate. Pollution, noise, crowding, and fear of crime add to the urban dwellers' experience, and people experience stress in association with each of these sources.

Pollution Although pollution of the environment has become an important concern, it is not a recent phenomenon. Both air and water pollution predate history (Eckholm, 1977). Modern technology has given us more pollutants and speeded their dispersion, but it did not originate the practice of adding harmful substances to the air, water, and soil.

Modern technology has increased not only the amount of pollution but also the potential for accidents in the storing or handling of dangerous nuclear or chemical pollutants. An accident with toxic chemicals could create extreme feelings of helplessness because such accidents are beyond the control of many of the affected people. Indeed, these accidents may occur quite randomly, as in a train derailment or a tank-car accident, and thus quite unpredictably. Furthermore, the fear of accidents may pervade the entire neighborhood near industries where dangerous chemicals are used or manufactured, providing long-lasting stress for residents (Baum, Gatchel, & Schaeffer, 1983; Moffatt, Phillimore, Bhopal, & Foy, 1995).

People tend to deal with problems produced by pollution in one of two ways—by ignoring the threat or by concentrating on the impact the pollution will have on them personally (Hatfield & Job, 2001). However, when neither of these strategies is possible, threats from environmental pollution can be a substantial source of stress. For example, a study that examined residents who lived in an area contaminated by industrial pollution showed that these people exhibited significantly more physical and psychological symptoms of stress than people who lived in an uncontaminated area (Matthies, Hoeger, & Guski, 2000). Therefore, pollution presents threats in the form of stress as well as in the form of toxins.

Noise Noise is considered a type of pollution because it is a noxious, unwanted stimulus that intrudes into a person's environment. Evidence also shows a relationship between noise and health problems, but again, the health effects of noise might be the direct influence of noise rather than an indirect effect produced by increased stress. In addition, noise is quite difficult to define in any objective way. Definitions are invariably subjective because noise is a sound that a person does not want to hear. Noise can be loud, soft, or somewhere between. One person's music is another person's noise.

The importance of subjective attitude toward noise was illustrated by a study (Nivision & Endresen, 1993) that asked residents living beside a busy street about their health, sleep, anxiety level, and attitude toward noise. No relationship appeared between objective noise levels and either health or sleep. However, the study showed a strong association between residents' subjective view of noise and the number of their health complaints.

Other studies have also indicated that noise is a source of stress that produces health problems as well as annoyance. Furthermore, the levels of noise need not be severe to produce these effects. For example, neighborhood noise (Evans, Lercher, Meis, Ising, & Kofler, 2001) and office-type noise (Evans & Johnson, 2000) produced effects on stress hormone levels, blood pressure, and heart rate. These effects apply to children as well as adults (Evans, Hygge, & Bullinger, 1995; Evans, Rhee, Forbes, Allen, & Lepore, 2000), and results indicated that persistent exposure to noise may have negative cognitive as well as physiological effects.

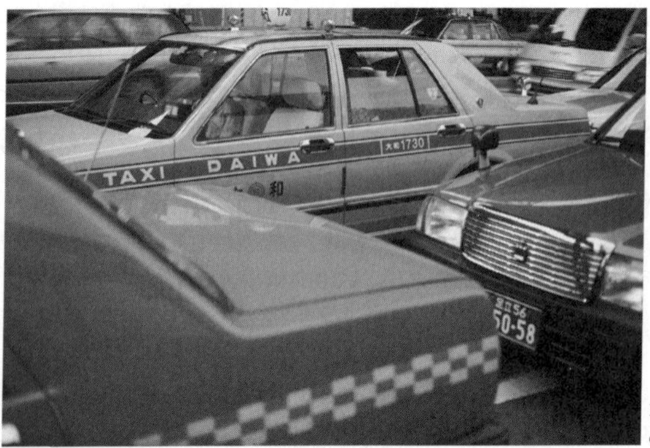

Corbis

Traffic and crowding are factors that combine to make urban living stressful.

Crowding Experiments with rats living in crowded conditions (Calhoun, 1956, 1962) have shown that crowding produces changes in social and sexual behavior that include increases in territoriality, aggression, and infant mortality but decreases in levels of social integration. These results suggest that crowding is a source of stress that affects behavior, but studies with humans are complicated by several factors, including a definition of crowding.

A distinction between the concepts of population density and crowding helps in understanding the effects of crowding on humans. In 1972, Daniel Stokols defined **population density** as a *physical* condition in which a large population occupies a limited space. **Crowding,** however, is a *psychological* condition that arises from a person's perception of the high-density environment in which that person is confined. Thus, density is necessary for crowding but does not automatically produce the feeling of being crowded. The crush of people in the lobby of a theater during intermission of a popular play may not be experienced as crowding, despite the extremely high population density. Conversely, however, a reclusive early American pioneer who migrated westward when a new resident came into his county would also not be crowded. He may have felt uncomfortable living within 10 miles of another person, but because the population was not dense, his experience would not meet Stokols's definition of being crowded. The distinction between density and crowding means that personal perceptions are critical in the definition of crowding, but the physical measurement and the perception tend to be related (Pandey, 1999).

Both density and crowding affect human behavior in negative ways. Living in crowded conditions leads to feelings of stress (Fuller, Edwards, Vorakitphokatorn, & Sermsri, 1996; Ruback, Pandey, & Begum, 1997) and a tendency to experience more physical symptoms (Ruback & Pandey, 1996). Crowding also prompts people to withdraw from social interactions as a strategy for coping (Evans et al., 2000), which may be a factor in promoting isolation. The negative effects of crowding can be offset by a feeling of control. People who feel crowded tend to feel that they have less control, but those who can retain a feeling of being in control decrease their stress (Pandey, 1999).

Gary Evans and Susan Saegert (2000) warned that considering the effects of crowding separate from its typical context misses the point of crowding as a stressor. Crowding often occurs in the circumstances of inner-city poverty, which combines crowding with noise, discrimination, and exposure to violence.

Violence Crime is not unique to urban life, and violence occurs in families far more often than on the streets. The effects of exposure to either family or community violence is well established as a stressor with developmental consequences for children (Margolin & Gordis, 2000). For adults, however, the threat of violence and fear of crime have become a part of the stress of modern urban life.

Crime victimization is unlikely for most individuals, but the fear of crime is much more common than its actual occurrence. These fears can affect behavior, such as installing locks on the doors and bars on the windows and avoiding locations perceived as high-crime areas.

Media coverage is a factor in the perception of crime. Reports of crime may create the impression that community violence is more common than it is, and one study (Williams & Dickinson, 1993) found a significant positive correlation between people's fear of crime and newspaper reporting of crime information. Another study (Koomen, Visser, & Stapel, 2000) indicated that the influence of newspaper reports depends on the credibility of the source, but reports from credible media sources influenced beliefs about vulnerability to crime. Such studies demonstrate the power of the press to increase or decrease the fear of crime.

When people fear victimization, their behavior changes, and withdrawal from their communities may be among the reactions (Taylor, Repetti, & Seeman, 1997). When people restrict activities that might take them into areas considered dangerous, they restrict their social interactions. For example, people who are concerned with increasing crime avoid walking alone at night (Forde, 1993). This change may seem like a small change in behavior, but becoming suspicious and limiting interactions with others fosters isolation. Such isolation makes communities increasingly vulnerable to crime.

The connection between fear of victimization and health appeared in the results of a survey of over 2,000 people varying in age from 18 to 90 years (Ross, 1993). People who were afraid of being assaulted, robbed, or physically injured reported worse health than people who had no such fears. One reason for this connection is that restriction from outdoor activities and exercise may contribute to poor health and fear of crime. Therefore, crime is not only a factor in the urban environment but fear of crime can also be a stressor that can have indirect effects on health.

WOULD YOU BELIEVE

The September 11 Attacks Did Not Produce Long-Term Stress

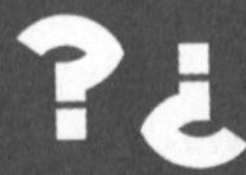

Would you believe that most of stress produced by the September 11 attacks on the World Trade Center and the Pentagon was short-lived?

Early research on the psychological reactions to the attacks found that a large number of both adults and children reacted to the attacks with concern, distress, and worry. A national survey 3 to 5 days after September 11 (Schuster et al., 2001) reported that 90% of Americans experienced some stress as a result of the attacks on the World Trade Center in New York City and the Pentagon in Washington, D.C. This survey also showed that nearly half of the sample said that they were greatly bothered by the events of September 11. In addition, 35% of the adults said that they had children who showed signs of stress. A similar survey, but one limited to people living close to the World Trade Center (Galea et al., 2002), found that people living closest to the attack were three times more likely to have experienced severe stress than those living farther away.

A nationwide survey conducted 1 to 2 months after September 11 (Schlenger et al., 2002) focused on the excess prevalence of **posttraumatic stress disorder (PTSD)** arising from the attacks in New York and Washington. Posttraumatic stress disorder is described by seven criteria: (1) threats of death to self or family members, (2) intense fear and helplessness, resulting in disorganized or agitated behavior, (3) persistent reexperiencing of the traumatic event, (4) avoidance of reminders of the event, (5) symptoms of emotional arousal, (6) persistence of symptoms for at least 1 month, and (7) impairment of regular daily activities (*Diagnostic and Statistical Manual of Mental Disorders,* 4th ed., text revision, American Psychiatric Association, 2000). (See Chapter 6 for more information on PTSD.) Results of the Schlenger et al. survey revealed that 11% of the people living in New York City showed signs of probable PTSD during the second month after the attacks. This rate was much higher in New York City than anywhere else. In Washington, where the Pentagon was attacked, only 2.7% of the population demonstrated probable PTSD. Rates in other metropolitan areas were 3.6%, whereas rates in the rest of the country were only 4.0%.

This study also addressed two interesting questions. First, why did people in Washington report lower levels of PTSD than people in other metropolitan areas? Second, why did survivors of the September 11 attacks and survivors of the April 19, 1995, bombing of the Murrah Federal Building in Oklahoma City experience more stress than did survivors of natural disasters, such as hurricanes and tornadoes?

At least two possibilities may provide answers to the question of why the attack on the Pentagon resulted in relatively low levels of stress among the people of Washington D.C. First, compared with the World Trade Center, the Pentagon is quite isolated, and the damage was limited to only a part of the building. Second, people in the Washington D.C. area regard the Pentagon as part of the military and therefore that attack could be seen as an act of war rather than an attack on civilians.

The second question can possibly be answered by the hypothesis that *intentional* acts produce more widespread stress than do natural disasters. More than one third of the survivors of the Oklahoma City blast suffered from PTSD 6 months after the bombing, a much higher level of stress than that experienced by survivors of hurricanes (North et al., 1999). In addition, intentional violence, such as that against the federal building in Oklahoma City or against the World Trade Center is experienced throughout the nation, whereas stress from natural disasters is more confined to those who lived through the event (Norris, Byrne, Diaz, & Kaniasty, 2001).

Therefore, several factors contribute to how much stress an event creates, including proximity, time, and intention. The September 11 attack on the World Trade Center included all three factors for those living in New York City, creating lingering trauma for those close to the site. For those not in New York City, stress associated with the attacks began to dissipate within weeks. The intentional nature of the attacks added to the stress, making these attacks more traumatic than natural disasters or even accidental airplane crashes.

In Summary

In summary, stress has a number of sources, which can be divided into those within the family, the workplace, and in the community. Although each of these areas may be considered separately, each person experiences combinations of these sources of stress.

Within the family, relationships such as spouse and parent present possibilities for conflict and stress. Within the workplace, jobs with high demands and little control create stress, and poor support adds to the stress. In addition, the conflict between family and work demands is a source of stress for many people. Differences in gender result in women feeling this conflict more strongly than men.

Stress from pollution, noise, crowding, and violence combine in urban settings with commuting hassles to create a situation described as urban press, but each of these sources of stress may be considered individually. Noise and crowding are annoyances, but there is some evidence that even low levels of these stressors can prompt stress responses, which suggests that long-term exposure may have negative health consequences. The combination of community stressors such as crowding, noise, and threat of violence is common in some neighborhoods, exerting negative effects on residents.

Measurement of Stress

Measuring stress is an important part of health psychology. This section discusses some of the more widely used methods and addresses the problems in determining their reliability and validity.

Methods of Measurement

Researchers have used a variety of approaches to measure stress, but most fall into two broad categories: physiological measures and self-reports. Physiological measures are associated with the view that stress is a response and concentrate on the biology of stress. Self-report measures are often used by health psychologists, who tend to take a transactional view of stress. Both approaches hold some potential for investigating the effects of stress on individuals' illness and health.

Physiological Measures One method of measuring stress uses various physiological and biochemical measures. Physiological indexes include blood pressure, heart rate, galvanic skin response, and respiration rate, whereas biochemical measures include increased secretion of glucocorticoids such as cortisol and catecholamines such as epinephrine.

The physiological indexes of blood pressure, heart rate, galvanic skin response, and respiration rate all change with activation of the sympathetic division of the autonomic nervous system. Therefore, stress and emotion produce changes in these responses. Indeed, these measures are the ones used in polygraphs, and their relationship with emotion is the basis for use of polygraphs as "lie detectors." This use is controversial (Iacono & Lykken, 1997), but these physiological indexes show some relationship to stress.

A more common approach to the physiological measurement of stress is through its association with the release of hormones. Epinephrine and norepinephrine are produced in the adrenal medulla in association with the experience of stress. Measurement of these two hormones can provide an index of stress, either through blood or urine samples (Baum & Grunberg, 1995). The levels of these hormones that circulate in the blood decrease within a few minutes after the stressful experience, so measurement must be quick to capture the changes. The levels of hormones persist longer in the urine, but factors other than stress contribute to urinary levels of these hormones. In addition, taking these measurements may be stressful experiences themselves, contaminating the assessment.

The problem of the measurement biasing the factor being studied is common to all physiological measurements of stress. A disadvantage of physiological measures is that the mechanical and electrical hardware and clinical settings that are frequently used may themselves produce stress. These measures of stress have the advantage of being direct, highly reliable, and easily quantified. Thus, this approach to measuring stress is useful but not the most widely used method. Self-report measures are far more common.

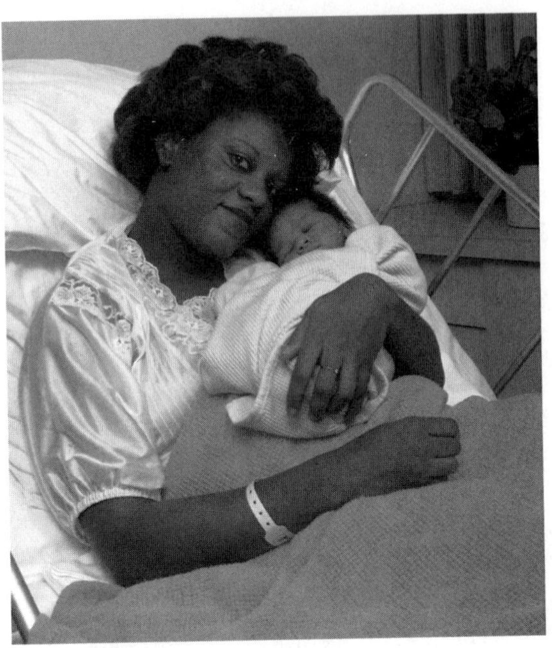

Positive life events can also be sources of stress that require adjustment.

Life Events Scales Since the late 1950s and early 1960s, researchers have developed a number of self-report instruments to measure stress. The earliest and best known of these self-report procedures is the Social Readjustment Rating Scale (SRRS), developed by Thomas H. Holmes and Richard Rahe in 1967. The scale is simply a list of 43 life events arranged in rank order from most to least stressful. Each event carries an assigned value, ranging from 100 points for death of a spouse to 11 points for minor violations of the law. Respondents check the items they have experienced during a recent period, usually the previous 6 to 24 months. Adding each item's point value and totaling scores yields a stress score for each person. These scores can then be correlated with future events, such as incidence of illness, to determine the relationship between this measure of stress and the occurrence of physical illness.

Because the SRRS has a deceptively simple format, it has often been misused by people looking for an easily administered scale to predict future health or illness. Life events scales like the SRRS have sometimes appeared in the popular press with the implication that people should count their stress points and use care to avoid additional stress that might put them beyond some critical total, usually 300 points on the SRRS. This advice ignores the fact that many people accumulate far more than 300 points in a year and never become ill. René, the subject of our case study, scored nearly 500 on the SRRS, but she did not develop any major illnesses during the year following her assessment.

Other stress inventories exist, including the Undergraduate Stress Questionnaire (USQ) (Crandall et al., 1992), the assessment that appears as Check Your Health Risks at the beginning of this chapter. This stress inventory is similar to the SRRS in providing a list of sources of stress and asking people to check the ones that have happened to them during the past two weeks. The USQ consists largely of events that are hassles rather than major life events. College students who check more stress situations tend to use health services more than students who check fewer events. Thus, the USQ represents a stress inventory tailored to college students.

The Perceived Stress Scale (PSS) (Cohen, Kamarck, & Mermelstein, 1983) emphasizes perception of events. The PSS is a 14-item scale that attempts to measure the degree to which situations in people's lives are appraised as "unpredictable, uncontrollable, and overloading" (Cohen et al., 1983, p. 387). The scale assesses three components of stress: (1) daily hassles, (2) major events, and (3) changes in coping resources. Respondents answer *never, almost never, sometimes, fairly often,* or *very often* to items that ask about their stressful situations during the past month. The PSS initially showed acceptable reliability but a low correlation between scores of a group of college students and their subsequent physiological ailments. Later research has shown greater ability of the PSS to predict symptoms, including headache, sore throat, and fatigue (Lacey et al., 2000), changes in immune system function (Maes et al., 1997), and levels of cortisol (Harrell, Kelly, & Stutts, 1996). Its brevity combined with good reliability and validity have led to use of this scale in a variety of research projects.

Everyday Hassles Scales Richard Lazarus and his associates pioneered an approach to stress measurement that looks at daily hassles rather than major life events. Daily hassles are "experiences and conditions of daily living that have been appraised as salient and harmful or threatening to the endorser's well-being" (Lazarus, 1984, p. 376). Recall from the discussion of theories of stress that Lazarus viewed stress as a transactional, dynamic complex shaped by people's *appraisal* of the environmental situation and their *perceived capabilities to cope* with this situation. Consistent with this view, Lazarus and his associates insisted that measurement instruments must not conceptualize stress as an objective environmental stimulus but instead must allow for subjective elements such as personal appraisal, beliefs, goals, and commitments (Lazarus, 2000; Lazarus, DeLongis, Folkman, & Gruen, 1985).

As a consequence, Lazarus and his associates (Kanner, Coyne, Schaefer, & Lazarus, 1981) developed the original Hassles Scale, which consisted of 117 items of annoying, irritating, or frustrating ways in which people may feel hassled. A companion inventory, the Uplifts Scale, contained 138 items that might make a person feel good. These scales required respondents to check any hassle or uplifting experience that happened to them during the past month and to indicate on a 3-point scale the degree to which each checked hassle or uplift was experienced. This second step was consistent with Lazarus's belief that an individual's *perception* of stress is more crucial than the objective event itself.

Research on the Hassles Scale (Kanner et al., 1981) indicated that hassles and life events were only modestly correlated, suggesting that these two types of stress are not the same thing. As a predictor of psychological health, the original Hassles Scale was more accurate than the life events scale (Lazarus, 1984). This finding suggests that the Hassles Scale supplements life events scales as a measure of stress and that the life events scale added little to the predictive value of the Hassles Scale.

Later, Anita DeLongis, Folkman, and Lazarus (1988) published a complete revision of the Hassles and Uplifts Scale. The revised Hassles and Uplifts Scale asks participants to think of how much of a hassle or uplift each of 53 items was to them that day. Respondents rate such items as "your spouse" or "the weather" on a 4-point scale, ranging from *none* to *a great deal*. The revised Hassles and Uplifts Scale has the advantage of being much shorter than the 255 items on the original Hassles and Uplifts Scales as well as the benefit of a better relationship to health outcomes. For example, research on the revised Hassles Scale indicated that this scale is superior to the Social Readjustment Rating Scale in predicting both the frequency and the intensity of headaches (Fernandez & Sheffield, 1996) and episodes of inflammatory bowel disease (Searle & Bennett, 2001). This study also suggested that perceived severity of hassles is a stronger predictor of headaches than the number of hassles, once again supporting Lazarus's contention that perception of an event is more important than the event itself.

Table 5.1 includes some of the many self-report inventories developed to measure stress. As this list reflects, the approach of asking people to report and assess their stressful events has spread to many types of situations and participants. Some of these instruments have been translated into different languages and norms established for the populations of different countries, including

TABLE 5.1 *Examples of Self-Report Stress Scales*

Scale Name	Author(s)	Goal	Number of Items and Scoring
Computer Hassles Scale	Richard A. Hudiburg	To define a measure for a specific type of stress	37 items rated on a 4-point scale of severity ranging from *not at all* to *extremely*
Daily Stress Inventory	Phillip J. Brantley Sheryl L. Catz Edwin Boudreaux	To determine the occurrence of daily stressors and the experience of symptoms	58 items rated on a 7-point scale ranging from *not stressful* to *caused panic*
Illness Effects Questionnaire	Glen D. Greenberg Rolf A. Peterson	To capture patients' illness experience and the impairment of daily function	20 items rated on an 8-point scale ranging from *agree* to *disagree*
Index of Teaching Stress	Richard R. Abidin Ross W. Greene	To measure the presence of teaching stress and the potential for problems with students	90 items rated on a 5-point scale ranging from *never stressful* to *very often stressful*
Mental Health Professionals Stress Scale	Delia Cushway Patrick A. Tyler Peter Nolan	To identify sources of stress for mental health professionals	42 items with 7 subscales
Nurse Stress Index	Stephen Williams Cary L. Cooper	To locate the main sources of stress in the daily work of nurses	30 items with 6 subscales
Occupational Stress Indicator	Stephen Williams Cary L. Cooper	To provide a comprehensive set of measurements for mental and physical health, sources of pressure, locus of control, and coping strategies	167 items rated on a 6-point scale, divided into 28 subscales
Parenting Stress Index	Richard R. Abidin	To measure the characteristics of parenting stress associated with the child, parent, and situation	120 items rated on a 5-point scale and yes/no format; a 36-item short form exists
Stress Schedule	Edmond Hallberg Kaylene Hallberg Loren Sauer	To provide a comprehensive measure of stress so that people with high stress get an "early warning"	60 items rated on a 5-point agree/disagree scale
Weekly Stress Inventory	Phillip J. Brantley Glen N. Jones Edwin Boudreaux	To assess minor stressors ("hassles") for the time span of a week	87 items rated on 7-point scale ranging from *not stressful* to *extremely stressful*

Source: *Evaluating stress: A book of resources*, 1997, edited by C. P. Zalaquett & R. J. Wood, Lanhan, MD: Scarecrow Press.

demonstrating the reliability and validity of the tests for those populations.

Reliability and Validity of Stress Measures

The usefulness of stress measures rests on their ability to predict some established criterion and to do so consistently. For our purposes, that criterion is illness. To predict future stress-related illness, these inventories must be both reliable and valid. Reliability is the consistency with which an instrument measures whatever it measures, and validity is the extent to which it measures what it is supposed to measure.

The *reliability* of self-report inventories is most frequently determined by either the paired-associate method or the test-retest technique. In the paired-associate method, close associates (usually a spouse) fill out the inventory, answering as if the item applied to their associate. Responses are then matched with those of the associate. The degree of agreement between the two associates is usually quite high for moderately or severely stressful events (Slater & Depue, 1981) but lower for less stressful experiences (Zimmerman, 1983).

The second approach to determining the reliability of self-report inventories is the test-retest technique, in which the same person completes the stress inventory at two different times. Inaccuracies in memory are the main reason for less than perfect agreement, and a review of test-retest reliability (Turner & Wheaton, 1995) indicated that the relationship is far from perfect. Techniques to improve memory such as cues and question wording to prompt recall can increase reliability scores for important events to a very high level for both the associate method and the individual test-retest approach.

To consider the *validity* of self-report inventories, we must begin with the question "What are these instruments supposed to measure?" At least three approaches to answering this question are possible. First, the scales should accurately represent all of the life events experienced by the respondents. Second, these scales are supposed to measure stress. Thus, scores on self-report inventories should correlate with some other measure of stress, such as judgments of a spouse or close associate or physical measurements of stress. Third, as they are most frequently used, self-report inventories are supposed to measure or predict the incidence of future illness. Let's consider these three approaches in more detail.

First, do self-report inventories accurately represent all experiences of stressful life events? Some investigators (Monroe, 1982; Turner & Wheaton, 1995) have suggested that many people tend to underreport (omit) life events, whereas other critics (Rabkin & Struening, 1976) contended that sick people overreport life events, providing a kind of justification for their illness. Other critics (Gorin & Stone, 2001) have argued that memory distortion and the biases of recall prevent self-reports from being valid indicators of past events. If people either overreport or underreport items on life events scales, then obviously the scales are not totally valid measures of life events.

The second approach asks how one can determine the degree to which a person is accurately reporting stressful events. One method is to compare reports from a spouse or close associate. But the result generally yields significant levels of disagreement between partners, especially when mildly distressful events are included.

The third and most useful type of validity for stress inventories is the extent to which they predict future illnesses or disorders. If self-report scales can demonstrate predictive validity, then they will play a valuable role in determining who may be at risk for stress-related illnesses. One problem in measuring the relationship between stress inventories and illness is the confounding of items on the major life events scales with the presence of physical disorders. Being ill can be stressful, of course, but it can also lead to answers that have been included in the Social Readjustment Rating Scale, such as sex difficulties, revision of personal habits, change in sleeping habits, and change in eating habits. Therefore, a high score on the SRRS or other similarly constructed life events scale may be a consequence rather than a cause of illness. The next chapter reviews several studies dealing with the relationship between stress and illness, but conclusions from this research must be tempered by a consideration of reliability, validity, and confounding problems of the various measures of stress.

In Summary

Stress can be measured by several methods, including physiological and biochemical measures and self-reports of stressful events. The most popular life events scale is the Social Readjustment Rating Scale, which emphasizes change in life events. Despite its popularity, the SRRS is not a good predictor of subsequent illness. Lazarus and his associates pioneered scales that measure daily hassles and uplifts. These inventories emphasize the perceived severity of importance of daily events. In general, the revised Hassles and Uplifts Scale is more accurate than the SRRS in predicting future illness.

Physiological and biochemical measures generally have acceptable levels of reliability, but their ability to predict illness has yet to be established. Self-report inventories of stress have only moderate levels of reliability and low levels of validity, when validity is defined as the ability to predict illness.

Answers

This chapter addressed four basic questions:

1. What is the physiology of stress?

The nervous system plays a central role in the physiology of stress. When a person perceives stress, the sympathetic division of the autonomic nervous system stimulates the adrenal medulla, producing catecholamines and arousing the person from a resting state. The perception of stress also prompts a second route of response through the pituitary gland, which releases adrenocorticotropic hormone (ACTH). This hormone, in turn, affects the adrenal cortex, which produces glucocorticoids. These hormones prepare the body to resist stress.

2. What theories explain stress?

Hans Selye and Richard Lazarus both proposed theories of stress. During his career, Selye defined stress first as a stimulus and then as a response. Whenever the body encounters a disruptive stimulus, it mobilizes itself in a generalized attempt to adapt to that stimulus. Selye called this mobilization the general adaptation syndrome. The GAS has three stages—alarm, resistance, and exhaustion—and the potential for trauma or illness exists at all three stages. Lazarus insisted that a person's perception of a situation is the most significant component of stress. To Lazarus, stress depends on one's appraisal of an event rather than the event itself. Whether or not stress produces illness is closely tied to one's vulnerability as well as to one's perceived ability to cope with the situation.

3. What sources produce stress?

Several possible sources of stress have been suggested, but the level of stress people experience depends in large part on their perception of these sources and on their perceived ability to cope, adding a transactional component. Stressors exist within the family, but family relationships also have the potential to buffer individuals against stress. Couples experience conflicts in maintaining their relationships, and the role of parent adds additional sources of stress (as well as satisfactions). However, dissolving a relationship is often more stressful than continuing them, and divorce adds stress for the divorcing couple as well as for children.

Some jobs are more stressful than others, but the number of decisions to be made on the job is not a valid indicator of stress. People who have some control over their work, such as executives of large corporations, have less stressful jobs than those who do not, such as food service workers and middle-level managers. Jobs with high demands, low control, and little support lead to stress, and when workplace problems spill over into the family, additional stress occurs. Contemporary couples experience problems when family demands come into conflict with work demands. Expectations that women will fulfill the majority of household and child care duties as well as be employed create conflicts that differ from those typically experienced by men. However, lack of support from partners is stressful for both genders.

Stressors from the community come from the combination of factors that occur in modern urban life—crowding, noise, pollution, and fear or crime are individual sources of stress. These stressors tend to occur more frequently in poor neighborhoods, making individuals who live in these neighborhoods subject to more stress than others. However, the combination of stressors in urban communities, described as urban press, affects individuals from all socioeconomic groups.

4. How has stress been measured?
Stress has been assessed by several methods, including physiological and biochemical measures and self-reports of stressful events. Most life events scales are patterned after Holmes and Rahe's Social Readjustment Rating Scale. Some of these instruments include only undesirable events, but the SRRS and other self-report inventories are based on the premise that any major change is stressful. Lazarus and his associates have pioneered scales that measure daily hassles and uplifts. These scales, which generally have better validity than the SRRS, emphasize the severity of the event as perceived by the person.

Physiological and biochemical measures have the advantage of good reliability, but self-report inventories of stress pose more problems in demonstrating reliability and validity. Although most self-report inventories have acceptable reliability, their ability to predict illness remains to be established. For these stress inventories to predict illness, two conditions must be met: first, they must be valid measures of stress; second, stress must be related to illness. Chapter 6 takes up the question of whether stress causes illness.

Suggested Readings

Dougall, A. L., & Baum, A. (2001). Stress, health, and illness. In A. Baum, T. A. Revenson, & J. E. Singer (Eds.), *Handbook of health psychology* (pp. 321–337). Mahwah, NJ: Erlbaum. This reading is relevant to both Chapters 5 and 6. Angela Dougall and Andrew Baum summarize the different definitions of stress and the issues involved in measuring stress in the first part of their article. The second part reviews connection between stress and disease.

Kasl, S. V. (1996). Theory of stress and health. In C. L. Cooper (Ed.), *Handbook of stress, medicine, and health* (pp. 13–26). Boca Raton, FL: CRC Press. Stanislav Kasl reviews the diverse theoretical conceptualization of stress, dividing these views into three categories: stress as a stimulus, as a response, or as a transaction. He also summarizes critical points in evaluating stress research and gives suggestions for methodology for future research.

Lazarus, R. S., & Folkman, S. (1984). *Stress, appraisal, and coping.* New York: Springer. In this classic book, Richard Lazarus and Susan Folkman present a comprehensive treatment of Lazarus's views of stress, cognitive appraisal, and coping. This book also discuses the relevant literature up to that time.

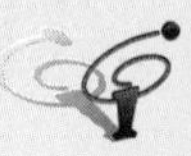

Search InfoTrac College Edition

Search these terms to learn more about topics in this chapter:

Allostasis
Nervous system and stress
Neuroendocrine and stress
Work related stress
Job demands and stress
Multiple roles and stress
Urban and stress
Crowding and stress
Fear of crime and health
Victimization and health
Assessment of stress

6

Understanding Stress and Disease

The Story of René—Continued

CHAPTER OUTLINE

Physiology of the Immune System

Psychoneuroimmunology

Does Stress Cause Disease?

QUESTIONS

This chapter focuses on three basic questions:

1. How does the immune system function?
2. How does the field of psychoneuroimmunology relate behavior to disease?
3. Does stress cause disease?

The Story of René—Continued

In Chapter 5, we introduced René, who was experiencing a high level of stress from trying to juggle her full-time job with being a full-time single mother and full-time college student. René has few friends she can call on for emotional support. Her former husband lives in another state, her mother holds two jobs, and her busy schedule precludes a relationship with a female friend who, at one time, was an important person in her life. René's most stressful relationship is with her 7-year-old son Michael who has been diagnosed as having attention-deficit/hyperactivity disorder (ADHD). René has recently moved back to her hometown after a bitter divorce from her second husband. That move, getting a new job, and returning to school have each presented major changes in her life. Do these changes in lifestyle increase René's chances of a stress-related diseases?

This chapter reviews the evidence relating to stress as a possible cause of disease and follows René to see whether her high levels of stress place her at an elevated risk for disease or death. If stress, a psychological factor, can influence physical disease, some mechanism must exist to allow this interaction. We begin with a discussion of the immune system, which protects the body against stress-related diseases and could provide the mechanism for stress to cause disease.

Physiology of the Immune System

The immune system consists of tissues, organs, and processes that protect the body from invasion by foreign material, such as bacteria, viruses, and fungi (Schindler, Kerrigan, & Kelly, 2002). In addition, the immune system performs housekeeping functions by removing worn-out or damaged cells and patrolling for mutant cells. Once the invaders and renegades are located, the immune system activates processes to eliminate them.

Organs of the Immune System

Rather than being a centralized system, the immune system is spread throughout the body in the form of the **lymphatic system.** The tissue of the lymphatic system is **lymph;** it consists of the tissue components of blood except red cells and platelets. In the process of vascular circulation, fluid and *leukocytes* (white blood cells) leak from the capillaries. These blood components routinely escape from the circulatory system, and body cells also secrete white blood cells. This tissue fluid is referred to as lymph when it enters the lymph vessels, which circulate lymph and eventually return it to the bloodstream.

The structure of the lymphatic system (see Figure 6.1) roughly parallels the circulatory system for blood. Lymph circulates by entering the lymphatic system and then reentering the bloodstream rather than staying exclusively in the lymphatic system. In its circulation, all lymph travels through at least one **lymph node.** The lymph nodes are round or oval capsules spaced throughout the lymphatic system that help clean lymph of cellular debris, bacteria, and even dust that has entered the body.

Lymphocytes are a type of white blood cell found in lymph. There are several types of lymphocytes, the most fully understood of which are T-lymphocytes, or **T-cells;** B-lymphocytes, or **B-cells;** and **natural killer (NK) cells.** Lymphocytes arise in the bone marrow, but they mature and differentiate in other structures of the immune system. In addition to lymphocytes, two other types of leukocytes exist, granulocytes and monocytes/macrophages. These leukocytes are involved in the nonspecific and specific immune system responses (discussed more fully later).

The **thymus,** which has endocrine functions, secretes a hormone called **thymosin.** This hormone seems to be involved in the maturation and differentiation of the T-cells. Interestingly, the thymus is

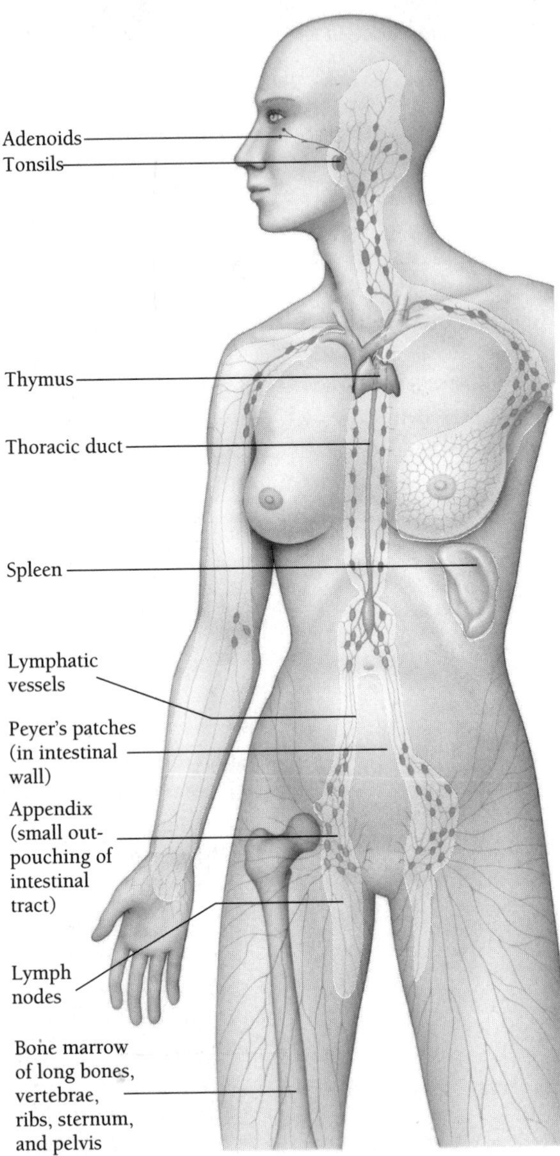

Figure 6.1 Lymphatic system.

Source: Introduction to Microbiology *(p. 407) by J. L. Ingraham & C. A. Ingraham, 1995, Belmont, CA: Wadsworth. Copyright 1995 by Wadsworth Publishing Company. Reprinted by permission.*

largest during infancy and childhood and then atrophies during adulthood. Its function is not entirely understood, but the thymus is clearly important in the immune system because its removal impairs immune function. Its atrophy also suggests that the immune system's production of T-cells is more efficient during childhood and that aging is related to lowered immune efficiency. The **tonsils** are masses of lymphatic tissue located in the throat. Their function seems to be similar to that of the lymph nodes: trapping and killing invading cells and particles. The **spleen,** an organ near the stomach in the abdominal cavity, is one site of lymphocyte maturation. In addition, it serves as a holding station for lymphocytes as well as a disposal site for worn-out blood cells.

The surveillance and protection that the immune system offers is not limited to the lymph nodes but takes place in other tissues of the body that contain lymphocytes. Therefore, the organs of the immune system may be considered all those structures that manufacture, differentiate, store, and circulate lymph; but immune function relies on more than these structures and is not confined to the lymphatic system. To protect the entire body, immune function must occur in all parts of the body.

Function of the Immune System

The immune system's function is generally to protect against injury and specifically to maintain vigilance against foreign substances that the body has encountered. The immune system must be extraordinarily effective to prevent 100% of the invading bacteria, viruses, and fungi from damaging our bodies. Few other body functions must operate at 100% efficiency, but the immune system must perform at that level for people (and other animals) to remain healthy.

Invading organisms have many ways to enter the body, and the immune system has a means to combat each type of entry. In general, immune system responses to invading foreign substances are of two types: general (nonspecific) and specific responses. Both may be involved in fighting an invader.

Nonspecific Immune System Responses Intact skin and mucous membranes are the first line of defense against foreign substances, but some invaders regularly bypass them and enter the body. Those that do face two general (nonspecific) mechanisms. One is **phagocytosis,** the attack of foreign particles by cells of the immune system. Two types of leukocytes perform this function. **Granulocytes** contain granules filled with chemicals. When these cells come into contact with invaders, they release their chemicals, which attack the invaders. **Macrophages** perform a variety of immune functions, including scavenging for worn-out cells and debris, assisting in the initiation of specific immune responses, and secreting a variety of chemicals involved in the immune response. Several chemical substances, called *complement,* are involved in breaking down the cell membranes of the invaders. Therefore, phagocytosis, which is part of the nonspecific immune system response, involves several mechanisms that can quickly result in the destruction of invading bacteria, viruses, and fungi. However, some invaders escape this nonspecific action.

Inflammation is a second type of nonspecific immune system response. Inflammation works to restore tissues that have been damaged by invaders. When an injury occurs, blood vessels in the area of injury contract temporarily. Later they dilate, increasing blood flow to the tissues and causing the warmth and redness that accompany inflammation. The damaged cells release enzymes that help destroy invading microorganisms; these enzymes can also aid in their own digestion, should the cells die. Both granulocytes and macrophages migrate to the site of injury to battle the invaders. Finally, tissue repair begins. Figure 6.2 illustrates the process of inflammation.

Specific Immune Systems Responses Two types of lymphocytes, T-cells and B-cells, carry out specific immune responses—that is, an immune response that is specific to one invader. When a lymphocyte encounters a foreign substance for the first time, both the general response and a specific response are initiated. Invading microorganisms are killed and eaten by macrophages, which present fragments of these invaders to T-cells that have moved to the area of inflammation. This contact sensitizes the T-cells; they acquire specific receptors on their surfaces so they can recognize the invader. An army of *cytotoxic T-cells* forms through this process, and it soon mobilizes a direct attack on the invaders. This process is referred to as *cell-mediated immunity* because it occurs at the level of the body cells rather than in the bloodstream. Cell-mediated immunity is especially effective against fungi,

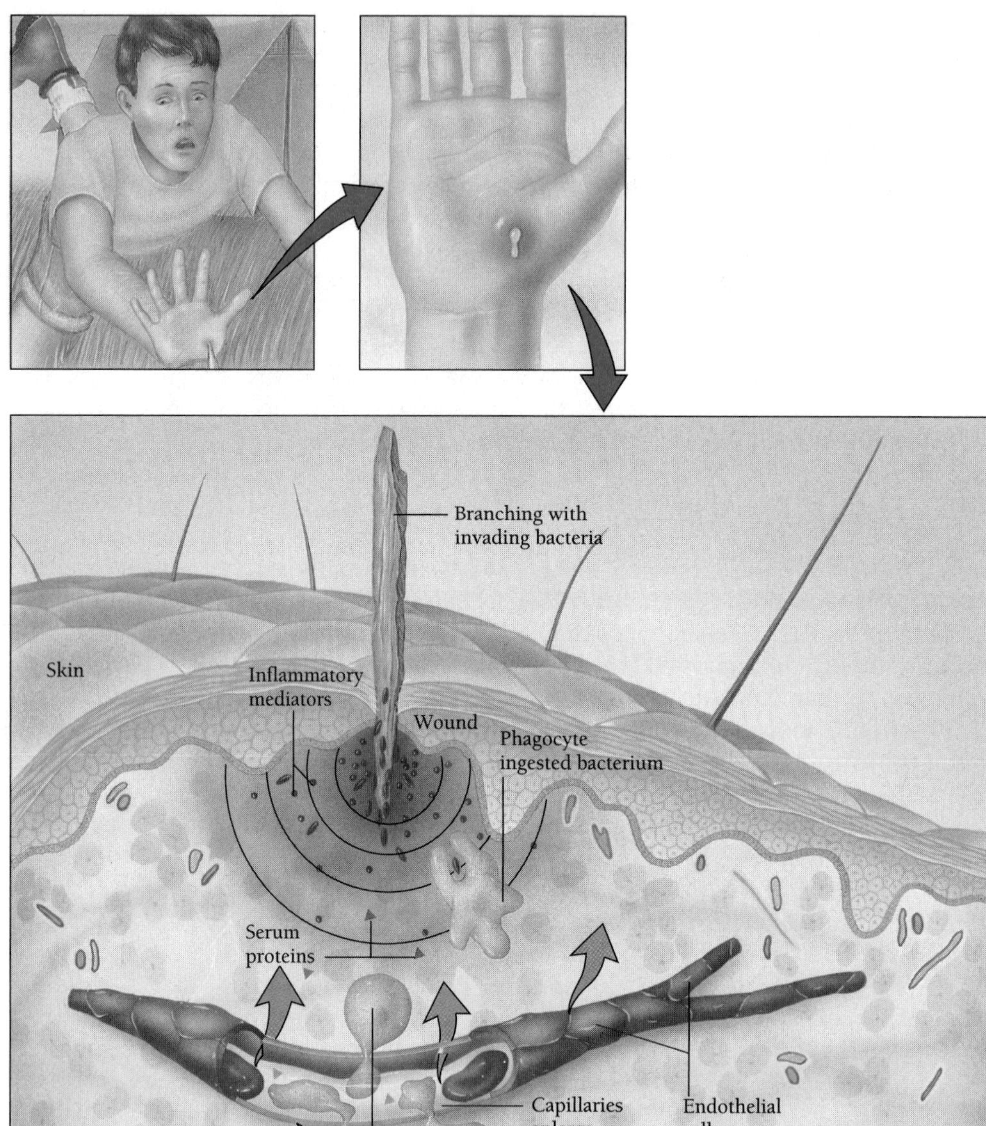

Figure 6.2 Acute inflammation is initiated by a stimulus such as injury or infection. Inflammatory mediators are produced at the site of the stimulus. They cause blood vessels to dilate and increase their permeability; they also attract phagocytes to the site of inflammation and activate them.

Source: Introduction to Microbiology *(p. 386) by J. L. Ingraham & C. A. Ingraham, 1995, Belmont, CA: Wadsworth. Copyright 1995 by Wadsworth Publishing Company. Reprinted by permission.*

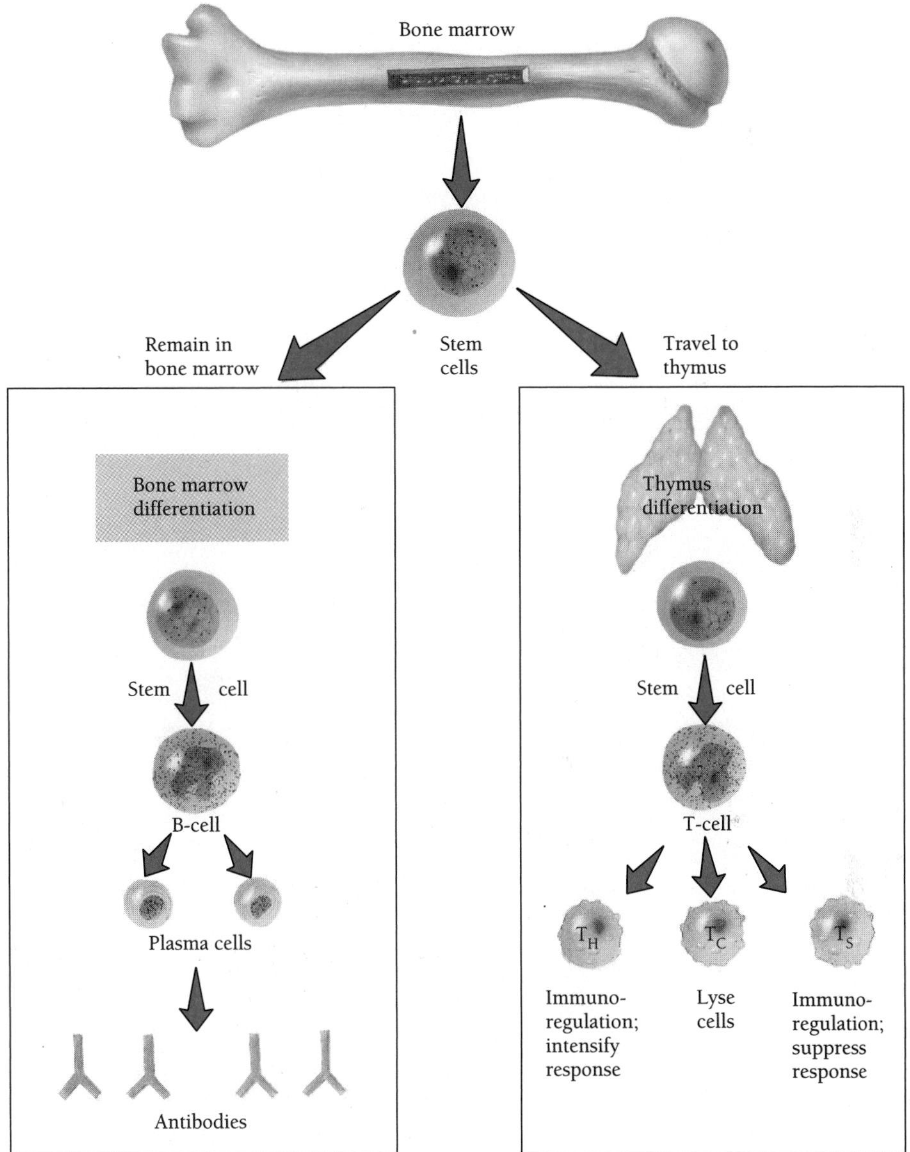

Figure 6.3 Origins of B-cells and T-cells.

Source: Introduction to Microbiology *(p. 406) by J. L. Ingraham & C. A. Ingraham, 1995, Belmont, CA: Wadsworth. Copyright 1995 by Wadsworth Publishing Company. Reprinted by permission.*

viruses that have already entered the cells, parasites, and mutations of body cells.

The other variety of lymphocyte, the B-cells, mobilizes an indirect attack on invading microorganisms. With the help of one variety of T-cell (the *helper T-cell*), B-cells differentiate into **plasma cells** and secrete **antibodies.** Each antibody is specifically manufactured in response to a specific invader. Foreign substances that provoke antibody manufacture are called **antigens** (for *anti*body *gen*erator). Antibodies circulate, find their antigens, bind to them, and mark them for later destruction. Figure 6.3 shows the differentiation of T- and B-cells.

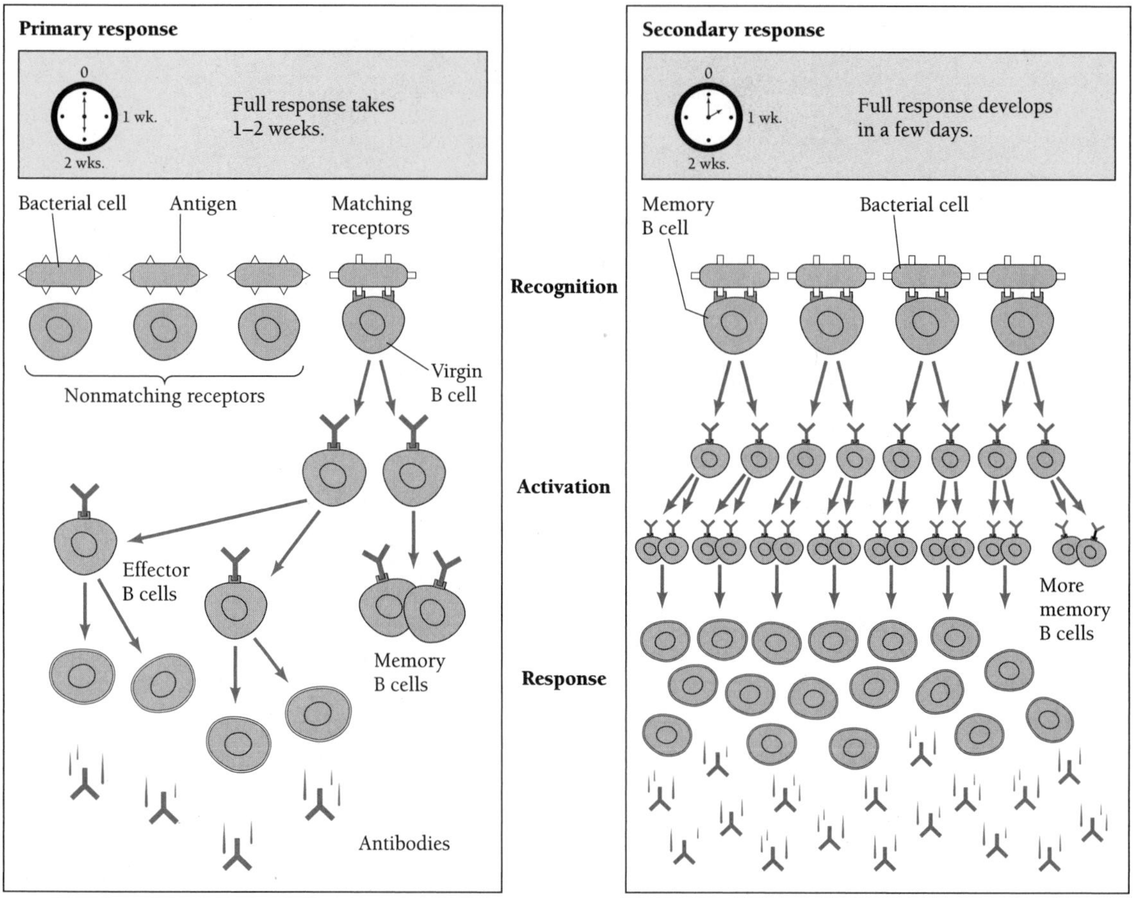

Figure 6.4 Primary and secondary immune pathways.

Source: Introduction to Microbiology *(p. 414) by J. L. Ingraham & C. A. Ingraham, 1995, Belmont, CA: Wadsworth. Copyright 1995 by Wadsworth Publishing Company. Reprinted by permission.*

The specific reactions of the immune system constitute the *primary immune response.* Figure 6.4 shows the development of the primary immune response and depicts how subsequent exposure activates the *secondary immune response.* During initial exposure to an invader, some of the sensitized T-cells and B-cells replicate, and rather than going into action, they are held in reserve. These *memory lymphocytes* form the basis for a rapid immune response on second exposure to the same invader. Memory lymphocytes can persist for years. They will not be activated unless the antigen invader reappears. If it does, then the memory lymphocytes initiate the same sort of direct and indirect attacks that occurred at the first exposure, but much more rapidly. This specifically tailored rapid response to foreign microorganisms that occurs with repeated exposure is what most people consider **immunity.**

This system of immune response through B-cell recognition of antigens and their manufacture of antibodies is called **humoral immunity,** because it happens in the bloodstream. The process is especially effective in fighting viruses that have already entered the cells, parasites, and mutations of body cells.

Creating Immunity One widely used method to induce immunity is **vaccination.** In vaccination, a weakened form of a virus or bacterium is introduced into the body, stimulating the production of antibodies. These antibodies then confer immunity for an extended period. Smallpox, which once killed thousands of people each year, has been eradicated through the use of vaccination. Now smallpox exists only in laboratory cultures; people are no longer vaccinated against smallpox. Concerns about smallpox as a biological weapon are based on the lack of immunity to this pathogen.

Other vaccines exist for a variety of diseases. They are especially useful in the prevention of viral infections. However, immunity must be created for each specific virus, and thousands of viruses exist. Even viral diseases that produce similar symptoms, such as the common cold, may be caused by many different viruses. Therefore, immunity for colds would require many vaccinations, and the development of these has not yet proven practical.

Immune System Disorders

Immune deficiency, an inadequate immune response, may occur for several reasons. For example, it is a side effect of most chemotherapy drugs used to treat cancer. Immune deficiency also occurs naturally. Although the immune system is not fully functional at birth, infants are protected by antibodies they have received from their mothers through the placenta, and infants who breastfeed receive antibodies from their mother's milk. These antibodies offer protection until the infant's own immune system develops during the first months of life.

In rare cases, the immune system fails to develop, leaving the child without immune protection. Physicians can try to boost immune function, but the well-publicized "children in plastic bubbles" still show the results of immune deficiency. Exposure to any virus or bacterium can be fatal to these children. They are sealed into sterile quarters to isolate them from the microorganisms that are part of the normal world.

A much more common type of immune deficiency is **acquired immune deficiency syndrome (AIDS).** This disease is caused by a virus, the human immunodeficiency virus (HIV), which acts to destroy the T-cells and macrophages in the immune system (O'Leary, 1990). Those who are infected with HIV usually progress to AIDS, and the destruction of their immune systems makes them vulnerable to a wide range of bacterial, viral, and malignant diseases. The disease is known to be contagious but not easily transmitted from person to person. The highest concentrations of the virus are found in blood and in semen. Blood transfusions from an infected person, injection with a contaminated needle, sexual intercourse, and transmission during the birth process seem to be the most common routes of infection. Treatment consists of controlling the proliferation of the virus through antiviral drugs and the management of the diseases that develop because of immune deficiency. As of 2003, a combination of antiviral drugs was capable of slowing the progress of HIV infection, but no treatment was capable of eliminating HIV from an infected person.

Allergies constitute another immune system disorder. An allergic response is an abnormal reaction to a foreign substance that normally elicits little or no immune reaction. People with allergies are hypersensitive to certain substances. A wide range of substances cause allergic reactions, and the severity of the reactions also varies widely. Some allergic reactions may be life threatening, whereas others merely cause runny noses. Some cases of allergy are treated by introducing regular, small doses of the allergen. This process desensitizes the person to the allergen, diminishing or alleviating the allergic response. Other cases of allergy are treated by teaching allergic individuals to recognize and avoid their allergens.

Autoimmune diseases occur when the immune system attacks the body, for reasons not well understood. Part of the function of the immune system is to recognize foreign invaders and mark them for destruction. In some people, the person's own body cells are marked for destruction. In these cases, the immune system appears to have lost the ability to distinguish the body from an invader, and it mounts the same vicious attack against itself that it would against an intruder. Lupus erythematosus, rheumatoid arthritis, and multiple sclerosis are autoimmune diseases.

Transplant rejection is not really an immune disorder, but it is a problem caused by the immune system's activity. When working efficiently, the immune system has the ability to detect foreign substances. With the exception of identical twins, no two humans have the same biochemistry. Therefore, the immune system normally recognizes any foreign tissue as an invader. A transplanted heart, liver, or kidney will be recognized as foreign tissue because the biochemical markers from its donor differ from those of its host. Thus the host's immune system will try to destroy the transplant. In an effort to prevent this reaction, drugs are administered that suppress immune system function. This strategy often works, but unfortunately, the suppression is not specific to the transplanted organ. The entire immune response is affected, leaving the person vulnerable to infection. Currently, people who have received successful organ transplants must adapt their lifestyles to minimize the risk of infection due to their weakened immune system. Modification of lifestyle and compliance with medical regimens are topics of interest to health psychologists and other health professionals who use them in the treatment of organ transplant patients.

According to the **immune surveillance theory,** cancer is also the result of an immune system dysfunction. This view holds that the cellular mutations that initiate cancer occur quite frequently, but that these mutations are normally identified and killed by the T-cells in the immune system. Cancer develops when the immune system fails to identify and destroy mutant cells. Researchers who are investigating this theory are interested in discovering methods of stimulating immune system function as a treatment for cancer. If this theory is supported by future research, a vaccine against cancer may be possible. As in the case of smallpox, cancer could someday become an object of laboratory study rather than the killer of hundreds of thousands.

In Summary

If stress can cause a disease, it can do so only by affecting biological processes (see Figure 6.4). The most likely candidate for this interaction is the immune system, which is made up of tissues, organs, and processes that protect the body from invasion by foreign material such as bacteria, viruses, and fungi. The immune system also protects the body by eliminating damaged cells. Immune system responses can be either specific or nonspecific. Specific responses attack one particular invader, whereas nonspecific immunity is capable of attacking any invader. Immune system problems can stem from several sources, including organ transplants, allergies, drugs used for cancer chemotherapy, and immune deficiency. Acquired immune deficiency syndrome (AIDS) is a type of immune deficiency that gradually destroys the immune system and leaves the person vulnerable to a variety of viral and malignant diseases.

Psychoneuroimmunology

The previous section examined the function of the immune system as well as its tissues, structure, and disorders. Physiologists have traditionally taken a similar approach, studying the immune system as separate and independent of other body systems. About 30 years ago, however, evidence began to accumulate suggesting that the immune system interacts with the central nervous system (CNS) and the endocrine system and that the CNS, endocrine system, and immune system can be affected by psychological and social factors. In addition, immune function can affect neural function, providing the potential for the immune system to alter behavior and thought (Maier & Watkins, 1998). This recognition has led to the founding and rapid growth of the field of **psychoneuroimmunology,** a multidisciplinary field that focuses on the interactions among behavior, the nervous system, the endocrine system, and the immune system.

History of Psychoneuroimmunology

George Solomon and Rudolph Moos first used the term *psychoneuroimmunology* in a publication in 1964. In that article and in his research in the 1960s, Solomon laid the groundwork for the field of psychoneuroimmunology (Kiecolt-Glaser & Glaser, 1989).

An event that dramatically shaped the field of psychoneuroimmunology was the 1975 publication of an article by Robert Ader and Nicholas Cohen on classical conditioning of the immune system. This research demonstrated how the nervous system, the immune system, and behavior could interact. Ader and Cohen conditioned rats to associate a novel, conditioning stimulus (CS)—a saccharine and water solution—with an unconditioned stimulus (UCS) that naturally produces an unconditioned response (UCR). In Ader and Cohen's procedure, a drug that suppresses the immune system was the UCS. The rats were allowed to drink the saccharin solution and then were injected with the drug. The response was the expected suppression of the immune system. However, the rats later showed immune suppression when they were given the saccharin solution alone. That is, their immune systems had been conditioned to respond to the saccharin solution in much the same manner that it reacted to the drug. This type of conditioning is not so surprising when one recalls Pavlov's classical experiment in which dogs learned to associate ringing bells with meat powder. But Ader and Cohen demonstrated that the immune system was subject to the same type of associative learning as other body systems.

Until Ader and Cohen's 1975 report, most physiologists believed that the immune system and the nervous system did not interact, and their results were not immediately accepted (Kiecolt-Glaser & Glaser, 1989). After many replications of their findings, physiologists now believe that the immune system and other body systems exchange information in a variety of ways. One mechanism is through **cytokines,** chemical messengers secreted by cells in the immune system (Ader, 2001). These chemical messengers are also known as *interleukins,* and they may underlie a number of states, including feelings associated with sickness and depression (Maier & Watkins, 1998).

The developing knowledge of the connections between the immune and nervous systems spurred researchers to explore the physical mechanisms by which interactions occur. Psychologists began to use measures of immune function to test the effects of behavior on the immune system. During the 1980s, the AIDS epidemic focused public attention (and federal funding) on how behavior influences the immune system and therefore health. The vitality of the new field of psychoneuroimmunology was demonstrated by the appearance in 1987 of a journal, *Brain, Behavior, and Immunity,* devoted to reporting psychoneuroimmunology research.

Research in Psychoneuroimmunology

Research in psychoneuroimmunology strives to develop an understanding of the role of behavior in changes in the immune system and the development of disease. To reach this goal, researchers must establish a connection between psychological factors and changes in immune function and also demonstrate a relationship between this impaired immune function and changes in health status. Ideally, research should include all three components—psychological distress, immune system malfunction, and development of disease—in order to establish the connection between stress and disease (Keller, Shiflett, Schleifer, & Bartlett, 1994). This task is difficult for several reasons.

One reason for the difficulty is the less-than-perfect relationship between immune system malfunction and disease. Not all people with impaired immune systems become ill (Cohen, 1996). Disease is a function of both the immune system's competence and the person's exposure to pathogens, the agents that produce illness. The best approach in psychoneuroimmunology comes from longitudinal studies that follow people for a period of time after they have 1) experienced stress that 2) prompted a decline in immunocompetence and then 3) assessed changes in their health status. Only a few studies have included all three components, and most such studies have been restricted to nonhuman animals.

The majority of research in psychoneuroimmunology has focused on the relationship between various stressors and altered immune system function. Also, most studies measure the immune system's function by testing blood samples rather than by testing immune function in people's bodies (Cohen & Herbert, 1996). Some research has concentrated on the relationship between altered immune system function and the development of disease or spread of cancer, but such studies are in the minority. Furthermore, the types of stressors, the species of animals, and the facet of immune system function studied have varied, resulting in a variety of findings (Baum & Posluszny, 1999).

Some researchers have manipulated short-term stressors such as electric shock, loud noises, or complex cognitive tasks in a laboratory situation; others have used naturally occurring stress in people's lives to test the effect of stress on immune system function. Laboratory studies allow researchers to investigate the physical changes that accompany stress, and such studies have shown correlations between sympathetic nervous system activation and immune responses (Cohen & Herbert, 1996). This research suggests that sympathetic activation may be a pathway through which stress can affect the immune system.

The naturally occurring stress of school exams provided an opportunity to study immune function in medical students (Kiecolt-Glaser, Malarkey, Cacioppo, & Glaser, 1994). A series of studies showed differences in immunocompetence measured by numbers of natural killer cells, percentages of T-cells, and percentages of total lymphocytes. A longitudinal assessment of these medical students revealed a trend toward more symptoms of infectious disease before and after exams.

Exam stress is typically a short-term stress, but chronic stress has also been related to decreases in immune competence. Relationship conflict has been shown to relate to immune system suppression for couples who experience marital conflict (Kiecolt-Glaser et al., 1996; Kiecolt-Glaser et al., 1997), for women who had recently separated (Kiecolt-Glaser, Fisher, et al., 1987), and for men who had recently engaged in an argument with their wives (Miller, Dopp, Myers, Stevens, & Fahey, 1999). In addition, stressful living conditions can affect immune system function. For example, residents who lived near the Three Mile Island nuclear plant at the time of a major accident at that facility had fewer B-cells, T-cells, and natural killer cells than matched controls (McKinnon, Weisse, Reynolds, Bowles, & Baum, 1989).

Chronic stress can also come from caring for someone with Alzheimer's disease (see Chapter 11 for more about the disease and the stress of caregiving). Janice Kiecolt-Glaser and her colleagues (Kiecolt-Glaser, 1999; Kiecolt-Glaser, Dura, Speicher, Trask, & Glaser, 1991; Kiecolt-Glaser, Marucha, Malarkey, Mercado, & Glaser, 1995) have studied a group of Alzheimer's caregivers over a period of years. These researchers found that, compared to a control group who were not caregivers for someone with a chronic illness, Alzheimer's caregivers had poorer psychological and physical health, longer healing times for wounds, and lowered immune function. Furthermore, the death of the Alzheimer's patient did not improve the caregivers' psychological health or immune system functioning (Robinson-Whelen,

Tada, MacCallum, McGuire, & Kiecolt-Glaser, 2001). Both caregivers and former caregivers were more depressed and showed lowered immune system functioning, suggesting that this stress continues after the caregiving is over. Thus, chronic stress can affect not only immune system function but also physical and psychological health.

Chronic stress can also influence immune system reaction to acute stressors. For example, a laboratory stressor produced more distress and stronger immune reactions in young men who were chronically stressed compared to young men who had not experienced chronic stress (Pike, Smith, Hauger, Nicassio, & Irwin, 1994). These results suggest that chronic stress sensitizes people so that their responses to other stressors are exaggerated.

After conducting a meta-analysis of studies on stress and immunity, Tracy Herbert and Sheldon Cohen (1993b) concluded that substantial evidence exists for a relationship between stress and decreased immune function. This meta-analysis showed that many types of immune system function are related to stress and that immune suppression varies with the duration and intensity of the stressor.

Some of the psychoneuroimmunology research that has most clearly demonstrated the three-way link among stress, immune function, and disease has used stressed rats as subjects, injecting material that provokes an immune system response and observing the resulting changes in immune function and disease (Ben-Eliyahu, Yirmiya, Liebeskind, Taylor, & Gale, 1991). Some research with human participants has also demonstrated the link among stress, immune function, and disease (Marucha, Kiecolt-Glaser, & Favagehi, 1998). This experimental study measured healing time after receiving a standardized wound either during vacation or during exams; thus, the stress component varied. Immune system function was measured during the two time periods, and the time for healing provided a physical outcome measurement. The results indicated that students under exam stress showed a decline in a specific immune function related to wound healing and that they healed 40% slower than the same students during vacation. Thus, some research on human as well as nonhuman subjects has demonstrated that stress can affect immune function and disease processes.

If behavioral and social factors can decrease immune system function, is it possible to *boost* immunocompetence through changes in behavior? Would such an increase enhance health? A number of researchers have conducted interventions designed to increase the effectiveness of the immune system. A meta-analysis of these studies (Miller & Cohen, 2001) indicated only modest effects. Hypnosis demonstrated more success than relaxation training and stress management, but all types of interventions showed some effects. Even small improvements could make a difference for some people with immune systems compromised through infection or multiple sources of distress.

Although behavioral interventions have demonstrated only limited usefulness in boosting immune function, their benefits in maintaining healthy functioning may be more promising. In a study of exam stress (Kiecolt-Glaser, Marucha, Atkinson, & Glaser, 2001), medical and dental students who participated in hypnosis maintained normal levels of immune function, whereas students in a comparison groups showed decreases in immune function. These findings suggest that behavioral interventions may be useful in helping stressed individuals maintain a healthy immune system.

Physical Mechanisms of Influence

"Psychosocial factors do not influence disease in some mystic fashion. Rather, the physiological status of the host is altered in some way" (Plaut & Friedman, 1981, p. 5). The previous section presented studies showing that such influence occurs but did not explore the physiology underlying that influence.

The effects of stress can occur through the relationship of the nervous system to the immune system through two routes—the peripheral nervous system and the secretion of hormones. Evidence exists for connection through both routes (Maier, Watkins, & Fleshner, 1994). The connection between the nervous system and the immune system occurs through the peripheral nervous system, which has connections to immune system organs such as the thymus, spleen, and lymph nodes. The brain can also communicate with the immune system through the production of *releasing factors,* hormones that stimulate endocrine glands to secrete hormones. These hormones travel through the bloodstream and affect target organs, such as the adrenal glands. (Chapter 5 included a description of these systems and the endocrine component of the stress response.) T-cells and B-cells have receptors for the glucocorticoid hormones.

When the sympathetic nervous system is activated, the adrenal glands release several hormones. The adrenal medulla releases epinephrine and norepinephrine, and the adrenal cortex releases cortisol. The modulation of immunity by epinephrine and norepinephrine seems to come about through the autonomic nervous system (Dougall & Baum, 2001).

The release of cortisol from the adrenal cortex results from the release of adrenocorticotropic hormone (ACTH) by the pituitary in the brain. Another brain structure, the hypothalamus, stimulates the pituitary to release ACTH. Elevated cortisol is associated with a number of physical and emotional distress conditions (Sapolsky, 1998), and it exerts an anti-inflammatory effect. Cortisol and the glucocorticoids tend to depress immune responses, phagocytosis, and macrophage activation. The nervous system can influence the immune system through either the sympathetic nervous system or through neuroendocrine response to stress.

Communication also occurs in the other direction: the immune system can signal the nervous system by way of cytokines, chemicals secreted by immune system cells (Maier & Watkins, 1998). Cytokines communicate with the brain, probably by way of the peripheral nervous system. This interconnection provides the possibility for bidirectional interactions of immune and nervous systems. Steven Maier and Linda Watkins (1998) argued that both stressors and the immune system rely on the same underlying physiology, resulting in equivalent responses from both immune and nervous system. Thus, the interrelationship between nervous system and immune system allows possibilities for each to influence the other to produce the symptoms associated with stress and disease.

In addition to affecting physiological responses in ways that promote disease, stress may alter health-related behaviors and affect health through this route (Baum & Posluszny, 1999). For example, people under stress may smoke more cigarettes, drink more alcohol, use illicit drugs, change their eating habits, and engage in risky sexual behaviors. Each of these behaviors increases risk for a variety of diseases.

In Summary

Researchers in the field of psychoneuroimmunology have demonstrated that various functions of the immune system respond to both short-term and long-term psychological stress. The field of psychoneuroimmunology has therefore made progress toward linking psychological factors, immune system function, and disease, but few studies have included all three elements.

Some research has been successful in linking immune system changes to changes in health status; this link is necessary to complete the chain between psychological factors and disease. In addition to establishing links between psychological factors and immune system changes, theorists and researchers in the field of psychoneuroimmunology have attempted to specify the physical mechanisms through which these changes occur. The possibilities for the mechanisms include direct connections between nervous and immune systems and an indirect connection through the neuroendocrine system; evidence exists for both.

In addition, stress may prompt people to change their behaviors, adopting less healthy habits that are risk factors for disease.

Does Stress Cause Disease?

Disease is caused by many factors, and stress may be one of those factors. In any consideration of the association between disease and major life events or daily hassles, remember that most people at risk from stressful experiences do *not* develop a disease. Furthermore, in contrast to other risk factors—such as having high cholesterol levels, smoking cigarettes, or drinking alcohol—the risks conferred by life events are usually temporary. Even temporary stress affects some people more than others.

Why does stress affect some people, apparently causing them to get sick, and leave others unaffected? Some high-stress individuals become sick and others remain healthy. Then, too, some low-stress people develop a disease and others do not. Why do some people fall ill from stress and other people stay well? The diathesis-stress model offers a possible answer to this question.

The Diathesis-Stress Model

The **diathesis-stress model** suggests that some individuals are vulnerable to stress-related diseases because either genetic weakness or biochemical imbalance inherently predisposes them to those diseases. The diathesis-stress model has a long history in psychology, particularly in explaining the development of psychological disorders. During the 1960s and 1970s, the concept was used as an explanation for the development of psychophysiological disorders (Levi, 1974) as well as schizophrenic episodes, depression, and anxiety disorders (Zubin & Spring, 1977).

Applied to either psychological or physiological disorders, the diathesis-stress model holds that some people are predisposed to react abnormally to environmental stressors. This predisposition (diathesis) is usually thought to be inherited through biochemical or organ system weakness, but some theorists (Zubin & Spring, 1977) also have included acquired propensities as components of vulnerability. Whether inherited or acquired, the vulnerability is relatively permanent. What varies over time is the presence of environmental stressors, which may account for the waxing and waning of illnesses.

Thus, the diathesis-stress model assumes that two factors are necessary to produce disease. First, the person must have a relatively permanent predisposition to the disease, and second, that person must experience some sort of stress. Diathetic individuals respond pathologically to the same stressful conditions with which most people can easily cope. For those people with a strong predisposition to a disease, even a mild environmental stressor may be sufficient to produce an illness episode. The disease does not flow from an interaction between personality and stress but from the interaction of *personal physiology* and stress (Cotton, 1990).

The diathesis-stress model may explain why life event scales (see Chapter 5) are so inconsistent in predicting illness. The number of points accumulated on the Holmes and Rahe's Social Readjustment Rating Scale or the number of items checked on the Undergraduate Stress Questionnaire is only a weak predictor of illness. The diathesis-stress model holds that a person's diathesis (vulnerability) must be considered along with stressful life events in predicting who will get sick and who will stay well and allows for a great deal of individual variability in who get sick and who stays well under conditions of stress (Marsland, Bachen, Cohen, & Manuck, 2001).

In this section, we review the evidence concerning the link between stress and several diseases, including headache, infectious disease, cardiovascular disease, diabetes mellitus, premature birth, asthma, and rheumatoid arthritis. In addition, stress shows some relationship to negative moods and mood disorders such as depression and anxiety disorders.

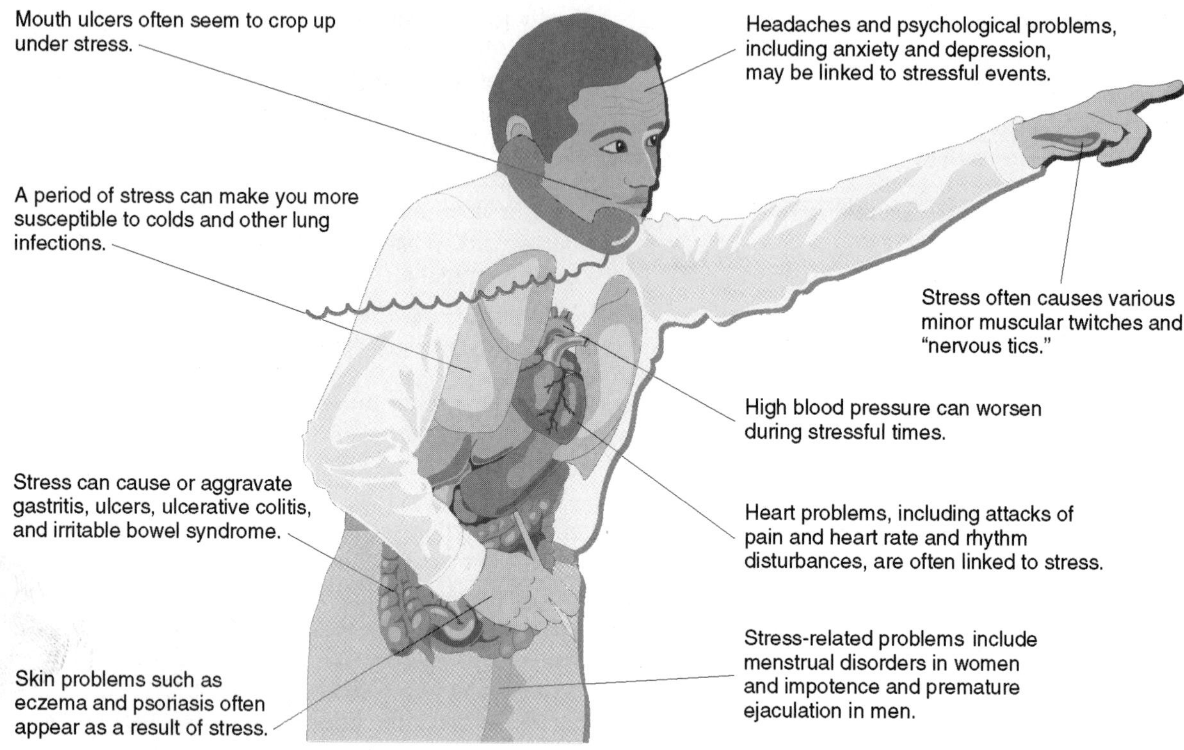

Figure 6.5 Effects of long-term stress.

Source: An Invitation to Health *(7th ed. p. 58) by D. Hales, 1997, Pacific Grove, CA: Brooks/Cole. Copyright 1997 by Brooks/Cole Publishing Company. Reprinted by permission.*

Stress and Disease

What is the evidence linking stress to disease? Which diseases have been implicated? What physiological mechanism might mediate the connection between stress and disease?

Selye's concept of stress (see Chapter 5) included suppression of the immune response, and now a growing body of evidence supports this hypothesis. Now a growing body of evidence suggests interactions among the nervous, endocrine, and immune systems. This interaction is similar to the responses hypothesized by Selye and provides strong evidence that stress could be involved in a variety of physical ailments. Figure 6.5 shows some possibilities for these effects.

Several possibilities exist for pathways through which stress could produce disease (Herbert & Cohen, 1994). Direct influence could occur through the effects of stress on the nervous, endocrine, and immune systems. Because any or all of these systems can create disease, sufficient physiological foundations exist to provide a link between stress and disease. In addition, indirect effects could occur through changes in health practices that increase risks; that is, stress tends to be related to increases in drinking, smoking, drug use, and sleep problems, all of which can increase the risk for disease. Thus, possibilities exist for both direct and indirect effects of stress on disease. Does the evidence support these hypothesized relationships?

Headaches Headaches are a common problem that most people experience; about 75% of people have headaches at least occasionally (Holroyd

& Lipchik, 1999). For most people, headaches are an uncomfortable occurrence, but others experience serious, chronic pain. Headache can signal serious medical conditions, but most often the pain associated with the headache is the problem. The majority of people who seek medical assistance for headaches are plagued by the same sorts of headaches as those who do not; the difference stems from the frequency and severity of the headaches or from personal factors involved in seeking assistance.

Although over 100 types of headaches exist, distinguishing among them has become controversial, and the underlying causes for the most common types remain unclear (Andrasik, 2001). Nevertheless, diagnostic criteria have been devised for several types of headaches. The most frequent type of headache is *tension headache,* usually associated with increased muscle tension in the head and neck region. Tension is also a factor in vascular headache, and many tension headaches have a vascular component. The most notorious of the vascular headaches are *migraine headaches,* hypothesized to be caused by changes in constriction of the vascular arteries and associated with throbbing pain localized in one side of the head.

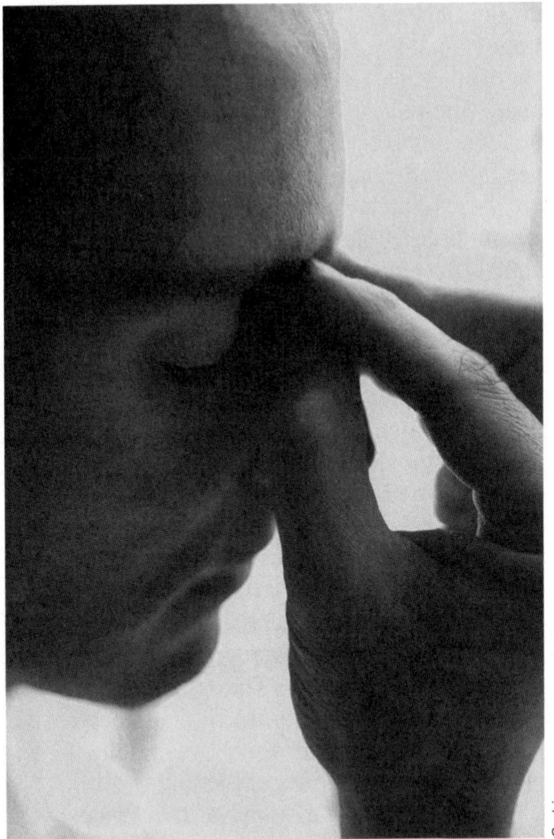
Corbis

Stress is a factor in chronic headaches.

Stress is recognized as a factor in headaches; people with either tension or vascular headache named stress as one of the leading precipitating factors (Spierings, Ranke, Honkoop, 2001). However, the type of stress associated with headaches tends not to be traumatic life events but rather small daily hassles (Fernandez & Sheffield, 1996). People with tension headaches were more likely than those with migraines to report more daily hassles as well as more intense daily hassles. In addition, stressful events precede periods of headache more often than they precede times with no headache, and stress during a headache intensified the attack (Marlowe, 1998).

A longitudinal study of headache pain (Aromaa, Sillanpaa, Rautava, & Helenius, 2000) illustrated how vulnerability and stress interact to produce disease. This study followed a representative group of families expecting their first child. When the children were 6 years old, the researchers screened them for headaches and found that over 10% suffered from headaches. When the researchers assessed the pain sensitivity of the children, the results indicated that children with chronic headaches were the ones who exhibited high sensitivity to pain in other circumstances and a tendency to react strongly to events in their environments. The children with tension headaches also tended to live in unhappy or stressful family environments, which provided the stress component of the diathesis-stress model. Their sensitivity to pain made them vulnerable to headaches, and their circumstances provided the stress.

Like most people, René had experienced occasional headaches during most of her life, but during her first marriage, she began to experience frequent and severe tension headaches, which she describes as a steady ache on both sides of her head. She believes that the stress related to her unhappy marriage is the basis for her current headaches. She also believes that these headaches are exacerbated by the stress she feels while watching after her two children and not being able to devote enough time to her school work.

Infectious Disease Are people who are under stress more likely than nonstressed individuals to develop infectious diseases such as the common cold? Research suggests that the answer is yes. An early study (Stone, Reed, & Neale, 1987) followed married couples who kept diaries on their own and their spouse's desirable and undesirable daily life experiences. Results indicated that participants who experienced a decline in desirable events or an increase in undesirable events developed somewhat more infectious diseases (colds or flu) 3 and 4 days later. The association was not strong, but this study was the first prospective design to show a relationship between daily life experiences and subsequent disease.

Later studies used a more direct approach; intentionally inoculating healthy volunteers with common cold viruses to see who would develop a cold and who would not. Sheldon Cohen and his colleagues (Cohen et al., 1998; Cohen, Tyrrell, & Smith, 1991, 1993) intentionally exposed healthy volunteers to various common cold viruses. Cohen et al. (1991) assessed the level of psychological stress in nearly 400 healthy male and female participants. Next, they gave varying levels of nasal drops to some participants and placebo saline nasal drops to other participants. They found that the degree of psychological stress was related in a dose-response manner to the number of both respiratory infections and clinical colds the participants developed. In other words, the higher the person's stress, the more likely it was that the person would become ill. The associations were similar for five different doses of viruses. Later, Cohen and his colleagues (Cohen et al., 1993) analyzed the relationship between the common cold and three individual measures of stress, which they had combined in their earlier study. Each of the three measures independently predicted a person's risk of developing a cold.

Later, Cohen et al. (1998) used the same inoculation procedure to see what types of stressors induce cold symptoms in people exposed to a cold virus. They found that duration of a stressful life event was more important than severity. Acute severe stress of less than 1 month did not lead to the development of colds, but severe chronic stress (more than 1 month) led to a substantial increase in colds. This association between stress and cold symptoms could not be explained by increases in epinephrine, norepinephrine, or cortisol or by such factors as social support, personality, or health practices. A naturalistic study of stress and colds (Takkouche, Regueira, & Gestal-Otero, 2001) showed that high levels of stress were related to increases in infection. Those people in the upper 25% of perceived stress were about twice as likely as those in the lowest 25% to get a cold.

The findings of these studies suggest that stress may be a more important contributor to the common cold than diet, lack of sleep, or even white cell count. To develop a cold, one must be exposed to a cold virus, but exposure alone cannot predict who will develop a cold and who will not. Psychological stress seems to be an important predictor.

Stress may also affect the progression of infectious disease. Many of these studies have tested nonhuman animals (Bonneau, Padgett, & Sheridan, 2001), and results have demonstrated the effects of stress on viral and bacterial infections. For example, activation of the adrenal glands and the release of glucocorticoids affect the activation of the bacterium that produces tuberculosis in previously infected mice. Steve Cole and his colleagues (2001) explored the effect of stress on HIV infection, demonstrating that stress affects both the progression of HIV infection and the infected persons' immune response to antiviral drug treatment. Therefore,

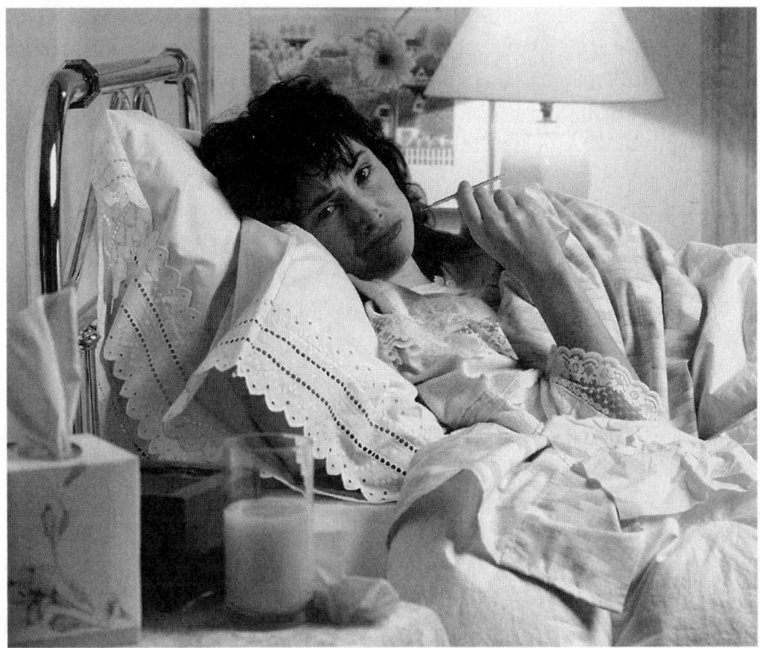
Corbis

Research has shown that stress can influence development of infectious disease.

stress is a significant factor in susceptibility, severity, and progression of infection.

Cardiovascular Disease Cardiovascular disease (CVD) has a number of behavioral risk factors, some of which are related to stress. Chapter 9 examines these behavioral risk factors in more detail; in this section, we look only at stress as a contributor to CVD. Although some people assume that stress is a major cause of heart disease, the evidence is less clear than people imagine. Two lines of research relate to stress and CVD: research that evaluates stress as a precipitating factor in heart attack or stroke and studies that investigate stress as a cause in the development of CVD.

Evidence for the role of stress as a precipitating factor for heart attack or stroke in people with CVD is clear; stress increases the risks. One study (Gullette et al., 1997) found that stress can serve as a trigger for heart attacks. This study looked at negative emotions of outpatients with coronary heart disease during the hour immediately preceding a heart attack and discovered that feelings of sadness, frustration, or tension can more than double the risk for heart attack. Stress increases the chances of chest pain as well as heart attacks in people with existing CVD (Krantz, Sheps, Carney, & Natelson, 2000). For women with CVD, the stress of marital conflict more than tripled their chances of unstable chest pain or heart attack (Orth-Gomér et al., 2000).

David Phillips and his colleagues (2001) investigated the relationship between stress and heart disease in an unusual way: they studied the relationship between death rates and the perception that some situations are unlucky. Several Asian cultures consider the number 4 to be unlucky, but few European Americans do. Phillips et al. made use of these cultural differences by hypothesizing that Japanese Americans and Chinese Americans, in contrast to European Americans, would be more likely to die of heart disease on the fourth day of the month than on other days. They examined death certificates and ethnicity and found significantly higher heart disease deaths on the fourth day of each month among Asian Americans but not European Americans. These findings are intriguing, but more research is clearly needed before investigators can claim that superstitions can affect cardiovascular deaths.

Thus, some evidence exists that stress may play a role in CVD for those who are already affected by this disease. But what role does stress play in the development of cardiovascular disease in healthy individuals?

The answer to this question is that stress may play a minor role in the development of heart disease. For example, a longitudinal study of middle-aged men with no history of coronary heart disease (Rosengren, Tibblin, & Wilhelmsen, 1991) noted different rates of coronary artery disease for six different levels of stress. Men in the lowest categories differed from those in the higher categories in risk for coronary artery disease, but the difference was significant only for the extremes, suggesting that only *substantial* psychological stress contributes to coronary artery disease.

A review of psychosocial factors related to the development of heart disease (Hemingway & Marmot, 1999) concluded that job-related stress is a significant factor. As we discussed in Chapter 5, the combination of high demands and low control tends to make for stressful working conditions. Using both self-evaluations of job stress and analysis of jobs for high demands and low control, prospective studies have demonstrated that people with high-stress jobs are at increased risk for developing heart disease. A study that examined blood pressure provides an example of the selective effects of workplace stress (Fauvel, 2001). This study measured blood pressure during a 24-hour period and found that individuals with the combination of high work demands and low job decision latitude showed higher blood pressure during working hours, but their blood pressure at home was not higher than that of other workers. This finding demonstrates that stressful situations can affect blood pressure and thus the cardiovascular system. René, our case study, does not have high blood pressure, but she does experience chest pains quite regularly. These chest pains usually occur in the evening when she is trying to balance school work with watching her baby and trying to control her 7-year-old son. Although the duration her pains is usually short, in recent weeks they have been getting longer, and occasionally she wakes up with chest pains.

Hypertension "Contrary to the implication of its name, hypertension is not a high level of nervous tension, in terms either of its causes or its manifestations" (Jenkins, 1998, p. 604). Although high blood pressure would seem to be the result of stress, no simple relationship exists between stress and blood pressure. Situational factors such as noise can elevate blood pressure, but most studies have shown that blood pressure returns to normal when the situational stimulus is removed.

A possible link between hypertension and stress is sodium retention. Some early research (Light, Kopke, Obrist, & Willis, 1983) suggested that stress can cause sodium retention in people whose nervous systems respond strongly in stress situations. Further research (Miller et al., 1998) showed that men high in hostility tended to consume more salt than men lower in hostility, suggesting that certain individuals are vulnerable to developing hypertension. For those individuals, stress may be a significant factor in the development of hypertension.

Reactivity The idea that some people react more strongly to stress than others is another possibility for the link between stress and cardiovascular disease. This response is called *reactivity,* which may play a role in the development of cardiovascular disease if the response is relatively stable within an individual and prompted by events that occur frequently in the individual's life. Researchers have investigated the stability of reactivity and have also tried to discover those events that prompt it. An array of situations has been considered as stressors as well as a variety of cardiac responses as reactions.

A factor analysis of the many stress-related measures of reactivity (Kamarck, Jennings, Pogue-Geile, & Manuck, 1994) revealed two factors, vascular reactivity and cardiac reactivity. This research showed that the patterns of responses for these factors were stable over time for the same people and for similar tasks on different people. This research demonstrated one of the necessary conditions for a relationship between reactivity and cardiovascular disease: a stable pattern of responding to similar stresses over time for the same individual.

Another study (Everson et al., 2001) showed that reactivity is related to incidence of stroke. Those men with higher systolic blood pressure reactivity were at greater risk for stroke than men with less blood pressure reactivity. In this study, educational level was also a factor that raised the risk of stroke. Hostility is another factor that relates to cardiac reactivity in men (Suarez, Kuhn, Schanberg, Williams, & Zimmermann, 1998).

Other studies have identified several characteristics that relate to higher reactivity, with a focus on gender and ethnicity. Because men develop cardiovascular disease at a younger age than women, researchers expected to find gender differences in reactivity, and some did so (Voegele, Jarvis, & Cheeseman, 1997). These gender differences appear during childhood (Treiber et al., 1993) and persist over time from childhood to adolescence (Murphy, Stoney, Alpert, & Walker, 1995). Boys and men seem to show higher reactivity than girls and women, and these gender-related differences may relate to the development of cardiovascular disease.

The higher rates of cardiovascular disease for African Americans compared to European Americans has led researchers to examine differences in reactivity between these two ethnic groups as well as the stressors that prompt such reaction. Beginning during childhood and continuing into adolescence, African Americans showed greater reactivity than European Americans (Murphy et al., 1995), and such differences appeared among

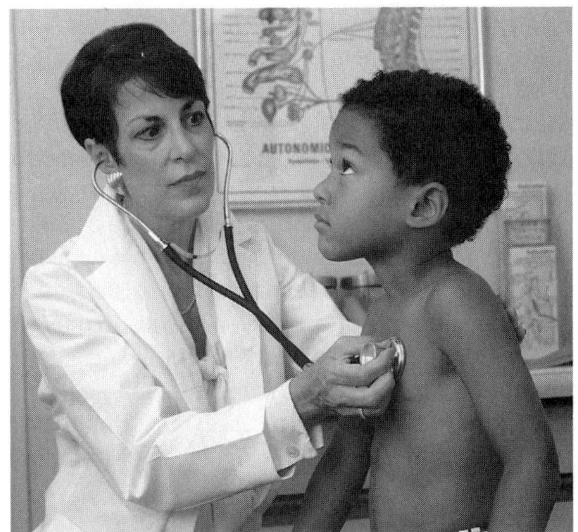

Corbis

Beginning during childhood, African Americans show higher cardiac reactivity than other ethnic groups, which may relate to their higher levels of cardiovascular disease.

children as young as 6 years of age (Treiber et al., 1993). In addition, African American children with a family history of cardiovascular disease showed significantly greater reactivity than any other group of children in the study.

Research on the experience of discrimination shows that racist provocations produce reactivity. A study comparing the reactions of African American and European American women (Guyll, Matthews, & Bromberger, 2001) showed that African American women who attributed mistreatment to discrimination exhibited greater blood pressure reactivity to a stressor than did the other participants. Both European American and African American men who viewed a racist film clip experienced increased blood pressure compared to the increases while viewing emotionally neutral films (Fang & Myers, 2001).

Another type of stressor that may relate to reactivity is *stereotype threat.* Claude Steele (1997) originated this term to describe situations in which individuals identified with some group are threatened by the negative stereotype associated with that group. Steele and his colleagues (Blascovich,

Spencer, Quinn, & Steele, 2001) have demonstrated that members of stereotyped groups such as African Americans, Hispanic Americans, and women perform more poorly when they believe that their performance is a reflection of their ethnicity or gender In addition, African Americans showed higher blood pressure reactivity under conditions of stereotype threat than European Americans, and these elevations persisted even during rest periods. People's tendencies to experience cardiac changes and the circumstances that prompt these changes may underlie the development of cardiovascular disease. Discrimination and stereotype threat may provide such situations to African Americans.

Other Physical Disorders Besides headache, infectious disease, and cardiovascular disease, stress has been linked to several other physical disorders, including diabetes, premature delivery for pregnant women, asthma, and rheumatoid arthritis. **Diabetes mellitus** is a chronic disease that may be related to stress. Two kinds of diabetes mellitus are Type 1, or insulin-dependent diabetes mellitus, and Type 2, or non-insulin-dependent diabetes mellitus. Type 1 diabetes usually begins in childhood and requires insulin injections for its control. Type 2 diabetes usually appears during adulthood and can most often be controlled by dietary changes. (The lifestyle adjustments and behavioral management required by diabetes mellitus are discussed in Chapter 11.)

Stress may contribute to the development of both types of diabetes through several routes (Cox & Gonder-Frederick, 1992). First, stress may contribute directly to the *development* of insulin-dependent diabetes through the disruption of the immune system. In general, retrospective studies have found that insulin-dependent diabetics had somewhat more stressful life events than people who were not diabetic. However, prospective investigations of this issue are extremely difficult to conduct on humans. Second, stress may contribute directly to Type 2 through its effect on the sympathetic nervous system; and third, stress may contribute to Type 2 through its possible effects on obesity. Research on stress and non-insulin-dependent diabetics has shown that stress can be a triggering factor and thus play a role in the age at which people develop Type 2 diabetes.

In addition, stress may affect to the *management* of diabetes mellitus through its direct effects of raising blood glucose (Wylie-Rosett, 1998) and through the indirect route of hindering people's compliance with controlling glucose levels (Herschbach et al., 1997). Indeed, compliance is a major problem for this disorder, as discussed in Chapter 4.

Stress during pregnancy has been the topic of research for both human and nonhuman subjects (Dunkel-Schetter & Lobel, 1998). Research with nonhuman subjects has conclusively demonstrated that stressful environments relate to lower birth weight and developmental delays in the infants of stressed mothers. Research with human participants cannot experimentally manipulate stress, so the results are not as conclusive, but a review of studies on stress during pregnancy (Adler & Matthews, 1994) revealed a tendency for stress to make preterm deliveries more likely and to result in babies with lower birth weights. Both factors are related to a number of problems for the infants. The importance of type and timing of stress remains unclear, but there is some indication that chronic stress may be more damaging than acute stress, and stress late in pregnancy is more risky than earlier stress (Dunkel-Schetter & Lobel, 1998).

Asthma is a respiratory disorder characterized by difficulty in breathing due to reversible airway obstruction, airway inflammation, and increase in airway responsiveness to a variety of stimuli (Creer & Bender, 1993). The prevalence and mortality rate of asthma have increased in recent years for both European American and African American women, men, and children, but poor African Americans living in urban environments are disproportionately affected (Weil et al., 1999).

Physical stimuli such as smoke can trigger an attack, but stressors, such as emotional events and pain, can also stimulate an asthma attack (Sandberg et al., 2000). Both acute and

WOULD YOU BELIEVE

Stress and Ulcers

Would you believe that stress is not the major factor in the development of ulcers? Stress was widely accepted as the cause of ulcers, but during the 1980s, two Australian researchers, Barry Marshall and J. Robin Warren, proposed that ulcers were the result of a bacterial infection rather than stress (Alper, 1993). At the time, their hypothesis seemed somewhat unlikely because most physicians believed that bacteria could not live in the stomach environment with its extreme acidity. Marshall (1995) reported that he had trouble receiving funding to research the possibility of a bacterial basis for ulcers.

With no funding for his research and the belief that he was correct, Marshall infected himself with the bacterium to demonstrate its gastric effects. He developed severe gastritis and took antibiotics to cure himself, providing further evidence that this bacterium has gastric effects. Results of a clinical trial comparing the traditional treatment of acid suppressants and antibiotics (Alper, 1993) revealed that stomach ulcers returned in 50% to 95% of patients who received the acid suppressant, but only 29% of the patients treated with antibiotics experienced a recurrence of ulcers. Positive results for antibiotic treatment changed not only the treatment strategy but also the thinking about ulcers.

Recently, the psychological component has returned to explanations for the development and reoccurrence of ulcers (Levenstein, 2000). This change has occurred because *H. pylori* infection does not seem to account for all ulcers. This infection is very common and related to a variety of gastric problems, yet most infected people do not develop ulcers (Weiner & Shapiro, 2001). Thus, *H. pylori* infection may create a vulnerability to ulcers, which stress or other psychosocial conditions then precipitate. For example, smoking, heavy drinking, caffeine consumption, and use of nonsteroidal anti-inflammatory drugs all relate to ulcer formation. Stress may be a factor in any of these behaviors, providing an indirect link between stress and ulcer formation in infected individuals. In addition, the hormones and altered immune function associated with the experience of chronic stress may be a more direct link. Therefore, behavioral factors play a role in the development of ulcers, but so do *H. pylori* infection, creating a complex interaction of factors in the formation of ulcers.

chronic stress increase the risk of asthma attacks in children with asthma. Children living in inner-city neighborhoods with parents who have mental problems are at sharply heightened risk (Weil et al., 1999). In addition, family discord, school problems, and being the target of bullying multiply the risk for asthma attack as much as eight times (Sandberg et al., 2000). Controlling the conditions that can precipitate an attack can be stressful, adding to the problems of management (Schmaling, 1998). Therefore, stress is a significant factor in triggering asthma attacks.

Rheumatoid arthritis, a chronic inflammatory disease of the joints, may also be related to stress. Rheumatoid arthritis is believed to be an autoimmune disorder in which a person's own immune system attacks itself (Ligier & Sternberg, 2001). The attack produces inflammation and damage to the tissue lining of the joints, resulting in pain and loss of flexibility and mobility.

A growing body of evidence (Zautra, 1998) indicates that stress can make arthritis worse by increasing sensitivity to pain, reducing coping efforts, and possibly affecting the process of inflammation itself. Direct effects of stress on inflammation could occur through neuroendocrine responses to stress (Ligier & Sternberg, 2001). People with rheumatoid arthritis show lower responding of stress hormones and lower levels of cortisol than healthy people, suggesting a role for stress in this disease. Other factors are important for the development of rheumatoid arthritis, but the stress that results from rheumatoid arthritis brings about negative changes in people's lives and requires extensive coping efforts.

Stress and Psychological Disorders

The relationship between stress and mood seems obvious—stress puts people in a bad mood. Being in a bad mood can change immune function. One group of researchers (Futterman, Kemeny, Shapiro, & Fahey, 1994) investigated the effect of mood change on immune function by inducing positive and negative mood states in a group of actors and measuring their immune function afterward. They found that mood changes of both types affected immune function. Thus, even daily normal mood swings can influence the function of the immune system.

Mood, however, may also be a somewhat permanent trait, that is, a stable way of looking at the world. *Negative affectivity* is a general tendency to experience distress and dissatisfaction in a variety of situations. Individuals high in negative affectivity focus on the negative aspects of self, others, and situations; the result is a pessimistic view of life. They complain about their health even when they are not sick.

Earlier, we saw that Sheldon Cohen and his colleagues inoculated healthy people with cold viruses to learn of the effects of stress on the common cold. Cohen et al. (1995) also measured negative affectivity in these volunteers and found that those high in negative affectivity who got sick complained more than those lower in negative affectivity, even though they were not objectively sicker. A study of college students (Gunthert, Cohen, & Armeli, 1999) found that those students high in negative affectivity tended to see more events as stressful and to report more stress than students with lower negative affectivity. This suggests that people with negative affectivity feel more stress and feel worse than other people when they are ill. Negative affectivity may also influence people's responses to stress (Wofford, 2001). Therefore, negative affectivity may produce a vulnerability to stress and stress-related conditions, including depression and anxiety disorders.

Depression The evidence that stressful life events cause depression is less than overwhelming. In general, research suggests some relationship between stress and depressive symptoms (Kessler, 1997). Chronic workplace stress is related to the development of depression (Tennant, 2001). Illness is another type of stress that shows a relationship to depression. Experiencing health problems produces stress both for the sick person and for caregivers. Heart disease (Guck, Navan, Elsasser, & Barone, 2001), cancer (Livneh, 2000), AIDS (Fleishman & Fogel, 1994), and Alzheimer's disease (Rabins, 1989) have all been related to increased incidence of depression. In addition, some research (Robinson-Whelen et al., 2001) indicated that the depression of caring for an Alzheimer's patient persists even after the caregiving has ended with the patient's death. In general, caregivers are two to three times more likely than other people to become depressed (Wright, 1997). Also, the incidence of depression seems to be directly proportional to amount of caregiving; that is, wives have the highest burden for caregiving, and caregiving wives have the highest rates for depression, followed by caregiving daughters, sons, and husbands, in that order (Wright, 1997).

People who can cope effectively are able to avoid depression, even with many stressful events in their lives. Richard Lazarus and his colleagues (Kanner et al., 1981; Lazarus & DeLongis, 1983; Lazarus & Folkman, 1984) regarded stress as the combination of an environmental stimulus plus the person's appraisal, vulnerability, and perceived coping strength. According to this theory, people become ill not merely because they had too many stressful experiences but because they evaluate these experiences as threatening or damaging, because they are physically or socially vulnerable at that time, or because they lack the ability to cope with the stressful event.

Research has supported the hypothesis that depression results from a complex of interrelated factors, especially the notion that stress produces depression in those who are vulnerable to the disorder. Several characteristics create a vulnerability. A negative outlook or the tendency to dwell on problems may exacerbate stress, making people more likely to think in ways that increase depression (Nolen-Hoeksema, 2000). In support of this view, adolescents with high levels of unrealistic, perfectionistic attitudes were more vulnerable to depression than adolescents with more reasonable attitudes and goals (Lewinsohn, Rohde, & Joiner, 2001). These dysfunctional attitudes provided a type of vulnerability such that adolescents who hold these views develop depression when they also experience a high level of negative events. Consistent with the diathesis-stress view, fewer negative events or more positive ways of thinking resulted in lower risk for depression.

Genetic vulnerability is another type of risk factor for depression. In a longitudinal study of twins (Kendler, Thornton, & Gardner, 2001), stress appeared as a significant factor in depression only under some circumstances. Stress had a higher relationship to depression for early episodes rather than later ones and for people with low rather than high genetic risk. This study also suggests that depression can occur through a complex interaction of factors, including vulnerability and stress.

The relationship between stress and depression is complex, but depression has a relationship to immune function (Herbert & Cohen, 1993a). Depression that meets the diagnostic criteria for clinical depression (American Psychiatric Association, 2000) is associated with several measures of immune function, with larger effects for older and for hospitalized patients. In addition, the more severe the depression, the greater will be the alteration of immune function. A meta-analysis of depression and immune function (Zorrilla et al., 2001) indicated that depression was significantly related to many facets of immune system function, including reduced T-cells and decreased activity of natural killer cells. Therefore, not only are stress and depression related to each other, but also the immune system responds to both.

Anxiety Disorders Anxiety disorders include a variety of fears and phobias, often leading to avoidance behaviors. Included in this definition are such conditions as panic attack, **agoraphobia,** generalized anxiety, obsessive-compulsive disorders, and posttraumatic stress (American Psychiatric Association, 2000). This section looks at stress as a possible contributor to anxiety states.

One anxiety disorder that, by definition, is related to stress is **posttraumatic stress disorder (PTSD).** The *Diagnostic and Statistical Manual of Mental Disorders* (4th ed., text revision, American Psychiatric Association, 2000) defines PTSD as "the development of characteristic symptoms following exposure to an extreme traumatic stressor involving direct personal experience of an event that involves actual or threatened death or serious injury" (p. 463). PTSD can also stem from experiencing threats to one's physical integrity; witnessing another person's serious injury, death, or threatened physical integrity; and learning about death or injury to family members or friends. The traumatic events often include military combat, but sexual assault, physical attack, robbery, mugging, and other personal violent assaults can trigger posttraumatic stress disorder.

Symptoms of PTSD include recurrent and intrusive memories of the traumatic event, recurrent distressing dreams that replay the event, and extreme psychological and physiological distress. Events that resemble or symbolize the original traumatic event as well as anniversaries of that event may also trigger symptoms. People with posttraumatic stress disorder attempt to avoid thoughts, feelings, or conversations about the event and to avoid any person or place that might trigger acute distress. A review of several studies on PTSD (Friedman, Clark, & Gershon, 1992) found support for the underlying assumption of the posttraumatic stress disorder; that is, PTSD symptoms are triggered by stressful events.

Lifetime prevalence of PTSD in the general population of the United States is around 8% (American Psychiatric Association, 2000), but particular stressful experiences raise the risk to over 50% (Foa & Meadows, 1997). The original conceptualization of PTSD as the result of combat stress was too limited; research has confirmed

BECOMING HEALTHIER

Stress may erode people's good intentions to maintain a healthy lifestyle. Under stress, people may eat an unhealthy diet, smoke, drink, use drugs, miss sleep, or avoid exercise. According to Dianne Tice and her colleagues (2001), distressed people tend to behave more impulsively. These researchers demonstrated that when distressed, people do things oriented toward making them feel better, and some of those things are health threatening, such as eating high-fat and high-sugar snacks. Stress is also the rationalization that some people use to smoke (or not quit), have a few drinks, or use drugs.

Some of these indulgences may make people feel better temporarily, but others are poor choices, even in the short run. Smoking, for example, may not reduce stress. Andy Parrott (1999) argued that just the opposite is true—smoking produces stress by involving smokers in nicotine addiction. Alcohol and drug use may present similar situations. People who engage in these risky behaviors do not decrease their stress.

Maintaining a healthy lifestyle is a good way to manage stress. People feel better when they eat a healthy diet, engage in physical exercise, and get enough sleep. When you are feeling a lot of stress, try to withstand the temptation to indulge in unhealthy behaviors. Instead, prepare to treat yourself with healthy indulgences, such a time with friends or family, more (rather than less) sleep, or time to play sports or other physical activity.

that many types of experiences are related to the development of this disorder. People who are the victims of crime (Resnick, Kilpatrick, Best, & Kramer, 1992), attacks by terrorists (Schlenger et al., 2002), domestic violence (Golding, 1999), sexual abuse (Roth, Newman, Pelcovitz, van der Kolk, & Mandel, 1997), and natural disasters (Norris et al., 2001; Wang et al., 2000) are vulnerable. The list of experiences the make people vulnerable to PTSD includes more events that happen to women than to men, and women are more likely to show symptoms of this disorder (Stein, Walker, & Forde, 2000). The disorder is not limited to adults, and children and adolescents who are the victims of violence or who observe violence are at increased risk (Silva et al., 2000). PTSD increases the risk for medical disorders, and its effects on the immune system may be the underlying reason; PTSD produces long-lasting suppression of the immune system (Kawamura, Kim, & Asukai, 2001).

The relationship between stress and other anxiety disorders is less clear. In retrospective investigations in which phobic patients are asked whether they identify any stressful event as the trigger for their anxiety disorder, most patients implicate one or more stressful events. Rabkin (1993) found that about two thirds of phobic patients reported some precipitating stressor. However, these subjective claims fall far short of proving that stress causes anxiety disorders. In her review of the literature, Rabkin (1993) reached a generally negative view of the possible connection between stress and anxiety or phobic reactions, concluding that "despite both clinical and lay expectations that phobic disorders are triggered, if not caused, by a particular stressor, investigators have not found a strong association" (p. 486). However, she noted that well-designed studies on the relationship between phobic disorders and stress remain to be conducted.

In Summary

Much evidence points to a relationship between stress and disease, but claims that stressful life events and daily hassles cause various somatic disorders are still premature. The diathesis-stress model hypothesizes that without some vulnerability, stress does not produce disease. Much of the research on stress and various diseases is consistent with this view. Stress plays a role in the development of several physical disorders, including headache and infectious disease. The evidence for a relationship between stress and heart disease is complex, with the possibility that stress may be involved in hypertension. Differential reactivity to stress may also contribute to the development of cardiovascular disease, and discrimination has been implicated as a factor in reactivity. Stress is also a factor in other diseases, including diabetes, asthma, and rheumatoid arthritis, as well as some premature deliveries.

The concept of negative affectivity relates both to a person's tendency to report negative life events and to a style of perceiving and dealing with stress that increases psychological problems. People with a pessimistic view of life and the tendency to ruminate over their problems increase their chances of becoming depressed, and the heightened sensitivity to negative aspects of life can increase their anxiety. Furthermore, their pessimistic outlook decreases their ability to cope actively, heightening their vulnerability to stressful events.

Stress is not as strong a contributor to psychological disorders as most people imagine. Depression is related to the experience of stressful life events in people who are vulnerable but not others. With the exception of posttraumatic stress disorder, little evidence exists that a stressful life event, or even an accumulation of events, contributes significantly to the onset of anxiety disorders.

Answers

This chapter addressed three basic questions:

1. **How does the immune system function?**
   The immune system consists of tissues, organs, and processes that protect the body from invasion by foreign material such as bacteria, viruses, and fungi. The immune system marshals both a nonspecific response capable of attacking any invader and a specific response tailored to specific invaders. The immune system can also be a source of problems when it is deficient (as in AIDS) or when it is too active (as in allergies and organ transplants).

2. **How does the field of psychoneuroimmunology relate behavior to disease?**
   The field of psychoneuroimmunology relates behavior to illness by finding relationships among behavior, the immune system, the central nervous system, and the endocrine system. Psychological factors can depress immune function, and some research has linked these factors with immune system depression and severity of physiological symptoms.

3. **Does stress cause disease?**
   Research indicates that stress and illness are related, but as the diathesis-stress model holds, individuals must have some vulnerability for stress to cause disease. Stress is a moderate risk factor for headache and infectious disease. The role of stress in heart disease is complex, and reactivity to stress may be involved in hypertension and the development of cardiovascular disease. Stress is one of the many factors that contribute to negative mood and mood disorders. Negative affectivity applies to a trait that describes a pessimistic life outlook that is related to stress and health problems.

Suggested Readings

Baum, A., & Posluszny, D. M. (1999). Health psychology: Mapping biobehavioral contributions to health and illness. *Annual Review of Psychology, 50,* 137–164. In this comprehensive review, Andrew Baum and Donna Posluszny examine the relationship between behavior and the development of disease. This article includes an examination of stress and the immune system and how stress affects health-related behaviors.

Kiecolt-Glaser, J. K., McGuire, L., Robles, T. F., & Glaser, R. (2002). Psychoneuroimmunology: Psychological influences on immune function and health. *Journal of Consulting and Clinical Psychology, 70,* 537–547. Beginning in 1982, Janice Kiecolt-Glaser, Ronald Glaser, and their associates collaborated to produce some of the most important research in the field of psychoneuroimmunology. In this article, Kiecolt-Glaser and her colleagues review research that links psychological factors and immune system function, concentrating on research within the past decade.

Sapolsky, R. M. (1998). *Why zebras don't get ulcers.* New York: Freeman. Neuroendocrinologist Robert Sapolsky reviews and integrates many lines of stress research in this popular book, including the complexities of the stress response and how stress may act to create disease.

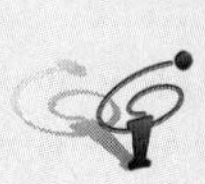

Search InfoTrac College Edition

Search these terms to learn more about topics in this chapter:

- Immune system and stress
- Stress and immunological aspects
- Psychoneuroimmunology
- Disease susceptibility and stress
- Stress and health habits
- Racism and stress
- Cardiovascular reactivity
- Stress and ulcers
- Stress and depression
- Stress and negative affect

7

Understanding Pain

The Story of Barb

CHAPTER OUTLINE

Pain and the Nervous System

The Meaning of Pain

Pain Syndromes

The Measurement of Pain

Pain Control through Prevention and Physical Treatments

QUESTIONS

This chapter focuses on five basic questions:

1. How does the nervous system register pain?
2. What is the meaning of pain?
3. What types of pain present the biggest problems?
4. How can pain be measured?
5. How can pain be controlled?

The Story of Barb

Barb was 24 when she sustained a back injury in a serious automobile crash. Her injuries included a ruptured disc in her spinal column and torn muscles. Her physician recommended back surgery, but Barb was afraid of such surgery and did not consent. Her treatment consisted of pain medication and physical therapy to allow her to regain the use of her muscles. After several months, Barb's pain was not so bad; she did not experience pain every day.

Barb got a job in a factory on an assembly line. This job required some lifting, which led to another back injury. This injury ruptured three discs and left her unable to walk or stand. After 9 months, she agreed to undergo back surgery to treat the damaged discs and nerves that were causing her pain. The surgery was only partially successful. She was in terrible pain and walked with a noticeable limp. Barb went through several physical therapy programs. The one that worked best helped her to develop muscle tone and improve her walking. During the 2 years after her surgery, Barb took prescription drugs to control her almost constant pain, but the drugs were only partially successful. In addition to the prescription drugs, she drank alcohol. That combination proved to be a problem: Barb began having hallucinations, and she decided that it was time to do something different. She asked her doctor to help her get off the drugs, and the doctor referred her to a pain specialist who put her in a program that included a variety of behavioral techniques to help manage her pain. Barb was successful in this program: she discontinued the drugs and learned how to cope with her pain.

Now, 10 years after her accident, Barb still has bad days during which hot, shooting pain courses up her back and down her legs. Despite this sharp pain, she strictly limits her medication so that she does not take a drug for more than 3 days. Accepting that her pain was a permanent part of her life allowed Barb to find ways to cope. She limited her physical ability, a difficult accomplishment because she greatly enjoyed playing softball and other sports.

Barb's experience is all too common. Chronic pain is a serious health problem in all countries (Gureje, Von Korff, Simon, & Gater, 1996), with as many as 20% of the people suffering from some type of persistent pain. These pain experiences account for lost work days and diminished productivity, with financial costs in the billions of dollars each year. Additionally, financial costs to the individual include money spent for surgery, loss of income, medication, hospitalization, disability payments, and litigation settlements (Clay, 2002). Personal suffering as well as family and relationship distress are additional costs with no dollar estimates.

Pain and the Nervous System

All sensory information, including pain, begins with sense receptors on or near the surface of the body. These receptors change physical energy—such as light, sound, heat, and pressure—into neural impulses. We can feel pain through any of our senses, but most of what we think of as pain originates as stimulation to the skin and muscles.

Neural impulses that originate in the skin and muscles are part of the peripheral nervous system (PNS); all neurons outside the brain and spinal cord, the central nervous system (CNS), are part of the PNS. Neural impulses that originate in the PNS travel toward the spinal cord and brain. Therefore, it is possible to trace the path of neural impulses from the receptors to the brain. Tracing this path is a way to understand the physiology of pain.

The Somatosensory System

The **somatosensory system** conveys sensory information from the body to the brain. The word *soma* means body in Greek; the somatic division of the PNS exists in and serves the body. All the PNS neurons from the skin's surface and muscles are part of the somatic nervous system. For example, a neural impulse that originates in the right index finger travels through the somatic nervous system to the spinal cord. The interpretation of this information in the brain results in a person's perception of sensations about the body and its movements. The somatosensory system

SCALE YOUR PAIN

Pain is practically a universal experience but not a uniform one. The following questions allow you to understand the role pain plays in your life. To complete the exercise, think of the most significant pain that you have experienced within the past month, or if you have chronic pain, make your ratings with that pain problem in mind.

1. How long did your pain persist? _____ hours and _____ minutes
2. If this pain is chronic, how often does it occur?
   - ☐ less than once a month
   - ☐ once a month
   - ☐ several times a month
   - ☐ throughout most of every day
   - ☐ about once a week
   - ☐ several times a week
   - ☐ daily
3. What did you do to alleviate your pain? (Check all that apply.)
   - ☐ took a prescription drug
   - ☐ tried to relax
   - ☐ did something to distract you from the pain
   - ☐ took an over-the-counter drug
   - ☐ tried to ignore the pain
4. Place a mark on the line below to indicate how serious your pain was.

   Not at all — Unbearable

   0 10 20 30 40 50 60 70 80 90 100
5. Place a mark on the line below to indicate how much this pain interfered with your daily routine.

   Not at all — Completely disrupted

   0 10 20 30 40 50 60 70 80 90 100
6. During your pain, what did people around you do? (Check all that apply.)
   - ☐ gave me a lot of sympathy
   - ☐ did my work for me
   - ☐ complained when I could not fulfill my normal responsibilities
   - ☐ ignored me
   - ☐ relieved me of my normal responsibilities

Completing this assessment will show you something about your own pain experience. Some of the items on this assessment are similar to those on some of the standardized pain scales that are described in "The Measurement of Pain" later in the chapter.

consists of several senses, including touch, light and deep pressure, cold, warmth, tickling, movement, and body position.

Afferent Neurons Afferent neurons are one of the three types of neurons. *Afferent (sensory) neurons* relay information from the sense organs toward the brain. The action of *efferent (motor) neurons* results in the movement of muscles or the stimulation of organs or glands. *Interneurons* connect sensory to motor neurons.

The sense organs contain afferent neurons, called **primary afferents,** with specialized receptors that convert physical energy into neural impulses. By way of these receptors, we gain information about the world in the form of neural impulses. Afferent neurons convey this information to the spinal cord and then to the brain, where that information is processed and interpreted.

The action of neurons is a combination of electrical and chemical activation. An electrical impulse forms in the receptors when the sense organs are stimulated. Sufficient stimulation will result in the formation of an **action potential,** a discharge of the neuron's electrical potential, and the neuron will "fire." But the stimulation must exceed the neuron's threshold to create an action potential. The action of each individual neuron is simple: each neuron is sufficiently stimulated either to fire or not. However, the events that lead up to the firing (or failure to fire) are not simple. Neurotransmitters convey the neural message between neurons, and the action of these transmitters is complex. The number of afferent neurons and the pattern of their responses permit them to relay enormously complex information.

Involvement in Pain The skin is the largest of the sense organs, and its numerous receptors provide sensation for the skin. The process of perceiving pain is called *nociception,* and receptors in the skin and organs, called **nociceptors,** are capable to responding to various types of stimulation that may cause tissue damage, such as heat, cold, crushing, cutting, and burning.

Some neurons that convey sensory information (including nociception) are covered with **myelin,** a fatty substance that acts as insulation. Myelinated afferent neurons are called A fibers, which conduct neural impulses faster than the unmyelinated **C fibers** do. In addition, neurons differ in size, and larger ones conduct impulses faster than smaller ones. Two types of A fibers are important in pain perception—the large **A-beta fibers** and the smaller **A-delta fibers.** The large, myelinated A-beta fibers conduct impulses over 100 times faster than small, unmyelinated C fibers (Melzack, 1973). A-beta fibers are easily stimulated, whereas C fibers require more stimulation. C fibers are much more common, however, with over 60% of all sensory afferents being C fibers (Melzack & Wall, 1982). Thus, these different types of fibers respond to different stimulation (Slugg, Meyer, & Campbell, 2000). Stimulation of A-delta fibers produces sharp, pricking pain, whereas the stimulation of C fibers often results in burning sensations (Chapman, Nakamura, & Flores, 1999).

The stimulation of A and C fibers creates neural impulses and starts the sensory message on its path to the brain. If the sensory information originates in the head and neck region, it will go to the brain by way of the 12 cranial nerves that emanate from the head and neck region. If the impulses originate in the rest of the body, the information will travel to the brain by way of the spinal cord.

The Spinal Cord

Protected by the vertebrae, the spinal cord is an avenue for sensory information traveling toward the brain and motor information coming from it. The spinal cord also produces the spinal reflexes. However, the most important role of the spinal cord is to provide a pathway for ascending sensory information and descending motor messages.

Damage to the spinal cord may interrupt the flow of sensory information, motor messages, or both. The type and extent of the loss of function depends on the extent and location of damage. If the cord is completely cut, incoming sensory messages cannot reach the brain for interpretation. The region of the body below the break loses feeling. Motor impulses from the brain are also blocked when the cord is cut, resulting in paralysis from the point of injury downward, yet the function of the spinal cord above and below the injury may remain intact. For example, the spinal reflexes (such as the patellar reflex) still occur, but people with spinal cord damage cannot move their calves voluntarily.

The afferent fibers group together after leaving the skin, and this grouping forms a nerve. Nerves may be entirely afferent, entirely efferent, or a mixture of both. Just outside the spinal cord, each nerve bundle divides into two branches (see Figure 7.1). The sensory tracts, which funnel information toward the brain, enter the dorsal (toward the back) side of the spinal cord. The motor tracts, which come from the brain, exit the ventral (toward the stomach) side of the cord. On each side of the spinal cord, the dorsal root swells into

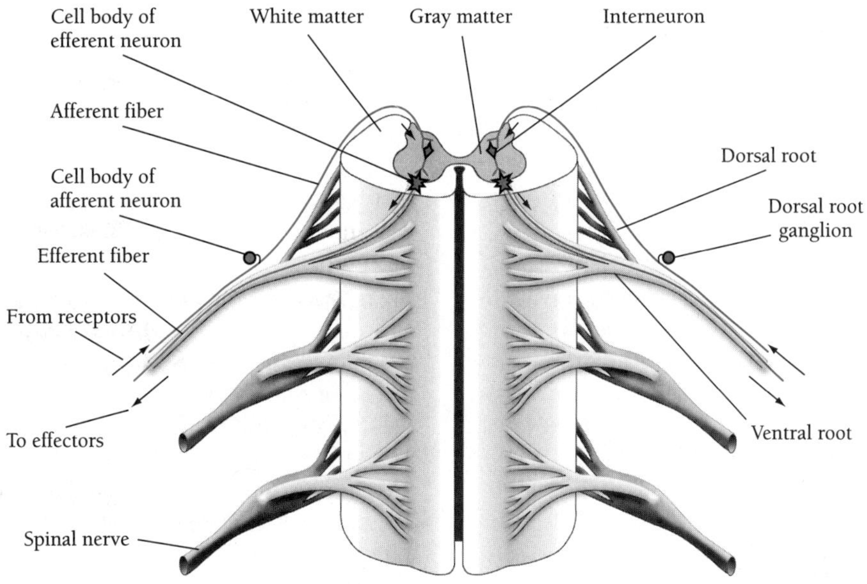

Figure 7.1 Cross section through the spinal cord.

Source: "Human Physiology: From Cells to Systems" (4th ed., p. 164) by L. Sherwood, 2001, Belmont, CA: Brooks/Cole. Reprinted by permission.

a dorsal root ganglion, which contains the cell bodies of the primary afferent neurons. The neuron fibers extend into the **dorsal horns** of the spinal cord. In the spinal cord, some afferent neurons connect to other neurons, called *secondary afferents* or **transmission cells,** and others continue to the lower part of the brain (Turk, 2001).

The dorsal horns contain several layers, or **laminae.** Each lamina receives incoming messages from afferent neurons. In general, the larger fibers penetrate more deeply into the laminae than the smaller fibers do (Melzack & Wall, 1982). The cells in laminae 1 and 2 receive information from the small A-delta and C fibers, and these two laminae form the **substantia gelatinosa.** Ronald Melzack and Peter Wall (1965) hypothesized that the substantia gelatinosa modulates sensory input information, and subsequent research has indicated that they were correct (Chapman et al., 1999). Other laminae also receive projections from A and C fibers as well as fibers descending from the brain and fibers from other laminae. Such reciprocal connections allow for elaborate interactions between sensory input and the central processing of neural information in the brain.

The Brain

The **thalamus** receives information from afferent neurons in the spinal cord. After making connections in the thalamus, the information is relayed to other parts of the brain.

Neural impulses go to the **somatosensory cortex** in the cerebral cortex, the structure that is the topmost part of the brain. The *primary somatosensory cortex* receives information from the thalamus that allows the entire surface of the skin to be mapped onto the somatosensory cortex. However, not all areas of the skin are equally represented. The top part of Figure 7.2 shows the area of the primary somatosensory cortex allotted to various regions of the body. Areas that are particularly rich in receptors occupy more of the somatosensory cortex than those areas that are poorer in receptors. For example, the hands take

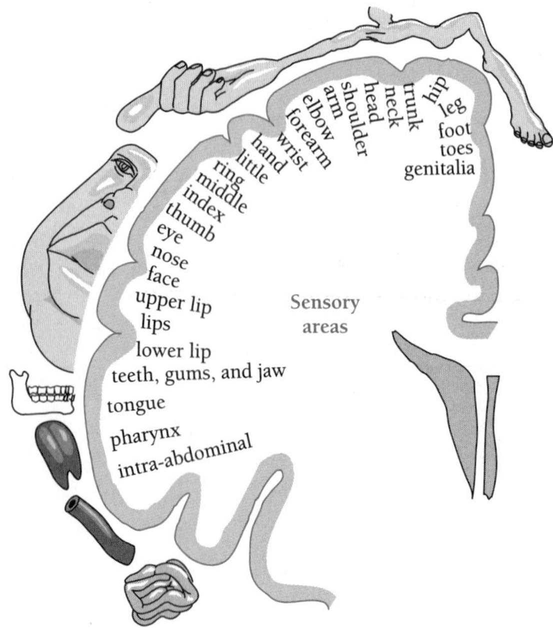

Figure 7.2 Somatosensory areas of the cortex.

up more of the somatosensory cortex than the back does. Even though the back has more skin, the hands have more receptors, and therefore more area of the brain is devoted to interpreting the information these receptors supply. This abundance of receptors also means that the hands are more sensitive; hands are capable of sensing stimuli that the back can not.

The person's ability to localize pain on the skin's surface is more precise than it is for internal organs. The viscera are not mapped in the brain in the same way as the skin. Internal stimulation can also give rise to sensations, including pain, but localizing internal sensation is much harder. In fact, intense stimulation of internal organs can result in the spread of neural stimulation to the pathways serving skin senses. Thus, visceral pain may be perceived as originating on the skin's surface. For example, a person who feels pain in the upper arm may not associate this sensation with the heart, but that type of pain is commonly produced by a heart attack.

The development of positron emission tomography (PET) and functional magnetic resonance imaging (fMRI) has allowed researchers to study what happens in the brain during the experience of pain. These techniques have confirmed neurological activity during the activation of nociceptors, but they paint a complex picture of how pain activates the brain (Rainville, Bushnell, & Duncan, 2000). Studies of brain responses to specific pain stimuli have shown activation in many areas of the brain, including the primary somatosensory cortex, but also in various regions of the frontal cortex, the thalamus, and even the cerebellum in the lower part of the brain (Davis, 2000). Adding to the complexity, an emotional reaction usually accompanies the experience of pain, and the brain imaging studies indicate activation in areas of the brain associated with emotion when people experience pain (Rainville et al., 2000). Therefore, the brain imaging studies using PET and fMRI have not revealed a "pain center" in the brain. Rather, these studies have shown that the experience of pain produces a variety of activation in the brain, ranging from the lower brain to several centers in the cerebral cortex.

Neurotransmitters and Pain

Neurotransmitters are chemicals that are synthesized and stored in neurons. The release of neurotransmitters carries neural impulses across the synaptic cleft, the space between neurons. The electrical action potential causes the release of neurotransmitters from the ends of neurons. After flowing across the synaptic cleft, neurotransmitters act on other neurons by occupying specialized receptor sites. Sufficient amounts of neurotransmitters will prompt the formation of an action potential in the stimulated neuron. Each occupies a specialized receptor site in the same way that a key fits into a lock. Without the proper fit, the neurotransmitter will not affect the neuron. Many different neurotransmitters exist, and each one is capable of causing an action.

In the 1970s, researchers (Pert & Snyder, 1973; Snyder, 1977) demonstrated that the neurochemistry of the brain plays a role in the perception of pain. This realization came about through an examination of how drugs affect the brain to alter pain perception. Receptors in the brain are sensitive to opiate drugs; that is, some neurons have receptor sites that opiate drugs are capable of occupying. This discovery explained how opiates reduce pain by fitting into brain receptors, modulating neuron activity, and producing pain relief.

The discovery of opiate receptors in the brain raised another question: Why does the brain respond to the resin of the opium poppy? In general, the brain is selective about the types of molecules that it allows to enter; only substances similar to naturally occurring neurochemicals can enter the brain. This reasoning led to the search for naturally occurring chemicals in the brain that affect pain perception. That search succeeded in finding naturally occurring neurochemicals that have properties similar to those of the opiate drugs (Goldstein, 1976; Hughes, 1975). This discovery prompted a flurry of research that identified more neurochemicals with opiate-like effects, including the **endorphins,** the *enkephalins,* and *dynorphin.*

These neurochemicals seem to be one of the brain's mechanisms for relieving pain. They can be activated by electrical stimulation of the brain as well as by the experiences of stress and by suggestion (Turk, 2001). The pain-relieving properties of drugs such as morphine may be coincidental. Perhaps they are effective only because the brain contains its own system for pain relief, which the opiates stimulate.

Neurochemicals also seem to be involved in producing pain. The neurotransmitters *glutamate* and *substance P* as well as the chemicals *bradykinin* and *prostaglandins* sensitize or excite the neurons that relay pain messages (Sherwood, 2001). Glutamate and substance P act in the spinal cord to increase neural firings related to pain. Bradykinin and prostaglandins are substances released by tissue damage, and they prolong the experience of pain by continuing to stimulate the nociceptors.

In addition, proteins produced by the immune system, *proinflammatory cytokines,* are involved in pain (Watkins & Maier, 2000). Infection and inflammation prompt the immune system to release these cytokines, which signal the nervous system and produce a range of responses associated with sickness, including decreased activity, increased fatigue, and increased pain sensitivity. These responses cause glia in the spinal cord to release these cytokines. Linda Watkins and her colleagues (Watkins, Milligan, & Maier, 2001) hypothesized that these cytokines are involved in the development of chronic pain by sensitizing the structures in the dorsal horn of the spinal cord that modulate the sensory message from the primary afferents. Therefore, the action of neurotransmitters and other chemicals produced by the body is complex, with the potentials to both increase and decrease the experience of pain.

The Modulation of Pain

Research directed toward finding the brain structures involved in pain led to the discovery that one area of the brain, the **periaqueductal gray,** is involved in modulating pain. This brain structure is in the midbrain, close to the center. If it is stimulated, pain is relieved, and the relief continues after stimulation of the area ceases (Sherwood, 2001). Neurons in the periaqueductal gray run down into the reticular formation and **medulla,** a structure in the lower part of the brain. These neurons descend into the spinal cord and make connections with neurons in the substantia gelatinosa. The result is that the dorsal horn neurons are kept from carrying pain information to the thalamus.

The inhibition of transmission also involves some familiar neurotransmitters. Endorphins act in the periaqueductal gray where they initiate activity in this descending inhibitory system. Figure 7.3 illustrates this type of modulation. The substantia gelatinosa contains synapses that use enkephalin as a transmitter. Indeed, neurons that contain enkephalin seem to be concentrated in the same parts of the brain that contain substance P,

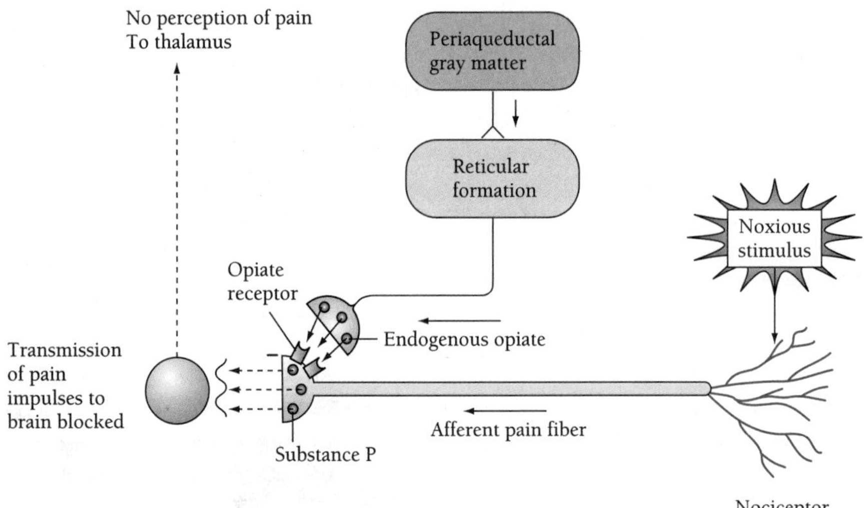

Figure 7.3 Descending pathways from the periaqueductal gray prompt the release of endogenous opiates (endorphins) that block the transmission of pain impulses to the brain.

Source: "Human Physiology: From Cells to Systems" (4th ed., p. 181), by L. Sherwood, 2001, Belmont, CA: Brooks/Cole. Reprinted by permission.

the transmitter that activates pain messages (McLean, Skirboll, & Pert, 1985).

These elaborate physical and chemical systems are the body's way to modulate the neural impulses of pain. The value of pain is obvious: pain signals tissue damage and provides a built-in motivation to discontinue activity that produces it. Pain after injury is also adaptive, furnishing a reminder of injury and discouraging activity that adds to the damage. In some situations, however, pain modulation is also adaptive. When people or other animals are fighting or fleeing, being able to ignore pain can be an advantage. Thus, the nervous system has complex systems that allow not only for the perception but also for the modulation of pain.

In Summary

The activation of receptors in the skin results in neural impulses that move along afferent pathways to the spinal cord by way of the dorsal root. In the spinal cord, the afferent impulses proceed along one of three systems to the thalamus in the brain. Impulses from two of the three systems arrive in the somatosensory cortex in the cerebral cortex. Impulses from the third system also reach the cerebral cortex, but by a less direct route. The primary somatosensory cortex includes a map of the skin, with more cortex devoted to areas of the body richer in skin receptors. Some types of nerve fibers, the A-delta and C fibers, are involved in pain, and the dorsal root of the spinal cord is part of the pain pathway.

The brain and spinal cord also contain mechanisms for modulating sensory input and thereby affecting the perception of pain. One mechanism is through the naturally occurring neurochemicals that relieve pain and mimic the action of opiate drugs. These neurochemicals exist in many places in the central and peripheral nervous systems. The second mechanism is a system of descending control through the periaqueductal gray and the medulla. This system affects the activity of the spinal cord and provides a descending modulation of activity in the spinal cord.

The Meaning of Pain

Until about 100 years ago, pain was most frequently considered a direct consequence of physical injury, and its intensity was generally thought to be proportional to the degree of tissue damage. Near the end of the 19th century, C. A. Strong and others began to think of pain in a new light. Strong (1895) hypothesized that pain was due to two factors: the sensation and the person's reaction to that sensation. In other words, psychological factors and organic causes were of equal importance. This attention to psychological factors in pain signaled the beginning of a new definition, an altered view of the experience, and new theories of pain.

Definition of Pain

Although pain is an almost universal experience, it is remarkably difficult to define. Some define pain as "perhaps the most universal from of stress" (Turk, Meichenbaum, & Genest, 1983, p. 73). Others (Covington, 2000) concentrate on the physiology that underlies the perception of pain. Still others (Wall, 2000) emphasize the subjective nature of pain. These different views reflect the multidimensional nature of pain, which the International Association for the Study of Pain (IASP) incorporated into their definition. The IASP Subcommittee on Taxonomy (1979, p. 250) defined pain as "an unpleasant sensory and emotional experience associated with actual or potential tissue damage, or described in terms of such damage." The essence of this definition continues to be acceptable to most pain researchers (Turk, 2001).

Another way to understand the meaning of pain is according to stages, classified by duration of the pain. Francis J. Keefe (1982) identified three stages of pain: acute, chronic, and prechronic. **Acute pain** is the type of pain that most people experience when injured; it includes pains from cuts, burns, surgery, dental work, childbirth, and other injuries. Its duration is normally brief. This type of pain is ordinarily adaptive; it signals the person to avoid further injury. In contrast, **chronic pain** endures over several months or even years. This type of pain may be due to a chronic condition such as rheumatoid arthritis, or it may be the result of an injury that persists beyond the time of healing (Turk & Melzack, 2001). Chronic pain is frequently experienced in the absence of any detectable tissue damage. It is not adaptive, but rather can be both debilitating and demoralizing and often leads to feelings of helpless and hopelessness. Chronic pain never has a biological benefit, but life without pain produces even more problems (see the Would You Believe . . . ? box, "Life without pain.").

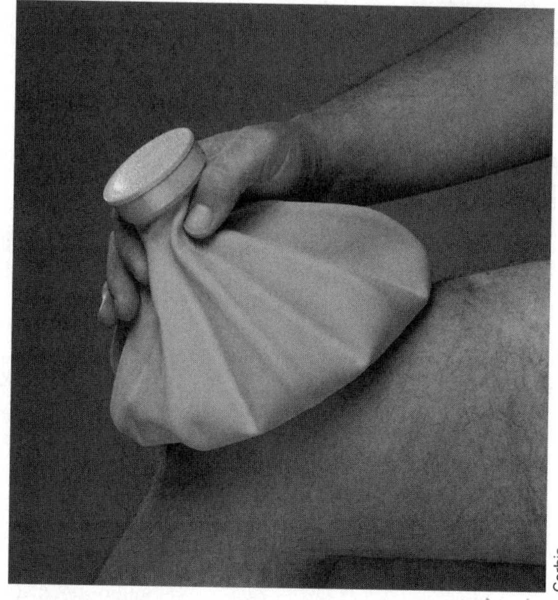

Corbis

Acute pain is typically the result of injury and does not progress to the stage of chronic pain.

Perhaps the most crucial stage of pain is the **prechronic pain stage,** which comes between the acute and the chronic stages. This period is critical because the person either overcomes the pain at this time or develops the feelings of helplessness that lead to chronic pain. These three stages do not exhaust all possibilities of pain: several other types of pain have been identified, the most common of which is *chronic recurrent pain,* or

WOULD YOU BELIEVE

Life without Pain

Would you believe that a life with pain is preferable to one without pain? Although pain is always unpleasant, a person who feels no pain has anything but a pleasant life. Some people might imagine that a life without pain would be serene and enjoyable, but such is not the case. The consequences of the inability to feel pain are enormous and potentially life threatening.

Medical science has identified a few people who have been unable to feel pain, and studies of those people show that a life without pain is not enviable.

A young western Canadian woman, Miss C, was described by Ronald Melzack (1973) as unfamiliar with the experience of pain. The daughter of a physician, Miss C was an intelligent young woman who attended college at McGill University in Montreal. Her father alerted his colleagues in Montreal about her condition, and these physicians studied her inability to feel pain.

Miss C was apparently normal in all respects except that she had never reported feeling pain. Once as a child she sustained third-degree burns because she had climbed on a hot radiator to look out of a window. Without the ability to feel pain, she was unaware of the damage that she was doing to her knees and legs. She could not remember ever sneezing or coughing. The gag reflex was difficult to elicit from her, and the corneal reflex that protects the eye was absent.

The physicians who tested Miss C in Montreal subjected her to various stimuli that would have been horrible for a normal person. They administered electric shock to different parts of her body, applied hot water, immersed her limbs in cold water for prolonged periods, pinched tendons, and injected histamine under her skin. She felt no pain. In addition, her heart rate, blood pressure, and respiration remained normal throughout these tortures.

Without pain to alert her, Miss C sustained many injuries and failed to protect damaged tissues, thus making them worse. Her insensitivity to pain caused serious medical problems, especially in the joints and spine. Melzack and Peter Wall (1982) explained that insensitivity to pain can lead people to remain in one position too long, causing inflammation of the joints. Even worse, the failure to feel pain leads one to neglect injuries and thus healing is obstructed. Injured tissue can easily become infected, and these infections are very difficult to treat if they extend into bone.

Miss C died when she was only 29 years old, and her death was from a failure to bring massive infections under control. During the last month of her life, Miss C finally complained of pain, which was relieved with aspirin. Although she felt practically no pain during her life, neither did she gain the benefits of feeling pain. Her insensitivity to pain directly contributed to the infections that killed her.

The story of Miss C provides ample evidence that a life without pain is not preferable to one with pain, and that pain provides us with a useful signal that we should take action to avoid potentially life-threatening damage to our bodies.

pain marked by alternating episodes of intense pain and no pain. A common example of chronic recurrent pain is headache pain, especially the pain of migraine headache.

The Experience of Pain

The experience of pain is individual and subjective, but situational and cultural factors have a critical impact on that experience. Acknowledgment of the situational influences on the experience of pain began with reports by Henry Beecher (1946), an anesthesiologist, who observed soldiers wounded at the Anzio beachhead during World War II. Beecher noted that, despite their serious battle injuries, many of these men reported very little pain. What made the experience of pain different in this situation? These men had been removed from the battlefront and thus from the threat of death or further injury. Under these conditions, the wounded soldiers were in a cheerful, optimistic state of mind.

Additional confirmation for the notion that a person's reaction to the physical sensation of pain strongly influences the degree of suffering came 10 years later from another study by Beecher (1956). In this report, injured civilians were found to have experienced more pain and requested more pain-killing drugs than did the wounded World War II soldiers, even though the civilians' injuries were less severe. These findings prompted Beecher (1956) to conclude that "the intensity of suffering is largely determined by what the pain means to the patient" (p. 1609) and that "the extent of wound bears only a slight relationship, if any (often none at all), to the pain experienced" (p. 1612). Finally, Beecher (1957) described pain as a two-dimensional experience consisting of both a sensory stimulus and an emotional component. Despite the methodological shortcomings of Beecher's studies, his view of pain as a psychological and physical phenomenon came to be accepted by others working in this field.

Battle wounds are an extreme example of sudden injury, but other injured also feel variable amounts of pain. For example, most—but not all—people admitted to an emergency room for treatment of injury reported pain (Wall, 2000). Pain was more common among people with injuries such as broken bones, sprains, and stabs than among people with injuries to the skin. Indeed, 53% of those with cuts, burns, or scrapes reported that they felt no pain for at least some time after their injury, whereas only 28% of those with deep tissue injury failed to feel immediate pain. These individual variations of pain contrast with people who have been tortured, all of whom feel pain, even though their injuries may not be as serious as those of people reporting to an emergency room. The threat, intent to inflict pain, and lack of control give torture a very different meaning from unintentional injury and thus produces a different pain experience.

In addition to situational aspects, individual factors also make a difference for the experience of pain. People learn to associate stimuli related to a painful experience with the pain and thus develop classically conditioned responses to the associated stimuli. For example, many people dislike the smell of hospitals or become anxious when they hear the dentist's drill because they have had experiences associating these stimuli with pain. Operant conditioning may also play an important role in pain by providing a means for acute pain to develop into chronic pain. John J. Bonica (1990) contended that psychological or environmental factors play a central role in chronic pain. He believed that tissue damage is a direct cause of acute pain, whereas chronic pain is a result of tissue damage plus one's experience of being rewarded for pain behaviors. Bonica emphasized the role of operant conditioning in pain, viewing differences in behavior as a result of varying experiences with rewards for pain behaviors. According to Bonica, people who receive attention, sympathy, relief from normal responsibilities, and disability compensation for their injuries and pain behaviors are more likely to develop chronic pain than are people who have similar injury but receive fewer rewards.

People's belief about individual variability in pain is more myth than reality. Some people stoically endure pain, but nevertheless, these individuals perceive discomfort. They display no sign of their pain because of situational factors, cultural sanctions against the display of emotion, or some combination of these two factors. For example, some Native American, African, and South Pacific island cultures have initiation rituals that involve the silent endurance of pain. These rituals often involve the passage from child to adult status and may include body piercing, cutting, tattooing, burning, or beating. To show signs of pain would result in failure, so individuals are strongly motivated to hide their pain. Individuals may withstand these injuries with no visible sign of distress yet react with an obvious display of pain behavior to an unintentional injury in a situation outside the ritual (Wall, 2000). Other than individuals with chronic pain insensitivity, all people perceive pain. However, some people's behaviors reflect their pain, whereas others' behaviors hide their discomfort. Despite these variations in expressions of pain, little evidence exists for pain-resistant personality.

If a pain-resistant personality does not exist, then could there be evidence for a *pain-prone* personality? The concept of a pain-prone personality is also poorly supported (Turk, 2001), but chronic pain is often associated with some type of psychological problems. People with severe chronic pain are much more likely than other people to suffer from some type of psychopathology, but the direction of the cause and effect is not always clear (Gatchel & Epker, 1999). Patients suffering from chronic pain are more likely to be depressed, to abuse alcohol and other drugs, and to suffer from personality disorders. For Barb, alcohol was a way to cope with her pain, and she abused alcohol and her prescription drugs. Like Barb, some chronic pain patients develop these disorders as a result of their chronic pain; others have some form of psychopathology prior to the beginning of their pain (Gatchel & Epker, 1999).

Another common belief about individual differences in pain is that women are more sensitive to pain than men. Women report pain more readily than men do, but this difference may reflect behavior that is consistent with gender roles rather than differences in perception. A study on women and men who had dental surgery (Averbuch & Katzper, 2000) indicated very small differences between pain reports for men and women and no difference in their responses to analgesic drugs. However, more women than men said that their pain was severe, providing limited support for the existence of gender differences in pain perception.

Cultural variations in pain sensitivity and expression show large differences. Cultural background and social context affect the experience, expression, and even treatment of pain (Gureje et al., 1996). These differences come from varying meanings that different cultures attach to pain and from stereotypes associated with various cultural groups.

Cultural expectations for pain are apparent in the pain women experience during childbirth (Streltzer, 1997). Some cultures hold birth as a dangerous and painful process, and women in these cultures reflect these expectations by experiencing great pain. Other cultures expect quiet acceptance during the experience of giving birth, and women in those cultures tend not to show much evidence of pain. Their failure to display signs of pain, however, does not mean that they do not feel pain (Wall, 2000). When questioned about their apparent lack of pain, these women reported that they felt pain but their culture did not expect women to show pain under these circumstances, so they did not.

Since the 1950s, studies have compared pain expression for people from various ethnic backgrounds (Streltzer, 1997). Some studies have shown differences whereas others have not, but the studies all suffer from the criticism of stereotyping. For example, Italians are stereotyped as people who show a lot of emotion. Consistent with this stereotype, studies have found that Italian Americans express more distress and demand more pain medication than "Yankees" (White Anglo-Saxons who had lived in the United States for generations), who have the reputation for stoically ignoring pain. These variations in pain behaviors among different cultures may reflect behavioral differences in learning and modeling, differences in sensitivity to pain, or some combination of these factors.

Laboratory studies of pain perception confirm differences between African Americans and Whites in sensitivity to painful stimuli; African Americans rated the stimuli as both more intense and more unpleasant (Sheffield, Biles, Orom, Maixner, & Sheps, 2000). These sensitivities carry over to clinical pain; African Americans reported higher levels (Edwards, Fillingim, & Keefe, 2001). Greater sensitivity to pain in African Americans is doubly unfortunate because they tend to receive less analgesia than Whites as outpatients, in hospitals, and in nursing homes, despite similar complaints about pain (Bonham, 2001). Hispanics received similar treatment—less analgesia in many types of medical settings. This differential treatment is a source of needless pain for ethnic minority patients.

Theories of Pain

How people experience pain is the subject of a number of theories. Of the several models of pain, two capture the divergent ways of conceptualizing pain: the specificity theory and the gate control theory.

Specificity Theory Specificity theory explains pain by hypothesizing that specific pain fibers and pain pathways exist, making the experience of pain virtually equal to the amount of tissue damage or injury (Chapman et al., 1999). The view that pain is the result of transmission of pain signals from the body to a "pain center" in the brain can be traced back to Descartes, who in the 1600s proposed that the body works mechanically. This mechanistic action of the body is consistent with the notion that transmission of pain signals is a relaying of information about body damage. Descartes hypothesized that the mind works by a different set of principles, and body and mind interact in a limited way. According to Ronald Melzack (1993), Descartes's view influenced not only the development of a science of physiology and medicine but also the view that pain is a physical experience largely uninfluenced by psychological factors.

Working under the assumption that pain was the transmission of one type of sensory information, researchers tried to determine which type of receptor conveyed what type of sensory information (Melzack, 1973). For example, they tried to determine which type of receptor relayed information about heat, cold, and other types of pain. The attempt to tie specific somatic sensations to specific types of receptors did not succeed. Researchers found that some parts of the body (like the cornea of the eye) contain only one type of receptor, yet those areas feel a full range of sensations. Some receptors seem specialized to react to specific types of stimulation, but these specialized receptors can also respond to other types of stimuli as well. The specificity of skin receptors is therefore limited, and any simple version of specificity theory is not valid.

Specificity does exist in the different types of receptors and nerve fibers. The different types of receptors in the skin allow us to sense light touch, pressure, itching, pricking, warmth, and cold. In addition, we can perceive texture, shape, and vibration and can localize the source of these stimuli on the surface of the skin. We can also sense pain, but pain can come through any of these stimuli.

More important, specificity theory fails to integrate the variability of the experience of pain with the physiology of the somatosensory system. Even if specific skin receptors are devoted to relaying pain, the existence of pain without injury (phantom limb pain), injury without pain (as experienced by the soldiers at Anzio beach and some emergency room patients) makes a simple, physiological theory of pain untenable. Contemporary theorists who believe in the specificity of pain acknowledge that specificity is limited and that pain is a complex, multidimensional phenomenon.

The Gate Control Theory In 1965, Ronald Melzack and Peter Wall formulated a new theory of pain, which suggests that pain is *not* the result of a linear process that begins with sensory stimulation of pain pathways and ends with the experience of pain. Rather, pain perception is subject to a number of modulations that can influence the experience of pain. These modulations begin in the spinal cord.

Melzack and Wall hypothesized that structures in the spinal cord act as a gate for the sensory input that the brain interprets as pain. Melzack and Wall's theory is thus known as the **gate control theory** (see Figure 7.4). It is based on physiology but explains both sensory and psychological aspects of pain perception.

Melzack and Wall (1965, 1982, 1988) pointed out that the nervous system is never at rest; the patterns of neural activation constantly change. When sensory information from the body reaches the dorsal horns of the spinal cord, that neural activation enters a system that is already active. The existing activity in the spinal

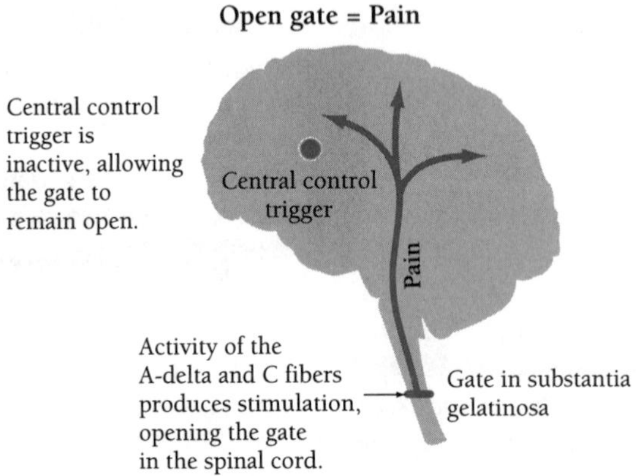

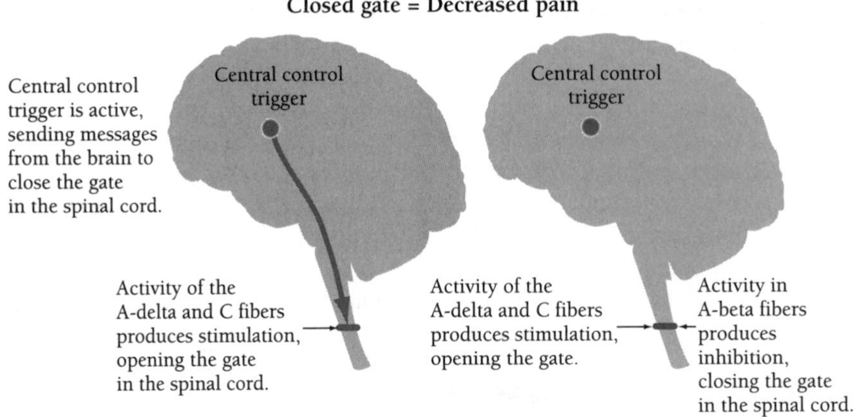

Figure 7.4 Gate control theory of pain.

cord and brain influences the fate of incoming sensory information, sometimes amplifying and sometimes decreasing the incoming neural signals. The gate control theory hypothesizes that these complex modulations in the spinal cord and in the brain are critical factors in the perception of pain.

According to the gate control theory, neural mechanisms in the spinal cord act like a gate that can either increase (open the gate) or decrease (close the gate) the flow of neural impulses. Figure 7.4 shows the results of opening and closing the gate. With the gate open, impulses flow through the spinal cord toward the brain, neural messages reach the brain, and the person feels pain. With the gate closed, impulses are inhibited from ascending through the spinal cord, messages do not reach the brain, and the person does not feel pain. Moreover, sensory input is subject to modulation, depending on the activity of the large A-beta fibers, the small A-delta fibers, and the small C fibers that enter the spinal cord and synapse in the dorsal horns.

The dorsal horns of the spinal cord are composed of several layers (laminae). Two of those laminae make up the substantia gelatinosa, which is the hypothesized location of the gate (Melzack & Wall, 1965). Both the small A-delta and C fibers and the large A-beta fibers travel through the substantia gelatinosa, which also receives projections from other laminae (Melzack

& Wall, 1982, 1988). This arrangement of neurons provides the physiological basis for the modulation of incoming sensory impulses. When Melzack and Wall formulated the gate control theory, these mechanisms were hypothetical, but later research has confirmed the modulation of afferent messages in the dorsal horns of the spinal cord.

Melzack and Wall (1982) proposed that activity in the small A-delta and C fibers causes prolonged activity in the spinal cord. This type of activity would promote sensitivity, which produces pain. Activity of these small fibers would thus open the gate. On the other hand, activity of the large A-beta fibers produces an initial burst of activity in the spinal cord, followed by inhibition. Activity of these fibers closes the gate. Subsequent research has not confirmed this feature of the gate control theory in a clear way (Turk, 2001). Activity of A-delta and C fibers seems to be related to the experience of pain, but under conditions of inflammation, increased activity of A-beta fibers can exacerbate rather than decrease pain.

The gate may be closed by activity in the spinal cord and also by messages that descend from the brain. Melzack and Wall (1965, 1982, 1988) proposed the concept of a **central control trigger** consisting of nerve impulses that descend from the brain and influence the gating mechanism. They hypothesized that this system consists of large neurons that conduct impulses rapidly. These impulses from the brain affect the opening and closing of the gate in the spinal cord and are affected by cognitive processes. That is, Melzack and Wall proposed that the experience of pain is influenced by beliefs and prior experience, and they also hypothesized a physiological mechanism that would account for such factors in pain perception. As we discussed, the periaqueductal gray matter furnishes descending controls, confirming this aspect of the gate control theory.

According to the gate control theory then, pain has not only sensory components but also motivational and emotional components. That aspect of the theory revolutionized conceptualizations of pain (Turk, 2001). The gate control theory explains the influence of cognitive aspects of pain and allows for learning and experience to affect the experience of pain. Anxiety, worry, depression, and focusing on an injury can increase pain by affecting the central control trigger, thus opening the gate. Distraction, relaxation, and positive emotions can cause the gate to close, thereby decreasing pain. The gate control theory is not specific about how these experiences affect pain, and other theorists have elaborated on how such psychological factors influence pain perception (Chapman et al., 1999; Turk, 2001).

Many personal experiences with pain are consistent with the gate control theory. When you accidentally hit your finger with a hammer, many of the small fibers are activated, opening the gate. An emotional reaction accompanies your perception of acute pain. You may then grasp your injured finger and rub it. According to the gate control theory, rubbing stimulates the large fibers that close the gate, thus blocking stimulation from the small fibers and decreasing pain.

The gate control theory also explains how injuries can go virtually unnoticed. If sensory input is sent into a heavily activated nervous system, then the stimulation may not be perceived as pain. A tennis player may turn an ankle during a game but not notice the acute pain because of excitement and concentration on the game. After the game is finished, however, the player may notice the pain because the nervous system is functioning at a different level of activation and the gate is more easily opened.

Although it is not universally accepted, the gate control theory is the most influential theory of pain. It allows for the complexities of pain experiences. Melzack and Wall proposed the gate control theory before the discovery of the body's own opiates or of the descending control mechanisms through the periaqueductal gray and the medulla. The gate control theory has been and continues to be successful in

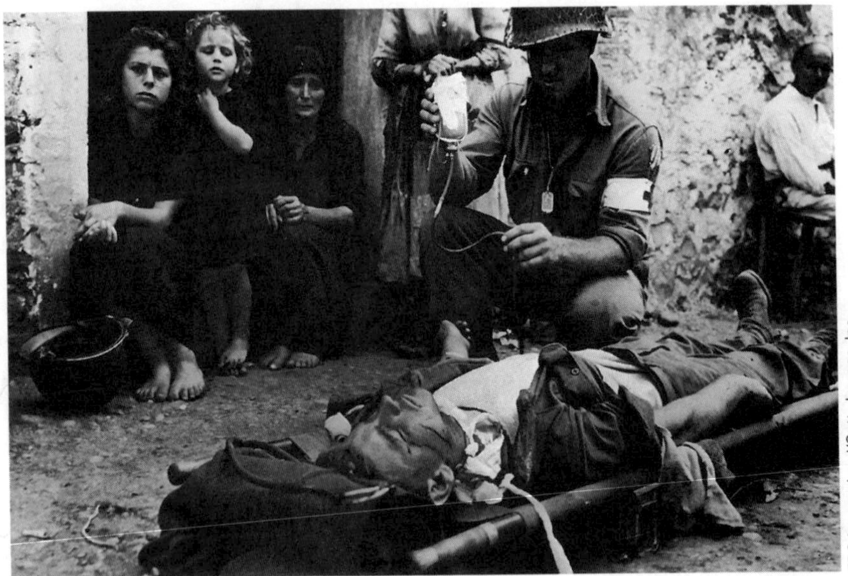

The experience of pain varies with the situation. Wounded soldiers removed from front lines may feel little pain despite extreme injuries.

spurring research and generating interest in the psychological and perceptual factors involved in pain.

Melzack (1993, 1999) proposed an extension to the gate control theory called the neuromatrix theory, which places a stronger emphasis on the brain's role in pain perception. He hypothesized a network of brain neurons that he called the neuromatrix, which is "distributed throughout many areas of the brain, comprises a widespread network of neurons which generates patterns, processes information that flows through it, and ultimately produces the pattern that is felt as a whole body" (Melzack, 1993, p. 623). Normally, the neuromatrix acts to process incoming sensory information, including pain, but the neuromatrix acts even in the absence of sensory input, such as with phantom limbs. Melzack's neuromatrix theory extends gate control theory but maintains that pain perception is part of a complex process affected not only by sensory input but also by activity of the nervous system and by experience and expectation.

In Summary

Although the extent of damage is important in the pain experience, personal perception is also important. Pain can be classified as acute, prechronic, or chronic, depending on the length of time that the pain has persisted. Acute pain is usually adaptive and lasts for less than 6 months. Chronic pain continues beyond the time of healing, and often in the absence of detectable tissue damage. Prechronic pain occurs between acute and chronic pain. All of these stages of pain appear in pain syndromes, such as headache pain, low back pain, arthritic pain, cancer pain, and phantom limb pain.

Several models have been proposed to explain pain, but specificity theory does not capture the complexity of the pain experience. The gate control theory has been the most influential model of pain. This theory holds that pain can be increased or diminished by mechanisms in the spinal cord and the brain. Since its formulation, increased knowledge of the physiology of the brain and spinal cord has supported this theory.

Pain Syndromes

Pain can also be categorized according to **syndrome,** symptoms that occur together and characterize a condition. This classification is not used for acute pain but is applied to chronic pain. Headache and low back pain are the two most frequently treated pain syndromes, but people also seek treatment for several other common pain syndromes.

Headache Pain

Headache pain is the most common of all types of pain, with a lifetime incidence of more than 99% (Smetana, 2000). Until the 1980s, no reliable classification of headache pain was available to researchers and therapists. Then in 1988, the Headache Classification Committee of the International Headache Society (HIS) published a classification system that standardized definitions of various headache pains (Olesen, 1988). Although the HIS identifies many different kinds of headache, the three primary pain syndromes are migraine, tension, and cluster headaches.

Migraine headaches are characterized by recurrent attacks of pain that vary widely in intensity, frequency, and duration. Originally conceptualized as originating in the blood vessels in the head, migraine headaches are now considered to originate in neurons in the brain stem (Holroyd, 2002). The attacks are associated with loss of appetite, nausea, vomiting, and exaggerated sensitivity to light and sound. Migraine headaches also often involve sensory, motor, or mood disturbances. The two most frequent kinds of migraine are those with aura and those without aura. Migraine with aura is characterized by identifiable sensory disturbances that precede the headache pain; migraine without aura has a sudden onset and an intense throbbing, usually (but not always) restricted to one side of the head (Smetana, 2000).

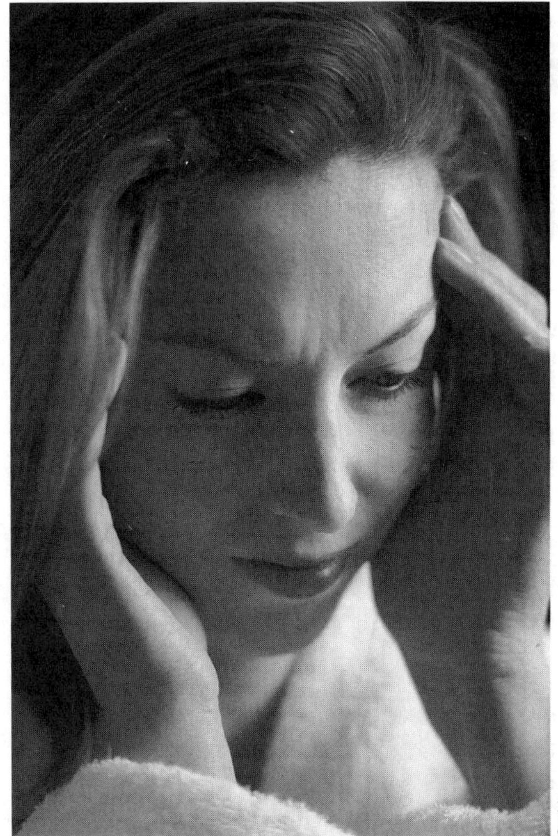

Corbis

Headache is a frequent pain syndrome, accounting for substantial loss of work days and decreased effectiveness.

Women are about three times more likely than men to have migraine headaches (Miaskowski, 1999), but men and women who have chronic migraines experience similar migraine symptoms, frequency, and severity (Marcus, 2001). Most migraine patients experience their first headache before age 30 and some before the age of 10. However, the period for the greatest frequency of migraines is between ages 35 and 45 (Pearce, 1994). Few patients have a first migraine after age

40, but people who have migraines continue to do so, often throughout their lives. Also, low-income people have significantly more migraines than people in the highest income brackets, and women 30 to 49 from low-income households have the greatest risk for migraine headache. However, disability from migraines is not related to gender, age, income, or urban/rural background (Stewart, Lipton, Celentano, & Reed, 1992).

Tension headaches have been described as muscular in origin, accompanied by sustained contractions of the muscles of the neck, shoulders, scalp, and face, but current explanations (Holroyd, 2002) include mechanisms within the central nervous system. These headaches are characterized by a gradual onset; sensations of tightness; constriction or pressure; highly variable intensity, frequency, and duration; and a dull, steady ache on both sides of the head. Nearly 40% of the U.S. population experiences tension headaches (Schwartz, Stewart, Simon, & Lipton, 1998), and people with this pain syndrome reported lost workdays and decreased effectiveness at work, home, and school because of their pain.

A third type of headache is the **cluster headache,** a severe headache that occurs in daily or nearly daily clusters for 4 to 16 weeks (Pearce, 1994). Some symptoms are similar to migraine, including severe pain and vomiting, but cluster headaches are much briefer, rarely lasting longer than 2 hours. The headache is localized on one side of the head, and often the eye on the other side becomes bloodshot and waters. In addition, cluster headaches are much more common in men than women, with a ratio of 10:1. These headaches appear in a cluster and disappear, only to recur every year or two (Smetana, 2000).

Low Back Pain

Low back pain is also very common, with as many as 80% of people in the United States experiencing this type of pain at some time (Deyo, 1998). More than 2.6 million men and women incur back injuries at work and another 4.5 million develop low back pain from performing repeated job activities (Behrens, Seligman, Cameron, Mathias, & Fine, 1994). Barb is a good example of the millions of people who sustain injuries at work. Even more people experience back pain from activities not associated with work, making the problem extensive but not necessarily serious: most injuries are not permanent, and most people recover quickly.

Low back pain has many potential causes, including infections, degenerative diseases, and malignancies, but the most frequent cause is probably injury or stress resulting in musculoskeletal, ligament, and neurological problems in the lower back. Pregnancy is also a contributor to low back pain, with nearly 90% of pregnant women suffering from low back pain (Hayes et al., 2000). Aging is yet another factor in back pain, because the fluid content and elasticity of the intervertebral disks decrease as one grows older. In addition, stress and psychological factors may play roles in back pain (Power, Frank, Hertzman, Schierhout, & Li, 2001). These many potential causes, combined with problems in diagnosis, result in many back pain patients without a definite diagnosis for the physical cause of their pain.

Many people experience back pain, but only a small percentage of these people develop chronic low back pain (Deyo, 1998). At any specific time, as few as 1% of U.S. workers are disabled by back pain. The high percentage of people who experience back pain and the low percentage of chronic disability points to the large number of people who recover from acute back pain. Those who do not quickly recover have a poor prognosis and are likely to develop chronic pain problems.

Arthritis Pain

Rheumatoid arthritis is an autoimmune disorder characterized by swelling and inflammation of the joints as well as destruction of cartilage, bone, and tendons. These changes alter the joint, producing direct pain, and the changes in joint structure lead to change in movement, which may result in additional pain through this indirect

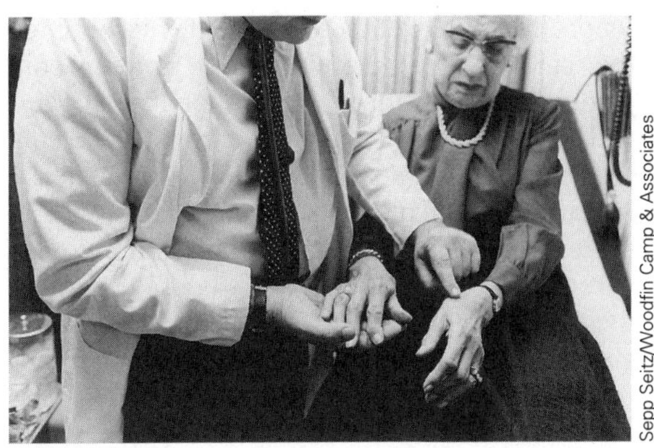

Sepp Seitz/Woodfin Camp & Associates

Arthritis is a source of pain and disability for over 20 million Americans.

route (Young, 1993). Rheumatoid arthritis can occur at any age, even during adolescence and young adulthood, but it is most prevalent among people 40 to 70 years old. Also, women are about 2.5 times more likely than men to develop this disease (Lee & Weinblatt, 2001). The symptoms of rheumatoid arthritis are extremely variable, with some people experiencing steady progression of increasing symptoms and most facing remissions and intensifications.

In contrast, **osteoarthritis** is a progressive inflammation of the joints affecting mostly older people and characterized by a dull ache in the joint area, which is exacerbated by movement. Osteoarthritis is the most common form of arthritis. Arthritis is one of the primary causes of disability in older people, with about 50% of those over age 70 affected by arthritis (Keefe et al., 2002). Older women make up a disproportionate number of those affected. The joint stiffness and pain prevent people with arthritis from engaging in basic self-care and enjoyable activities. People with arthritis often experience feelings of helplessness, depression, and anxiety, which exacerbates their pain.

Cancer Pain

Over a million people were diagnosed with cancer in the United States in the year 2000 (USBC, 2001). Cancer can produce pain in two ways: through its growth and progression and through the various treatments to control its growth. Studies have shown that pain is present in about 30% to 40% of all cancer cases and 60% to 90% of all terminal cancer cases (Fife, Irick, & Painter, 1993). Some cancers are much more likely than others to produce pain. For example, nearly all patients suffering from head, neck, and cervical cancer experience pain, about half the patients with breast and lung cancer experience at least moderate pain, but pain is quite rare among leukemia patients (Anderson, Syrjala, & Cleeland, 2001). In addition, treatments for cancer may also produce pain; surgery, chemotherapy, and radiation therapy each have painful effects. Thus, either the disease or its treatment creates pain for most cancer patients (Syrjala & Abrams, 1999). Many suffer from emotional distress, fear, anxiety, irritability, feelings of hopelessness and helplessness, changes in their relationships with spouses and other family members, or some combination of these conditions (Syrjala & Abrams, 1999).

Phantom Limb Pain

Just as injury can occur without producing pain, pain can occur in the absence of injury. One such type of pain is **phantom limb pain,** the experience of chronic pain in an absent body part. Amputation removes the nerves that produce the impulses leading to the experience of pain. Despite removal of the physical basis for pain, phantom limb pain is not an unusual experience for amputees.

Estimates of the proportion of amputees who experience phantom limb pain have varied. Until the 1970s, phantom pain was believed to be rare, with less than 1% of amputees experiencing a painful phantom limb, but more recent research has indicated that the percentage may be as high as 67% (Wall, 2000). Most commonly, amputees feel sensations from their amputated limbs soon after surgery. These sensations often start as a tingling sensation and then develop into other sensations that resemble actual feelings in the missing limb. Nor are the sensations of a phantom pain limited to limbs. Women who have undergone breast removal also perceive sensations from the amputated breast, and people who have had teeth pulled sometimes continue to experience feelings from those teeth.

Amputees who experience unpleasant sensations from their amputated limbs may feel that the phantom limb is of an abnormal size or in an uncomfortable position (Melzack & Wall, 1982). Phantom limbs can also produce painful feelings of cramping, shooting, burning, or crushing. These pains vary from mild and infrequent to severe and continuous. The pain may start shortly after amputation or not begin until years later. Melzack and Wall (1988) reported that 72% of amputees have pain in their phantom limb 8 days after their surgery, 65% have pain 6 months afterward, and 60% have pain 2 years later. The severity and frequency of the pain tend to decrease over time.

The underlying cause of phantom limb pain has been the subject of bitter controversy (Melzack, 1992; Melzack & Wall, 1988). Because surgery rarely relieves the pain, some have hypothesized that phantom limb pain has an emotional basis. Melzack (1992) argued that phantom limb sensation arises within the brain as a result of the generation of a characteristic pattern of neural activity, which he called a *neuromatrix.* Melzack contended that this brain activity constituted "a characteristic pattern of impulses indicating that the body is intact and unequivocally one's own" (p. 123). This neuromatrix pattern continues to operate, even if the neurons in the peripheral nervous system do not furnish input to the brain. Melzack believed that this brain activity is the basis for phantom limb sensations, which may include pain.

In Summary

Acute pain may result from hundreds of different types of injuries and diseases, but chronic pain can be classified according to a limited number of syndromes. A few of these syndromes account for the majority of people who suffer from chronic pain. Headache is the most common type of pain, and some people experience chronic problems with migraine, tension, or cluster headaches. Most people's experience of low back pain is acute, but for some people, the pain becomes chronic and debilitating. Arthritis is a degenerative disease that affects the joints, producing chronic pain. Rheumatoid arthritis is an autoimmune disease that may affect people of any age, but osteoarthritis is the result of progressive inflammation of the joints that affects mostly older people. Pain is not an inevitable consequence of cancer, but most people with cancer experience pain either as a result of the progression of the disease or due to the various treatments for cancer. One of the most puzzling pain syndromes is phantom limb pain, which constitutes pain without any physical basis. A majority of people with amputations experience this pain syndrome.

The Measurement of Pain

We have seen that pain has physical and psychological elements, both of which can be quantified and measured. The measurement of pain is important because it allows clinicians to quantify their patients' pain and allows researchers to evaluate different pain-reducing techniques.

The most simple and direct way to measure people's pain is to ask them to rate their pain on a scale. This type of pain assessment would seem to be reliable and valid. Who knows better than patients themselves how much pain they are feeling? However, some pain experts (Turk & Melzack, 2001) have questioned both the reliability and validity of this procedure, stating that people do not reliably remember how they rated an earlier pain. For this reason, pain researchers have developed a number of other techniques for measuring pain, including (1) self-reports, (2) behavioral assessments, and (3) physiological measures.

Self-Reports

Self-reports of pain include simple rating scales, standardized pain inventories, and standardized personality tests.

Rating Scales Although pain researchers have developed a number of other self-reports, as well as behavioral and physiological assessments, the simple rating scale remains an important part of the pain measurement arsenal. On this rating scale, patients are asked to rate their intensity of pain on a scale from 0 to 10 (or 0 to 100), with 10 being the most excruciating pain possible and 0 being the complete absence of pain. A similar technique is the Visual Analog Scale (VAS), which is simply a line anchored on the left by a phrase such as "no pain" and on the right by a phrase such as "worst pain imaginable."

Both the VAS and the numerical rating scales are easy to use, but they have been criticized as sometimes being confusing to patients not accustomed to quantifying their experience. They are also more time consuming to score than rating scales that include numbers on the scale. Another rating scale is the face scales, 8 to 10 drawing of faces expressing emotions from intense joy to intense pain. Again, patients merely indicate which illustration best fits their level of pain (Jensen & Karoly, 2001). A limitation of each of these rating scales is that they measure only the intensity of pain: they do not tap in to patients' verbal description of their pain.

Pain Questionnaires Ronald Melzack (1975, p. 278) contended that describing pain on a single dimension was "like specifying the visual world only in terms of light flux without regard to pattern, color, texture, and the many other dimensions of visual experience." Rating scales make no distinction, for example, among pains that are pounding, shooting, stabbing, or hot. In an attempt to rectify the weakness in single-dimensional measurement scales, Melzack (1975) developed the McGill Pain Questionnaire (MPQ).

The McGill Pain Questionnaire provides a subjective report of pain and categorizes it in three dimensions: sensory, affective, and evaluative. *Sensory* qualities of pain are its temporal, spatial, pressure, and thermal properties; *affective* qualities are its fear, tension, and autonomic properties that are part of the pain experience; and *evaluative* qualities are the words that describe the subjective overall intensity of the pain experience.

In addition to these three dimensions of pain, the MPQ has four parts. Part 1 consists of front and back drawings of the human body. Patients mark on these drawings, indicating the areas where they feel pain. Part 2 consists of 20 sets of words describing pain, and patients draw a circle around the one word in each set that most accurately describes their pain. These adjectives are ordered from least to most painful—for example, *nagging, nauseating, agonizing, dreadful,* and *torturing.* Part 3 asks how patients' pain has changed with time. Part 4 measures the intensity of pain on a 5-point scale from *mild* to *excruciating.* This fourth part yields a Present Pain Intensity (PPI) score.

The MPQ is the most frequently used pain questionnaire (Piotrowski, 1998). It has been used to assess pain relief in a variety of treatment programs and has demonstrated some validity in assessing multiple pain syndromes (Melzack & Katz, 2001). The MPQ shows considerable promise as a multidimensional pain assessment inventory, but it has a difficult vocabulary and lacks a standard scoring format (Syrjala & Chapman, 1984). A short form of the McGill Pain Questionnaire (Melzack, 1987) preserves the multidimensional assessment and correlates highly with scores on the standard MPQ.

The Multidimensional Pain Inventory (MPI), also known as the West Haven-Yale Multidimensional Pain Inventory (WHYMPI) is another assessment tool specifically designed for pain patients (Kerns, Turk, & Rudy, 1985). The 52-item MPI is divided into three sections. The first rates (1) pain severity, (2) pain's interference with patients' lives, (3) patients' dissatisfaction with their present functioning, (4) patients' view of the support they receive from others, (5) patients' perceived life control, and (6) patients' negative mood states. The second section rates the patients' perceptions of the responses of significant others, and the third measures how often patients engage in each of 30 different daily activities.

Using this scale allowed researchers (Kerns et al., 1985) to develop 13 different scales that captured different dimensions of the lives of pain patients. Turk and Rudy (1988) have used the statistical technique of cluster analysis to group pain patients into three clusters: (1) dysfunctional, (2) interpersonally distressed, and (3) adaptive copers. Patients in the dysfunctional cluster tend to report higher levels of pain, greater psychological distress, lower perceived control, greater interference with their lives, lower levels of activity, and lower levels of perceived control over their lives. The second cluster of patients perceive that their families and significant others did not support them, so this group was called *interpersonally distressed*. The people in this profile had problems because they perceived that those around them were failing to provide necessary support. The third cluster—*adaptive copers*—tend to report lower levels of pain severity, lower interference with their lives, lower personal distress, and higher levels of activity and control. These patients are less troubled by their pain and appear to be coping with it.

Other research (Turk et al., 1998; Walter & Brannon, 1991) has obtained similar clusters using different populations of pain patients. However, another team of researchers (Burns, Kubilus, Bruehl, & Harden (2001) found evidence for a fourth cluster, that is, a repressor group. Repressors report high pain, but low activity and low distress. They are defensive and tend to repress emotional distress.

Standardized Psychological Tests The McGill Pain Questionnaire and the Multidimensional Pain Inventory are the most commonly used pain inventories. but clinicians also use a variety of standardized psychological tests in assessing pain patients. The most frequently used of these tests is the Minnesota Multiphasic Personality Inventory (MMPI) (Piotrowski, 1998) and the MMPI-2 (Vendrig, Derksen, & de Mey, 1999). The MMPI was not originally designed to assess pain but rather to measure such clinical diagnoses as hypochondriasis, depression, paranoia, schizophrenia, and other psychopathologies. Research from the early 1950s (Hanvik, 1951) found that different types of pain patients could be differentiated on several MMPI scales. Since that time, other researchers have used this inventory for pain measurement. Research (Bradley, Prokop, Gentry, Van der Heide, & Prieto, 1981; Bradley & Van der Heide, 1984) has found that the so-called neurotic triad—a cluster of elevated scores on hypochondriasis, depression, and hysteria—consistently relates to reports of pain.

In addition to the MMPI, the Beck Depression Inventory (Beck, Ward, Mendelson, Mock, & Erbaugh, 1961) and the Symptom Checklist-90 (Derogatis, 1977) have been used to measure pain. The Beck Depression Inventory is a short self-report questionnaire that assesses depression, and the Symptom Checklist-90 measures symptoms related to various types of behavioral problems. A comparative analysis self-report measures of chronic pain (Mikail, DuBreuil, & D'Eon, 1993) revealed that the McGill Pain Questionnaire, the Multidimensional Pain Inventory, and the Beck Depression Inventory measured the pain experience with very little overlap, a result suggesting that each of these three has something unique to offer.

Behavioral Assessments

A second major approach to pain measurement is observation of patients' behavior. Nearly 30 years ago, Wilbert Fordyce (1974) reported that people in pain often groan, grimace, rub, sigh, limp, miss work, remain in bed, or engage in other behaviors that signify to observers that they may be suffering from pain. Other observable behaviors include lowered levels of activity, use of pain medication, body posture, and facial expressions. Each of these behaviors has potential reward value; that is, pain patients are frequently reinforced by some sort of disability compensation, avoidance of responsibility, and sympathy and attention from other people. Environmental reinforcers increase the tendency for pain behaviors to recur and to become more important in people's lives. The use of operant conditioning techniques to decrease these learned behaviors is discussed in Chapter 8.

Spouses and others close to the pain patient can be trained to make careful observations of pain behaviors without further reinforcing these behaviors. For example, Fordyce (1976) trained significant others by first asking them to list 5 to 10 items indicating that the patient is in pain. This list might include such behaviors as requesting medication, moaning, or verbalizing pain. Fordyce recommended a list of this length because more than 10 items might prompt too much attention to pain behaviors, and fewer than 5 items would probably not be enough to make reliable observations. Once the list is complete, the significant other is asked to record the amount of time the patient spends exhibiting each of these behaviors. Next, the significant other records his or her own behaviors immediately following the patient's pain behaviors.

People have the ability to both assess and exacerbate their partner's pain (Romano, Jensen, Turner, Good, & Hops, 2000). These researchers videotaped chronic pain patients and their partners interacting in seven common household activities. They found that partner's demonstration of attention, care, and concern was closely associated with the increase of patient's pain behaviors. This study adds more support for the behavioral approach to both measuring pain and to identifying environmental triggers for pain.

Some researchers have relied on trained observers in a clinic or laboratory to assess such pain behaviors (Fordyce, 1990; Keefe, 1982). Investigators have used both direct observations and videotape recordings (carried out surreptitiously) to assess pain. One study (Keefe & Block, 1982) used two trained observers to independently view and record videotapes of patients with low back pain. The two observers had very high categories of agreement on each of five nonverbal pain behaviors: sighing, grimacing, rubbing, bracing, and guarding, indicating strong reliability for this technique. Patients also rated their intensity of pain, thus allowing a validity check of the observers' ratings. For all behaviors except grimacing, the correlation was significant, a result suggesting that the ratings of trained observers have some validity. Moreover, the frequency of pain behaviors tended to decrease with behaviorally oriented treatment, and these decreases in pain behaviors correlated with changes in pain ratings.

Physiological Measures

A third approach to pain assessment is the use of physiological measures (Flor, 2001; Turk & Melzack, 2001). Electromyography (EMG) is frequently used to measure the level of muscle tension experienced by a pain patient. If muscle tension is greater in one part of the body than in adjoining parts, then the clinician can assume that the patient is experiencing pain in the area of increased muscle tension. Electromyography is most often used to measure low back pain, headache pain, and neck and jaw pain.

Although electromyography devices can be reliable measures of muscle tension, their ability to assess self-reports of pain has not yet been proven. For example, Herta Flor (2001) reported little consistency between self-reports of pain and EMG levels. Thus, muscle tension, as measured by electromyography, may not be a valid measure of pain.

Researchers have also attempted to assess pain through several autonomic indices, including such involuntary processes as hyperventilation, blood flow in the temporal artery, heart rate, hand surface temperature, finger pulse volume, and skin resistance level. Again, most of these attempts have met with only limited success. One exception to these generally negative results has been the use of thermography to measure skin temperature (LeRoy & Filasky, 1990). Thermographic instruments measure minute changes in skin temperature and provide an estimate of autonomic nervous system functioning. This procedure has demonstrated some success in measuring some types of pain, but pain is only one of many factors contributing to changes in skin temperature.

In Summary

Pain measurement techniques can be grouped into three general categories: (1) self-reports. (2) behavioral assessments, and (3) physiological measures. Self-reports include rating scales; pain questionnaires such as the McGill Pain Questionnaire and the Multidimensional Pain Inventory; and standardized objective tests such as the Minnesota Multiphasic Personality Inventory, the Beck Depression Inventory, and the Symptom Checklist-90. Clinicians who treat pain patients often use a combination of assessments, relying most often on self-report inventories. Behavioral assessments of pain include ratings by significant others as well as ratings by clinicians in therapeutic or laboratory settings. Observations of pain-related behavior show some reliability and validity. Physiological measures include muscle tension and autonomic indices, but these devices do not reliably predict self-reports of pain.

Pain Control through Prevention and Physical Treatment

Both acute and chronic pain create problems, making control an urgent goal. Although acute pain has adaptive properties, it also produces suffering for those recovering from injuries. Chronic pain has no adaptive advantages and causes misery and disability for millions of people worldwide. Some chronic pain can be prevented, and physical treatment can control most types of acute and some types of chronic pain. In addition, an array of coping strategies and interventions can help people with chronic pain deal with their pains in more effective ways. We examine strategies to prevent pain and physical treatments next, and these latter techniques appear in Chapter 8.

Preventing Pain

Preventing problems is generally preferable to solving them once they have occurred; pain is no exception. Chronic pain can be prevented by avoiding injury or by physical or psychological treatment that keeps acute pain from becoming chronic. This section examines the possibility of preventing pain, the next section looks at physical treatments, and Chapter 8 discusses behavioral treatments for pain.

Several programs have targeted the prevention of low back pain, the type of pain that most often causes lost work days. One such program, called Back to Balance (Donaldson, Stanger, Donaldson, Cram, & Skubick, 1993), attempted to minimize work-related back injuries by educating workers about causes of pain. Participants of this study were nursing aides, orderlies, and other employees at a health care facility who had a very high rate of lost work time due to chronic repetitive lifting injuries to the back. Some of the participants were assigned to the treatment group and some were placed in control group. The Back to Balance procedure consists of an easy-to-read booklet containing information on the anatomy of the back and guidelines on how to keep the back balanced while engaging in repetitive lifting.

Results from this study indicated that participants in the treatment group reported significantly less pain (as measured by the McGill Pain Questionnaire) than participants in the control group, and that these differences remained after a 12-month follow-up. Moreover, treatment par-

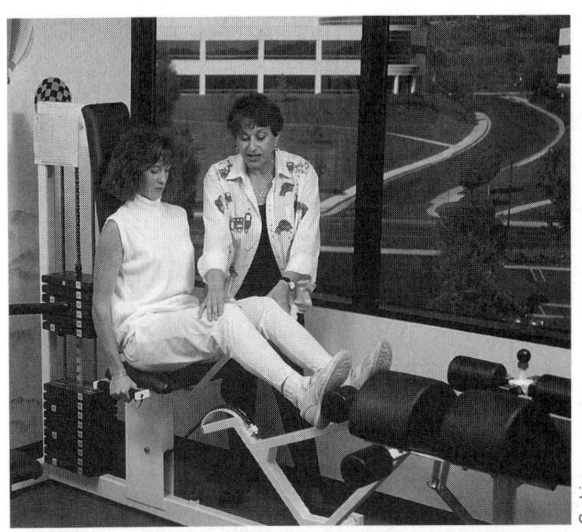
Corbis

Physical activity can help to diminish pain and prevent injury from becoming chronic pain.

ticipants generalized their knowledge beyond the workplace and had fewer back injuries at home.

A similar program, the Active Back School (Lonn, 1999), also showed that at least some back pain can be prevented through education plus exercise. Using previous episodes of back pain as a criterion, the experimenter divided the participants into two groups; a treatment group and a control group. The Active Back School treatment consisted of a series of 20-minute theoretical sessions and 40-minute activity sessions. A 1-year follow-up showed that the Active Back School program was effective in reducing the severity of back injuries and increasing the time between back pain episodes.

Although the results of these two studies indicated that knowledge can translate into action and that information about the anatomy of the back can help prevent low back pain, most educational programs have not been very effective in preventing pain. Steven Linton (1999) reviewed a variety of strategies, including educational programs, and found that most of these strategies were not very effective. "Back schools" may help workers avoid situations that lead to musculoskeletal pain, but they are not sufficient to prevent pain. Primary prevention aimed at changing the workplace is even less effective. For example, decreasing heavy work loads does not reduce pain problems, but cutting back on repetitive movements, even light repetitive movements such as typing at a keyboard, can be an effective means of avoiding chronic pain. Linton's review also found very limited benefit for increasing exercise. Programs that showed more promise included training supervisors to contact workers who are absent from work and using cognitive behavioral strategies to keep workers from viewing their pain as a terrible catastrophe.

Finally, results from a study in Finland (Malmivaara et al., 1995) suggest that doing nothing out of the ordinary is probably the best approach to preventing additional pain in pain patients. The researchers divided city workers with back pain into three groups: a control group that was told to continue their ordinary activities as well as they could, one experimental group that was prescribed 2 days of bed rest, and a second experimental group that was taught special back exercises. Results indicated that the control group—the workers who continued their everyday activities—returned to work sooner and visited the pain clinic fewer times than either the bed rest group or the exercise group.

Physical Treatments for Pain

In 2001, a jury found a physician guilty of allowing a patient to be in pain when he could have treated that pain (Wilson, 2001). The U.S. Congress passed legislation making the years beginning with 2001 the Decade of Pain Control and Research. Patients' pain now must be monitored like other vital signs such as blood pressure and fever. Funding for pain research has increased. These events signal an increased interest in pain management. However, pain treatment presents complex problems. Treatment for acute pain is usually more straightforward than management of chronic pain. Approaches to both kinds of pain may involve a multidisciplinary treatment team including both physical and behavioral

BECOMING HEALTHIER

One technique that helps people manage and minimize pain is guided imagery. This technique involves creating an image and being guided (or guiding yourself) through it. The process can be helpful in dealing with both chronic pain and acute pain such as medical or dental procedures. Those who are not experienced at guided imagery will benefit from putting the guided imagery instructions on an audiotape.

To practice guided imagery, choose a quiet place where you will not be disturbed and where you will be comfortable. Prepare for the experience by placing the tape player where you can turn it on, seating yourself in a comfortable chair, and taking a few deep breaths. Turn on the tape, close your eyes, and follow the instructions you have recorded.

The tape should include a description of a special place, one that you either imagine or have experienced, where you feel utterly safe and at peace. Tailor the place to fit with your life and experiences—one person's magic place may not be so attractive to another person, so think about what will be appealing to you. Many people enjoy a beach scene, but others like woods, fields, or special rooms. The goal is to imagine somewhere that you will feel relaxed and at peace.

Put instructions on your tape concerning this place and its description. Spend time in this place and experience it in detail. Pay attention to the sights and sounds, but do not neglect the smells and skin senses associated with the place. Spend time imagining each of these sensory experiences, and include instructions to yourself about the feelings. You should feel relaxed and peaceful as you go though this scene. Linger over the details and aim to allow yourself to become completely absorbed in the experience.

Include some instructions for relaxed breathing in your tour of your special place. Your goal is to achieve peace and relaxation that will replace the anxiety and pain that you have felt. As you repeat the guided imagery exercise, you may want to revise the tape to include more details. The tape should include at least 10 minutes of guided instructions, and you may want to redo the tape into a longer version as you become more proficient in the exercise. Eventually, you will not need the tape, and you will be able to take this technique with you wherever you go.

techniques. Behavioral treatments are discussed in the next chapter; this section looks at physical treatments for pain.

A study conducted over a decade ago highlights how health care professionals can allow patients' pain to go untreated. This study (Krokosky & Reardon, 1989) assessed pain in patients who were recuperating from surgery and then asked the patients' nurses and physicians to measure their perception of each patient's pain. A comparison of the three sets of pain scores revealed many discrepancies. The correlations between the patients' ratings of their pain and the nurses' ratings of the patients' pain failed to show a statistically significant relationship, as did the correlation between physicians' and patients' ratings. The lack of correlation shows that neither nurses nor physicians perceived the amount and duration of their patients' pain. Both nurses and physicians generally underestimated the pain their patients experienced. Thus, health care workers may undermedicate patients, leaving them to experience serious pain.

In most cases of acute pain such as postoperative pain, drugs are available to control pain. Managing chronic pain presents much more of a challenge, and drug treatment carries greater risks. Both acute and chronic pain have been treated by stimulation to the skin, using electrical impulses (transcutaneous electrical nerve stimulation), needles (acupuncture), or pressure (acupressure or massage). Chronic pain that has not responded to other methods of management is sometimes treated by surgery.

Drugs **Analgesic drugs** relieve pain without causing loss of consciousness. Hundreds of different analgesic drugs are available, but almost all fall into two major groups: the opiates and the nonnarcotic analgesics (Polatin, 1996). Both types exist naturally as derivatives of plants, and both have many synthetic variations. Of the two, the opium type is stronger and has a longer history of use.

The nonnarcotic analgesics include a variety of nonsteroidal anti-inflammatory drugs (NSAIDs) as well as acetaminophen. *Aspirin,* one of the NSAIDs, comes from an extract of willow bark. The active component is salicin, a compound isolated in 1827 (Wall, 2000). The Bayer Company used the name aspirin as a trade name beginning in 1899. In addition to having analgesic properties, aspirin acts against inflammation and fever.

NSAIDs, such as aspirin, ibuprofen, and naproxen sodium, appear to block the synthesis of prostaglandins (Winter, 1994), a class of chemicals released by damaged tissue and involved in inflammation. Their presence sensitizes neurons and increases pain. These drugs act at the site of injury instead of crossing into the brain, but they change neurochemical activity in the nervous system and affect pain perception. As a result of their mechanism of action, NSAIDs do not alter pain perception when no injury is present, for example in laboratory situations with people who receive experimental pain stimuli.

Aspirin and the NSAIDs have many uses in pain relief. Because these drugs appear to work by influencing the effects of injury, they are especially useful for pain in which injury has occurred. This description takes in a wide variety of pain, including minor cuts and scratches as well as more severe injuries such as broken bones. But pain that occurs without inflammation is not so readily relieved by NSAIDs. In addition, NSAIDs have the capability of irritating and damaging the stomach lining, even producing ulcers (Huang, Sridhar, & Hunt, 2002). A new type of NSAID, the Cox-2 inhibitor, affects prostaglandins but does not produce gastric toxicity. This analgesic has advantages for people who are sensitive to the gastric irritation that accompanies NSAID use or for people who take large doses of analgesics. For most people, the analgesic effects of aspirin or other NSAIDS are more beneficial than their side effects are damaging, but these drugs have risks.

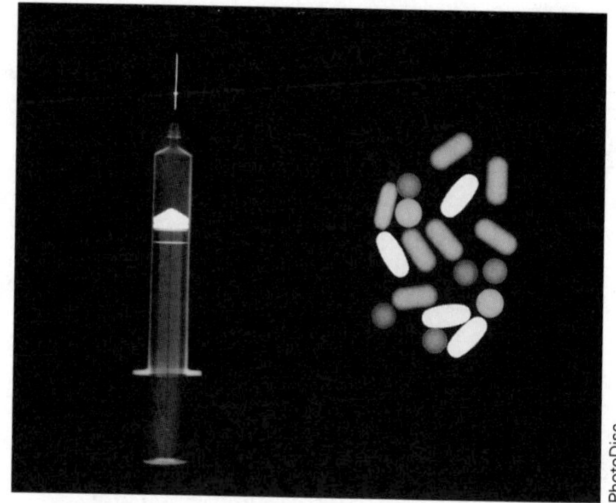

PhotoDisc

Drugs offer effective treatment for acute pain but are not a good choice to treat chronic pain.

Another of aspirin's side effects is the alteration of blood-clotting time, a condition that can be either an advantage (as in patients who are at risk for forming internal blood clots) or a disadvantage (as in patients who are candidates for surgery). This side effect makes aspirin unsuitable for some people who are in pain. Aspirin and other NSAIDs are also toxic in large doses and can cause damage to the liver and kidneys. People who take an overdose of these drugs sometimes do so by taking a combination of over-the-counter analgesics without recognizing the similarity of many of them (Winter, 1994).

Acetaminophen, another nonnarcotic analgesic, is not one of the NSAIDs. It has no anti-inflammatory properties but has a pain-relieving capability that is similar to aspirin but somewhat weaker. Under brand names such as Tylenol, acetaminophen has become the most frequently used drug for pain relief (DeNitto, 1993). Acetaminophen does not have the gastric side effects of aspirin, so people who cannot tolerate aspirin find it a good substitute. Despite the lack of gastric effects, acetaminophen is not harmless. Large quantities of acetaminophen can be fatal, but even nonlethal doses can do serious damage to the liver, especially when combined with alcohol (Australian Consumers' Association, 2002).

The most powerful analgesics are of the *opium* type. The extract of the opium poppy has been in use for at least 5,000 years, and its analgesic properties were known to the ancient Romans (Melzack & Wall, 1982). In 1803, morphine was isolated. Many synthetic compounds have structures and actions similar to those of morphine, and several neurotransmitters produce analgesia in the same way that the opiates do (Pert & Snyder, 1973). This mechanism is responsible for the pain-relieving effect of opiates and explains why these drugs can alleviate even strong pain.

Between 1996 and 2000, the market for prescription analgesic drugs tripled (Raymond et al., 2001). Much of this increase was for the drugs oxycodone and hydrocodone. Both are opiates with a potential for abuse, and physicians are wary about prescribing opiates in amounts that reduce intense pain; many patients fear the possibility of addiction and are reluctant to take sufficient doses to obtain relief. Thus, many acute pain patients and people with chronic cancer pain do not receive sufficient relief. This problem was not part of Barb's experience. Instead, Barb's physician continued for several years to prescribe opiates, which Barb (unwisely) combined with alcohol. This pattern of drug use posed problems, and Barb finally discontinued opiates as a way to manage her pain.

One procedure that has overcome the undermedication problem is a system of self-paced administration. Patients can activate a pump attached to their intravenous lines and deliver a dose of medication whenever they wish, within limits that are programmed into the delivery device (Siwek, 1997). Such systems began to appear in the late 1970s and have since gained wide acceptance. The initial fears that patients would overmedicate if allowed free access to self-administered opiate analgesics has proven unfounded. In fact, the average amount of medication consumed is often lower than with the traditional type of delivery. Because an intravenous line is necessary for this system of drug delivery, it is most common in postsurgical patients. The system is effective for children (Dunbar, 1995) as well as adults (Carpenter, 1997).

How realistic are the fears of drug abuse as a consequence of prescribed opiate drugs? Do patients become addicted while recovering from surgery? What about the dangers to patients with terminal illnesses? According to one study (Porter & Jick, 1980), the risk of addiction is less than 1%. During the late 1990s, prescriptions for opiate analgesics increased dramatically, and publicity about an epidemic of analgesic abuse fueled the fear that increased prescriptions for these drugs led to widespread addiction. A study on the topic (Joranson, Ryan, Gilson, & Dahl, 2000) indicated that, during the period in which opiate prescriptions showed an increase, opiate abuse showed a decrease.

The advantages of opiate drugs outweigh their dangers. No other type of drug produces more complete pain relief. However, their potential for abuse and their side effects make them more suitable for treating acute pain than for managing chronic pain. The opiate drugs remain an essential part of pain management for the most severe, acute injuries, for recovery from surgery, and for terminal illnesses.

Skin Stimulation As Melzack and Wall (1982) pointed out, skin stimulation is one of the activities that can "close the gate" that relays pain impulses. Several techniques furnish such stimulation, including electrical stimulation of nerves, acupuncture, acupressure, application of heat and cold, and massage. Manipulations of the skin to relieve pain have a long and successful history (Field, 1998).

Transcutaneous electrical nerve stimulation (TENS), however, has a short history, dating only to the early 1970s (Walsh, 1997). Electrical stimulation, which affects all nerves within about 4 centimeters of the skin's surface, can be accomplished by placing an electrode on the surface of the skin. Developed as a result of the gate control theory of pain, this type of stimulation should "close the gate" to incoming pain stimulation. The TENS system typically consists of electrodes that attach to the skin and are connected to a unit that supplies electrical stimulation. TENS has been used for both acute pain, such as postsurgical pain, and chronic pain, such as back pain. A variation on TENS is percutaneous electrical nerve stimulation (PENS), which involves insertion of needles that receive electrical stimulation (Ghoname et al., 1999). This approach combines the electrical stimulation of the skin with insertion of needles, the basis for acupuncture.

Acupuncture is an ancient Chinese form of analgesia that consists of inserting needles into specific points on the skin and continuously stimulating the needles (Loitman, 2000). The stimulation can be accomplished electrically or by twirling the needles. **Acupressure** is the application of pressure rather than needles to the points used in acupuncture. Inherent in the use of acupuncture and acupressure is a philosophy of the body and illness not accepted by many Westerners. Acupuncture has been used as an anesthetic for surgery, and some patients in China have undergone surgery with acupuncture as their only anesthetic.

The U.S. National Institutes of Health convened a panel that found acupuncture to be effective in the treatment of some conditions, including postoperative pain and low back pain (Morey, 1998). The British Medical Association's Board of Science and Education endorsed acupuncture as an effective treatment (Silvert, 2000). In addition to its effectiveness in managing several types of pain, acupuncture is also helpful in controlling nausea and not as likely to produce side effects as is drug therapy. About 10,000 licensed acupuncturist practice in the United States (Rosenfeld, 1998), and acupuncture is one of the most frequently sought alternative therapies in Great Britain (Silvert, 2000).

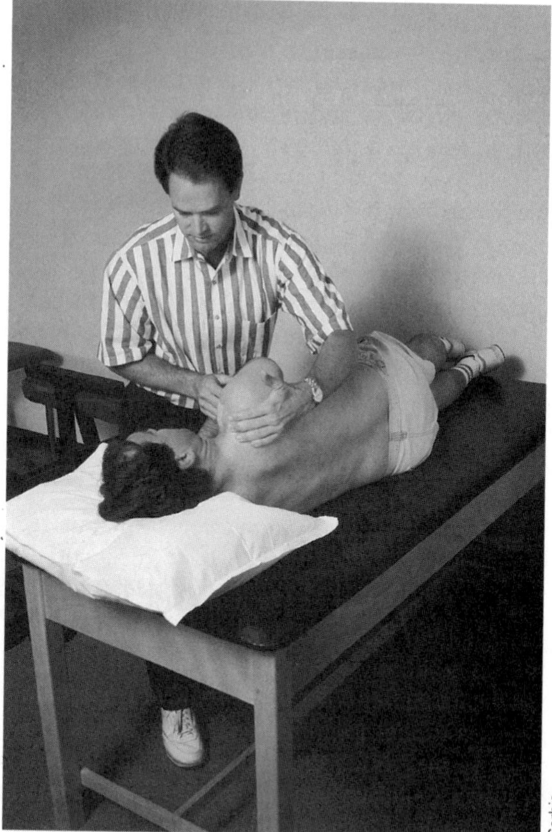
Corbis

Manipulating muscles is one of the alternative therapies that can be effective in relieving pain.

Considered a luxury a few years ago, massage is another alternative therapy now used to control pain (Bower, Rubik, Weiss, & Starr, 1997). Several different types of therapeutic massage can be applied to a variety of pain problems. Benefits come from direct manipulation of soft tissue as well as from relaxation and stress relief (Field, 1998). This therapy can decrease muscle tension, ease muscle pain, disperse fluid to decrease swelling, and relieve anxiety. Massage can be useful in easing not only muscle pain but also migraine, postoperative pain, and pain resulting from spinal cord injuries (Field, 1998).

In summary, a variety of therapies involve manipulation of the skin to relieve pain. A growing body of research indicates that these therapies can be effective, and an increasing number of people seek such therapies.

Surgery A third physical treatment for pain is surgery, which is most commonly used to alleviate chronic low back pain. For any pain syndrome, surgery is the most extreme approach and is usually recommended only when other means have failed. Some evidence (BenDebba et al., 2002) suggests that delaying surgery may not be the most successful approach: patients who have surgery immediately fare better than those who wait.

Surgery to control pain can occur at any level of the nervous system. The least radical surgery involves destroying the peripheral nerves close to the site of the pain or destroying the dorsal root ganglion, just outside the spinal cord (Carson, 1987). Both approaches involve loss of sensory function, which may be a more distressing sensation than pain. In addition, this type of surgery may not provide permanent relief.

Other possible sites for surgical intervention to control pain include the spinal cord and the brain itself. Severing spinal cord tracts and even destruction of brain sites were once approaches for pain control (Melzack & Wall, 1982), but advances in understanding pain physiology have allowed a more selective approach. One strategy involves destroying the neurons in the spinal cord that transmit pain by selectively destroying the neurons that have receptors for substance P, a pain neurotransmitter (Nichols et al., 1999).

Another approach involves stimulation of the spinal cord and brain to block pain messages (Stojanovic, 2001). Surgery is required for this approach, which involves implanting devices that can deliver electrical stimulation to either the spinal cord or brain. Activation of the system produces pain relief by activating neurons and by releasing neurotransmitters that block pain. This process does not destroy neural tissue; thus, it offers advantages over destruction of brain or spinal cord tissue. Spinal stimulation is a promising technique in controlling back pain (Van Buyten, Van Zundert, Vueghs, Vanduffel, 2001), but stimulation of brain centers is limited to a few patients (Stojanovic, 2001).

Limitations of Physical Treatments Drugs, skin stimulation, and surgery can all be effective means of controlling pain. However, all these physical treatments have limitations.

One limitation of opiate drugs is the tolerance and dependence they produce in patients. **Tolerance** is the body's decreased responsiveness to a drug. When tolerance occurs, larger and larger doses of a drug are required to bring about the same effect. **Dependence** occurs when the drug's removal produces withdrawal symptoms. Because opiates produce both tolerance and dependence, they are potentially dangerous and subject to abuse. As a result, health care professionals are reluctant to prescribe these drugs, and many pain patients are afraid to use them, even when they could relieve intractable pain (Donovan, 1989; Melzack & Wall, 1982).

Because of these concerns, patients are often undermedicated and do not receive sufficiently large or frequent doses of medication to produce relief. The average dose of opiate drugs is often below the therapeutic level, and many patients take only one-fourth to one-third of the medication that their physicians order (Donovan, 1989). Physicians also hold misconceptions about the use of opiates (Siwek, 1997), making their patients more likely to suffer needlessly as a result.

Whereas undermedication may be a problem for cancer pain patients, overmedication is often a problem for patients suffering from low back pain. Barb's physician continued to prescribe opiates for her back pain and referred her to a pain specialist only when Barb requested help in getting off the drugs. One team of investigators (Von Korff, Barlow, Cherkin, & Deyo, 1994) grouped primary care physicians into low, moderate, and high frequency of prescribing pain medication and bed rest for back pain patients. A 1- and 2-year follow-up found that patients who took less medication and who remained active did just as well as back pain patients who were told to take more medication and to rest. In addition, patients with the least medication were the most satisfied with their treatment. Moreover, patients whose physicians rated low in prescription of medication and bed rest spent only about half as much money on treatment as patients whose doctors rated high on medication and bed rest.

All forms of skin stimulation also have limitations. Transcutaneous electrical nerve stimulation (TENS), despite some promising early results, has not proven to provide long-term relief for chronic pain patients (Samanta & Beardsley, 1999). Barb's many treatments for pain included TENS, which she believes provided relief by distracting her from her pain rather than through the nerve stimulation. Like drug treatment, massage has effects that do not last beyond the treatments (Field, 1998) but produces significant benefits during the duration of treatments (Cherkin et al., 2001). In addition, massage is not suitable for arthritis or other pain problems related to joints (Bower et al., 1997). Acupuncture and acupressure do not work for everyone. Some people do not respond, some types of manipulation of the needles are more effective than others, and some placements for needles work better than other placements (Martindale, 2001).

Surgery has at least two limitations as a treatment for pain. First, it does not always repair damaged tissue, and second, it does not provide all patients with sufficient pain relief. Surgery is not a successful treatment for many people with chronic back pain (Deyo, 1998). Despite the popularity of surgical interventions, some back pain patients fail to obtain relief from surgery, and the pain returns for many who experienced initial relief, making this approach an expensive but unreliable approach to controlling this pain syndrome (Wetzel, Phillips, Aprill, Bernard, & LaRocca, 1997). Also, surgery has its own potential dangers and possibilities for complications. These limitations of surgery as a treatment for pain were reflected in Barb's experience. Her two back surgeries were only partially successful in repairing tissue damage and not very successful in controlling her pain.

In Summary

Prevention is the ideal way to approach pain, and several educational programs that train workers to avoid low back injuries have demonstrated some effectiveness. Early attention and treatment are important in preventing injury from developing into chronic pain, and continuing with regular activities is an effective approach in achieving this goal.

A variety of medical treatments for pain have demonstrated uses but also limitations. Analgesic drugs offer pain relief for acute pain and can be of use for chronic pain. These drugs include non-narcotic and opiate drugs. Non-narcotic drugs include aspirin, nonsteroidal anti-inflammatory drugs (NSAIDs), and acetaminophen. These drugs are effective in managing mild to moderate acute pain and have some uses in managing chronic pain. Opiates are effective in managing severe pain, but their tolerance and dependence properties pose problems for use by chronic pain patients. Indeed, both health care professionals and patients are so cautious concerning the use of opiates that physicians are reluctant to prescribe and patients may be reluctant to use these drugs in sufficient doses to achieve adequate pain control.

Other medical treatments include skin stimulation such as transcutaneous electrical nerve stimulation (TENS), acupuncture and acupressure, and massage. TENS shows few benefits for managing severe or chronic pain. Acupuncture, accupressure, and massage therapy are among the alternative approaches that are increasing in popularity and recognition, and each has benefits. Surgery can alter either peripheral nerves or the central nervous system. Surgical procedures are often done as a last resort in controlling chronic pain, and procedures that involve destruction of nerve pathways are often unsuccessful. Procedures that allow for stimulation of the spinal cord show more promise in pain management.

Answers

This chapter addressed five basic questions.

1. **How does the nervous system register pain?**
   Receptors near the skin's surface react to stimulation, and the nerve impulses from this stimulation relay the message to the spinal cord. The spinal cord includes laminae (layers) that modulate the sensory message and relay it toward the brain. The somatosensory cortex in the brain receives and interprets sensory input, and neurochemicals and the periaqueductal gray can also modulate the information and change the perception of pain.
2. **What is the meaning of pain?**
   Pain is difficult to define, but it can be classified as acute (resulting from specific injury and lasting less than 6 months), chronic (continuing beyond the time of healing), or prechronic (the critical stage between acute and chronic). The personal experience of pain is affected by situational and cultural factors as well as individual variation and learning history. The meaning of pain can also be understood through theories, the gate control theory of pain being the leading model. This view takes both physical and psychological factors into account in the experience of pain.
3. **What types of pain present the biggest problems?**
   The individual experience of pain can also be defined in terms of syndromes that classify chronic pain according to their symptoms. These syndromes include headache pain, low back pain, arthritic pain, cancer pain, and phantom limb pain; the first two are the most common sources of chronic pain and lead to the most time lost from work or school.
4. **How can pain be measured?**
   Pain can be measured physiologically by assessing muscle tension or autonomic arousal, but these measurements do not have high validity. Observations of pain-related behaviors (such as limping, grimacing, complaining) have some reliability and validity. Self-reports are the most common approach to pain measurement and include rating scales, pain questionnaires, and standardized psychological tests.
5. **How can pain be controlled?**
   Pain can be controlled by avoiding injury or by preventing acute pain from becoming chronic pain. Severals programs aimed at preventing low back pain through training workers safe lifting techniques have demonstrated some effectiveness, and research indicates that continuing with normal activities is an effective way to prevent acute back pain from becoming chronic.

   Analgesic drugs are used to control acute pain, but fears about addiction to opiates prevent their use for controlling chronic pain. In addition to drugs, other approaches to pain control exist. Skin stimulation techniques include transcutaneous electrical nerve stimulation (TENS), acupuncture, acupressure, and massage. TENS has limited effectiveness, but acupuncture and massage can be effective for some types of pain. Surgery is often used when other methods have failed, but this approach is unsuccessful for many people with chronic pain.

Suggested Readings

Fordyce, W. E. (1990). Learned pain: Pain as behavior. In J. J. Bonica (Ed.), *The management of pain* (2nd ed., pp. 291–299). Malvern, PA: Lea & Febiger. One of the foremost authorities on pain discusses the influence of learning on pain behavior. Fordyce points out that the consequences of pain behaviors are often reinforcing to the pain patient.

Gatchel, R. J. (1999). Perspectives on pain: A historical overview. In R. J. Gatchel & D. C. Turk (Eds.), *Psychosocial factors in pain: Critical perspectives* (pp. 3–17). New York; Guilford Press. Gatchel reviews pain from a historical point of view, considering views of pain from other cultures, past and present theories of pain, and the development of the current, multidisciplinary approach to pain and its management.

Melzack, R. (1999). Pain and stress: A new perspective. In R. J. Gatchel & D. C. Turk (Eds.), *Psychosocial factors in pain: Critical perspectives* (pp. 89–106). New York; Guilford Press. Melzack was one of the originators of the gate control theory of pain and subsequently expanded this theory into a more comprehensive view of pain and perception of the body. In this article, Melzack again expands his view of pain, this time focusing on the contribution of stress to pain perception.

Wall, P. (2000). *Pain: The science of suffering.* New York: Columbia University Press. Peter Wall, the other originator of the gate control theory of pain, tells about his extensive experience in trying to understand this phenomenon. He provides a nontechnical examination of the experience of pain, considering the cultural and individual factors that contribute.

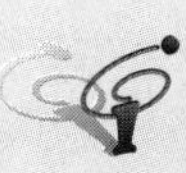

Search InfoTrac College Edition

Search these terms to learn more about topics in this chapter:

- Pain and physiology
- Brain imaging and pain
- Neurotransmitters and pain
- Cytokines and pain
- Pain and demographic aspects
- Gender and pain perception
- Gate control and pain
- Migraine headache
- Tension headache
- Cluster headache
- Low back pain and causes
- Low back pain and treatment
- Arthritis pain
- Pain and assessment and measurement
- Pain and alternative treatment
- Analgesics and pain treatment
- Acupuncture and effectiveness
- Massage and pain

8

Coping with Stress and Pain

The Stories of René and Barb—Continued

CHAPTER OUTLINE

Personal Resources that Influence Coping

Personal Coping Strategies

Techniques for Coping with Stress and Pain

QUESTIONS

This chapter focuses on three basic questions:

1. What personal resources influence coping?
2. What strategies do people use to cope with stress?
3. What techniques do health psychologists use to teach people to cope with stress and pain?

The Stories of René and Barb—Continued

Chapter 5 introduced René, a single parent juggling multiple roles, including student, worker, and parent. In Chapter 6, we saw that René believed that most of her physical symptoms were a result of the many stressors she experiences on a daily basis. In this chapter, we will look at some of the ways she has used to cope with her stress. None of these methods included medical or psychological techniques: all were strategies she seems to have discovered on her own.

In Chapter 7, we considered the case of Barb, a young woman experiencing chronic pain from a back injury incurred in an automobile crash. When surgery was not completely successful, Barb turned to a variety of physical therapies, including transcutaneous electrical nerve stimulation and opiate drugs. After none of these therapies were successful, Barb sought treatment from a pain specialist who prescribed such behavioral techniques as biofeedback and relaxation training. In this chapter, we reconsider the problems of René, Barb, and the millions of other Americans who suffer from elevated stress and chronic pain.

Personal Resources that Influence Coping

Stress and chronic pain are common conditions for humans—common but not normal. The normal tendency is toward health, and any inclination away from health sets up a state of "disease." People fight against distress and disease in a variety of ways. One way is through the immune system, the body's natural protection from invasion by foreign material, as discussed in Chapter 6. People sometimes adjust to pain through medical treatments, such as drugs and surgery, which are discussed in Chapter 7. Still other ways of seeking relief from stress and chronic pain include taking recreational drugs, overeating, abusing alcohol, smoking, and exercising. Exercising usually promotes health, but the other behaviors are ultimately unhealthy, and even exercise can be carried to an unhealthy extreme. The health-related effects of smoking, eating, drinking, and exercising are discussed in Chapters 13 through 16.

This chapter looks at several psychological strategies for coping with stress and chronic pain. These strategies are used in programs oriented toward helping people cope with stress and pain problems. Such formal programs offer help to people who seek treatment, but personal resources, such as social support, feelings of personal control, and personal hardiness can help nearly everyone to cope.

Social Support

During the 1980s, evidence began to emerge suggesting that people who receive social support from friends, family members, and health care providers tended to live longer and healthier lives than people who lacked support. A review led by James House (House, Landis, & Umberson, 1988) concluded that people who have high levels of social support are more able than other people to cope with stress and chronic pain. Indeed, lack of social support rivaled other well-established risk factors—such as cigarette smoking, high blood pressure, obesity, and sedentary lifestyle—as a risk for poor health. This section discusses the meaning of social support and suggests possible reasons why social support seems to protect against disease and death.

The Meaning of Social Support What is social support? Although social support has been widely researched, no single definition of the concept has emerged, and researchers have used dozens of inventories to measure social

CHECK YOUR HEALTH RISKS

Check the items that apply to you.

- ☐ 1. I live alone.
- ☐ 2. If I needed a favor, I would have a friend or relative to call.
- ☐ 3. I would like to talk to someone about my personal problems, but I don't have anyone I can trust to keep a secret.
- ☐ 4. I feel isolated from my family.
- ☐ 5. My job offers many opportunities to make meaningful decisions.
- ☐ 6. I believe strongly in fate—whatever will be will be.
- ☐ 7. I feel responsible for nearly everything that happens around me.
- ☐ 8. I have a lot of stress in my life, but I don't know how to reduce it.
- ☐ 9. When I feel a lot of stress, I have a confidant I can talk to.
- ☐ 10. I suffer from chronic pain and believe that pain-killing drugs are the only way to control it.
- ☐ 11. When I'm in pain, I find that alcohol is a good way to forget about it.
- ☐ 12. I suffer from back pain, and when it becomes too intense, I stay in bed for a couple of days.

Items 2, 5, and 9 are healthy means of coping with stress and pain, but each of the other items represents an attitude, situation, or behavior that may increase your risk for a stress-related illness or lead you to unhealthy or ineffective ways of coping with stress and pain. As you read this chapter, you will see the advantages of adopting other attitudes or behaviors to minimize your chances of developing a stress-related illness and to enhance your health and well-being.

support, many of them with questionable reliability and validity. The term **social support** refers to a variety of material and emotional supports a person receives from others. The related concepts of **social contacts** and **social network** are sometimes used interchangeably, and both refer to the number and types of people with whom one associates. The opposite of social contacts is **social isolation,** which refers to an absence of specific meaningful interpersonal relations. People with a high level of social support ordinarily have a broad social network and many social contacts; socially isolated people have neither.

Social support may be measured in terms of either the structure or the function of social relationships (Wills, 1998). Structural support includes the number of social relationships and the configuration of interconnections among these relationships. Functional support includes emotional support, information or advice, and companionship, as well as assistance with financial or material needs. These two measures are not strongly related to each other, but both are related to health.

The Link Between Social Support and Health

Stress researchers generally agree that a link exists between social support and health. That is, people who receive high levels of social support are usually healthier than those who do not. Evidence from studies done in California, Georgia, Michigan, and Scandinavia (Wills, 1998) demonstrates that people with higher levels of social support have lower rates of mortality and better health than people with lower levels of support.

The Alameda County Study (Berkman & Syme, 1979) was the first to establish a strong link between social support and longevity. This study indicated that lack of social support was as strongly linked to mortality as cigarette smoking and a sedentary lifestyle. Figure 8.1 shows that women in all age groups had lower mortality rates than men (as indicated by the height of the bar in the graph). However, for both men and

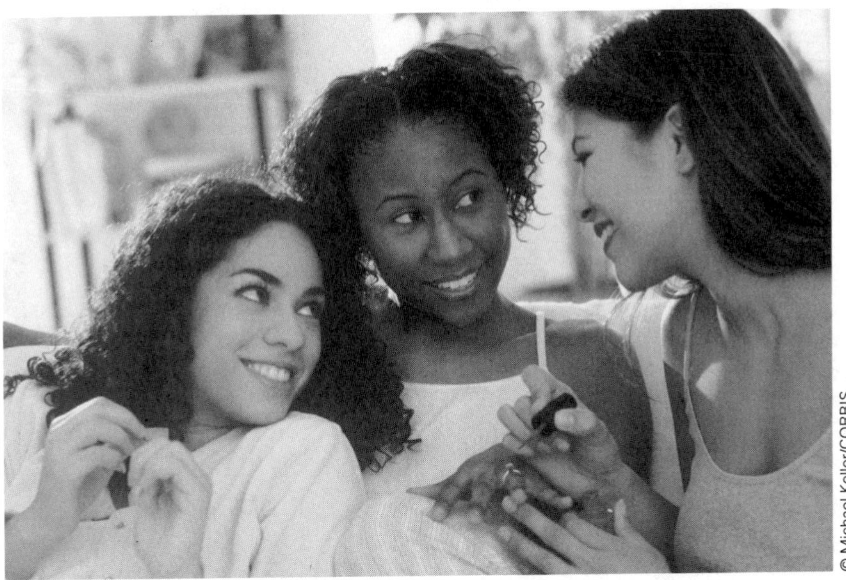
© Michael Keller/CORBIS

Emotional support and companionship are both beneficial to health.

women, as the number of social ties decreased, the death rate increased. In general, participants with the fewest social ties were two to four times more likely to die than participants with the most social ties. For men, this trend was most pronounced from age 50 to 59 (relative risk = 3.2), whereas for women, the trend was greatest at ages 30 to 49 (relative risk = 4.6).

Marriage, Gender, Ethnicity, and Social Support Marriage (or at least happy marriage) would seem to provide excellent social support for both partners, but the benefits of marriage are not equal for women and men. Marriage benefits men more than women (Kiecolt-Glaser & Newton, 2001). The reason for men's advantage is not clear, but both direct and indirect influences are likely. Marital conflict is a major source of stress, and women may have stronger physiological reactions to marital stress than do men. This hypothesis suggests the possibility that women suffer more direct damage to their bodies as a consequence of marital conflict. In addition to this indirect damage, women may be more vulnerable to indirect influences, because their role as caregivers puts them in the position of providing more care than they receive, especially for women who ignore their own health to take care of spouse and children. For older people, marriage may not be as important as having a confidant. A survey of people age 65 and older (Oxman, Berkman, Kasl, Freeman, & Barrett, 1992) showed that both men and women who never had a confidant were more likely to become depressed than were those who had never been married. Also, long-standing confidants provided more social support than newly acquired confidants.

The health benefits of having a wife would suggest that husbands would be more affected by the death of their spouse than would wives. Indeed, research (Martikainen & Valkomen, 1996) indicates that death of a spouse increased mortality risk for the surviving spouse, but men were at greater risk than women. The risk was higher not only for men but also for younger persons of either gender. In addition, the risk was higher during the 6 months following the spouse's death. Death from heart disease and cancer increased, but the greatest mortality risks were

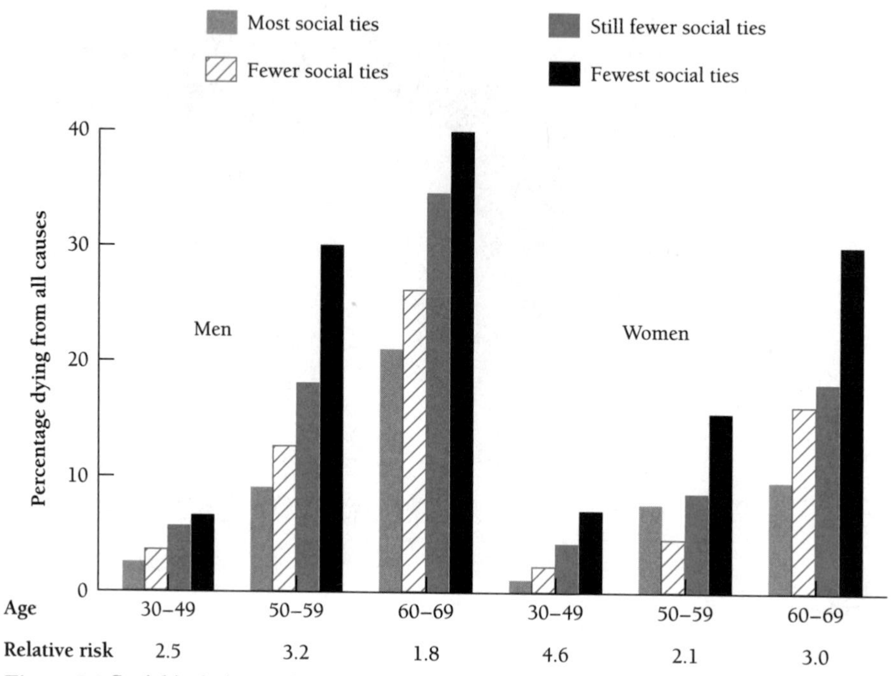

Figure 8.1 Social isolation and 9-year mortality in Alameda County, California, 1965–1974

Source: From "Social Networks, Host Resistance, and Mortality: A Nine-Year Follow-up of Alameda County Residents," by L. F. Berkman & S. L. Syme, 1979, American Journal of Epidemiology, 109, *p. 190. Copyright © 1979 by the Johns Hopkins University School of Hygiene and Public Health. Reprinted by permission of the publisher and the senior author.*

from accidental and violent deaths, especially suicide. Again, these risks may relate to typical gender roles in which men depend on their wives for support, but women cultivate a larger social network of family members and friends and are thus more likely to receive support after the death of a husband.

Although men gain more from marriage, women gain more from social support, at least up to a point. In the Alameda County Study (Berkman & Syme, 1979), women with few social ties had a substantially higher relative risk for mortality than men (see Figure 8.1). However, when women have a great many social contacts, they lose their advantage over men and may even have a disadvantage (Orth-Gomér, 1998). A possible explanation for this finding is that women with many social contacts are overextended, receiving demands for support that may add to rather than detract from their stress.

Does ethnic background play a role in social support? African American and Hispanic American families have traditions of close extended family relationships that can provide stronger social support than those of many European American families. Analyses of African American families (Neighbors, 1997) and Mexican American (Phillips, Torres de Ardon, Komnenich, Killeen, & Rusinak, 2000) families indicated that these relationships can be sources of stress as well as support. Indeed, the people who provide support at one time are those who cause problems at other times.

In the United States, older women of all ethnic groups have more extensive social networks than their male counterparts (Barker, Morrow & Mitteness, 1998; Berkman, 1986; Phillips et al., 2000), but the size of these social networks differs little among various ethnic groups (Pugliese & Shook, 1998). Lisa Berkman (1986) found that European American men not only had smaller social networks, but they used social support less than others. Berkman also found an interaction among gender, ethnicity, and employment. European American men who were employed tended to have smaller social networks than those who were not employed, but employment was not a factor in network size for men from other ethnic groups or for women. This suggests that the structure and use of social networks are complex and influenced by a number of factors, including marriage, gender, ethnicity, and employment.

How Does Social Support Contribute to Health? In Chapter 6, we examined the link between stress and illness. If stress causes illness, then social support may offer some buffer against stress-related illnesses. What does social support provide that is helpful? What is stressful, even life threatening, about social isolation? At least three explanations are possible for the health benefits of a large social support system (Wills, 1998).

First, highly stressed individuals may benefit from a strong support network that encourages them to stop smoking, begin exercising. and start healthy eating practices. People who are isolated are less likely to have friends and acquaintances who encourage them to protect their health or who insist that they go to the doctor when they are sick. However, persistent and overt attempts to offer social support may have negative consequences. For example, insisting that highly hostile people engage in healthy behaviors may not be wise. One study (Allen, Markovitz, Jacobs, & Knox, 2001) found that, whereas social support is generally helpful in increasing physical activity, encouraging hostile men to exercise is not an effective strategy. Also, social support need not be obvious to be beneficial. Partners who received "invisible," that is, subtle and discreet, social support were helped more than partners who received obvious support (Bolger, Zuckerman, & Kessler, 2000).

A second possibility is through appraisal and coping. When people know that they have a large network of friends, they may gain confidence in their ability to handle stressful situations, so when they experience stress, they may appraise the stressor as less threatening than people who have fewer coping resources (Wills, 1998). Indeed, knowledge of the availability of support (even if that support is not used) can reduce the magnitude of the stress response (Uchino & Garvey, 1997). Social support may also provide more knowledge about coping strategies, thus giving people with more sources of support useful information on solving problems and implementing solutions.

A third explanation is that social support may alter the physiological responses to stress (Chesney & Darbes, 1998; Kiecolt-Glaser & Newton, 2001). This view is referred to as the *buffering hypothesis,* which suggests that social support lessens or eliminates the harmful effects of stress and therefore protects against disease and death. Another view of this explanation is that people who have little social support may react more strongly to stress, showing higher levels of neurohormones and more physical damage than people with strong social support networks. A study of the effects of religious involvement (Schnittker, 2001) supported the stress-buffering hypothesis. In this study, people who sought spiritual help and who held religion as an important experience in their lives received significant stress-buffering effects against depression arising from multiple negative events. (For the potential health benefits of religious involvement, see the Would You Believe . . . ? box "Religious Involvement May Lengthen Your Life.")

Mobilizing Social Support If social support provides health advantages, can people improve their social support through specific efforts? Perhaps so, but increasing social support is not as easy as increasing the number of social contacts. For example, people who are high in hostility may profit from more social support, but they receive less than those who are lower in hostility (Allen et al., 2001). Even if hostile people—those who are unpleasant and difficult to befriend—could

WOULD YOU BELIEVE

Religious Involvement May Lengthen Your Life

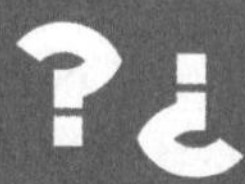

Beginning with Emile Durkheim (1912/1954) nearly a century ago, social scientists have pondered and debated the health benefits of religious involvement. When researchers began to study this issue, they generally produced mixed results; some studies found that people involved with religion were both physically and psychologically sicker than other people, whereas other studies reported opposite results. In the 1960s, Gordon Allport (1966) offered a possible explanation for this paradox. He suggested two distinctive types of churchgoers—people with an extrinsic religious orientation and those with an intrinsic religious orientation. People with an extrinsic orientation are not deeply religious but see attendance at religious functions as a means to an end, for example a way of meeting people. In contrast, people with an intrinsic orientation have deeply felt religious beliefs and regard religion as a central part of their lives. They have an internalized creed and follow it fully. Allport further suggested that researchers must consider these two distinct religious orientations, otherwise they are quite likely to get mixed results. For example, his own research showed that people with an extrinsic religious orientation are quite prejudiced and narrow minded, whereas those with an intrinsic orientation have very little prejudice.

More recently, researchers have looked at the relationship between religious involvement and health consequences. Jason Schnittker (2001) examined three types of religious involvement: (1) attendance at religious services, (2) religious salience; that is, the importance of religion in one's life, and (3) spiritual help seeking. Using a large U.S. sample of participants, Schnittker found that attendance at religious services by itself was not related to levels of depression. He also found a U-shaped effect of religious salience on depression, which may have resulted from a dichotomy between an extrinsic religious orientation and an intrinsic orientation. Finally, Schnittker found that people who sought spiritual guidance tended to have low levels of depression. These findings are consistent with Allport's assumptions, but they do not prove that an intrinsic religious orientation leads to lower levels of depression.

A major meta-analytic study by Michael McCullough and his associates (McCullough, Hoyt, Larson, Koenig, & Thoresen, 2000) examined previous studies that had found religious involvement to be related to lower rates of hypertension, heart disease, stroke, and cancer. Such a relationship, of course, does not establish a causal relationship between religious involvement and lower rates of death. The link between religion and health could just as well be due to psychosocial resources provided by religious involvement. For example, religious involvement is likely to expand one's circle of friends and thus increase the social support these friends provide.

McCullough et al. were interested in a different question. Does involvement in religion per se decrease mortality? In their analysis, they gave more weight to the most reliable studies and those that had controlled for age, ethnicity, gender, health, social support, psychological well-being, and other possible confounders. Results of their meta-analysis revealed a small but highly reliable association between religious involvement and lower rates of all-cause mortality; that is, people high in religious involvement were somewhat more likely to be alive at follow-up than were people low in religious involvement. These findings indicate that religious activity—independent of the social support it provides—is associated with a slight increase in one's span of life.

increase the number of their social contacts, they may not increase their social support.

One hint concerning increased social support comes from the gender difference in support: women tend to have larger and more active support networks than men. The reason for this difference can be seen in women's friendship style, which tends to rely on emotional sharing, cooperation, and positive nonverbal signals (Argyle, 1992). Indeed, both men and women prefer to have women as confidants, but men are less likely than women to have a female confidant, whereas women are more likely to be part of a support network that is comprised mostly of women.

Are people who are lacking in social support destined to remain so? Two strategies exist to improve social support (Gottlieb, 1996). One strategy involves enhancing existing support sources. This might include seeking the help of a health care professional, becoming more self-disclosing, or supporting others who are in need of support.

The second strategy is to join a support group, that is, a social network consisting of people with similar stressful circumstances, such as those caring for an Alzheimer's disease patient. Meeting with others in similar circumstances can give people many valuable experiences, including emotional support, information, and practical help. A huge array of support groups exists to serve people with a variety of conditions and to help their families cope.

Personal Control

A second factor that may affect a person's ability to cope with stressful life events is a feeling of personal control. Many investigators believe that people who feel that they have some control over the events of their lives are better able to cope with stress than are people who feel that their lives are determined by forces outside themselves. René felt that her hectic life was beyond her control and that there was little she could do to gain control of her life.

Research in the area of personal control was given an impetus in 1966 when Julian Rotter published a scale for measuring internal and external control of reinforcement. Rotter hypothesized that people can be placed along a continuum according to the extent to which they believe they are in control of the important events in their lives. Those who believe they control their own lives score in the direction of *internal locus of control,* whereas those people who believe that luck, fate, or the acts of others are the determinants of their lives score high on *external locus of control.*

Psychologists have applied the locus of control concept to health problems in order to learn if a sense of personal control affects people's health. A classic example of the effects of personal control was reported by Ellen Langer and Judith Rodin (1976) in a study that demonstrated the importance of a sense of personal control for health. These researchers studied older nursing home residents, some of whom were encouraged to assume more responsibility and control over their daily lives and some of whom had decisions made for them. The type of control was fairly minor: rearranging their furniture, choosing when and with whom to visit in the home, deciding what leisure activities to pursue, and so on. In addition, these residents were offered a small growing plant, which they were free to accept or reject and to care for as they wished. A comparison group of residents received information that emphasized the responsibility of the nursing staff, and each of them also received a plant.

The two groups of residents were approximately equal in age, gender, physical and psychological health, and prior socioeconomic status. The main difference was in the amount of control they had, and that factor made a substantial difference in health. Residents in the responsibility-induced group were happier, more active and more alert; they had a higher level of general well-being. In just 3 weeks, most of the comparison group (71%) had become more debilitated, whereas nearly all the responsibility-induced group (93%) showed some overall mental and physical improvement.

An 18-month follow-up of these same residents (Rodin & Langer, 1977) showed that residents in the original responsibility-induced group retained their advantage. They were more healthy, active, sociable, vigorous, and self-initiating than residents in the original comparison group. In addition, the mortality rate in the original responsibility-induced group was lower than expected and also lower than that for the original comparison group. The significance of these findings is obvious: older people (and perhaps others as well) seem to thrive on personal control and responsibility.

How much control does a person need in order to feel in control? The Langer and Rodin studies suggest that control over relatively minor matters can have major consequences in the life of the individual. People need to be able to make choices and to assume responsibility for these choices.

Personal Hardiness

Are psychologically healthy people buffered against the kind of stress that might lead to disease in less healthy individuals? Do these psychologically hardy individuals have a greater ability to cope with harmful stress than do other individuals? In 1977, Suzanne Kobasa and her mentor Salvatore Maddi proposed the notion of the hardy personality as an explanation for why stress relates to disease in some people but not others. The **hardy personality model** grew out of existential personality theory, which emphasizes the idea that authentic, psychologically healthy people do not passively accept their fate, but rather they seize and maintain control of their life.

Kobasa and Maddi (1977) hypothesized that hardiness buffers the harmful effects of stress and thus protects the hardy personality from stress-related illness. In her original study, Kobasa (1979) looked at middle-aged, mostly White Protestant executives who had filled out Holmes and Rahe's (1967) Social Readjustment Rating Scale. She followed these middle- and upper-level managers for 3 years and found that some of them were able to withstand stress and not succumb to disease. Kobasa used the term *hardiness* to describe these people. Hardy executives differed from those who became sick in three important ways. First, they expressed a stronger sense of *commitment* to self; second, they demonstrated an internal locus of *control* over their lives; and third, they were more likely to view necessary readjustments as a *challenge* rather than a stress. These three factors—commitment, control, and challenge—separated the hardy executives from those who became sick, even though both groups experienced equal amounts of stress. Executives who became sick were those who lacked purpose in life, felt powerless, had a sense of alienation from self, lacked vigor, and believed that their lives were beyond their personal control. These findings suggest that hardiness may help people cope with the harmful effects of stress.

To measure the validity of the hardiness concept, a number of researchers have constructed scales to measure this concept (Kobasa, Maddi, & Kahn, 1982; Maddi, 1990). Research findings on the health-protective power of hardiness have been mixed. In general, those studies that used college students have failed to support the model, whereas those that included older employees have found that commitment, control, and challenge—the essence of the hardiness construct—can provide a buffer against job-related stress. For example, one recent study (Soderstrom, Dolbier, Leiferman, & Steinhardt, 2000) found that hardiness related to coping strategies, perceived stress, and symptoms of illness for middle-aged men and women but not for introductory psychology students. A later report from this same research team (Dolbier et al., 2001) indicated that high-hardy employees had stronger immune responses than low-hardy individuals. In addition, other studies have found that high-hardy health care workers, compared with those who scored low on hardiness, showed less stress and lower levels of exhaustion and job burnout (Constantini, Solano, Di-Napoli, & Bosco, 1997; Duquette, Kerouac, Sandhu, Ducharme, & Saulnier, 1995; Sciacchitano, Goldstein, & DiPlacido, 2001). However, another study of health care professionals (Rowe, 1997) found that hardiness—independent of temperament and coping skills—was only weakly associated with burnout.

The notion that some people possess personal traits that help protect them against the harmful effects of stress is an appealing one. Nevertheless, Kobasa's conception of hardiness has been widely criticized. Some researchers (Benishek, 1996) have suggested the three factors of commitment, control, and challenge do not constitute the essence of hardiness, and others (Funk, 1992) have contended that *neuroticism,* or general maladjustment, may account for any relationship between hardiness and self-reports of illness; that is, neuroticism overlaps substantially with measures of hardiness and probably accounts for most of the correlation between hardiness scores and subsequent illness.

However, Kobasa (who has also published under the names S. C. Ouellette and S. C. Ouellette Kobasa) has pointed out that many of the inconsistent findings on hardiness are the result of different measures of the hardy personality (Ouellette, 1993; Ouellette & DiPlacido, 2001). She contended that many investigators have attempted to extend the concept to inappropriate populations—for example, college undergraduates. Hardiness, with its origins embedded in existential philosophy and psychology, is probably most applicable to people who are searching for a sense of meaning or purpose in life, who are motivated by responsibility and freedom, who view subjective experience as reality, and who believe that they are capable of significantly shaping society.

In Summary

Humans have a natural tendency toward health and away from distress, disease, and pain. When "diseases" become part of our lives, we attempt to cope with them in order to restore our health. Some attempts at coping, such as self-medication with alcohol and drugs, have long-term disadvantages rather than benefits, but other methods of coping provide ways to manage these problems.

Some people cope successfully with stress and chronic pain because they possess sufficient personal resources such as social support, a strong feeling of personal control, and hardy personality. Social support, defined as the emotional quality of one's social contacts, is inversely related to disease and death. In general, people with high levels of social support, compared to those with low levels, are only about half as likely to die within a designated period of time. These findings are most pronounced for European American men, but other groups also show some benefit from a network of quality relationships. People with adequate social support probably receive more encouragement and advice regarding good health practices, have advantages in coping skills, and may react less strongly to stress than people who are socially isolated. All of these factors can contribute to greater health and lower mortality.

Adequate feelings of personal control also seem to enable people to cope better with stress and illness. People who believe that their lives are controlled by fate or outside forces have greater difficulty changing health-related behaviors than do those who believe that the locus of control resides with themselves. The classic study by Langer and Rodin (1976) demonstrated that when people are allowed to assume even small amounts of personal control and responsibility, they seem to live longer and healthier lives.

People who have high personal hardiness are probably better able to cope with stress than are people with low hardiness scores. Research on the concept of hardiness has yielded mixed results, but this may be a result of researchers having inadequate measures of personal hardiness and/or using inappropriate participants, such as young college students. Those studies that looked at older employees generally have confirmed the notion that personal hardiness buffers against stress-related illness and reduces job burnout, especially among health care workers.

Personal Coping Strategies

People experience an almost constant attempt to manage the problems and stresses of their lives, and most of these attempts may be considered as coping (Coyne & Racioppo, 2000). However, the term **coping** is usually applied to strategies that individuals use to manage the distressing problems and emotions in their lives. The term first appeared in psychology research in the 1960s, and the 1970s were a time of explosive growth on the topic. Researchers have conducted thousands of studies on coping, exploring the personal and situational characteristics as well as the effectiveness of various coping strategies.

As the previous section described, personal factors such as a feeling of control, social support, and hardiness affect people's coping resources and their appraisal of stressful situations. As Richard Lazarus and Susan Folkman (1984) emphasized, appraisal is a critical factor in individuals' approaches to dealing with stress. People who view a situation as a threat will behave differently than people who see the situation as a challenge.

Coping strategies can be categorized in many ways, but Folkman and Lazarus's (1980) conceptualization of coping strategies as emotion focused or problem focused has been influential. **Problem-focused coping** is aimed at changing the source of the stress, whereas **emotion-focused coping** is oriented toward managing the emotions that accompany the perception of stress. Several different strategies exist within each of these categories. For example, taking action to try to get rid of the problem in a problem-focused strategy, but so is making a plan of the steps to take or asking someone to help you in solving the problem. Getting upset and venting emotions is clearly emotion focused, but seeking the company of friends or family for comfort and reassurance and refusing to accept the situation are also oriented toward managing the negative emotions associated with stress.

If an upcoming exam is a source of stress, a problem-focused way to cope is to make (and follow) a plan to devote time to studying. Calling up a friend and complaining about the test or going out to a movie might help manage the distress would be emotion-focused ways of coping. The problem-focused strategy clearly sounds like a better choice, and problem-focused strategies are often more effective than emotion-focused approaches. However, in some situations, emotion-focused coping can be effective. For example, if a person needs to keep a job with a supervisor who is unpleasant, finding ways to deal with the emotional aspects of the situation can be effective in managing this stress, whereas confronting the supervisor to discuss the problem may make the situation worse. René generally used emotion-focused strategies to cope with stress. After finishing her final class about 1:00 P.M., she headed to the recreation complex where she swam, lifted weights, and ran around the indoor track. René found that this heavy schedule of physical activity reduced her stress level—while she worked out. Unfortunately, physical activity was merely a diversion; once she finished, she immediately returned to thinking about her children, job, and academic work.

The differences in problem-focused and emotion-focused coping evoke stereotypical images of men and women—"emotional" women and "rational" men. However, research has failed to substantiate these gender stereotypes (Sigmon, Stanton, & Snyder, 1995). Some stress situations produced differences in coping strategies in women and men, but these differences failed to fall into the emotion- versus problem-focused categories. Indeed, men and women used problem-focused coping equally often. Both used emotion-focused coping strategies but different ones: women tended to seek social support, and men avoided the situation. These results suggest that people use a variety of strategies to manage stress and that the gender differences do not match the stereotypes.

Later research (Tennen, Afflect, Armeli, & Carney, 2000) confirmed the use of both types of coping strategies, suggesting that the same individuals use both types of coping. This longitudinal study followed rheumatoid arthritis patients, tracking their use of emotion-focused and problem-focused coping. A pattern of coping emerged that reflected problem-focused coping as a first choice. When these efforts were unsuccessful, emotion-focused strategies followed.

Susan Folkman and Judith Moskowitz (2000) also explored the intersection of problem- and emotion-focused coping, emphasizing the value of gaining positive emotions as a result of coping. They studied people coping with AIDS, both as caregivers and as patients, and found that people attempt to derive meaning from their distress and to experience positive emotion even in the face of enormous stress. Emotion-focused coping is an obvious way to do so, but Folkman and Moskowitz also discovered that successful problem-focused coping engenders positive emotion. Therefore, the relationship between these two types of coping is complex, and the choice of one strategy does not prohibit the use of the other.

A meta-analysis of the effects of coping strategies on psychological and physical health (Penley, Tomaka, & Wiebe, 2002) revealed benefits for some coping strategies and risks for some others. However, the relationships between coping strategies and health outcomes were moderated by the type of stressor and whether the impact was on psychological or physical health. In general, problem-focused coping showed positive associations with good health, whereas emotion-focused coping strategies tended to show negative associations. Use of problem solving strategies showed the strongest positive relationship to both psychological and physical health for a variety of stressors. The negative effects of emotion-focused coping tended to relate to psychological rather than physical health. For example, people who used avoidance-oriented coping, such as eating more, drinking, sleeping, or using drugs, reported poorer overall health. Therefore, choice of coping strategy may have effects for both psychological and physical health.

Thus, people attempt to manage stressful situations, choosing a way to try to cope that focuses on the problem. If those efforts are successful, they also eliminate some of the distress they experience, which manages their emotional distress. If the problem-focused strategy does not work, then they may turn to another problem-focused strategy or to an emotion-focused approach that allows them to manage their distress. When people exhaust their personal strategies for coping, they may choose to turn to therapies that teach them additional coping skills.

Techniques for Coping with Stress and Pain

People who seek professional assistance in coping with stress and pain are typically individuals whose personal strategies have proven ineffective in managing their problems. Psychologists have been prominent in devising therapies that teach people how to improve their coping. Psychological interventions for stress and pain management include relaxation training, hypnotic techniques, biofeedback, behavior modification, cognitive therapy, and various combinations of these techniques—that is, multimodal approaches (Turk, 2001).

Relaxation Training

Relaxation training is perhaps the simplest and easiest to use of all psychological interventions, and relaxation may be the key ingredient in other types of therapeutic techniques for coping with stress and pain.

What Is Relaxation Training? During the 1930s, Edmond Jacobson (1938) discussed a type of relaxation he called *progressive muscle relaxation.* With this procedure, patients first receive a rationale for the procedure, including an explanation that their present tension is mostly a physical state resulting from tense muscles. While reclining in a comfortable chair, often with eyes closed and with no distracting lights or sounds, patients first breathe deeply and exhale slowly. After this, the series of deep muscle relaxation exercises begins, a process described in the box, Becoming Healthier.

Once patients learn the relaxation technique, they may practice independently at home. If independent practice is too difficult, prerecorded audiotapes are available that allow patients to listen to the soothing voice of a professional instructor without returning to the clinic. Length of relaxation training programs varies, but 6 to 8 weeks and about 10 sessions with an instructor are usually sufficient to allow patients to easily and independently enter a state of deep relaxation (Blanchard & Andrasik, 1985).

Another frequently used relaxation technique is *meditative relaxation,* developed by Herbert Benson and his colleagues (Benson, 1975; Benson, Beary, & Carol, 1974). This approach derives from various religious meditative practices, but as used by psychologists, it has no religious connotations. Bensonian relaxation combines muscle relaxation with a quiet environment, comfortable position, repetitive sound, and passive attitude. Participants usually sit with eyes closed and muscles relaxed. They then focus attention on their breathing and repeat silently a sound, such as "om" or "one" with each breath for about 20 minutes. Repetition of the single word prevents distracting thoughts and sustains muscle relaxation. Meditation requires a conscious motivation to focus attention on a single thought or image along with effort not to be distracted by other thoughts.

Mindfulness meditation is a third type of meditation, one that has its roots in ancient Buddhist practice. Nevertheless, mindfulness mediation is applicable to anyone suffering from stress, anxiety, or pain (Kabat-Zinn, 1993). In mindfulness meditation, people do not try to ignore unpleasant thoughts or sensations by focusing on their breathing or on a single sound. Rather, they take the opposite approach, focusing on any thoughts or sensations as they occur. However, they should observe these thoughts nonjudgmentally. By noting thoughts objectively, without censoring or editing them, people can gain insight into how they see the world and what motivates them.

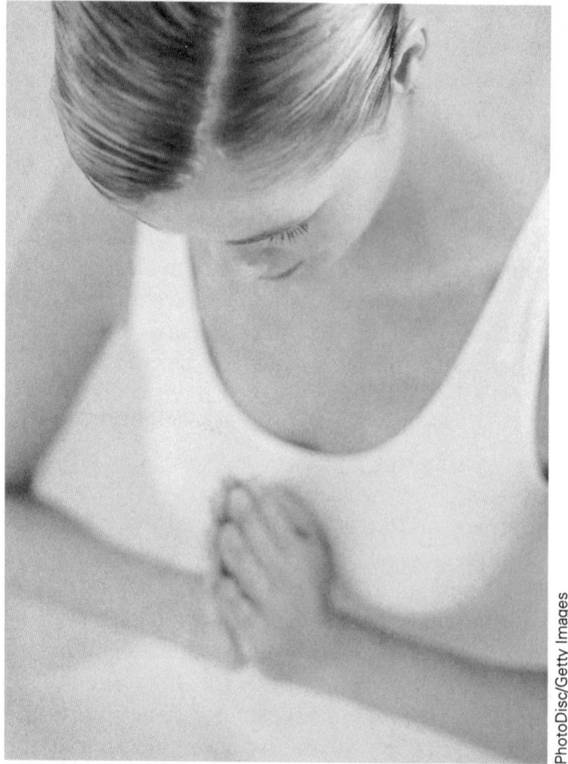

PhotoDisc/Getty Images

Meditation is one relaxation technique that can help people cope with a variety of stress-related problems.

Guided imagery has some elements in common with meditative relaxation, but it also has important differences. In guided imagery, patients conjure up a calm, peaceful image such as the repetitive rhythmic roar of an ocean or the quiet beauty of a pastoral scene. Patients then concentrate on that image for the duration of a painful or anxiety-filled situation. The assumption underlying guided imagery is that a person cannot concentrate on more than one thing at a time. Therefore, a patient must imagine an especially powerful or delightful scene—one so pleasant or powerful that it averts attention from the painful experience.

BECOMING HEALTHIER

Progressive muscle relaxation is a technique that you may be able to use to cope with stress and pain. Although some people may need the help of a trained therapist to master this approach, others are able to train themselves. To learn progressive muscle relaxation, recline in a comfortable chair in a room with no distractions. You may wish to remove your shoes and either dim the lights or close your eyes to enhance relaxation. Next, breathe deeply and exhale slowly. Repeat this deep breathing exercise several times until you begin to feel your body becoming more and more relaxed. The next step is to select a muscle group (for example, your left hand) and deliberately tense that group of muscles. If you begin with your hand, make a fist and squeeze the fingers into your hand as hard as you can. Hold that tension for about 10 seconds and then slowly release the tension, concentrating on the relaxing, soothing sensations in your hand as the tension gradually drains away. Once the left hand is relaxed, shift to the right hand and repeat the procedure, while keeping your left hand as relaxed as possible. After both hands are relaxed, go through the same tensing and relaxing sequence progressively with other muscle groups, including the arms, shoulders, neck, mouth, tongue, forehead, eyes, toes, feet, calves, thighs, back, and stomach. Then repeat the deep breathing exercises until you achieve a complete feeling of relaxation. Focus on the enjoyable sensation of relaxation, restricting your attention to the pleasant internal events and away from irritating external sources of pain or stress. You will probably need to practice this procedure several times to learn to quickly place your body into a state of deep relaxation.

How Effective Is Relaxation Training? Like other psychological interventions, relaxation can be regarded as effective only if it proves more powerful than a control situation, or placebo. Research generally indicates that relaxation techniques are more effective than placebos. In addition, relaxation is at least equal to biofeedback in reducing pain and alleviating stress, and it may be an essential part of both biofeedback and hypnotic therapies.

Relaxation techniques have been used successfully to treat both tension and migraine headaches. A meta-analysis of research on migraine headache in children (Hermann, Kim, & Blanchard, 1995) found that when progressive muscle relaxation was added to thermal biofeedback, the combination was superior to psychological and drug placebos and more effective than medication. A later study (Sartory, Muller, & Pothmann 1998) found that stress management and relaxation training were more effective than drugs in reducing both the frequency and the intensity of migraine headaches in children, and the effects remained after an 8-month follow-up.

Although relaxation procedures are effective in reducing the frequency and intensity of migraine headaches, their most successful use is with tension headache (Lehrer, Carr, Sargunaraj, & Woolfolk, 1994; Syrjala & Chapman, 1984). Relaxation training alone can significantly reduce a substantial number of tension headaches, is more effective than a placebo, and is at least equal to biofeedback in decreasing tension headache pain.

Progressive muscle relaxation can also be an effective treatment for such stress-related disorders as depression, hypertension, low back pain, and the stressful effects of cancer chemotherapy as well as reducing both tension and migraine headache. A meta-analysis of studies (Carlson & Hoyle, 1993) found that an abbreviated form of progressive muscle relaxation was generally helpful in coping with each of these disorders, although the effect size varied substantially from study to study. However, progressive relaxation training is no panacea for pain reduction. Perhaps as many as 50% of tension headache patients do not experience significant relief through relaxation. For this reason, Edward Blanchard and Frank Andrasik (1985) viewed relaxation as a necessary first step in a pain management program, but one that may not be effective for all pain sufferers.

Can listening to classical music bring about as much relaxation as progressive muscle relaxation? To answer this question, Peter Scheufele (2000) exposed male participants to a simple but stressful task—crossing out all the sixes on a page with several hundred digits. After 15 minutes of the stressor test, participants received one of four conditions—progressive muscle relaxation, classical music by Mozart, attention control, or silence control. Participants in the progressive relaxation group had the highest relaxation scores, followed by the music group and the two control groups. These results suggest that listening to classical music can help reduce stress, but progressive muscle relaxation may be a better choice.

Meditation is a second form of relaxation used to help people to cope with pain, stress, and anxiety. Jon Kabat-Zinn and his colleagues (Kabat-Zinn et al., 1992) studied the effectiveness of mindfulness meditation on chronic pain patients and found it to be more effective than a traditional intervention that included physical therapy, analgesics, and antidepressants. Patients decreased their use of pain medications, improved their activity levels, and increased their feelings of self-esteem. Kabat-Zinn and colleagues (Miller, Fletcher, & Kabat-Zinn, 1995) later found a meditation-based stress-reduction program to be effective for treating anxiety disorders. Patients taught meditation techniques had significant reductions in anxiety and depression, and they maintained these gains at a 3-year follow-up.

What is the effective ingredient in mindfulness meditation? Some evidence (Astin, 1997) suggests that meditation may be simply a powerful cognitive behavioral strategy for changing the way people respond to stressful life events. In any event, mindfulness meditation can be considered as an effective therapy for at least some stress-related disorders, and it may be at least as powerful as any other behavioral intervention.

A third relaxation strategy is guided imagery. A growing number of studies have demonstrated the effectiveness of guided imagery in coping with pain, anxiety, and stress. This approach is effective for reducing postoperative pain (Lambert, 1996) and the anxiety and pain of cancer surgery (Tusek, Church, & Fazio, 1997). Other studies have found that guided imagery is more effective than either a therapist-attention group or a no-treatment control group in reducing anxiety and nausea both during and after chemotherapy (Lyles, Burish, Krozely, & Oldham, 1982). Also, guided imagery can help severely burned patients cope with pain (Achterberg, Kenner, & Lawlis, 1988), and it is superior to biofeedback in treating migraine headache (Ilacqua, 1994). These studies indicate that guided imagery is at least as effective as other forms of relaxation therapy in coping with stress, pain, and anxiety.

Barb learned relaxation as part of her pain program and continues to practice relaxation for her chronic pain. She was amazed at how difficult it was to relax and how much practice it took to do so. She believes that relaxation helped her take control of her pain, and she is now committed to this method of pain control. Table 8.1 summarizes the effectiveness of relaxation techniques.

Hypnotic Treatment

Although trancelike conditions are as old as human history, modern hypnosis is usually thought to have begun during the last part of the 18th century, when Franz Anton Mesmer, an Austrian physician, conducted elaborate demonstrations in Paris. Although Mesmer's work was heavily criticized, modifications of his technique, known as *mesmerism,* soon spread to other parts of the world. By the 1830s, mesmerism was being used

TABLE 8.1 *Effectiveness of Relaxation Techniques*

Problem	Findings	Studies
1. Migraine headache in children	Relaxation added to biofeedback is more effective than placebos or drugs.	Hermann et al., 1995; Sartory et al., 1998
2. Tension headache	Relaxation is superior to placebo and equal to biofeedback.	Blanchard & Andrasik, 1985; Lehrer et al., 1994;
3. Stress-related disorders	Progressive muscle relaxation helps in coping with headache, hypertension, and effects of chemotherapy in cancer patients.	Carlson & Hoyle, 1993
4. Laboratory stress	Progressive muscle relaxation is superior to classical music in coping with stress.	Scheufele, 2000
5. Anxiety disorders and chronic pain	Mindfulness meditation is better than physical therapy, analgesics, and antidepressants.	Kabat-Zinn et al., 1992; Miller et al., 1995
6. Laboratory stress	Progressive relaxation is more effective than music or placebo.	Scheufele, 2000
7. Postoperative pain	Guided imagery reduces surgery pain and shortens hospital stay.	Lambert, 1996; Tusek et al., 1997
8. Unpleasant effects of chemotherapy	Guided imagery is more effective than placebos.	Lyles et al., 1982
9. Burn pain	Guided imagery adds to other relaxation strategies.	Achterberg et al., 1988
10. Migraine headache	Guided imagery is superior to biofeedback.	Ilacqua, 1994

by some surgeons as an anesthetic during major operations (Hilgard & Hilgard, 1994).

With the discovery of chemical anesthetics, the popularity of hypnosis waned, but during the late 19th century, many European physicians, including Sigmund Freud, employed hypnotic procedures in the treatment of mental illness. Since the beginning of the 20th century, the popularity of hypnosis as a medical and psychological tool has continued to wax and wane. Its present position is still somewhat controversial, but a significant number of practitioners within medicine and psychology are using hypnotherapy to treat health-related problems, especially pain management.

What Is Hypnotic Treatment? Not only is the use of hypnotic processes still controversial, but the precise nature of hypnosis is also debatable. Some authorities, such as Joseph Barber (1996) and Ernest Hilgard (1978) regard hypnosis as an altered *state* of consciousness in which a person's stream of consciousness is divided or dissociated. Joseph Barber believes that hypnotic analgesia works through a process of negative hallucination, or simply not perceiving something that one would ordinarily perceive. To Hilgard, the process of **induction**—that is, being placed into a hypnotic state—is central to the hypnotic process. After induction, the responsive person enters a state of divided or dissociated consciousness that is essentially different from the normal state. This altered state of consciousness allows people to respond to suggestion and to control physiological processes that they cannot control in the normal state of consciousness.

In contrast, Theodore X. Barber (1982, 1984) views the hypnotic process as a more generalized *trait,* or a relatively permanent characteristic of people who respond well to suggestion. He insists that the hypnotic process involves something more than simple relaxation. In addition, he rejects the notion that induction is necessary and holds that the suggestive procedures can be just as effective without the person's entering a trancelike state. Regardless of some of these technical differences, most current hypnotherapists believe that all hypnosis is self-hypnosis.

Not everyone is equally subject to suggestion. Hypnotherapists frequently measure people's ability to be hypnotized by using the Stanford Hypnotic Susceptibility Scales. With the Stanford scales, the hypnotherapist may first relax subjects by speaking in a slow, soft, soothing voice and asking them to stare at a point on a wall. Next, subjects typically respond to 12 activities, which determine their level of suggestibility. With one activity, for example, the therapist suggests that a subject has no sense of smell and then waves a vial of ammonia past the subject's nose. If the subject shows no reaction, then that activity is "passed." Subjects who "pass" all 12 activities receive a score of 12 and are highly suggestible, whereas those who show no suggestibility and "fail" all activities receive a score of 0. Michael Nash (2001) claimed that 95% of the population score at least a 1 and that most people score between 5 and 7. Thus, suggestibility seems to be widely distributed among the population, almost following a normal, bell-shaped curve. For this reason, clinicians need to determine the level of suggestibility of their clients prior to employing hypnosis as an analgesic.

How Effective Is Hypnotic Treatment? Like other interventions, hypnotherapy can be regarded as effective only if it proves more powerful than a placebo. Although the placebo effect depends on suggestion, research (Jacobs, Kurtz, & Strube, 1995) has shown an advantage for hypnotic suggestion over the placebo effect, at least for highly suggestible patients. Thus, for people who are easily hypnotized, hypnotherapy is more effective than a simple placebo. However, people who are low in hypnotizability tend to respond to hypnotic suggestions of analgesia at rates comparable to their response to placebos (Miller, Barabasz, & Barabasz, 1991). Nevertheless, the pain-controlling effects of hypnosis are real and do not depend on one's expectations. Individual differences in susceptibility may mitigate hypnotherapy as a pain reducer for some individuals, but highly suggestible people can receive substantial analgesic benefits from this technique.

Thus, although authorities differ in their opinions concerning the nature of the mechanisms for hypnotic analgesia, few doubt that hypnosis works, at least with some pain patients. The list of pains that are responsive to hypnotic procedures is extensive, but headache, cancer pain, and burn pain have received the most attention. In addition, hypnotherapy has been used successfully to relieve the pain associated with sickle cell disease, surgery, childbirth, dental work, and low back treatment as well as experimental pain.

Hypnotherapy can be useful in helping people cope with migraine, tension, and cluster headaches. For example, in one experimental study (ter-Kuile et al., 1994), chronic headache patients were randomly assigned to a hypnotherapy group or a waiting-list control group. People receiving hypnotherapy reported greater reduction in headache pain compared with those in the control group. Consistent with many other studies, this investigation found that highly hypnotizable participants reported less pain at posttreatment and follow-up than participants who were low in hypnotizability.

A diagnosis of cancer almost always produces anxiety, and the progress of cancer often produces pain. Hypnotherapeutic techniques have helped children and adolescents with cancer cope with the anxiety, the pain, and the nausea and vomiting associated with cancer treatment (Genuis, 1995). According to the results from another study with pediatric cancer patients (Smith, Barabasz, & Barabasz, 1996), the benefits of hypnosis were restricted to highly hypnotizable children.

Hypnotherapy has also been used to treat burn pain. A review (Van der Does & Van Dyck, 1989) examined 28 studies that used hypnosis with burn patients and found consistent evidence that hypnotherapy is an effective analgesia for burn pain. However, this review found no evidence that hypnosis could speed the healing of burn wounds.

In addition to easing headache, cancer pain, and burn pain, hypnotic treatments have been successful in alleviating pain in patients with sickle cell disease (Dinges, et al., 1997); to stabi-

TABLE 8.2 *Effectiveness of Hypnotic Techniques*

Problem	Findings	Studies
1. Headache	Hypnosis reduces pain, especially for highly hypnotizable patients.	ter-Kuile et al., 1994
2. Cancer pain in children	Hypnosis reduces pain and anxiety in pediatric cancer patients, especially for hypnotizable children.	Genuis, 1995; Smith et al., 1996
3. Burn pain	Hypnosis is better than placebo for severe pain, but does not speed healing.	Van der Dose & Van Dyck, 1989
4. Pain from sickle cell disease	Hypnosis improves sleep, reduces medication, and lessens pain.	Dinges et al., 1997
5. Surgery pain	Self-hypnosis stabilizes surgery pain and reduces the need for drugs.	Lang et al., 2000
6. Childbirth discomfort	Hypnosis reduces pain and stress during childbirth and after delivery.	Mairs, 1995
7. Dental pain	Hypnosis reduces the need for medication and lessens pain.	Enqvist & Fischer, 1997
8. Low back pain	Hypnosis lessens pain and suffering.	Burte et al., 1994
9. Experimental pain	Hypnotic suggestion is equally effective in clinical or experimental settings.	Montgomery et al., 2000

lize the pain of invasive surgical procedures and to reduce surgery patients' need for analgesic drugs (Lang et al., 2000); to lessen both pain and stress during childbirth and after delivery (Mairs, 1995); to reduce medication and lessen dental pain (Enqvist & Fischer, 1997); and to reduce the suffering in patients with low back pain (Burte, Burte, & Araoz, 1994). In addition, a recent meta-analysis (Montgomery, DuHamel, & Redd, 2000) showed that hypnotic suggestion is equally effective in reducing clinical as well as experimental pain; in both situations, hypnotic suggestion reduced pain in about 75% of participants.

Despite strong evidence that hypnosis can decrease acute pain and manage chronic pain, many health care providers have gross misunderstandings of this form of analgesia. A survey of a large number of burn therapists and rehabilitation therapists (Bryant, 1993) found that many of them were not aware of research on the efficacy of hypnotherapy and that some expressed many of the same misconceptions of hypnosis that nonprofessionals have. For example, some believed that hypnosis is an altered state of consciousness in which patients are not aware of their surroundings and possess an enhanced ability to recall past events. Such misconceptions discourage the use of hypnosis in situations in which it could be effective.

As Table 8.2 shows, the hypnotic process can be an effective tool for coping with pain. Nevertheless, more research is needed to identify those people who will respond favorably to hypnosis, the conditions under which they will respond, and the types of pain problems that will be alleviated.

Biofeedback

Until the 1960s, most people in the Western world assumed that conscious control of such physiological processes as heart rate, the secretion of digestive juices, and the constriction of blood vessels was impossible. These biological functions do not require conscious attention for their regulation, and conscious attempts at regulation seem to have little effect on these functions controlled by the autonomic nervous system. Then, during the late 1960s, a number of researchers began to explore the possibility of controlling biological processes traditionally believed to be beyond conscious control. Their efforts culminated in the development of **biofeedback,** the process of providing feedback information about the status of biological systems. Early experiments indicated that biofeedback made possible the control of some otherwise automatic functions. In 1969, Neal E. Miller reported a series of experiments in which he and his colleagues altered the levels of animals' visceral response through reinforcement. Some subjects received rewards for raising their heart rate and others for lowering it. Within a few hours, significant differences in heart rate appeared. After other investigators (Brown, 1970; Kamiya, 1969) proved that biofeedback could be used with humans, interest in this procedure became widespread, and soon a variety of biofeedback machines appeared on the market.

What Is Biofeedback? In biofeedback, biological responses are measured by electronic instruments, and the status of those responses is immediately available to the person being tested. In other words, a person gains information about changes in biological responses as they are taking place. This feedback allows the person to alter physiological responses that cannot be voluntarily controlled without the biofeedback information.

The type of biofeedback most commonly found in clinical use is **electromyograph (EMG) biofeedback.** EMG biofeedback reflects the activity of the skeletal muscles by measuring the electrical discharge in muscle fibers. The measurement is taken by attaching electrodes to the surface of the skin over the muscles to be monitored. The level of electrical activity reflects the degree of tension or relaxation of the muscles. The machine responds with a signal that varies according to the electrical activity of the muscle. The electrodes may be placed over any muscle group; the choice of placement depends on the type of problem. Biofeedback can be used to increase muscle tension in rehabilitation or to decrease muscle tension in stress management. The most common use of EMG biofeedback is in the control of low back pain and headaches. Barb's pain program included a EMG biofeedback component, and she believes that monitoring her level of muscle tension helped her learn when she was tense and when she was more relaxed.

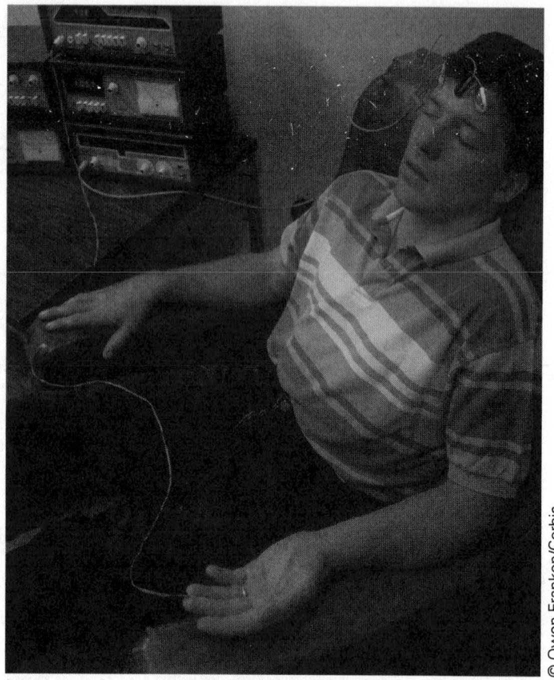

Electromyograph (EMG) biofeedback can help people lower muscle tension.

Thermal biofeedback, which is also frequently used to help people cope with stress and pain, is based on the principle that skin temperature varies in relation to levels of stress. High stress tends to constrict blood vessels, whereas relaxation opens them. Therefore, cool surface skin temperature may indicate stress and tension; warm skin temperature suggests calm and relaxation.

Thermal biofeedback involves placing a **thermister**—a temperature-sensitive resistor—on the skin's surface. The thermister signals changes in skin temperature, thereby furnishing the information that allows control. The feedback signal, as with EMG biofeedback, may be auditory, visual, or both. The goal of thermal biofeedback is almost always to raise skin temperature and thereby increase relaxation. Migraine headache and **Raynaud's disease** are the disorders most commonly treated with thermal biofeedback. Raynaud's disease is a vasoconstrictive disorder in which the fingers (and less often the toes) suf-

TABLE 8.3 *Effectiveness of Biofeedback Techniques*

Problem	Findings	Studies
1. Migraine and tension headache	Thermal biofeedback plus relaxation produces a 45% to 50% reduction in headache activity.	Blanchard et al., 1990; Holroyd & Penzien, 1990; Compas et al., 1998
2. Migraine headache	EMG biofeedback is more effective than a placebo and about as effective as thermal biofeedback.	Compas et al., 1998
3. Low back pain	EMG biofeedback has no immediate advantage over other interventions but may have a more lasting effect.	Bush et al., 1985; Flor & Birbaumer, 1993
4. Hypertension	Biofeedback-induced relaxation is moderately successful in temporally controlling blood pressure.	Paran et al., 1996; McGrady, 1994; Nakao et al., 1997

fer from restricted blood flow. Medical treatment involves surgery or drugs that dilate blood vessels, but both treatments have unwanted side effects. Biofeedback may offer an alternative treatment (Sedlacek, & Taub, 1996).

How Effective Is Biofeedback? To be considered an effective coping technique, biofeedback must not only be superior to a placebo, but it should also produce better results than relaxation training, hypnosis, or any other behavioral intervention that does not require expensive technology. During the past decade, interest in the effectiveness of biofeedback has waned as research has failed to uncover a specific advantage for this procedure. Research during the 1990s used biofeedback techniques for a wide range of disorders, including migraine and tension headaches, low back pain, and hypertension.

Edward Blanchard and his colleagues (Blanchard et al., 1990) reported that thermal biofeedback with relaxation could be an effective treatment for migraine and tension headaches. This combination of biofeedback and relaxation resulted in about a 50% reduction in pain—an improvement greater than that produced by a headache monitoring placebo but no more effective than a drug placebo. Similar results appeared in a meta-analysis of psychological interventions combining thermal biofeedback with relaxation training to produce a 43% reduction in headache activity (Holroyd & Penzien, 1990). A later summary of research (Compas, Haaga, Keefe, Leitenberg, & Williams, 1998) concluded that thermal biofeedback plus relaxation is more effective than a headache monitoring placebo, but no more effective than relaxation alone.

EMG biofeedback has demonstrated some effectiveness for several problems but few advantages over relaxation or hypnosis. EMG biofeedback improves headache, but no more so than thermal biofeedback plus relaxation training, relaxation, or hypnosis (Compas et al., 1998). For low back pain, EMG biofeedback showed a small advantage (Bush, Ditto, & Feuerstein, 1985; Flor & Birbaumer, 1993), but no more than a placebo. Psychologists have also applied biofeedback techniques to the management of hypertension, or high blood pressure. Biofeedback is capable of decreasing hypertension in laboratory demonstrations (Nakao et al., 1997), but people with hypertension experienced only a slight decrease in blood pressure and the need for hypertension drugs (Paran, Amir, & Yaniv, 1996). A larger study (McGrady, 1994) showed some initial effectiveness for a combination of thermal biofeedback and relaxation training but no maintenance of this reduction in blood pressure 10 months later. Thus, biofeedback shows little promise as a treatment for low back pain or hypertension.

As summarized in Table 8.3, these studies do not indicate that biofeedback alone is sufficient for controlling headache pain, low back pain, or hypertension.

Behavior Modification

Health psychologists also use **behavior modification** to help people cope. Behavior modification is aimed at changing behavior through the application of operant conditioning principles. The goal of behavior modification is to shape *behavior,* not to alleviate *feelings* of stress or *sensations* of pain. Because stress is difficult to define in terms of specific behaviors, behavior modification is not often used for coping with stress. However, pain behaviors can be more clearly identified and thus lend themselves more easily to modification by operant conditioning techniques.

What Is Behavior Modification? People in pain usually communicate their discomfort to others. They complain, moan, sigh, limp, rub, grimace, miss work, or behave in a variety of other ways that indicate to other people that they are suffering. Many of these behaviors have been reinforced by the environment—that is, other people have in some manner rewarded these verbal and nonverbal expressions of pain.

Behavior modification strategies for coping with stress and pain are based on B. F. Skinner's (1953, 1987) notion that positive and negative reinforcers are central to operant conditioning. A **positive reinforcer** is any stimulus that, when added to a situation, increases the probability that the behavior it follows will recur. Positive reinforcers are also known as rewards. An example might be the attention and sympathy a person receives from family and friends when exhibiting pain behaviors. A **negative reinforcer** is any aversive or painful stimulus that, when removed from a situation, increases the probability that the behavior it follows will recur. Examples include the relief from pain a person experiences after taking pain medication or the avoidance of work or school responsibilities that can occur when a person shows pain.

Wilbert E. Fordyce (1974) was among the first to emphasize the role of operant conditioning in the perpetuation of pain behaviors. He recognized the *reward* value of increased attention and sympathy, financial compensation, and other positive reinforcers that frequently follow pain behaviors. Behavior modification techniques of pain management assume that pain behaviors are observable and can be reliably measured. Indeed, there is good evidence for these assumptions (McCracken, 1997). Once pain behaviors and their reinforcers have been identified, the process of behavior modification can begin. Nursing staff and patients' spouses can be trained to use praise and attention to reinforce more desirable behaviors and to withhold reinforcement when patients exhibit less desired pain behaviors. In other words, the inappropriate groans and complaints are now ignored, whereas efforts toward greater physical activity and other positive behaviors are reinforced. Progress is noted by such criteria as amount of medication taken, absences from work, time in bed or off one's feet, number of pain complaints, physical activity, range of motion, and length of sitting tolerance.

Using the case study method, Fordyce and his colleagues (Fordyce, Shelton, & Dundore, 1982) illustrated how behavior modification works. The pain patient was a young man suffering abdominal pain, dizziness, and disturbances in walking. The therapists gave the young man a choice of either walking an assigned distance at a predetermined speed or walking twice that distance at his own pace. They also instructed the patient's mother to ignore him when he failed to walk and to encourage him when he showed progress in walking. The treatment intervention, which also included vocational counseling, was successful. At the end of treatment, the young man was walking more freely and complaining less of severe pain. After more than 2 years, the patient had maintained his gains despite no further treatment. Single-subject studies such as this show that behavior modification can work in individual cases, but they do not demonstrate the treatment's general efficacy.

How Effective Is Behavior Modification? The effectiveness of behavior modification in controlling pain is difficult to judge because many studies using behavior modification techniques have been

TABLE 8.4 *Effectiveness of Behavior Modification Techniques*

Problem	Findings	Studies
1. Low back pain	Behavior therapy improves physical activity and decreases medication.	Turner & Chapman, 1982; Nicholas et al., 1991
2. Workers' low back pain	Operant conditioning speeds workers' return to work.	Lindstrom et al., 1992; Vendrig, 1999
3. Chronic low back pain	Behavior therapy may be better than traditional physical therapy methods.	Fordyce et al., 1986
4. Chronic low back pain	Behavior therapy is initially more effective than cognitive treatments, but this advantage is lost during follow-up.	Nicholas et al., 1991; Turner & Clancy, 1988

embedded within a variety of other strategies. An early review (Turner & Chapman, 1982) found some consistent trends for more than a dozen studies that used behavior modification to control a variety of pain syndromes (mostly low back pain). A later study of low back pain patients (Vendrig, 1999) demonstrated that a largely behavioral approach enabled 87% of low back pain workers to gain confidence in their physical mobility and to return to work. Although these studies suggest that behavioral techniques have some initial effectiveness, other studies (Nicholas, Wilson, & Goyen, 1991; Turner & Clancy, 1988) found that the early advantage of behavior modification may not continue after treatment.

How do behavior modification methods compare with traditional medical treatments for chronic low back pain? Fordyce and his associates (Fordyce, Brockway, Bergman, & Spengler, 1986) found some evidence to support the superiority of behavior methods over traditional medical treatment. Patients in the traditional management group received medication on an "as needed" basis and with the possibility of prescription renewal, whereas patients in the behavior therapy group were given medication on a time-contingent basis and with no renewal of the original prescription. In addition, the traditional treatment patients could stop their activity and exercises whenever they wished. For the behavior treatment patients, activity and exercises were completed on a predetermined basis. After 9 to 12 months, patients in the behavior management group were doing better than those treated with traditional procedures.

Fordyce and a group of colleagues headed by Lindstrom (Lindstrom et al., 1992) reported on a study in Sweden that found operant conditioning principles were effective in helping workers with low back pain regain normal physical activity and return to work much earlier than workers who received a standard treatment. Beginning with the principle that exercise is more effective than rest, these researchers randomly assigned half the pain patients to a graded activity program and half to a control group. Prior to assignment, workers in both groups were examined by an orthopedic surgeon and a social worker to assure them that an increase in physical activity would not be harmful. Physical therapists praised nonpain behaviors of workers in the experimental group and ignored pain behaviors. Participants in the control group received only traditional care. Results easily favored the experimental group; they returned to work an average of almost 6 weeks earlier than those in the control group, they gained more confidence in their ability to work even while feeling pain, and they were more active after a 1-year follow-up.

Currently, few researchers limit their studies to behavioral techniques alone. Most combine behavior modification programs with one or more other techniques, making an evaluation of behavioral methods problematic. However, most multimodal psychological approaches to pain management include a behavior modification component. The strength of the operant conditioning technique is its ability to increase levels of physical activity and decrease the use of medication—two important targets in any pain treatment regimen. Table 8.4 shows the effectiveness of behavior modification.

Cognitive Therapy

Cognitive therapy also uses reinforcement but places more emphasis on intrinsic or self-reinforcers than on reinforcers from therapists or other external sources. Cognitive therapy is based on the principle that people's beliefs, personal standards, and feelings of self-efficacy strongly affect their behavior (Bandura, 1986, 2001; Beck, 1976; Ellis, 1962). Cognitive therapies concentrate on techniques designed to change cognitions rather than on the immediate reinforcement of overt behavior.

What Is Cognitive Therapy? Cognitive therapy includes a variety of therapeutic strategies for changing behavior by changing thoughts. It rests on the assumption that a change in the interpretation of an event can change people's emotional and physiological reaction to that event. Although this approach typically uses operant conditioning techniques, it adds an emphasis on patients' ability to think about and evaluate their own behaviors. Pain patients frequently exaggerate their pain-engendering thoughts, thus exacerbating their subjective feelings of pain and ultimately adding a psychological component to the physical experience of pain.

Although he did not originally use the term *cognitive,* Albert Ellis (1962) evolved an approach called *rational emotive therapy* that became the precursor of modern cognitive therapies. According to Ellis, thoughts, especially irrational thoughts, are the root of behavior problems. He contends that irrational beliefs form the basis for a variety of problems, and that these problems are self-reinforced by an internal monologue in which people perpetuate and "catastrophize" their misery with continued self-statements of irrational beliefs and unreasonable expectations.

Ellis believes that the most effective way to alleviate stressful problems is to dispute a person's catastrophic thoughts and to change them into rational beliefs. An irrational, catastrophizing statement would be, "I didn't get the raise that I deserved, so everyone will be disappointed in me, and I'll never get the recognition that I deserve." The therapist would teach the person to substitute rational self-statements for irrational ones, decreasing the tendency to catastrophize. A rational statement might be, "Even though I didn't get this raise, I can work to get others. If I am not as successful as I want to be in this job, I can succeed in other ways, and there are other jobs." Thus, the emotional element of the stress response is averted or minimized, and the person has a greater opportunity to cope rationally and positively with stress.

The experience of pain is one that can easily be turned into a catastrophe, and any exaggeration of feelings of pain can lead to maladaptive behaviors and further exacerbation of irrational beliefs. One early report (Keefe, Brown, Wallston, & Caldwell, 1989) showed that rheumatoid arthritis pain sufferers who catastrophized their pain tended to report more intense pain, increased functional impairments, and greater depression. This finding supports Ellis's contention that magnifying an event into a catastrophe will lead to increased emotional distress and elevated levels of pain.

Once irrational cognitions have been identified, the therapist actively attacks these beliefs, with the goal of eliminating or changing them into more rational beliefs. Ellis's cognitive therapy, then, is based on the assumption that people possess the ability to examine their belief systems logically and to change irrational beliefs into rational ones.

Psychologists have developed a variety of other cognitive strategies for coping with pain and stress. Two of these strategies are the pain inoculation program designed by Dennis Turk and Donald Meichenbaum (Meichenbaum & Turk, 1976; Turk, 1978, 2001) and the parallel stress inoculation program of Meichenbaum and Roy Cameron (1983). Both procedures rely on inoculation techniques; that is, they work in a manner analogous to vaccination. By introducing a weakened dose of a pathogen (in this case, the pathogen is either pain or stress), the therapist attempts to build some immunity against high levels of pain and stress.

Because pain is a perception influenced by expectation and situation, therapists who use inoculation techniques work first at getting patients to think differently about the source of their pain experience. The first step in pain inoculation is the *reconceptualization* stage. During this stage, patients are encouraged to accept the importance of psychological factors for at least some of their pain. Once patients accept the potential effectiveness of psychologically based treatment, they are ready to enter the second stage—*acquisition and rehearsal of skills.* During this phase, patients learn relaxation and controlled breathing skills. Because relaxation is incompatible with tension and anxiety, learning to relax can be a valuable tool in managing pain. Patients also learn to direct their attention away from the pain experience by concentrating on a pleasant scene, such as a cool waterfall, or by focusing their attention outside themselves—for example, by counting spots on ceiling tiles or by thinking about a funny movie they have seen recently.

After patients have acquired and consolidated these skills, they are ready to enter the final, or *follow-through,* phase of treatment. During this follow-through stage, therapists give instructions to spouses and other family members to ignore patients' pain behaviors and to reinforce such healthy behaviors as greater levels of physical activity, decreased use of medication, fewer visits to the pain clinic, or an increased number of days at work. With the help of their therapists, patients construct a posttreatment plan for coping with future pain, and finally, they apply their coping skills to everyday situations outside the pain clinic.

The stress inoculation program of Meichenbaum and Cameron (1983) is quite similar to Turk and Meichenbaum's method for coping with pain. Stress inoculation includes three stages: conceptualization, skills acquisition and rehearsal, and follow-through or application.

The *conceptualization* stage is a cognitive intervention in which the therapist works with clients to identify and clarify their problems. During this overtly educational stage, patients learn about stress inoculation and how this technique can reduce their stress. The *skills acquisition and rehearsal* stage involves both educational and behavioral components to enhance patients' repertoire of coping skills. At this time, patients learn and practice new ways of coping with stress. One of the goals of this stage is to improve self-instruction by changing cognitions, a process that includes monitoring one's internal monologue—that is, self-talk. During the *application and follow-through* stage, patients put into practice the cognitive changes they achieved in the two previous stages.

How Effective Is Cognitive Therapy? Evaluations of the effectiveness of cognitive therapy programs are difficult because widely diverse procedures have been placed under the rubric of cognitive therapy. Moreover, cognitive programs often are embedded in multimodal programs that also include relaxation training, biofeedback, behavior modification, systematic desensitization, and other techniques that are not strictly cognitive. Nevertheless, researchers have tested the effectiveness of cognitive therapy for a wide variety of stress and pain problems.

One review (Compas et al., 1998) reported that cognitive therapy for low back pain increased patients' physical activity and also improved their psychological functioning. This review suggested that cognitive behavioral group therapy may be able to reduce reliance on medication. In addition, a study of low back pain patients in the Netherlands (Kole-Snijders et al., 1999) compared a combined cognitive and relaxation procedure with a combination of an operant behavioral treatment group discussion. Both strategies were also compared to a wait-list control group. In general, pain patients receiving cognitive coping skills did better than the behavior modification group, and both groups did better than the wait-list group.

Combined cognitive and behavioral approaches are effective with a variety of pain syndromes. A study with children suffering recurrent abdominal pain (Sanders, Shepherd, Cleghorn, & Woolford, 1994) compared a cognitive-behavioral approach with a standard pediatric care program and found that the cognitive-behavioral intervention was more effective in reducing pain, both at the end of treatment and after a 12-month follow-up. Another multimodal program (Mishra, Gatchel, & Gardea, 2000) found that temporomandibular pain patients who received a treatment program consisting of cognitive-behavioral therapy and biofeedback experienced significant decreases in pain, whereas those in the no-treatment group did not. Moreover, these differences remained significant after a 1-year follow-up (Gardea, Gatchel, & Mishra, 2001).

In addition, cognitive-based therapies have been found to help people cope with myriad painful and stressful symptoms. For example, cognitive-behavioral strategies are effective in helping people deal with rheumatoid arthritis pain (Keefe & Van Horn, 1993; Sharpe et al., 2001), cancer and AIDS pain (Breibart & Payne, 2001), headache pain (Blanchard et al., 1990) and the stressors associated with terminal illness (Turk & Feldman, 2001). Moreover, cognitive-behavioral therapy is cost effective in a program to alleviate the pain of sickle cell disease (Thomas, Gruen, & Shu, 2001).

Is inoculation training effective for coping with pain and stress? Research on the efficacy that these forms of cognitive therapy shows promise in helping people cope with pain and stress. A meta-analysis (Saunders, Driskell, Johnston, & Sales, 1996) of nearly 40 studies found that inoculation training was effective in decreasing anxiety and raising performance under stress. Additional research has confirmed the usefulness of pain and stress inoculation training. One study (Ross & Berger, 1996) found that pain inoculation procedures were effective with athletes recovering from knee-injury pain. A later study (Foa et al., 1999) looked at the efficacy of inoculation training and **exposure therapy** for lessening the negative effects of posttraumatic stress disorder in female assault victims. Exposure therapy called for the women to relive their traumatic experience in vivo, that is, in their imagination, and to speak of the event in the present tense. Assault victims were randomly assigned to four groups: (1) in vivo exposure, (2) stress inoculation training, (3) a combination of in vivo exposure and stress inoculation, and (4) a wait-list control. Each of the three active therapy groups did better than the control, but no posttest differences emerged among the three therapy groups.

In summary, these studies show that inoculation training, either alone or in combination with other procedures, can be an effective intervention for pain and stress management for a variety of people in many painful and stressful situations. They also suggest that traumatic events can become less stressful when victims face their experience rather than shunning it. A possible advantage of cognitive approaches over other strategies is their ability to change patients' self-perceived efficacy to cope with a range of stresses and pains. Table 8.5 summarizes the effectiveness of cognitive therapy and the problems it can be used to treat.

Emotional Disclosure

In recent years, James Pennebaker has provided evidence that emotional self-disclosure improves both psychological and physical health. Moreover, these positive effects of emotional disclosure extend to a variety of people, in myriad settings, and among diverse cultures.

What Is Emotional Disclosure? **Emotional disclosure** is a therapeutic technique whereby people express their strong emotions by talking or writing about negative events that precipitated those emotions. For centuries, confession of sinful deeds has been part of personal healing in many religious rituals. Then, during the late 19th century, Joseph Breuer and Sigmund Freud (1895/1955) recognized the cathartic value of the "talking cure," and **catharsis,** or the verbal expression of emotions, became an important part of psychotherapy. Pennebaker has taken the notion of catharsis beyond Breuer and Freud and has been able to demonstrate the health benefits of talking or writing about traumatic life events.

TABLE 8.5 *Effectiveness of Cognitive Therapy Techniques*

Problem	Findings	Studies
1. Chronic low back pain	Cognitive therapy increases physical activity and improves psychological functioning.	Compas et al., 1998
2. Severe low back pain	Cognitive therapy is more effective than a behavioral approach.	Kole-Snijders et al., 1999
3. Temporomandibular pain	Cognitive behavior therapy and biofeedback is more effective than standard care.	Mishra et al., 2000; Gardea et al., 2001
4. Rheumatoid arthritis	Cognitive behavior therapy can relieve some pain.	Keefe & Van Horn, 1993; Sharpe et al., 2001
5. Cancer and AIDS pain	Cognitive-based therapies help people cope with pain.	Breibart & Payne, 2000
6. Headache pain	Cognitive therapy combined with biofeedback and relaxation is more effective than a placebo.	Blanchard et al., 1990
7. Stress of terminal illness	Cognitive-based therapy can enhance quality of life.	Turk & Feldman, 2001
8. Pain of sickle cell disease	Cognitive behavioral therapy alleviates pain and is cost effective.	Thomas et al., 2001
9. Performance anxiety	Inoculation training reduces performance anxiety and boosts performance under stress.	Saunders et al., 1996
10. Athletes with knee-injury pain	Pain inoculation training reduces pain.	Ross & Berger, 1996
11. Posttraumatic stress of female assault victims	Inoculation procedures lessen negative effects of posttraumatic stress.	Foa et al., 1999

The general pattern of Pennebaker's research is to ask people to write or talk about traumatic events for 15 to 20 minutes, three or four times a week. The physical and psychological changes in these people are typically compared with those of a control group, who are asked to write or talk about superficial events. This relatively simple procedure seems to be responsible for such physiological changes as fewer physician visits, improved immune functioning, and lower rates of asthma, arthritis, cancer, and heart disease. In addition, disclosure has produced psychological and behavioral changes, such as better grades among college students, increased ability to find new jobs, and an enhanced sense of well-being (Pennebaker & Graybeal, 2001).

Emotional disclosure should be distinguished from emotional expression. The latter term simply refers to emotional outbursts or emotional venting, such as crying, laughing, yelling, or throwing objects. Emotional disclosure, in contrast, involves the transfer of emotions into language and thus requires a measure of self-reflection. Emotional outbursts are often unhealthy and may add more stress to an already unpleasant situation, whereas emotional disclosure can be healthy—both psychologically and physiologically (Smyth & Pennebaker, 2001).

In one of their early studies on emotional disclosure, Pennebaker and colleagues (Pennebaker, Barger, & Tiebout, 1989) asked survivors of the Holocaust to talk for 1 to 2 hours about their war experiences. Those survivors who disclosed the most personally traumatic experiences had better subsequent health than survivors who expressed less painful experiences. Since then, Pennebaker and his colleagues investigated other forms of emotional disclosure, such as asking people to talk into a tape recorder or to speak to a therapist about highly stressful events. With each of these techniques, the key ingredient is language—the emotions must be expressed through language.

How Effective Is Emotional Disclosure? A substantial number of studies by Pennebaker's team as well as by other researchers have demonstrated the effectiveness of disclosure in reducing a variety of illnesses. One study (Pennebaker, Colder, & Sharp, 1990) showed that students who disclosed

TABLE 8.6 *Effectiveness of Emotional Disclosure*

Problem	Findings	Studies
1. General health problems	Holocaust survivors who talked most about their experience had fewer health problems 14 months later.	Pennebaker et al., 1989
2. Anxiety about entering college	Students who disclosed had fewer illnesses.	Pennebaker et al., 1990
3. General health problems	Writing about traumatic events is more effective than writing about superficial events.	Francis & Pennebaker, 1992
4. Asthma and rheumatoid arthritis	Keeping a journal of stressful events reduces symptoms and and improves functioning.	Smyth et al., 1999
5. Visits to a health center for illness	Writing about the positive aspects of traumatic events is as effective as writing only about negative aspects of traumatic events.	King & Miner, 2000

feelings about entering college had fewer illnesses than those who merely wrote about superficial topics. A second study (Francis & Pennebaker, 1992) revealed that university employees age 22 to 70 who wrote about personal traumatic experiences had health advantages over those who wrote about nontraumatic experiences, thus supporting Pennebaker's hypothesis that expressing superficial events is less beneficial than disclosing more frightful events.

Writing about stressful experiences may reduce symptoms in patients with asthma and arthritis. Joshua Smyth, Arthur Stone, Adam Hurewitz, and Alan Kaell (1999) asked asthma patients and rheumatoid arthritis patients to keep a journal that described either stressful life events or emotionally neutral topics. After 4 months in which both groups also received standard care, nearly half the patients who wrote about highly emotional events were functioning better, whereas less than one fourth of the patients who wrote about nonemotional topics were functioning better.

Can health benefits accrue from writing about the positive aspects of a traumatic experience? Laura King and Kathi Miner (2000) asked college students to write about ways in which a traumatic life event had contributed to their personal growth. King and Miner found that these students received as much health benefit as participants who wrote about a traumatic experience without including episodes of personal growth. Both conditions were associated with fewer visits to health care facilities and greater subjective well-being when compared with a control group of students who wrote about their plans for the next day or about the appearance of their shoes. These findings extend Pennebaker's research on disclosure by suggesting that people who write about the positive outcomes of a traumatic experience can receive health benefits equal to those who simply write about a traumatic life event.

Pennebaker's research has added an effective and easily assessable tool to the arsenal of coping strategies. Expressing rather than denying negative experiences may benefit both psychological and physiological health. See Table 8.6 for a summary of the effectiveness of self-disclosure through writing or talking.

In Summary

Health psychologists help people cope with stress and chronic pain by using relaxation training, hypnotic procedures, biofeedback, behavior modification, cognitive therapy, and emotional disclosure.

Relaxation techniques include (1) progressive muscle relaxation, (2) meditative relaxation, (3) mindfulness meditation, and (4) guided imagery. All four approaches have demonstrated some success in helping patients cope with headache pain, anxiety disorder, dental pain, childbirth discomfort, postoperative pain, and stress-related disorders. Relaxation is generally more effective than a placebo.

Debate still exists over the exact nature of hypnotic treatment, but there is little disagreement that hypnosis can be a powerful analgesic for managing pain. The benefits of hypnotherapy vary individually, but for suggestible people, hypnotic processes are an effective means of treating headache, cancer pain, burn pain, surgery pain, childbirth discomfort, dental pain, and the pain that accompanies sickle cell disease.

Biofeedback can be an effective procedure—either alone or in combination with other techniques—for lessening some kinds of pain. EMG and thermal biofeedback are effective in alleviating migraine and tension headache, reducing low back pain, and controlling hypertension, but biofeedback is usually no more effective than relaxation or hypnosis.

Behavior modification, a technique based on the principles of operant conditioning, can help people cope with pain, or at least reduce the frequency of pain behaviors. Behavior modification is based on the assumption that withholding reinforcement for pain behaviors will decrease the likelihood that those behaviors will recur. When people are no longer rewarded for moaning, limping, missing work, or complaining, they tend to stop doing these things and begin to exhibit more nonpain behaviors. Behavior modification principles are most effective in reducing pain behaviors associated with low back pain and other musculoskeletal pains.

Cognitive therapy programs often rely on reinforcement techniques, but they also add other strategies such as self-talk, self-efficacy, and self-evaluation of behavior. Because pain is at least partially due to psychological factors, cognitive therapists attempt to get patients to think differently about their pain experiences. One goal of cognitive treatment for pain is to increase patients' confidence that they can cope with increases in pain. Cognitive therapy—either alone or in combination with other coping strategies—is effective for treating low back pain, headache pain, temporomandibular pain, rheumatoid arthritis pain, cancer pain, the pain that accompanies AIDS, and the pain of sickle cell disease. Pain and stress inoculation—types of cognitive therapy that introduce low levels of pain and stress and then gradually increase those levels—have been successful in treating performance anxiety, knee-injury pain of athletes, and posttraumatic stress.

Emotional disclosure calls for patients to disclose strong negative emotions either through writing or talking. Patients who write about traumatic life events do so for 15 to 20 minutes, three or four times a day. Those who talk frequently speak into a tape recorder or to a therapist. Emotional disclosure generally enhances good health, relieves anxiety, reduces visits to health care providers, and may reduce the symptoms of asthma and rheumatoid arthritis.

Answers

This chapter addressed three basic questions:

1. **What personal resources influence coping?** Two personal strategies for helping cope with pain and stress are social support and personal control. Social support, defined as the emotional quality of one's social contacts, is inversely related to disease and death. People with high levels of social support, compared to those with low levels, are only about half as likely to die within a designated period of time. People with social support receive more encouragement and advice to seek medical care, and social support may provide a buffer against the physical effects of stress. Second, people's beliefs that they have control over the events of their life seem to have a positive impact on health. Even a sense of control over small matters may improve health and prolong life.

2. What strategies do people use to cope with stress?
People use a variety of strategies to cope with stress, all of which may be successful. Problem-focused coping is often a better choice for coping attempts than emotion-focused efforts because problem-focused coping can change the source of the problem, eliminating the stress-producing situation. Emotion-focused coping is oriented toward managing the distress that accompanies stress. Research indicates that most people use both types of coping strategies, often in combination.

3. What techniques do health psychologists use to teach people to cope with stress and pain?
At least six techniques are available to health psychologists in helping people cope with stress and pain. First, relaxation training can help people cope with a variety of stress and pain problems such as headache, chemotherapy side effects, anxiety, dental pain, and hypertension. Second, for people who are suggestible, hypnosis can be effective in treating headache, cancer pain, burn pain, childbirth discomfort, dental pain, and hypertension. Third, biofeedback is effective in alleviating migraine and tension headache, anxiety, low back pain, and hypertension. Fourth, behavior modification is especially effective in decreasing pain behaviors, but whether or not it decreases actual pain is not clear. Fifth cognitive therapy—including stress inoculation—is effective in reducing both pain and stress, but in practice, it is typically combined with behavioral and other strategies. Sixth, emotional disclosure—including writing about traumatic events—shows some promise in helping people cope with those events.

Suggested Readings

Fordyce, W. E. (1990). Contingency management. In J. J. Bonica (Ed.), *The management of pain* (2nd ed., pp. 1702–1710). Malvern, PA: Lea & Febiger. Wilbert Fordyce discusses terminology and principles of behavioral management of pain. Contingency management procedures typically target some combination of problem behaviors that include overmedication, reduced activity levels, excessive pain behaviors, deficits in well behavior, and inappropriate responses to pain behavior.

Nash, M. R. (2001, July). The truth and the hype of hypnosis. *Scientific American, 285,* 47–55. Michael Nash discusses the nature of hypnosis and takes a scientific look at the evidence for what hypnosis can and cannot do.

Pennebaker, J. W., & Graybeal, A. (2001). Patterns of natural language use: Disclosure, personality, and social integration. *Current Directions in Psychological Science, 10,* 90–93. In this brief article, James Pennebaker and Anna Graybeal discuss the rationale of emotional disclosure, review some of the research on the topic, and hypothesize about the challenges for the future.

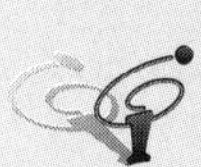

Search InfoTrac College Edition

Search these terms to learn more about topics in this chapter:

- Social support and health
- Personal control and health
- Hardy personality
- Hardiness and personality
- Stress and problem-focused coping
- Coping styles
- Relaxation training and stress
- Relaxation training and pain
- Hypnosis and treatment
- Biofeedback and pain
- Biofeedback and headache
- Behavior therapy and pain
- Cognitive therapy and stress
- Writing and therapeutic use

9

Cardiovascular Disease

The Story of Jason

CHAPTER OUTLINE

The Cardiovascular System

Measures of Cardiovascular Function

The Changing Rates of Cardiovascular Disease

Risk Factors in Cardiovascular Disease

Reducing Cardiovascular Risks

QUESTIONS

This chapter focuses on five basic questions:

1. What are the structures, functions, and disorders of the cardiovascular system?
2. What measurements of cardiovascular function can reveal damage?
3. How does lifestyle relate to cardiovascular health?
4. What are the risk factors for cardiovascular disease?
5. What approaches allow people to lower their cardiovascular risks?

The Story of Jason

Jason was determined that he would never undergo coronary bypass surgery, saying, "They're not going to take a vein out of my leg and put it in my heart. No way. I don't care if I die." However, Jason was not an immediate candidate for cardiac surgery; he was 15 years old, and his 42-year-old father had undergone this procedure. The details of that surgery made a dramatic impression on Jason and gave him a better acquaintance with the risk factors for cardiovascular disease than most 15-year-olds.

Despite Jason's determination to avoid cardiovascular disease, he is at increased risk for several reasons. Jason's father developed heart disease in his early 40s, and this hereditary factor places Jason at increased risk. His African American ethnic background is another factor that increases his risk; African Americans experience cardiovascular disease and death at higher rates than European Americans. His gender is yet another risk factor for heart disease—men in the United States develop cardiovascular disease at earlier ages than women.

Although Jason knew that changing certain behaviors would lower his risk for heart disease, at age 15 he refused to consider such options. He said that he had no intention of restricting his diet by avoiding high-fat or salty foods. He planned to eat what he wanted, and if he has a heart attack, then he has a heart attack. At age 21, Jason's feelings are somewhat different. He accepts his risks for heart disease, and he does watch his diet.

Jason was strongly opposed to smoking, felt no urge to experiment with cigarettes, and ridiculed those who did. His attitudes about drinking were not as extreme, but he did not drink as a teenager and felt that he would never be a smoker or a drinker. As a young adult, Jason is not a smoker and is a moderate drinker, and both of these behaviors help to decrease his risk.

Jason was competitive and impatient. His competitive attitude appeared in his interactions with his peers and in his motivation for success. He was outgoing and, as a teenager, liked to be the center of attention, and his wit allowed him to achieve this goal often. However, he sometimes used his wit to score points at others' expense. Jason also tended to have trouble getting along with others due to his impatience, which extended to himself as well as others. When he failed to meet his own high standards, he became annoyed. He was as critical of himself as he was of others, but he was openly critical of others who were less intellectually capable than he was and who could not keep up with his verbal wit. These tendencies restricted his circle of friends to a few who enjoyed his intelligence and sense of humor.

Jason was also very oriented toward success, which he defined as making a lot of money. At age 15, he had not chosen a career, and his academic performance was not always excellent. At age 21, Jason is less abrasive, more acceptant of others and himself, and more academically focused. He says that he knows that he has a strong hereditary risk for heart disease and is not sure that he can avoid a heart attack, even if he is careful about diet and exercise.

This chapter examines the behavioral risks for cardiovascular disease—the most frequent cause of death in the United States and other industrialized nations—and looks at Jason's risk from both inherent and behavioral factors. But first it describes the cardiovascular system and methods of measuring cardiovascular function.

The Cardiovascular System

The **cardiovascular system** is the part of the body that contains the heart, arteries, and veins. Its purpose is to pump blood throughout the body, providing a rapid-transport system for oxygen and nutrients and for the disposal of wastes. During normal functioning, the cardiovascular, respiratory, and digestive systems are integrated: the digestive system produces nutrients and the respiratory system furnishes oxygen, both of which circulate through the blood to various parts of the body. In addition, the endocrine system affects the cardiovascular system by stimulating or depressing the rate of cardiovascular activity. Although the cardiovascular system can be analyzed in isolation, it does not function that way.

CHECK YOUR HEALTH RISKS

Check the items that apply to you.

- ☐ 1. Someone in my immediate family (a parent, sibling, aunt, uncle, or grandparent) died of heart disease before the age of 55.
- ☐ 2. I am diabetic.
- ☐ 3. I am female.
- ☐ 4. I am African American.
- ☐ 5. My blood pressure is less than 135 over 80.
- ☐ 6. My total cholesterol level is between 170 and 200.
- ☐ 7. My HDL is less than 40
- ☐ 8. The ratio of my total cholesterol to HDL is 6 to 1 or higher.
- ☐ 9. I have never been a smoker.
- ☐ 10. I am less than 30 years old.
- ☐ 11. I eat three or four servings of fruits and vegetables every day.
- ☐ 12. My diet contains lots of red meat.
- ☐ 13. I almost never eat fish.
- ☐ 14. My diet is high in fiber.
- ☐ 15. I am an unmarried man.
- ☐ 16. I frequently get angry, and when I do I let everyone around me know about it.
- ☐ 17. I frequently get angry, and when I do I keep my anger to myself.

Each of these topics is either a known risk factor for some type of cardiovascular disease or has the potential to protect against it. Conditions consistent with items 3, 5, 6, 9, 10, 11, and 14 may offer some protection against cardiovascular disease. If you checked none or only a few of these items and a large number of the remaining items, you may be at risk for heart disease or stroke.

This section briefly considers the functioning of the cardiovascular system, concentrating on the physiology underlying **cardiovascular disease (CVD),** a general term that includes coronary artery disease, coronary heart disease, and stroke. The cardiovascular system consists of the heart and the blood vessels. By contracting and relaxing, the heart muscle pumps blood that circulates through the body. The circulation of blood allows the transport of oxygen to body cells and the removal of carbon dioxide and other wastes from cells. The entire circuit takes about 20 seconds when the body is at rest, but exertion speeds the process.

The blood's route through the body is pictured in Figure 9.1. Blood travels from the right ventricle of the heart to the lungs, where hemoglobin (one of the components of blood) becomes saturated with oxygen. From the lungs, oxygenated blood travels back to the left atrium of the heart, then to the left ventricle, and finally out to the rest of the body. The **arteries** that carry the oxygenated blood branch into vessels of smaller and smaller diameter, called **arterioles,** and finally terminate in tiny **capillaries** that connect arteries and **veins.** Oxygen diffuses out to body cells, and carbon dioxide and other chemical wastes pass into the blood so they may be disposed. Blood that has been stripped of its oxygen returns to the heart by way of the system of veins, beginning with the tiny **venules** and ending with the two large veins that empty into the right atrium, the upper right chamber of the heart.

The Coronary Arteries

The coronary arteries supply blood to the heart muscle, the **myocardium** (see Figure 9.2). The two principal coronary arteries branch off from the aorta, the main artery that carries oxygenated blood from the heart. Left and right coronary

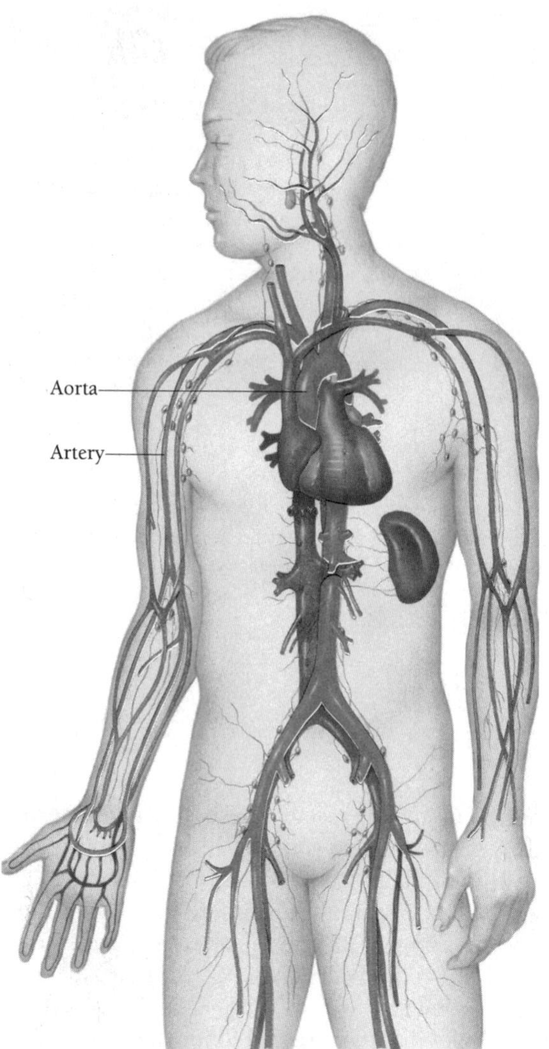

Figure 9.1 Cardiovascular circulation.

Source: Introduction to Microbiology *(p. 671) by J. L. Ingraham & C. A. Ingraham, 1995, Belmont, CA: Wadsworth. Copyright 1995 by Wadsworth Publishing Company. Reprinted by permission.*

arteries divide into smaller branches, providing the blood supply to the myocardium.

With each beat, the heart makes a slight twisting motion, which moves the coronary arteries. The coronary arteries, therefore, receive a great deal of strain as part of their normal function. This movement of the heart has been hypothesized to almost inevitably cause injury to the coronary arteries (Friedman & Rosenman, 1974). The damage can heal in two different ways. The preferable route involves the formation of small amounts of scar tissue and results in no serious problem. The second route involves the formation of **atheromatous plaques,** deposits composed of cholesterol and other lipids (fats), connective tissue, and muscle tissue. The plaques grow and calcify into a hard, bony substance that thickens the arterial walls. The formation of plaques and the resulting occlusion of the arteries is called **atherosclerosis,** shown in Figure 9.3.

A related but different problem is **arteriosclerosis,** or the loss of elasticity of the arteries. The beating of the heart pushes blood through the arteries with great force, and arterial elasticity allows adaptation to this pressure. Loss of elasticity tends to make the cardiovascular system less capable of tolerating increases in cardiac blood volume. Hence, a potential danger exists during strenuous exercise for people with arteriosclerosis.

The formation of arterial plaques (atherosclerosis) and the "hardening" of the arteries (arteriosclerosis) often occur together. Both can affect any artery in the cardiovascular system, but when the coronary arteries are affected, the heart's oxygen supply may be threatened.

Coronary Artery Disease

Coronary artery disease (CAD) arises as a result of atherosclerosis and arteriosclerosis in the coronary arteries. No clearly visible, outward symptoms accompany the buildup of plaques in the coronary arteries; CAD can be developing while a person remains totally unaware of its progress. However, the plaques narrow the arteries and restrict the supply of blood to the myocardium. In addition, blood platelets tend to stick to and blood clots to form around the plaques. These blood clots can transform the partially obstructed artery into a completely closed one. Restriction of blood flow is called **ischemia.** If the coronary arteries do not allow enough blood to reach the heart muscle, the

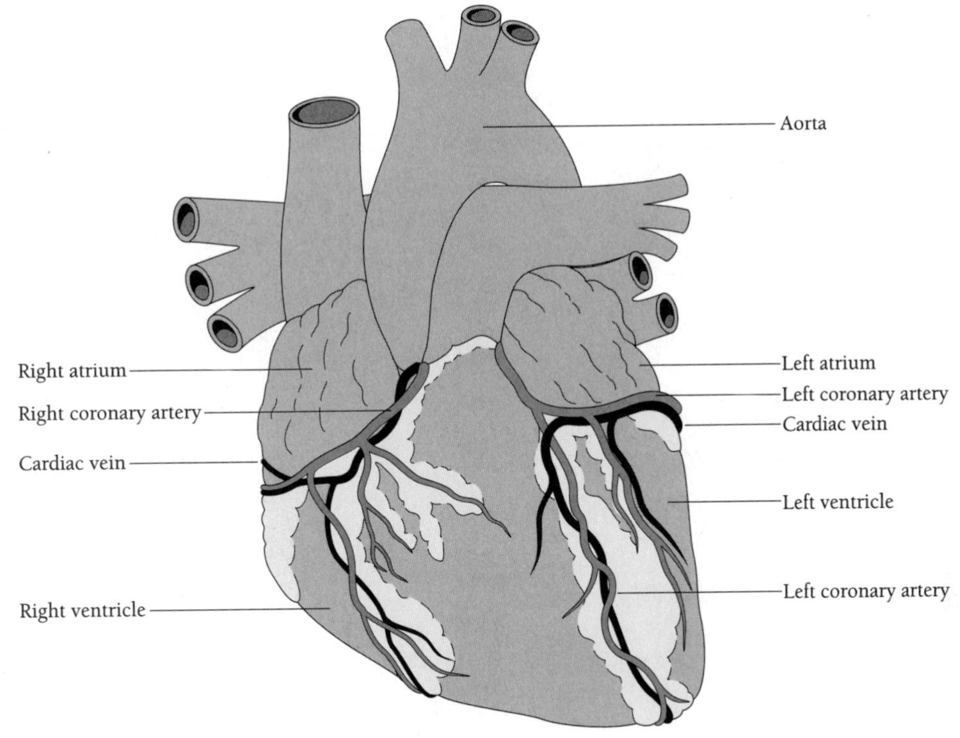

Figure 9.2 Heart with coronary arteries and veins.

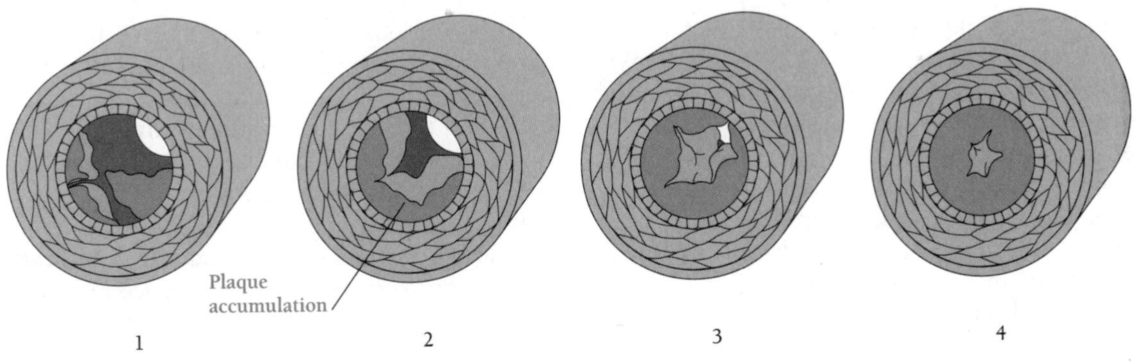

Figure 9.3 Progressive atherosclerosis.

heart, like any other organ or tissue deprived of oxygen, will not function properly.

The term **coronary heart disease (CHD)** is sometimes used interchangeably with coronary artery disease. Technically, coronary heart disease refers to any damage to the myocardium due to insufficient blood supply, whereas coronary artery disease refers to damage to the coronary arteries, typically through the processes of atherosclerosis and arteriosclerosis.

Complete blockage of either coronary artery shuts off the blood flow and thus the oxygen

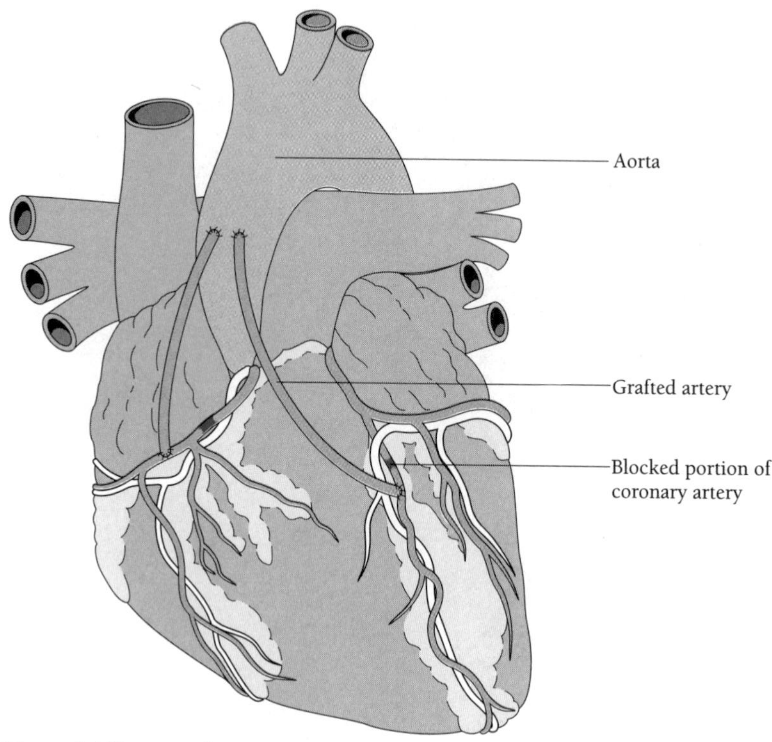

Figure 9.4 Coronary bypass.

supply to the myocardium. Like other tissue, the myocardium cannot survive without oxygen; therefore, coronary blockage results in the death of myocardial tissue, an infarction. **Myocardial infarction** is the medical term for the condition commonly referred to as a heart attack. During myocardial infarction, the damage may be so extensive as to completely disrupt the heartbeat. In less severe cases, heart contractions may become less effective. The signals for a myocardial infarction include a feeling of weakness or dizziness combined with nausea, cold sweating, difficulty in breathing, and a sensation of crushing or squeezing pain in the chest, arms, shoulders, jaw, or back. Rapid loss of consciousness or death may occur, but the victim sometimes remains quite alert throughout the experience. The severity of symptoms depends on the extent of damage to the heart muscle.

A less serious result of restriction of the blood supply to the myocardium is **angina pectoris,** a disorder with symptoms of crushing pain in the chest and difficulty in breathing. Angina is usually precipitated by exercise or stress because these conditions increase demand to the heart. With oxygen restriction, the reserve capacity of the cardiovascular system is reduced, and heart disease becomes evident. The uncomfortable symptoms of angina rarely last more than a few minutes, but angina is a sign of obstruction in the coronary arteries.

One approach to the treatment of CAD is surgery that replaces the blocked portion of the coronary artery (or arteries) with grafts of healthy sections of the coronary arteries (see Figure 9.4). Bypass surgery is expensive, carries some risk for death, and may not extend the patient's life significantly. This treatment is the procedure that Jason refused to consider, but it is generally successful in relieving angina and improving quality of life, as it was for his father.

Unfortunately, the disease processes that led to the initial blockage of the coronary arteries often lead to obstruction of the replacement vessels. Therefore, people who have coronary bypass surgery may redevelop CAD, and these patients must change their lifestyle if they are to prevent blockage of the replacement arteries.

Both myocardial infarction and angina pectoris are typically the result of atherosclerosis, which is most dangerous when it involves the coronary arteries. Continued thickening of the arterial walls restricts the flow of blood, causing angina. If the restriction is severe, heart tissue may die and the heartbeat will be disrupted; that is, the person will experience a myocardial infarction.

In those people who survive a myocardial infarction (somewhat more than half do), the damaged portion of the myocardium will not regrow or repair itself. Instead, scar tissue forms at the infarcted area. Scar tissue does not have the elasticity and function of healthy tissue, so a heart attack lessens the capacity of the heart to pump blood efficiently. A myocardial infarction can limit the type and vigor of activities that a person can safely do, prompting some lifestyle changes. Frequently, these changes result from cardiac patients' uncertainty about which activities are safe and from their fears about suffering another attack. Such fears have some basis. The coronary artery disease that caused a first attack can cause another, but future infarctions are not a certainty.

The process of **cardiac rehabilitation** often involves psychologists, who help cardiac patients adjust their lifestyle to minimize risk factors and lessen the chances of future attacks. Because heart disease is the most frequent cause of death in the United States, preventing heart attacks and furnishing cardiac rehabilitation is a major task for the health care system. This chapter discusses the development and prevention of cardiovascular disease and cardiac rehabilitation programs.

Stroke

Atherosclerosis and arteriosclerosis can also affect the arteries that serve the head and neck, thereby restricting the blood supply to the brain. Plaques may become detached from the artery wall, or one of the blood clots that tend to form on plaques may detach and flow through the circulatory system. Any obstruction in the arteries of the brain will restrict or completely stop the flow of blood to the area of the brain served by that portion of the system. A piece of material too small to obstruct an arteriole might completely block a capillary. Oxygen deprivation causes the death of brain tissue within 3 to 5 minutes. This damage to the brain resulting from lack of oxygen is called a **stroke,** the third most frequent cause of death in the United States. But strokes have other causes as well—for example, a bubble of air (air embolism) or infection that impedes blood flow in the brain may also result in a stroke. In addition, the weakening of artery walls associated with arteriosclerosis may lead to an *aneurysm,* a sac formed by the ballooning of a weakened artery wall. Aneurysms may burst, causing a *hemorrhagic stroke* or death (see Figure 9.5).

A stroke damages neurons in the brain, and these neurons have no capacity to replace themselves. Therefore, death of any neuron results in the permanent loss of its function. The brain, however, contains billions of neurons. Rarely do people suffer from strokes that kill *all* neurons controlling a particular function. More commonly, some of the neurons devoted to a particular function are lost, impairing brain function. Even though no neurons are replaced, the remaining healthy neural tissue compensates to some extent. For example, one specific area of the brain controls speech production. If this area is completely damaged by a stroke, the victim can no longer speak (but can still comprehend speech). A stroke that damages some of the neurons in this area results in partial loss of fluency and some difficulty in speaking. The extent of the loss is related to the amount of damage to the

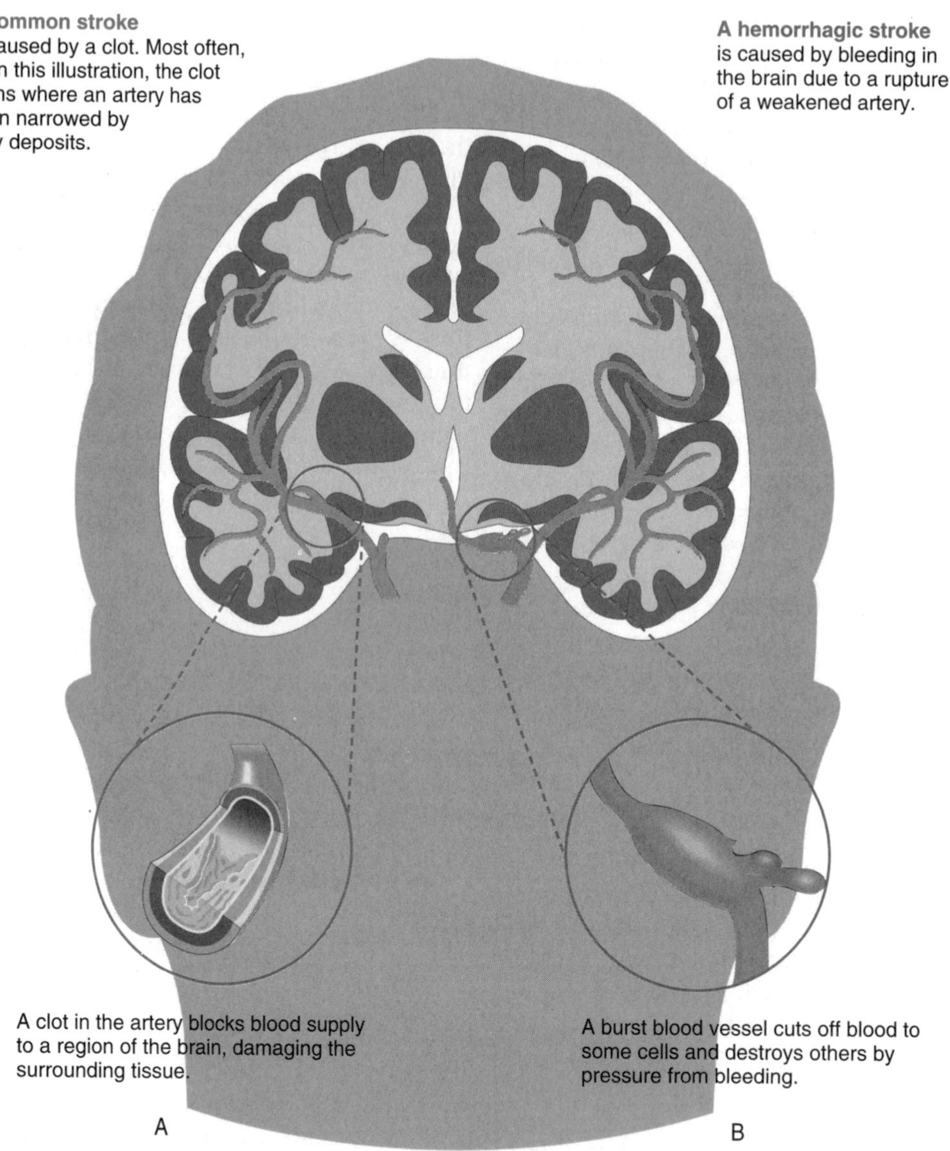

Figure 9.5 Two types of strokes. Common strokes are caused by blockage of an artery; hemorrhagic strokes are caused by the bursting of an artery in the brain.

Source: From Hales, 1997, p. 379.

area; more extensive damage results in greater impairment. This same principle applies to other types of disabilities caused by stroke. Damage may be so extensive—or in such a critical area—as to bring about immediate death; or damage may be so slight as to go unnoticed.

Degenerative diseases of the cardiovascular system, such as atherosclerosis and arteriosclerosis, are not the only cause of stroke. Blood clots can form around internal wounds in the process of healing and break away to float through the circulatory system. However, the most common cause of stroke is atherosclerosis. Blood clots can form around atheromatous plaques, and a plaque itself may detach from the artery wall, forming a floating hazard in the cardiovascular system that may result in a debilitating or deadly stroke.

Blood Pressure

When the heart pumps blood, the force must be substantial to power circulation for an entire cycle through the body and back to the heart. In a healthy cardiovascular system, the pressure in the arteries is not a problem because arteries are quite elastic. In a cardiovascular system diseased by atherosclerosis and arteriosclerosis, however, the pressure of the blood in the arteries can produce serious consequences. The narrowing of the arteries that occurs in atherosclerosis and the loss of elasticity that characterizes arteriosclerosis both tend to raise blood pressure and make the cardiovascular system less capable of adapting to the demands of heavy exercise and stress.

Blood pressure measurements are usually expressed by two numbers. The first number represents **systolic pressure,** the pressure generated by the heart's contraction. The second number represents **diastolic pressure,** or the pressure achieved between contractions, reflecting the elasticity of the vessel walls. Both numbers are measured by determining how high in millimeters (mm) a column of mercury (Hg) can be raised in a glass column.

Elevations of blood pressure can occur through several mechanisms. Some elevations in blood pressure are normal and even adaptive. Activation of the sympathetic nervous system, for example, increases heart rate and also causes constriction of the blood vessels, both of which raise blood pressure. The parasympathetic division blocks sympathetic action and returns blood pressure to its baseline rate, so sympathetic activation should not result in permanent increases in blood pressure. Other elevations in blood pressure, however, are neither normal nor adaptive; they are symptoms of cardiovascular disorder.

Millions of people in the United States have **hypertension**—that is, abnormally high blood pressure. This "silent" illness is the single best predictor of both heart attack and stroke, but it can also cause eye damage and kidney failure (see Figure 9.6). Hypertension is of two types—primary or essential hypertension and secondary hypertension. **Essential hypertension,** which accounts for 90% of the hypertension in the United States (Williams & Knight, 1994), refers to elevations of blood pressure that have no identified cause. It is positively related to such factors as age, African American ancestry, weight, sodium intake, tobacco use, and lack of exercise. **Secondary hypertension** is much less common than essential hypertension and stems from other diseases such as arteriosclerosis, kidney disorders, and some disorders of the endocrine system.

Table 9.1 shows the ranges for normal blood pressure, borderline hypertension, and hypertension. Despite beliefs to the contrary, people with hypertension are not able to diagnose their own blood pressure reliably (Meyer, Leventhal, & Gutman, 1985). Therefore, people can have dangerously elevated blood pressure and remain completely unaware of their vulnerability to heart attack and stroke.

Hypertension tends to progress from elevated systolic blood pressure coupled with normal or slightly elevated diastolic pressure to elevations of both systolic and diastolic blood pressure. Although systolic and diastolic hypertension may occur separately, people—especially older people—with hypertension typically experience elevations of both. Systolic pressure that exceeds 200 mm Hg presents a danger of rupture in the arterial walls (Berne & Levy, 2000). A rupture of the aorta is usually fatal; a rupture of a cerebral artery results in a stroke that may be fatal. Diastolic hypertension tends to result in vascular damage that may injure organs served by the affected vessels, most commonly the kidneys, liver, pancreas, brain, and retina.

Because the underlying cause of essential hypertension is unknown, no treatment exists

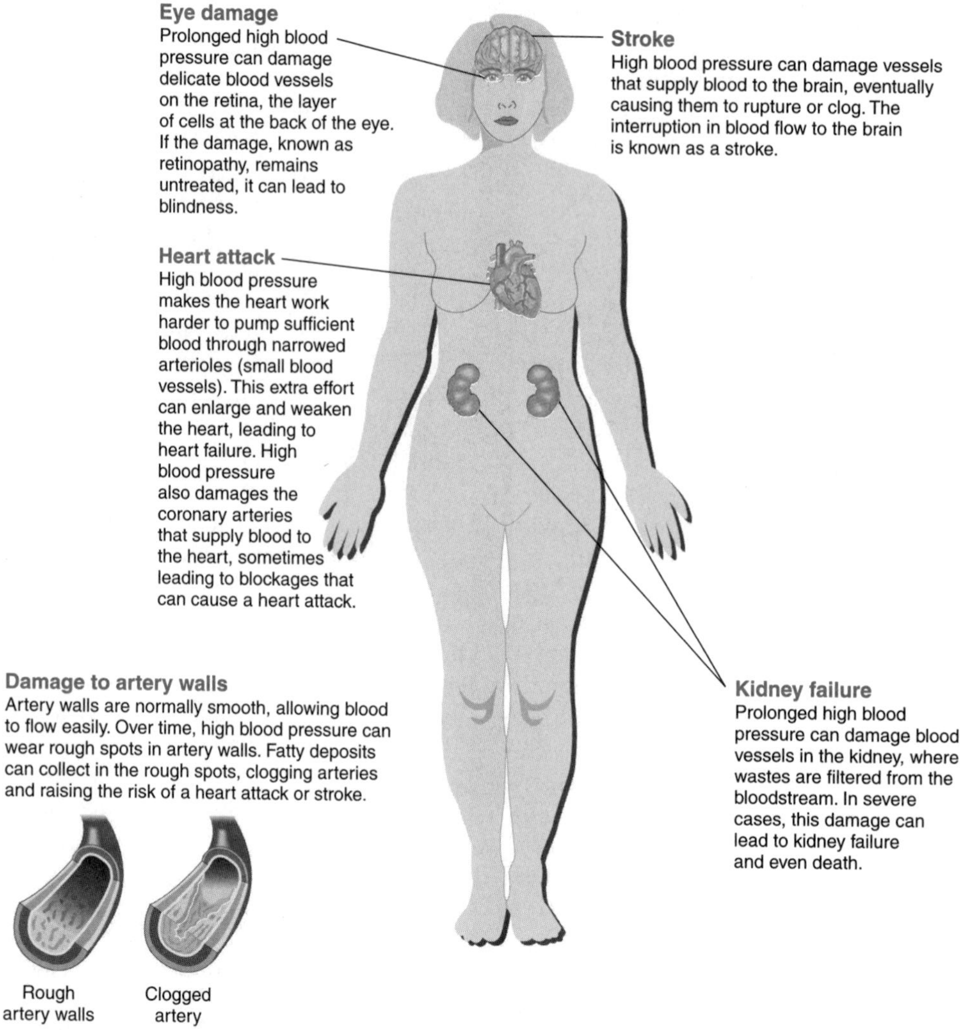

Eye damage
Prolonged high blood pressure can damage delicate blood vessels on the retina, the layer of cells at the back of the eye. If the damage, known as retinopathy, remains untreated, it can lead to blindness.

Stroke
High blood pressure can damage vessels that supply blood to the brain, eventually causing them to rupture or clog. The interruption in blood flow to the brain is known as a stroke.

Heart attack
High blood pressure makes the heart work harder to pump sufficient blood through narrowed arterioles (small blood vessels). This extra effort can enlarge and weaken the heart, leading to heart failure. High blood pressure also damages the coronary arteries that supply blood to the heart, sometimes leading to blockages that can cause a heart attack.

Damage to artery walls
Artery walls are normally smooth, allowing blood to flow easily. Over time, high blood pressure can wear rough spots in artery walls. Fatty deposits can collect in the rough spots, clogging arteries and raising the risk of a heart attack or stroke.

Rough artery walls

Clogged artery

Kidney failure
Prolonged high blood pressure can damage blood vessels in the kidney, where wastes are filtered from the bloodstream. In severe cases, this damage can lead to kidney failure and even death.

Figure 9.6 The consequences of high blood pressure.

Source: From Hales, 1997, p. 370.

TABLE 9.1 *Ranges of Blood Pressure (Expressed in mm of Hg)*

	Systolic	Diastolic
Normal	< 140	< 85
Borderline	140–159	85–104
Hypertensive	160 +	105 +

Sources: Adapted from the *1984 Report of the Joint National Committee on Detection, Evaluation and Treatment of High Blood Pressure* (p. 8) by the U.S. Department of Health and Human Services (USDHHS), 1984, Washington, DC: U.S. Government Printing Office.

that will remedy its basic cause. Treatment tends to be oriented toward drugs or changes in behavior or lifestyle that can lower blood pressure. Because part of the treatment of hypertension involves behavioral changes, health psychologists have a role to play in encouraging such behaviors as controlling weight, maintaining a regular exercise program, and restricting sodium intake.

In Summary

The cardiovascular system consists of the heart and blood vessels. The heart pumps blood, which circulates throughout the body, supplying oxygen and removing waste products. The coronary arteries supply blood to the heart itself, and when atherosclerosis affects these arteries, coronary artery disease (CAD) occurs. In this disease process, plaques form within the arteries, restricting the blood supply to the heart muscle. The restriction can cause angina pectoris, with symptoms of chest pain and difficulty in breathing. Blocked coronary arteries can also lead to a myocardial infarction (heart attack). When the oxygen supply to the brain is disrupted, stroke occurs. Stroke can affect any part of the brain and can vary in severity from minor to fatal. Hypertension—high blood pressure—is a predictor of both heart attack and stroke. Both behavioral and medical treatments can lower hypertension as well as other risk factors for cardiovascular disease.

Measures of Cardiovascular Function

For 55% of the people with coronary disease, a heart attack is the first symptom of a problem (Ellestad, 1996). Therefore, diagnosis of CAD is an urgent issue. Accurate diagnoses depend on reliable measures of both the functioning of the cardiovascular system and changes in that functioning.

The most common measurement of cardiovascular function is blood pressure. Blood pressure measurements suggest whether arteries have narrowed, lost elasticity, or both. Because high blood pressure has many causes, hypertension does not always signal heart disease. Other techniques can assess cardiovascular function more precisely than the measurement of blood pressure, but none of these other assessments are as simple or as available as blood pressure tests. Although there are no easy methods for the early diagnosis of CAD, several measures besides blood pressure are commonly used to detect potential cardiovascular problems.

Measurements of Electrical Activity in the Heart

An **electrocardiogram (ECG)** is a measurement of the electrical impulses produced by the heartbeat; this measurement is capable of revealing abnormalities in the resting heartbeat. People who show an abnormal ECG usually have some type of cardiovascular disorder. However, ECG readings cannot reveal the buildup of plaques in the coronary arteries. Consequently, dangerously advanced CAD may go undetected by an electrocardiogram.

A **stress test** measures the heart's electrical activity when stressed, usually during exercise. Exercise increases oxygen demand by the heart muscle, so blockage of arteries is more easily detectable during exercise. Therefore, this measure is more sensitive and useful than an electrocardiogram in diagnosing heart problems. For example, an ECG cannot detect coronary artery blockage of less than 75%, but a stress test can reveal blockage of around 50%. This level of blockage often fails to produce noticeable symptoms, thus stress testing is useful for discovering moderate yet significant levels of coronary artery blockage (Ellestad, 1996).

In a stress test, measuring electrodes are placed in a standard pattern on the torso, and then the person engages in progressively more strenuous exercise, typically either walking on a treadmill with an increasing slope or riding a stationary bicycle with increasing pedal resistance. As the exercise increases the body's demand for oxygen, the heart increases its action. If coronary arteries are partially blocked, the blood cannot be delivered fast enough to keep up with the increased demand. This restriction results in a pattern of electrical activity with a characteristic waveform that permits trained professionals to make a diagnosis of coronary artery disease.

Stress tests can provide additional diagnostic information about cardiovascular problems. People with angina pectoris may know that restriction of blood flow is the cause of their chest pains, but stress testing can inform them about the severity of the restriction. People with chest pains are sometimes given stress tests to determine whether their pains are a result of ischemia or some other cause. Stress tests are also recommended after myocardial infarction, as a way to measure damage to the heart, and after coronary bypass surgery, as a way to assess the effectiveness of the procedure (Ellestad, 1996). Stress tests are also recommended for previously sedentary people who decide to start an exercise program.

A range of new techniques measures the function of the heart and cardiovascular system, but none replaces stress testing (Lavie, Milani, & Mehra, 2000). These techniques include nuclear perfusion imaging and echocardiography. These tests are often added to rather than substituted for exercise stress testing. Each adds information, and a combination may substitute for angiography.

Angiography

The most definitive method of diagnosis for coronary artery disease is cardiac catheterization and **angiography.** Werner Forssmann was the first person to attempt cardiac angiography—on himself in 1929 (Ricciuti, 1997). The technique did not develop until the 1940s and 1950s, but it is now a routine diagnostic procedure. Angiography is used to determine the extent of coronary artery disease in cases of angina pectoris, after a positive result from a stress test, or after a myocardial infarction.

With cardiac angiography, the patient's heart is injected with a dye so that the coronary arteries are visible during X ray. Injecting the dye involves inserting a catheter into a blood vessel in either the patient's arm or groin and then threading it through the circulatory system to the heart. The heart pumps the released dye into the coronary arteries, allowing an X ray to reveal the extent of the blockage as well as the areas where blood flow is reduced. For a complete diagnostic procedure, several catheterizations are necessary, and the procedure takes a total time of 1 to 2 hours (Ricciuti, 1997).

Cardiac catheterization and angiography are invasive surgical procedures, but patients are awake and usually only lightly sedated. The procedure is uncomfortable and even painful, and patients are typically anxious about their health as well as the procedure itself. In addition, angiography carries some slight risk of injury or death. The chances of complications increase with patients who have more serious heart problems or diabetes (Ricciuti, 1997). Health psychologists can train patients in various techniques to relieve the stress and discomfort involved with this procedure.

Cardiac catheterization can be used in treatment as well as in diagnosis. Clot-dissolving drugs can be injected during a heart attack to dissolve the blood clot that precipitated the infarction, to minimize damage to the heart muscle. In addition, catheters with inflatable tips can reopen blocked arteries, helping to prevent heart attacks.

Angioplasty is the procedure of inserting a balloon-tipped catheter into blocked arteries and inflating the tip to reduce artery blockage. First used successfully in 1977, angioplasty has now become routine (Ricciuti, 1997). Although angioplasty involves an invasive surgical procedure, it is less risky than coronary bypass grafting. The success of angioplasty depends on the severity of the lesions, but the procedure is successful in at least 65% of cases. The main problem with angioplasty is the tendency for the blockage to reoccur, which occurs in 25 to 35% of patients.

Catheterization can also be used to install a stent in an artery (Ricciuti, 1997). A stent is a metal device that can open a blocked artery and keep it open. Catheterization is also part of the process of removing artery blockages by breaking up the plaque or removing it. Catheterization is necessary for these treatment procedures, but diagnosis without surgical intervention is a desirable goal. Several techniques allow diagnosis of various heart problems with less invasive technologies, but catheterization and angiography remain the "gold standard" of diagnosis (Lavie et al., 2000).

In Summary

Several techniques measure the functioning of the cardiovascular system. The simplest of these is a blood pressure reading, which does not offer a complete diagnosis. The ECG can determine cardiovascular abnormalities of a resting heartbeat. However, an exercise stress test is more valid and sensitive because it combines electrical measurement of the heart with the increased demands on the cardiovascular system that exercise produces. This technique can reveal blockage of the coronary arteries if substantial damage has occurred. Angiography, which involves x-raying the heart and coronary arteries, is currently considered the most precise diagnostic procedure. However, angiography requires placement of catheters in the heart, an invasive, uncomfortable, stressful procedure. All of these diagnostic procedures help health care professionals advise patients about the extent of damage and the possibility of surgery, angioplasty, and lifestyle changes.

The Changing Rates of Cardiovascular Disease

The current mortality rate from CVD for people in the United States is almost identical to the rate in 1920. However, between 1920 and 1998, the death rates changed dramatically. Figure 9.7 reveals a sharp rise in CVD deaths from 1920 until the 1950s and 1960s, followed by a decline that continued throughout the century. By 2000, the mortality rate was slightly lower than it was in 1920. Currently, 31% of all deaths in the United States are from heart disease and another 6.7% from stroke (USBC, 2001).

In 1920, the rate of deaths due to heart disease was similar for women and men. Overall, the rates of death from CVD are similar, but the pattern of deaths began to differ when CVD rates began to rise. During the middle of the 20th century, men died from CVD at younger ages than women, creating a gender gap in heart disease.

Reasons for the Decline in Death Rates

The decline in cardiac mortality in the United States is due largely to two causes—improved emergency coronary care and changes in lifestyle (CDC, 1999a; Wise, 2000). Beginning in the 1960s, many people in the United States began to change their lifestyle. They began to smoke less, be more aware of their blood pressure levels, control serum cholesterol levels, watch their weight, and follow a regular exercise program.

Many of these lifestyle changes were prompted by the publicity given to two monumental studies. The first was the Framingham Heart Study that began to issue reports during the 1960s, implicating cigarette smoking, high cholesterol, hypertension, a sedentary lifestyle, and obesity as risk factors in cardiovascular disease (Voelker, 1998). The second study was the highly publicized 1964 surgeon general's report (U.S. Public Health Service [USPHS], 1964), which found an unequivocal close association between cigarette smoking and heart disease. Many people became aware of these studies and began to alter their way of living.

Although these lifestyle changes closely parallel declining heart disease death rates, they offer no proof of a causal link between behavior changes and the drop in cardiovascular mortality. During this same period, medical care and technology continued to improve, and many cardiac patients who in earlier years would have died were saved by better and faster treatment. Which factor—lifestyle changes or better medical care—has

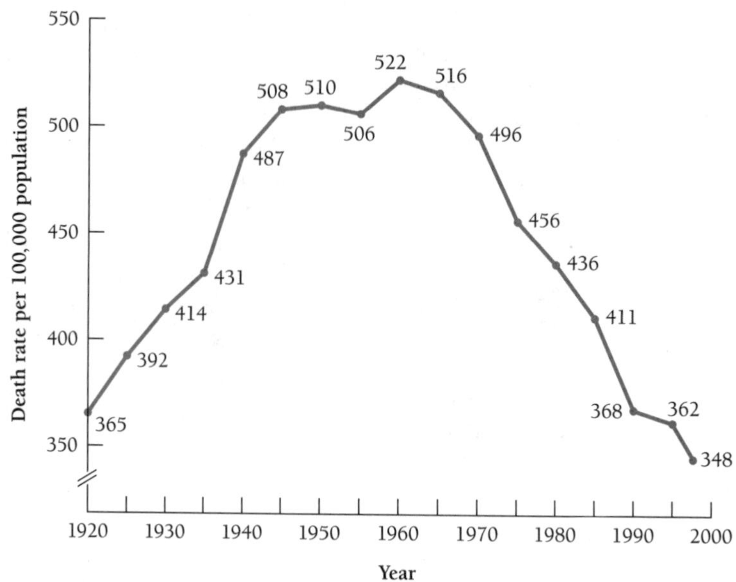

Figure 9.7 Death rates for cardiovascular disease per 100,000 population, United States, 1920–1998.

Sources: Data from Historical Statistics of the United States: Colonial Times to 1970 *(p. 58) by U.S. Bureau of the Census, 1975, Washington, D.C.: U.S. Government Printing Office; from* Statistical Abstracts of the United States; 1986 *(p. 73), by U.S. Bureau of the Census, 1985, Washington, D.C.: U.S. Government Printing Office; and from* Statistical Abstracts of the United States, 2001 *(121st ed., p. 79), by U.S. Bureau of the Census, 2001, Washington, D.C.: U.S. Government Printing Office.*

contributed most to the declining death rate from heart disease? One answer to this question comes from a review of studies published in the United States (Hunink et al., 1997) that found that more than 50% of the decline in death from coronary heart disease was explained by behavior and lifestyle changes that protected people against both first and subsequent heart attacks and that about 43% of decline in CHD was due to improvements in treatment. Thus, the declining rates of death from heart disease is due at least as much to changes in behavior and lifestyle as it is to improved medical care.

Heart Disease Mortality throughout the World

Heart disease is the leading cause of death, not only in the United States, but worldwide. This situation is not true for every country; in some countries, infectious diseases kill more people than CVD, but the number of total deaths for heart disease and stroke accounts for about 30% of all deaths (Martin, 1998). The United States is only one of many industrialized Western countries that have seen lifestyle changes and dramatic reductions in cardiovascular deaths among its population. Other countries, however, have experienced dramatic increases in CVD.

In Finland CVD rates have fallen over 70% from the 1970s through the 1990s (Puska, Vartiainen, Tuomilehto, Salomaa, & Nissinen, 1998). Part of this decrease is the result of a countrywide effort to change risk factors. That effort began with a community intervention that targeted an area of Finland with particularly high rates of CVD and attempted to change diet, hypertension, and smoking. That region of Finland experienced a sharper decline in CVD than the rest of the country, but CVD rates fell nationwide (as did cancer deaths).

In New Zealand and Australia, nonfatal myocardial infarctions declined for both men and women by about 3% per year from the mid-1980s to the mid-1990s (Beaglehole et al., 1997). The rate of prehospitalized deaths declined more than deaths after hospitalization, which means that lifestyle changes rather than medical treatment have reduced the number of first heart attack deaths in those countries.

A very different situation occurred in countries that had been part of the Soviet Union, many of which have experienced a dramatic increase in CVD over the past 10 years (Weidner, 2000). This epidemic affects middle-aged men more than other groups, and the gender gap in heart disease is larger in Russia than any other country. The risk of premature death from heart disease is four times more likely for a Russian man than one in the United States. In some countries in eastern Europe, coronary heart disease accounts for 80% of deaths, and the average life expectancy has decreased. The reasons for this plague of heart disease are not completely understood, but lack of social support and stress are implicated (Stone, 2000).

People associate CVD with industrialized countries, but heart disease and stroke are also leading causes of death in developing and undeveloped countries (Martin, 1998). These countries will not undergo a decline in CVD but an increase. In addition, the declines in CVD have been significant in many industrialized countries, but despite the decreased rates, CVD remains the leading cause of death in these countries. Thus, the burden of CVD is immense.

In Summary

Since the mid-1960s, deaths from coronary artery disease and stroke have steadily declined in the United States and most (but not all) other industrialized nations. Although some of that decline is a result of better and faster coronary care, most authorities believe that lifestyle changes account for 50% or more of this decrease. During the past 3 decades, millions of people in the United States quit smoking, became more aware of their blood pressure, watched their diet in order to control weight and cholesterol, and began an exercise program to lower their risk of heart disease.

Risk Factors in Cardiovascular Disease

Medical research has no exact answers as to what causes dangerous buildup of atheromatous plaques in the arteries of some people but not in others. However, research has linked several risk factors to cardiovascular disease. In Chapter 2, we defined a *risk factor* as any characteristic or condition that occurs with greater frequency in people with a disease than in people free from that disease. The risk factor approach does not reveal the underlying physiology in the development of the disorder; that is, it does not allow for the identification of a cause. Nor does it allow a precise prediction of who will be affected and who will remain healthy. The risk factor approach simply yields information concerning which conditions are associated—directly or indirectly—with a particular disease or disorder.

The risk factor approach to predicting heart disease began with the Framingham Heart Study in 1948, an investigation of more than 5,000 people in the town of Framingham, Massachusetts. The study was a prospective design; thus all participants were free of heart disease at the beginning of the study. The original plan was to follow these people for 20 years to study heart disease and the factors related to its development. The results proved so valuable that the study has continued now for more than 50 years and includes both second and third generation offspring of the original participants (Voelker, 1998).

During its early years, the Framingham study uncovered a number of risk factors for cardiovascular disease, including cigarette smoking, high cholesterol levels, elevated blood pressure, lack of physical activity, diet, and obesity. Other studies have found additional conditions that relate directly or indirectly to heart disease, and these include inherent risk factors such as old age, diabetes, family history, gender, and ethnic background as well as psychosocial factors such as phobic anxiety, marital status, employment, hostility, and anger. Despite this impressive list, some observers (Nieto, 1999) believe that we currently know only a fraction of all the risk factors and that the ones we do know contribute to only about half of all heart disease.

Cardiovascular risk factors include those that are inherent and cannot be changed, physiological conditions such as hypertension and high serum cholesterol level, behavioral factors such as smoking and diet, and a variety of psychosocial factors.

Inherent Risk Factors

Inherent risk factors result from genetic or physical conditions that cannot be modified through lifestyle changes. Although inherent risk factors cannot be changed, people with these risk factors are not necessarily destined to develop cardiovascular disease. Identifying people with inherent risk factors is important because such high-risk individuals can minimize their overall risk profile by controlling the things that they can: hypertension, smoking, and diet. Inherent risk factors for CVD include advancing age, diabetes, family history, gender, and ethnic background.

Advancing Age Advancing age is the primary risk factor for cardiovascular disease as well as for cancer and many other diseases. As people become older, their risk for cardiovascular death rises sharply. Figure 9.8 shows that for every 10-year increase in age, both men and women more than double their chances of dying of cardiovascular disease. For example, men 85 and older are about 2.8 times as likely to die of cardiovascular disease compared to men 75 to 84 years of age, and women 85 and older are about 3.7 times as likely as women 75 to 84 to die from cardiovascular disease.

Diabetes A second inherent risk factor for CVD is diabetes. People who have juvenile-onset (Type 1) diabetes are more likely to die of heart disease than those whose sugar metabolism is normal (Olson & Wilson, 2000). Type 2 diabetes also elevates the risk of CVD (Hu et al., 2001; Lotufo et al., 2001). People with either type of diabetes can decrease their risk by following a healthy lifestyle and by adhering to their medical regimen. (We discuss diabetes and cardiovascular disease more fully in Chapter 11.)

Family History Family history is also an inherent risk factor for CVD. People with a history of cardiovascular disease in their family are more likely to die of heart disease than those with no such history; Jason, our case study, is at risk because of his father's history of heart disease at an early age. Like other inherent risk factors, family history cannot be altered through lifestyle changes, but people with a family history of heart disease can lower their risk by changing those behaviors and lifestyles that can be altered.

Gender Gender is another inherent risk factor. Heart disease is the leading cause of death in the United States for both women and men. Men have a higher *rate* of death from CVD than women, and this discrepancy is strongest during the middle-age years. Figure 9.8 shows that the rate of men's death from cardiovascular disease is about double that of women for ages 35 to 74. After that age, the percentage of women's deaths due to CVD increases sharply but still does not equal that of men.

What factors explain this gender gap? Lifestyle alone cannot account for the gender gap. In the United States, research that adjusts for lifestyle factors such as smoking, education, physical activity, cholesterol levels, and blood

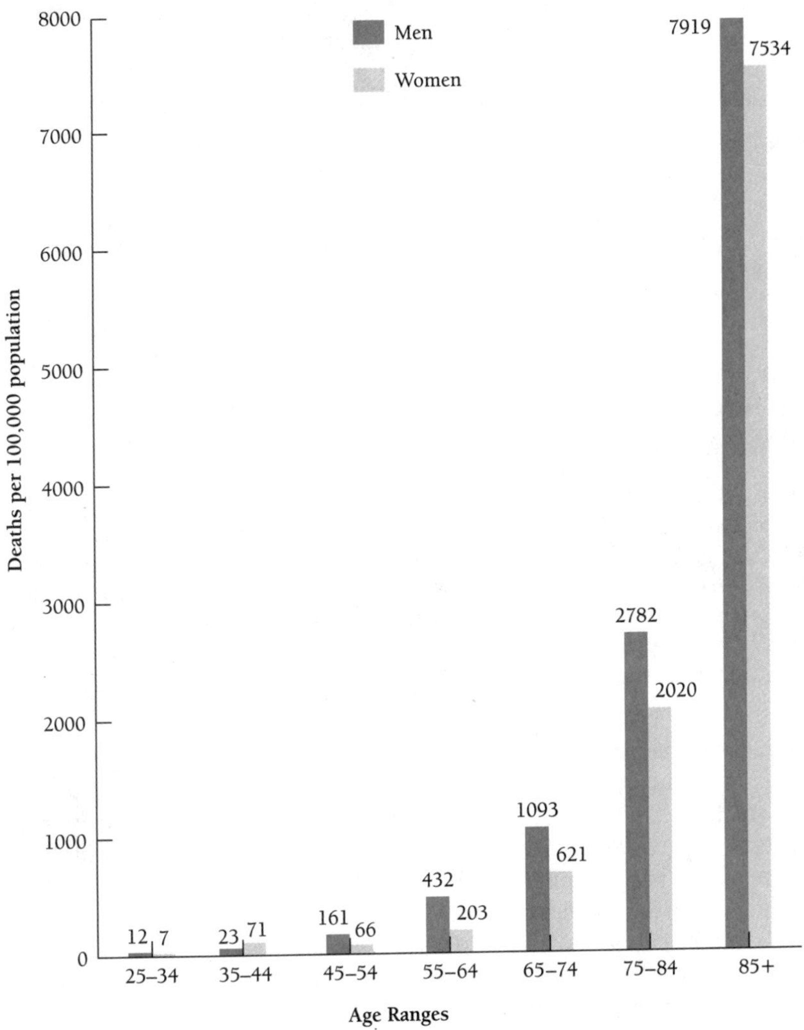

Figure 9.8 Cardiovascular disease mortality rates by age and gender, United States, 1999.

Source: Health United States, 2001, *by National Center for Health Statistics, 2001, Hyattsville, MD: U.S. Government Printing Office, pp. 189, 192.*

pressure do not change the risk, at least not for elderly men (Fried et al., 1998). Even with the same risk factors as women, men are still more than twice as likely to die from coronary artery disease. However, lifestyle must be responsible for some of the discrepancy, because differences among countries are greater than the difference between genders. For example, in Russia and in Beijing, China, men are 60% more likely to die of coronary heart disease than are women, but the added risk for men in Iceland is only about 10% (Wiedner, 2000). Also, Mexican American men have nearly three times the risk for CVD mortality compared with Mexican American women (Sundquist & Winkleby, 1999). The fact that gender differences in CVD mortality are much

WOULD YOU BELIEVE

Baldness Is a Risk for Heart Disease

Would you believe that bald men are at higher risk for heart disease than men with more hair? Several studies have indicated that they are, including one large, prospective study (Lotufo, Chae, Ajani, Hennekens, & Manson, 2000). The results from this study showed that men who have lost some of their hair by age 45 were at increased risk for heart disease during the next 11 years.

The risk is not equal for all balding men; some patterns of hair loss increased the risk more than others. Hair loss occurs in several patterns, including baldness beginning at the forehead and loss starting at the top of the head. Men who lost their hair in the front showed very little elevated risk for coronary heart disease, but those with even mild top-of-the-head baldness showed elevated risk. In addition, the severity of this type of baldness was related to the degree of risk; men with more extensive hair loss were at progressively increased risk. Men with severe hair loss had a risk three times greater than those with no hair loss.

The elevated risk held, even when the researchers controlled for risk factors such as age, parental history of heat attack, diabetes, smoking, physical activity, and hypertension. However, a subgroup of men with severe top-of-the-head baldness, plus high blood pressure, plus high cholesterol levels had higher than a threefold risk of CHD before age 60.

The relationship between hair loss and heart disease may be through testosterone. High levels of androgens may contribute both to baldness and to conditions that promote coronary heart disease, such as atherosclerosis and high cholesterol. Therefore, men who have more androgen receptors may be more likely to lose their hair and also to develop the underlying disease processes for heart disease.

greater in some countries than in others suggests that inherent gender differences, such as estrogen levels, play only a small role in the CVD mortality discrepancy between men and women.

In addition, if gender is truly an inherent risk factor for CVD, then the differences between men and women should be similar not only from country to country but throughout history. Evidence suggests that the gender gap in heart disease in the United States was small until the 1920s (Nikiforov & Mamaev, 1998). Until that time, CVD deaths for men ages 25 to 74 years were only about 20% higher than for women, and these differences remained modest until the 1960s. At that time, however, the gap between men and women began to expand as middle-aged men's rates increased while women's rates declined. As a consequence, men now have twice the cardiovascular mortality as women during middle age (see Figure 9.8). This historical perspective suggests that factors other than biology are at work in creating the gender gap, but it leaves the discrepancy unexplained.

Incidentally, although middle-age men are about twice as likely as middle-age women to die of CVD, they are more likely than women to *survive* a heart attack. One study (Vaccarino, Parsons, Every, Barron, & Krumholz, 1999) found that women less than 50 years old who had a heart attack were more than twice as likely to die as were male heart attack victims. However, these gender differences diminished with age so that, at age 74, women are as likely as men to survive a heart attack. The reason for these discrepancies remains unexplained.

Ethnic Background A fifth inherent risk for cardiovascular disease is ethnic background. African Americans have nearly a two-fold risk for cardiovascular deaths compared to European Americans (Harry Rosenberg, Centers for Disease Control and Prevention, personal communication, September 23, 1998). Whether this increased risk for African Americans is inherent or related to social, economic, or behavioral factors remains in question.

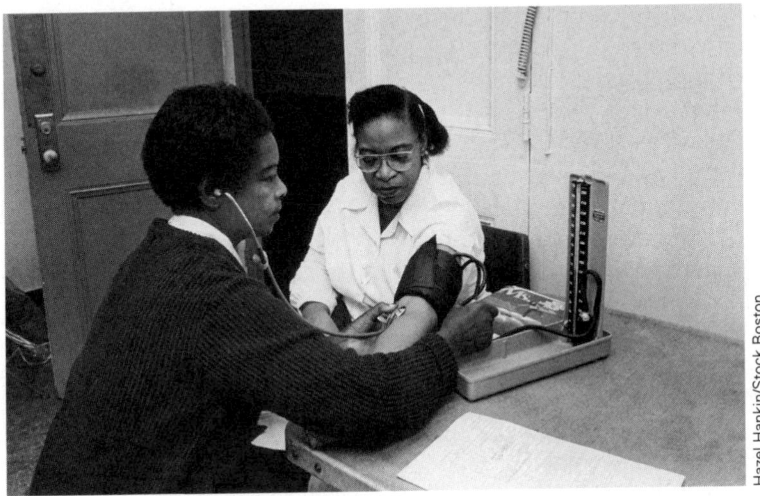

African Americans are more likely to have hypertension than European Americans.

African Americans tend to have the same category of risk factors for heart disease as do European Americans. However, the level of many of those risks is greater for African Americans, a discrepancy that exists even during childhood (Winkleby, Robinson, Sundquist, & Kraemer, 1999). The risks that are strongest for African Americans are high blood pressure, low income, and low educational level (Gillum, Mussolino, & Madans, 1998). The higher rates of cardiovascular death among African Americans may relate to their higher rate of hypertension, which may relate to greater cardiac reactivity, which in turn, may relate to racial discrimination. Even threats of discrimination can raise blood pressure in African Americans (Blascovich, Spencer, Quinn, & Steele, 2000). The tendency to react to stress and threats of stress with increased cardiac reactivity is probably not inherent, but rather it springs from years of racial discrimination, a discrimination most likely experienced by dark-skinned people. For example, Elizabeth Klonoff and Hope Landrine (2000) found that dark-skinned African Americans, compared with light-skinned African Americans, were 11 times more likely to experience frequent racial discrimination. This finding suggests that the high blood pressure ratings of African Americans may be a result of color discrimination. Racial discrimination is a factor in the increased blood pressure levels among African Americans, but the issue is complicated by gender, skin color, and social class (Krieger et al, 1998).

Physiological Conditions

A second category of risk factors in cardiovascular disease includes the physiological conditions of hypertension and serum cholesterol level.

Hypertension Other than advancing age, hypertension is the single most important risk factor in cardiovascular disease. Regardless of nationality or ethnic background, high blood pressure is an important risk factor (van den Hoogen et al., 2000). Yet millions of people with high blood pressure are not aware of their vulnerability. Unlike most disorders, hypertension produces no overt symptoms, and dangerously elevated blood pressure levels commonly occur with no signals or symptoms. Most people believe that if their blood pressure were high, they would be aware of the elevation (Meyer, Leventhal, & Gutman, 1985). They are wrong; hypertension ordinarily has no discernible symptoms. At 15, Jason did not monitor his blood pressure, but at 21, he knows that his blood pressure is in the normal range.

Although the Framingham Heart Study was not the first to suggest that people with high blood pressure have more cardiovascular problems than those with normal blood pressure, it provided solid evidence of the importance of hypertension. The Framingham study (Dawber, 1980) divided blood pressure into three categories: normotensive (normal blood pressure), borderline, and hypertensive. Regardless of people's age or gender, their risk of cardiovascular disease increased with increases in blood pressure, clearly indicating that high blood pressure is a risk factor. Since that time, many other studies (e.g., Fried et al., 1998; Stamler et al., 1999) have found an association between blood pressure and rate of cardiovascular disease.

Serum Cholesterol Level A second physiological condition related to cardiovascular disease is high serum cholesterol level. *Serum* or *blood cholesterol* is the level of cholesterol circulating through the blood stream; this level is related (but not perfectly related) to *dietary cholesterol,* or the amount of cholesterol in one's food. Cholesterol is a waxy, fat-like substance that is essential for human life as a component of cell membranes. Dietary cholesterol comes from animal fats and oils but not from vegetables or vegetable products. Although cholesterol is essential for life, too much may lead to cardiovascular disease.

After a person eats cholesterol, the bloodstream transports it as part of the process of digestion. A measurement of the amount of cholesterol carried in the serum (the liquid, cell-free part of the blood) is typically expressed in milligrams (mg) of cholesterol per deciliters (dl) of serum. This measurement is a ratio, but it is generally abbreviated to the cholesterol count. Thus, a cholesterol reading of 210 means 210 mg of cholesterol per deciliter of blood serum. But what does a cholesterol level of 210 mean? Is it good or bad?

Very high levels of cholesterol are associated with increased deaths from cardiovascular disease, but the relationship between total cholesterol and all-cause mortality is complex. Recent studies (Stamler et al., 1999; Stamler et al., 2000) continue to find that total cholesterol levels above 250 are significantly related to increased risk for death from CHD and CVD for both men and women. However, during the past 15 years evidence began to emerge that very low cholesterol levels do not lower total mortality rates (Holme, 1990; Iso, Jacobs, Wentworth, Neaton, & Cohn, 1989). A recent large-scale study of Korean men (Song, Sung, & Kim, 2000) found that cholesterol level below 165 was associated with increased risk of all-cause mortality and that the safest levels of total cholesterol ranged from about 210 to 250, a level higher than that of the average Korean man!

If people with low cholesterol levels, compared with those of average or high cholesterol, have a lower rate of death from cardiovascular disease but the same rate of all-cause mortality, then how are these people dying? Song et al. (2000) reported that Korean men with very low cholesterol (<135) had higher rates of death from liver and colon cancer than did men of average and above average cholesterol levels. Another possible culprit is violent deaths; that is, people with very low cholesterol seem to have an increased chance of dying from suicide or unintentional injuries.

Not all cholesterol is equally implicated in coronary heart disease. Cholesterol circulates in the blood in several forms of **lipoproteins,** which can be distinguished by analyzing their density. The Framingham researchers found that **low-density lipoprotein (LDL)** was positively related to cardiovascular disease, whereas **high-density lipoprotein (HDL)** was negatively related. That is, HDL seems to offer some protection against CVD, whereas LDL seems to promote atherosclerosis. For these reasons, LDL is sometimes referred to as "bad cholesterol" and HDL as "good cholesterol." Indeed, women's higher levels of HDL may be a partial explanation for the gender gap in heart disease (Davis et al., 1996).

Total cholesterol (TC) is determined by adding the values for HDL, LDL, and 20% of very low-density lipoprotein (VLDL), also called **triglycerides.** A low ratio of total cholesterol to HDL is more desirable than a high ratio. A ratio of less than 4.5 to 1 is healthier than a ratio of 6.0 to 1; that is, people whose HDL level is about 20% to 22% of total cholesterol have a reduced risk of CVD. Most authorities now believe that a favorable balance of total cholesterol to HDL is more critical than total cholesterol in avoiding cardiovascular disease.

However, neither total cholesterol nor the ratio of TC to HDL is important in older people. Data from the Framingham study (Kronmal, Cain, Ye, & Omenn, 1993) revealed that total cholesterol was a predictor of death from heart disease up to about age 60. From age 60 to 70, there was no significant relationship, and after age 80 total serum cholesterol levels may actually have a protective effect against death from cardiovascular disease, including stroke (Sacco et al., 2001). Therefore, cholesterol should be a concern through middle age, but older people can be less focused on attaining a low cholesterol level.

Research on cholesterol suggests several conclusions. First, cholesterol intake and blood cholesterol are related. Second, the relationship between dietary intake of cholesterol and blood cholesterol relates strongly to habitual diet—that is, eating habits maintained over many years. Lowering blood cholesterol level is possible, but the process is neither quick nor easy. Third, the ratio of total cholesterol to HDL is probably more important than total cholesterol alone. Fourth, the guidelines that apply to young and middle-aged people do not apply to older people.

Behavioral Factors

Behavioral correlates of cardiovascular disease constitute a third risk for CVD, and the most important of these lifestyle factors are smoking and diet. For example, women who do not smoke, eat a diet high in fiber and low in saturated fat, are not overweight, and are physically active have an 80% lower risk for coronary heart disease than other people (Stampfer, Hu, Manson, Rimm, & Willett, 2000).

Smoking Cigarette smoking is the leading behavioral risk factor for cardiovascular death in the United States, although cardiovascular deaths due to smoking have begun to decline (CDC, 2002). This decrease in smoking has closely paralleled the drop in CVD mortality, an association that does not prove cause and effect, but nevertheless is a necessary condition for a causal relationship. This positive relationship between declines in smoking and CHD is shown dramatically in a report from the Nurses' study (Hu, Stampfer, Manson et al., 2000), which showed a 41% decrease in smoking from the early 1980s to the mid-1990s. This decline was paralleled by a 31% decrease in incidence of coronary heart disease.

A study of lifestyle and biological risk factors for coronary artery disease (Twisk, Kemper, van Mechelen, & Post, 1997) looked at such factors as diet, physical activity, alcohol consumption, cholesterol levels, blood pressure, body fat, cardiopulmonary fitness, and smoking. Most lifestyle factors were relatively low risks, but cigarette smoking was a strong risk for coronary artery disease. The link between smoking and heart disease has been well established for more than 35 years, and few studies are currently being conducted to confirm this association. Studies designed to discover a variety of cardiovascular risk factors (for example, Fried et al., 1998) continue to find that high levels of cigarette smoking more than double one's chances of dying from cardiovascular disease. Passive smoking is not as dangerous, but exposure to environmental tobacco smoke raises the risk for cardiovascular disease by about 20% (Werner & Pearson, 1998).

Diet Diet may either increase or decrease one's chances of developing heart disease, depending on the foods people eat. Evidence is quite strong that diets heavy in saturated fats are positively related to CVD. Replacing saturated fat, including butter and stick margarine with other types of fat such as liquid margarine and soybean oil, is one strategy to reduce cholesterol, improve the ratio of TC to HDL, and lower the risk for heart disease (Lichtenstein, Ausman, Jalbert, & Schaefer, 1999). Moderate alcohol consumption can also improve the ratio of TC to HDL (Linn et al., 1993).

In addition to saturated fats, several other foods, including sodium and eggs, have been suspected of contributing to CVD. Jiang He and associates (He et al., 1999) divided participants aged 25 to 74 into an overweight group and a normal-weight group and measured the sodium intake for each group. A follow-up that averaged 19 years showed that sodium intake was significantly and independently associated with increased CHD, CVD, and stroke in overweight but not for normal- or below-average-weight participants. Thus, people who are overweight should be extra careful about eating lots of salt.

Eggs have long been suspected of raising cholesterol levels and increasing risks for CVD. Is this suspicion justified? A prospective study of egg consumption (Hu et al., 1999) found no added risk for CHD for either men or women who consumed as many as seven eggs per week. However, this study showed a slight increase for CHD for diabetic participants who ate that many eggs.

Can diet serve as protection against cardiovascular disease? For more than 2 decades, researchers have found that diets high in fiber are associated with lower CVD risks. For example, a report from the Nurses' Health Study (Wolk et al., 1999) showed that women in the highest group of dietary fiber consumption had only about half the risk for CHD as women in the lowest group. Other research (Liu et al., 2000) suggests that diets high in fiber can protect against stroke. Thus, diets high in fruits, vegetables, and whole-grain cereals offer some protection against CVD.

Can a diet high in fish protect against heart disease and stroke? Evidence on this question is not strong. Some studies (Albert et al., 1998; Daviglus et al., 1997) have shown that fish consumption seems to offer moderate protection against coronary heart disease. However, evidence from the Seven Countries Study (Oomen et al., 2000) found no benefit of eating lean fish, but a diet high in fatty fish may offer some protection against CHD. Other researchers (Iso et al., 2001) have also found some benefit from fatty fish, specifically fish high in omega-3 fatty acids, which may lower the risk of stroke in women.

Do certain vitamins protect against cardiovascular disease? Vitamin E, beta carotene, selenium, and riboflavin are referred to as antioxidants because they seem to protect LDL from oxidation and thus from its potential damaging effects on the cardiovascular system. Consuming high levels of vitamin E lowered the CVD risk for female nurses (Stampfer et al., 1993) and male health care professionals (Rimm et al., 1993). The protective effects were not immediate, but after 2 years of taking vitamin E supplements, risks decreased. A measure of antioxidants in the blood, called serum carotenoids, also seems to protect against coronary disease (Morris, Kritchevsky, & Davis, 1994). These studies suggest that regular consumption of vitamin E and beta carotene probably has some ability to protect against heart disease.

Is obesity an independent risk for cardiovascular disease? Complicating any answer to this question is the small number of obese individuals who have no other risks. Ample evidence exists that as weight goes up, so too do blood pressure, Type 2 diabetes, total cholesterol, LDL, and triglycerides (Ashton, Nanchahal, & Wood, 2001). For this reason, the question of obesity as an independent risk factor for CHD and stroke remains unanswered.

Psychosocial Factors

In addition to inherent factors, physiological conditions, and behaviors, researchers have identified a number of psychosocial factors that relate to heart disease (Smith & Ruiz, 2002). Included among these factors are anxiety, depression, education, income, marital status, social support, cynical hostility, and anger.

Anxiety and Depression Both anxiety and depression are related to cardiovascular disease, but the evidence is stronger for men than for women. A report from the Framingham study (Markovitz, Matthews, Kannel, Cobb, & D'Agostino, 1993) revealed that men, but not women, who had heightened anxiety were more than twice as likely as men with lower anxiety levels to develop hypertension during middle age. A prospective study that included only men (Kawachi et al., 1994) showed that phobic anxiety increased the likelihood of sudden death from heart disease by a factor of three.

Depression is also related to cardiovascular disease. Susan Everson and colleagues (Everson, Roberts, Goldberg, & Kaplan, 1998) found that people with five or more depressive symptoms had a higher level of death from stroke than nondepressed participants. Similarly, a 16-year follow-up study (Jonas & Mussolino, 2000) found that depressed people were about 70% more likely to develop stroke, but the risk was not the same for all ethnic groups. After controlling for all important risk factors for stroke, this study found that depressed European American men had higher rates of stroke than depressed European American women and that depressed African Americans generally had higher rates of stroke than depressed European Americans.

Educational Level and Income Low educational level and low income are two additional risk factors for heart disease. A prospective study (Eaker, Pinsky, & Castelli, 1992) found that women with little education, whether they worked in the home or outside the home, were at increased risk of myocardial infarction. Other studies (e.g., Fried et al., 1998) reported that both women and men with less than a high school education had nearly twice the rate of cardiovascular mortality as men and women with higher levels of education. Also, the National Health and Nutrition Examination Survey (Gillum et al., 1998) found that both African American and European American men and women with fewer than 12 years of school were at an increased risk for coronary artery disease, but the risk was greatest for African American men. For this group, low education was an even higher risk than elevated blood pressure. What factors link low levels of educational to high levels of heart disease? One possibility is that people with low education are much more likely to be overweight, have higher blood pressure, and have less access to the health care system (Molarius, Seidell, Sans, Tuomilehto, & Kuulasmaa, 2000).

Income level is another risk factor for cardiovascular disease; people with lower incomes have higher rates of heart disease than people in the higher income brackets. Redford Williams and his associates (1992) looked at the survival rates of male and female patients with coronary artery disease and found that high-income patients had nearly double the survival rate of low-income patients. Similarly, Linda Fried and her associates (1998) reported that older people with incomes of less than $50,000 a year were nearly twice as likely to die of cardiovascular disease as those with incomes of $50,000 or more. Also, a report from China (Yu et al., 2000) showed that socioeconomic level—defined as education, occupation, income, and marital status—related to such cardiovascular risk factors as blood pressure, body mass index, and cigarette smoking. These findings suggest that people who lack financial or educational resources are probably less able or less likely to seek medical care—conditions that place them at a greater risk for a variety of disorders, including heart disease.

Marriage and Social Support Being single and lacking social support are also coronary risk factors, at least for some people. Unmarried people who lack someone in whom they can confide are much more likely to die of coronary artery disease than people who have a spouse, a confidant, or both. For people who have already had a heart attack, living alone or having only a few confidants can be an independent risk for additional heart problems. Beverly Brummett and her colleagues (2001) found that CAD patients who had only one to three people in their social network were nearly two and half times more likely to die of coronary artery disease than were patients with four or more close

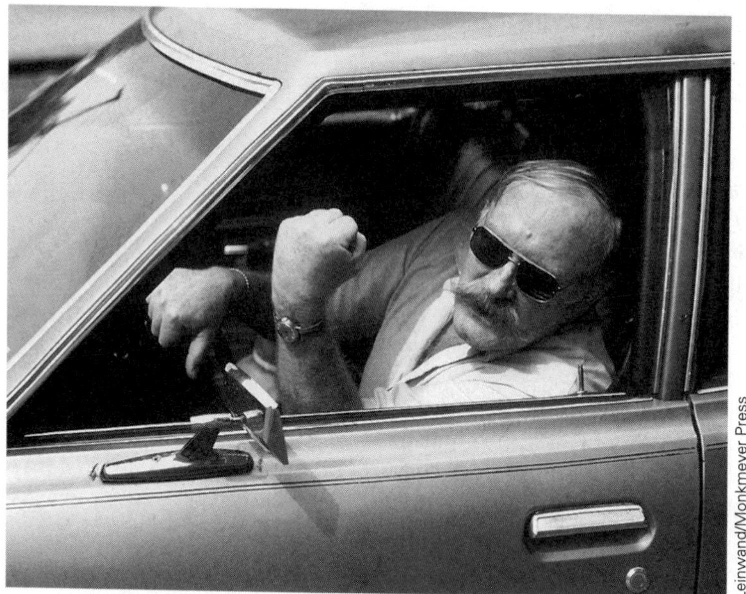

Leinwand/Monkmeyer Press

Hostility and expressed anger are risk factors for cardiovascular disease.

friends. Having more than four friends in one's social network provided no added benefit.

These studies confirm results from other research on social support discussed in Chapter 8, which indicated that people who have a wide circle of friends or who feel they can confide in another person are less likely to die of stress-related diseases. Social support may reduce risk of cardiovascular mortality when a spouse or friend encourages a patient to maintain a healthy lifestyle, to seek medical attention, and to comply with medical advice.

Cynical Hostility and Anger In recent years, researchers have found that some types of hostility and anger are risk factors for cardiovascular disease. Much of this research grew out of work on the Type A behavior pattern, originally proposed by **cardiologists** Meyer Friedman and Ray Rosenman, physicians who specialized in heart disease (Friedman & Rosenman, 1974: Rosenman et al., 1975). As conceived by Friedman and Rosenman, people with the Type A behavior pattern are hostile, competitive, concerned with numbers and the acquisition of objects, and possessed of an exaggerated sense of time urgency. During the early years of its history, the Type A behavior pattern demonstrated promise as a predictor of heart disease, but later researchers were unable to affirm a consistent link between the global Type A behavior pattern and incidence of heart disease

Redford Williams, Ted Dembroski, and Aron Siegman have led teams of investigators to analyze the component behaviors in the Type A pattern to determine whether some one behavior or some constellation of behaviors might yield a more valid predictor. In time, they began to focus on one possible toxic component of the Type A behavior pattern—namely hostility, including *cynical hostility* and *anger.*

In 1989, Williams presented evidence that one type of hostility—cynical hostility—is especially harmful to cardiovascular health, and he contended that people who mistrust others, think the worst of humanity, and interact with others with cynical hostility are harming themselves and their hearts. Furthermore, he suggested that people who use anger as a response to interpersonal problems have an elevated risk for heart disease.

To investigate the relationship between hostility and heart disease, researchers have used several measures of hostility, particularly the Cook-Medley Hostility (Ho) Index (Cook & Medley, 1954). The Cook-Medley consists of 50 items taken from the original Minnesota Multiphasic Personality Inventory (MMPI) and therefore offers the advantage of being part of a widely administered psychological test. The Ho scale of the Cook-Medley measures suspiciousness, resentment, frequent anger, and cynical mistrust of others more than it measures the tendency to behave violently. In addition, Erika Rosenberg and her associates (Rosenberg et al., 2001) found that facial expressions of anger and nonenjoyment smiles were significantly related to measures of ischemia in men with coronary artery disease.

Some research (Siegler, Peterson, Barefoot, & Williams, 1992) has found that hostility is not an independent predictor of heart disease. Rather, it is related to other behaviors that relate to heart disease. These include alcohol consumption, smoking, and body weight. When research controls for these conditions, the relationship between hostility and coronary artery disease tends to disappear, demonstrating that hostility is not an independent risk factor for heart disease (Everson et al., 1997). For this reason, some researchers have shifted their investigations to a specific component of hostility—anger.

Hostility and anger are related, but anger can be defined as an unpleasant *emotion* accompanied by physiological arousal and usually lasting for a relatively short duration (Smith, 1994). On the other hand, hostility involves a negative *attitude* toward others and may be of long duration. The *experience* of anger probably does not threaten cardiovascular functioning, but the *expression* of anger may well be a risk factor for coronary artery disease (Siegman, Dembroski, & Ringel, 1987). The expression of anger includes yelling back when someone yells at you, raising your voice when arguing, and throwing temper tantrums. This type of expression of anger is more dangerous than the mere experience of anger (Siegman et al., 1987).

Anger and Cardiovascular Reactivity Why should the expression of anger relate to coronary heart disease? To answer this question, researchers have begun to focus on **cardiovascular reactivity (CVR),** typically defined in laboratory settings as increases in blood pressure and heart rate due to frustration or harassment.

In one study, Aron Siegman and his associates (Siegman, Anderson, Herbst, Boyle, & Wilkinson, 1992) provoked male undergraduates and measured their cardiovascular reactivity. They found that participants' heart rate and diastolic and systolic blood pressure increased and that participants generally felt a great deal of anger after being provoked. In another study, Barbara Fredrickson and her associates (Fredrickson et al., 2000) measured heart rate and blood pressure of older men and women who were asked to relive an earlier anger experience. In this study, high-hostility participant had higher and longer-lasting blood pressure responses less hostile participants, and African Americans had more CVR than European Americans. Similarly, in a study in Singapore of Chinese and Indian men (Bishop & Robinson, 2000), some participants performed a difficult task while harassed and others performed the same task without harassment. As expected, the harassed men showed higher levels of reactivity than men who were allowed to finish their tasks without interruption. An earlier study (Smith & Brown, 1991) showed that women may not experience comparable reactivity when provoked. In this study, husbands experienced increases in heart rate and systolic blood pressure while attempting to control their wives, but the wives experienced no comparable reactivity while trying to control their husbands. Interestingly, the wives experienced an increase in systolic blood pressure only at the times their husbands were expressing cynical hostility.

This research suggests that provoked anger increases CVR in cynically hostile men but perhaps not in women. If psychosocial factors can cause heart disease, then these findings may partially explain the different between men and women in rates of early CHD.

Suppressed Anger If expressing anger can undermine cardiac health, then would it be better to suppress anger? Ted Dembroski and his colleagues (Dembroski, MacDougall, Williams, Haney, & Blumenthal, 1985; MacDougall, Dembroski, Dimsdale, & Hackett, 1985) found evidence suggesting that suppressed anger, or anger-in, was a toxic element in heart disease. Results of these studies suggest that cardiologists should not recommend to people (especially men) with early signs of heart disease that they keep their anger suppressed.

If avoiding the experience of anger is impossible and both the suppression and the violent expression of anger are potentially dangerous, then how can people handle anger situations? Siegman (1994) suggested that people learn to recognize their anger but to express it calmly and rationally. When people express anger in a soft, slow voice, as opposed to a loud, rapid voice, they may reduce their risk of developing coronary heart disease.

Presently, evidence is lacking that any component of the Type A behavior pattern, including hostility and anger, is a strong independent risk for cardiovascular disease in people generally. Personality factors do not appear to put people (men and women, Black and White, young and old) at the same elevated risk for heart disease as do traditional risk factors, such as cigarette smoking, hypertension, or high cholesterol levels. However, evidence suggests that cynical hostility and anger interact with high blood pressure to increase a person's risk for heart disease.

Figure 9.9 shows the evolution of the Type A behavior pattern to hostility, to anger, and finally to the calm expression of anger. Ample research evidence suggests that physical and/or verbal expression of anger may be a behavioral risk factor for the development of cardiovascular disease.

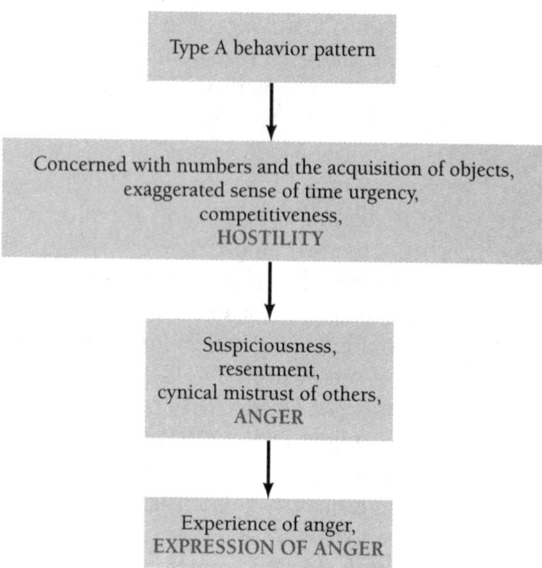

Figure 9.9 The evolution of expressed anger from the Type A behavior pattern.

In Summary

Although the exact causes of cardiovascular disease are not fully understood, an accumulating body of evidence points to certain risk factors. These factors include such inherent risks as advancing age, diabetes, family history of heart disease, gender, and ethnic background. Although none of these factors can be changed, people who are inherently at risk can modify other risks and thus lower their chances of developing heart disease.

Other risk factors include physiological conditions such as hypertension and high serum cholesterol levels. Other than age, hypertension is the best predictor of coronary artery disease, and a dose-response relationship exists between blood pressure level and risk for heart disease. Total cholesterol level is also related to coronary artery disease, but the *ratio* of total cholesterol to high-density lipoprotein (HDL) is a more critical risk factor.

Behavioral conditions such as smoking and imprudent eating also relate to heart disease. Cigarette smokers have a two- to threefold risk of developing heart disease, but nonsmokers exposed to other people's tobacco smoke probably have only a very slight risk. Eating foods high in saturated fat and consuming low levels of fiber and antioxidants (vitamin E, beta carotene, and selenium) add to one's risk of heart disease.

Psychosocial risk factors related to coronary artery disease include anxiety, depression, educational level, income, marriage, social support, and the hostility/anger component descended from the Type A behavior pattern. People with persistent anxiety and depression have elevated risks for CVD, as do people with low levels of education and income. However, being married and/or having a confidant can lower one's risk for heart disease. Hostility is a component of the Type A behavior pattern, but it is probably not an independent risk factor for heart disease. One of its dimensions—anger—has potentially lethal consequences. Moreover, the mere experience of anger seems to have no detrimental effect on cardiovascular functioning. Rather, both the violent expression and the suppression of anger may be the toxic agents underlying some CHD disease. Expressing anger in a soft, calm voice avoids any harmful effects of violently expressing anger or timidly holding it in.

Reducing Cardiovascular Risks

Psychology's main contribution to cardiovascular health has focused on changing unhealthy behaviors before these behaviors lead to heart disease. In addition, psychologists may also help people who have previously been diagnosed with heart disease, that is, they often help cardiac rehabilitation patients to adhere to an exercise program and to a healthy diet.

Before Diagnosis: Preventing First Heart Attacks

What can people do to lower their risks for cardiovascular disease? Coronary artery disease and stroke are closely associated with several unhealthy behaviors and living habits, and modifying these behaviors and life styles can help people avoid this disease. Cardiovascular risk factors begin during childhood and usually increase during adulthood. Keeping traditional risk factors low can pay substantial dividends in later years (Stamler et al., 1999). After people acquire high risks from behavioral factors such as smoking and unwise eating, the advice to stop smoking or to go on a diet is likely to be ineffective. People who enjoy eating red meats (and who have done so since they were children) often have quite a bit of trouble changing their eating patterns. People who have smoked two or three packs of cigarettes a day for 15 or 20 years may not find it easy to quit. But psychologists have traditionally been concerned with changing behavior, and many of their techniques can be used to modify behaviors that place people at risk for developing cardiovascular disease.

Before people will cooperate with programs to change their behavior, they must perceive that these behaviors place them in jeopardy. People's perceptions can be colored by potentially deadly biases that decrease their perceptions of risk. They may recognize established risk factors in calculating their personal risk, but they often display what Neil Weinstein (1984) called an **optimistic bias** in assessing their risk. That is, they tend to believe that they are immune from the risks that make other people vulnerable. This tendency to exempt oneself from risks, especially behavioral risks, is a strong influence on the perception of personal risk, and that perception can affect a person's willingness to change behavior. Accurate feedback about people's risk status can decrease optimistic bias (Weinstein, 1983) and enhance their belief that they do something about changing their risk factors for cardiovascular disease.

The most serious behavioral risk factor in cardiovascular disease is cigarette smoking, a behavior also implicated in a variety of other disorders, especially lung cancer. For this reason, all of Chapter 13 is devoted to a discussion of tobacco use. Although hypertension and serum cholesterol are not behaviors and thus cannot be directly modified through psychological interventions, both can be affected indirectly through changes in behavior (Linden, 2000).

Reducing Hypertension Lowering high blood pressure into the normal range is difficult because a number of physiological mechanisms act to keep blood pressure at a setpoint. At least eight different feedback systems either raise or lower blood pressure when the body senses that blood pressure is out of the critical zone. The body may perpetuate hypertension by means of these feedback mechanisms, regulating blood pressure to the hypertensive level instead of regulating it into the normal range (Linden, 1988). Because complex feedback systems work against rather than for the maintenance of appropriate blood pressure, hypertension tends to be difficult to control.

Interventions aimed toward reducing hypertension usually try to control blood pressure through antihypertensive drugs that require a physician's prescription. Patients receiving drug therapy should be periodically monitored to achieve the best control of blood pressure with the fewest side effects. Because hypertension presents no unpleasant symptoms, many patients are reluctant to continue with a daily medication that may cause unpleasant side effects. (The factors affecting adherence with this and other medical regimens are discussed in Chapter 4.)

Several behaviors relate to both the development and the treatment of hypertension. Obesity is correlated with hypertension, and many obese people who lose weight lower their blood pressure into the normal range. A regular physical activity program has also been found effective in controlling hypertension (We discuss exercise in Chapter 16). Although some research (He et al., 1999) has questioned the wisdom of recommending sodium restriction for everyone, hypertensive individuals should strive to lower their blood pressure by restricting sodium intake. People with high blood pressure can lower their risk for heart disease if they reduce alcohol consumption and lose weight. (We discuss strategies for modifying alcohol consumption in Chapter 14 and losing weight in Chapter 15.) Other techniques for reducing blood pressure are stress management and relaxation training, and we discuss both in Chapter 8.

Lowering Serum Cholesterol Interventions aimed at lowering cholesterol levels can include drugs, dietary changes, or both. Cholesterol-lowering drugs such as the *statin* drugs are frequently prescribed for patients with high total cholesterol levels. These drugs act by blocking an enzyme that the liver needs to manufacture cholesterol, and they lower LDL and raise HDL. These drugs are effective (Hebert, Gaziano, Chan, & Hennekens, 1997), but they require a prescription, cost money, and have side effects.

For postmenopausal women, estrogen-replacement therapy is also a strategy for cholesterol lowering. The difference in cardiovascular disease between women before and after menopause has led to the belief that estrogen can lower CVD risks. Many observational studies have shown such benefits, but an experimental study (Hulley et al., 1998) showed that although estrogen-replacement therapy lowered cholesterol, it provided no survival advantage for women who had already developed cardiovascular disease. Indeed, women who began this therapy had an elevated risk for other diseases, making estrogen replacement a bad choice for postmenopausal women with coronary disease.

For those with very high cholesterol levels, drugs may be a better choice than dietary restrictions (Knopp et al., 1997). However, as we discussed in Chapter 2, Andrew Steptoe and his colleagues (2000) found that people with very high levels of cholesterol can lower dietary fat through behavioral counseling and social support, thereby reducing total cholesterol. For people with moderately high cholesterol, a change in diet alone may reduce total cholesterol (Brunner et al., 1997).

The recommendations for cholesterol lowering are complex. First, the ratio of total cholesterol to HDL is more important than total cholesterol. Second, lowering total cholesterol

BECOMING HEALTHIER

1. Know about your family risk for heart disease. Although you cannot change this risk factor, knowing that you are at high risk can motivate you to change some of your modifiable risk factors.
2. Have your blood pressure checked. If it is in the normal range, you can keep it that way by exercising, controlling your weight, and moderating alcohol consumption. Also, try some of the relaxation techniques we discussed in Chapter 8. If your blood pressure is in the hypertensive range, consult a physician.
3. Know your cholesterol level, but be sure to ask for a complete profile, one that includes measures of both HDL and LDL as well as the ratio of total cholesterol to HDL.
4. If you are a smoker who has tried to quit but failed, keep trying. Many ex-smokers made multiple attempts before successfully quitting.
5. Keep a food diary for at least 1 week. Note the amount of saturated fat you ate, the approximate number of calories consumed per day, and the amount of fruits and vegetables you ate. A heart-healthy diet includes five servings of fruits and vegetables per day.
6. If you are persistently angry and react to anger-arousing events with loud, sudden explosions of anger, try to change your reactions by expressing your frustrations in a soft, quiet voice.

does not reduce all-cause mortality, and very low cholesterol (<140) is related to violent death. Third, men and women do not profit equally from cholesterol-lowering regimens. For men whose total cholesterol is over 240, lowering total cholesterol will probably result in a 15% to 20% reduction in CAD. For women with existing coronary artery disease, however, lowering cholesterol does not seem to produce the same benefits (Walsh & Grady, 1995). Psychological interventions can help both men and women adhere to a regular exercise program as well as a low-fat diet. Such adherence can lower LDL and improve the ratio of total cholesterol to HDL.

Ideally, modifying risk factors should take place before people have significant signs of CVD. A longitudinal study by Jerry Stamler and his colleagues (1999) indicated that it does. Stamler et al. looked at young adult and middle-aged men and women in five large cohorts to see if a low-risk profile prior to disease would reduce both CVD and other causes of mortality. They divided the participants into risk groups. After screening for as long as 57 years, Stamler et al. found that low-risk participants had not only lower rates of death from CHD and stroke but also from all causes. Thus, young and middle-aged men and women who can modify CVD risks will also lower their risk for all-cause mortality and can expect to live 6 to 10 years longer.

Modifying Psychosocial Risk Factors Earlier, we discussed research strongly suggestive that hostility and its anger component are the toxic elements in the Type A behavior pattern. If this is so, then a reduction in hostility and anger should prove therapeutic. Several years ago, Redford Williams (1989) suggested that becoming more trusting is the antidote to cynical hostility. He outlined a 12-step program through which people can decrease their cynicism and hostility and thus lower their risk of heart disease. The steps constitute a type of cognitive therapy in which people become aware of their attitudes, stop cynical thoughts, reason with themselves, and practice trust and relaxation. Consistent with Williams's concept, research on people who received angioplasty (Helgeson,

2003) indicated that those who had a more positive outlook about themselves and their future were less likely to experience a recurrence of cardiovascular disease.

Anger, too, can be dealt with in a therapeutic manner, and clinical health psychologists have recommended a variety of strategies for coping with anger. The goal of intervention strategies is not to eliminate anger but to cope with it. Aron Siegman and Selena Cappell Snow (1997) asked college students to participate in three experimental conditions: (1) Anger-out, in which anger-arousing events were expressed loudly and quickly; (2) Anger-in, in which students relived their anger inwardly, that is in their imagination; and (3) Mood-incongruent speech, in which students expressed their anger softly and slowly—that is, in a manner incongruent with their strong emotion. As hypothesized, only participants who expressed anger openly and loudly experienced significant cardiovascular reactivity. Participants who relived their anger-arousing experience in imagination or who expressed it in a soft, slow manner had almost no increase in reactivity. These results suggest that people may buffer the toxic elements of anger by reliving the event in imagination or by speaking softly and slowly about the event.

To reduce the toxic element in anger, perpetually angry people can learn to become aware of cues from others that typically provoke angry responses. They can also remove themselves from provocative situations before they become angry, or they can do something else. In interpersonal encounters, angry people can use self-talk as a reminder that the situation will not last forever. Humor is another potentially effective means of coping with anger, but one must be careful with its use. Sarcastic or hostile humor can incite additional anger, but silliness or mock exaggerations often defuse potentially volatile situations. Relaxation techniques can also be effective strategies for dealing with anger. These can include progressive relaxation, deep breathing exercises, tension-reduction training, relaxing to the slow repetition of the word "relax," and relaxation imagery, in which the person imagines a peaceful scene. Finally, angry people can lower their blood pressure by constructively discussing their feelings with other people (Davidson, MacGregor, Stuhr, Dixon, & MacLean, 2000).

After Diagnosis: Rehabilitating Cardiac Patients

After people have been diagnosed with cardiovascular disease, they typically enter a cardiac rehabilitation program to change their lifestyle and thereby avoid subsequent CVD. In addition to survival, the goals of cardiac rehabilitation programs is to help patients deal with psychological reactions to their diagnosis, to return as soon as possible to normal activities, such as work, hobbies, and sexual relations, and to change to a healthier lifestyle.

Patients recovering from heart disease, as well as their spouses, often experience a variety of psychological reactions that include depression, anxiety, anger, fear, guilt, and interpersonal conflict. For cardiac patients, the most common psychological reaction to a myocardial infraction is *depression.* Depressed survivors of a heart attack have a 3.5 greater risk of death than do nondepressed cardiac patients (Guck et al., 2001), with most of those deaths occurring during the first 6 months after diagnosis (Frasure-Smith, Lesperance, & Talijic, 2000). Another common psychological reaction to heart attack is *anxiety.* Patients with high anxiety levels often suffer additional complications, such as angina, heart spasms, another heart attack, or death (Moser & Dracup, 1996). One common source of anxiety among heart patients and their spouses is the resumption of sexual relations. The probable source of this anxiety is concern about the elevation of heart rate during sex, especially during orgasm. However, sexual activity poses little threat to those who have experienced a heart attack. Also, male CAD patients who take Viagra do not have an elevated risk of subsequent heart problems (Arruda-Onson, Mahoney, Nehra, Leckel, & Pellikka, 2002).

Cardiac rehabilitation programs usually include helping patients stop smoking, eat a low-fat and low-cholesterol diet, control weight, moderate alcohol intake, learn to manage stress and hostility, and adhere to a prescribed a medication regimen. Also, cardiac patients frequently participate in a graduated or structured exercise program in which they gradually increase their level of physical activity. In other words, the same lifestyle recommendations for avoiding a first cardiovascular event are also recommended to people who have survived a myocardial infraction or coronary artery bypass graft surgery. In addition, cardiac patients are often encouraged to join a social support group, participate in health education programs, and allow support from their primary caregiver.

Are rehabilitation programs effective in reducing cardiac mortality? An important obstacle to the effectiveness of a cardiac rehabilitation is adherence, with only 15% to 30% of cardiac patients completing their rehabilitation regimen (King, Humen, Smith, Pfan, & Teo, 2001). Nevertheless, a meta-analysis of studies on the effectiveness of two components of a cardiac rehabilitation (Dusseldrop, van Elderen, Maes, Meulman, & Kraaj, 1999) found that heart disease patients who followed a health education and stress management program had a 34% reduction in cardiac mortality and a 29% reduction in recurrence of a heart attack In addition, this rehabilitation program significantly reduced blood pressure, cholesterol, body weight, and smoking rates. It also increased patients' level of physical activity and improved their eating habits.

Increasing Physical Activity Physical activity should be a component of cardiac rehabilitation programs, but it is often underutilized. Paul Thompson (2001) believes that exercise is one of the few cardiac rehabilitation procedures that can make patients feel better, while at the same time, it can increase muscle strength and lower heart rate. Thompson listed three main goals of exercise after a diagnosis of heart problems. First, exercise can maintain or improve functional capacity; second, it can enhance a person's quality of life, and third, it can help prevent recurrent heart attacks.

Physical activity after a heart attack has some potential dangers, and some cardiac patients suffer subsequent cardiovascular problems during exercise. However, the risks are quite small and are greatly exceeded by the benefits. One study (Franklin, Bonzheim, Gordon, & Timmis, 1999) found only one cardiac complication for approximately every 50,000 hours of physical activity, and another study (Thompson, 2001) reported that 85% of cardiac rehabilitation patients who experience a heart attract while exercising are successfully resuscitated. These results also suggest that heart patients should avoid highly competitive sports, such as racquetball, basketball, singles tennis, or any other activity that incites a patient's competitive attitude.

Exercise can be safe even in patients who have had a heart transplant (Kolbashigawa et al, 1999). In addition, adhering to a physical activity program after a heart attack is associated with a variety of positive benefits. For example, a graded exercise program can enhance patients' self-efficacy for increasing levels of activity (Cheng & Boey, 2002) as well as increase self-esteem and physical mobility (Ng & Tam, 2000). Exercise also improves aerobic fitness and muscle strength in highly disabled patients (Ades, 1999). This evidence indicates that cardiac rehabilitation patients who follow a supervised exercise program can reap important physical and psychological benefits.

Changing Eating Habits Dean Ornish and his colleagues (Ornish et al., 1998) tested the possibility of *reversing* heart patients' coronary artery damage by introducing substantial changes in lifestyle, including diet. Although similar to the interventions that attempt to alter risk factors, this program was more comprehensive and imposed more stringent modifications, especially with regard to diet. The Ornish program recommends that cardiac patients should reduce their consumption of fat to only 10% of their total caloric intake. This compares with the American Heart Association's guidelines of no more than 30% and the average American's diet of about 40% of calories from fat. It also necessitates a careful vegetarian diet with no added fats from oils, eggs, butter, or nuts. Ornish (1995) contended that a diet in which 30% of calories come from fat is not sufficient to reverse coronary artery disease (CAD), although such a diet may be sufficient to *prevent* the development of CAD.

In addition to the dietary restrictions, participants in Ornish's program received stress management training and were encouraged to stop smoking, moderate alcohol intake, and start exercising. A control group in this study followed a typical program intended to lower risk factors for people with coronary heart disease, including eating a low-fat diet, quitting smoking, and increasing physical activity. After 1 year of the program, Ornish and his colleagues (1990) found that 82% of patients in the treatment group showed a regression of plaques in the coronary arteries, a truly difficult achievement. Compared with the control group, patients in the treatment group had significantly less blockage of their coronary arteries, and those who most faithfully followed the program showed the most dramatic changes. After 5 years, this program produced less artery blockage and fewer coronary events, which compared favorably with standard risk modification. These studies demonstrated that a change in the coronary arteries can occur without the use of drugs that alter cholesterol levels and without coronary bypass surgery.

Although the Ornish plan can be a successful cardiac rehabilitation program, it is not an easy one to follow. Perhaps its most difficult aspect is adhering to the 10% ratio of fat to total calorie intake. One recent study (American Dietetic Association, 2001) compared two procedures for reducing dietary fat to 10% of energy. The first procedure was to reduce fat incrementally until patients reached 10%, while the second method was to immediately restrict dietary fat. The results of the study showed that two approaches were equally ineffective; that is, neither group achieved the goal of reducing fat intake to 10% of energy intake. The authors suggested that 10% may not be a realistic target, even for people who have had a cardiac event. Despite the difficulty of reaching the 10% goal, most heart patients should strive to reduce dietary fat, lower LDL cholesterol, and lose weight. These changes in eating habits combined with a graduated exercise plan and a reduction in psychological factors such as anxiety, stress, and depression can help heart patients avoid subsequent heart attack.

In Summary

Health psychologists can help reduce risks for a first cardiovascular incident as well as contribute to rehabilitating people who have already been diagnosed with CVD. For example, behavioral interventions have been moderately successful in lowering high blood pressure. In addition, health psychologists can help people deal with such psychological reactions as anger, depression, anxiety, and guilt. Also, they may become involved, along with trained physical therapist and cardiologists, in increasing heart patients' level of physical activity. However, they must recognize the potential dangers of strenuous exercise, especially highly competitive physical activity. Finally, health psychologist can be involved in altering heart patients' diet and helping them avoid excessive consumption of foods that raise both blood pressure and cholesterol levels. Research suggests that long-term changes in diet can lower total cholesterol without reducing HDL.

Answers

This chapter addressed five basic questions:

1. **What are the structures, functions, and disorders of the cardiovascular system?**
   The cardiovascular system includes the heart and blood vessels (veins, venules, arteries, arterioles, and capillaries). The heart pumps blood throughout the body, delivering oxygen and removing wastes from body cells. Disorders of the cardiovascular system include (1) coronary artery disease (CAD), which occurs when the arteries that supply blood to the heart become clogged with plaque, restricting the blood supply to the heart muscle; (2) myocardial infarction (heart attack), caused by blockage of coronary arteries; (3) angina pectoris, a nonfatal disorder with symptoms of chest pain and difficulty in breathing; (4) stroke, which occurs when the oxygen supply to the brain is disrupted; and (5) hypertension (high blood pressure), a silent disorder but a good predictor of both heart attack and stroke. Heart attack and stroke account for over 30% of deaths in the United States.

2. **What measurements of cardiovascular function can reveal damage?**
   Two measurements that can reveal cardiovascular damage are blood pressure assessment and the electrocardiogram. However, neither can reveal blockage to the coronary arteries. An exercise electrocardiogram (stress test) can reveal coronary artery blockage for severe damage. The most accurate test for coronary artery blockage is angiography, imaging of the coronary arteries. This procedure has the disadvantage of requiring an invasive procedure, namely cardiac catheterization.

3. **How does lifestyle relate to cardiovascular health?**
   Lifestyle factors such as cigarette smoking, unwise eating, and a sedentary lifestyle all relate to cardiovascular health. During the past 3 decades, deaths from heart disease steadily decreased in the United states, with perhaps as much as 50% of that drop a result of changes in behavior and lifestyle. During this same time period, millions of people have quit smoking, altered their diet to control weight and cholesterol, and began an exercise program.

4. **What are the risk factors for cardiovascular disease?**
   Beginning with the Framingham study, researchers have discovered a number of cardiovascular risk factors. These include (1) inherent risk, (2) physiological risks, (3) behavioral and lifestyle risks, and (4) psychosocial risks. Inherent risk factors, such as advancing age, juvenile-onset diabetes, family history, gender, and ethnicity cannot be changed, but people with inherent risk can alter their other risks to lower their chances of developing heart disease.

   The two primary physiological risk factors are hypertension and high cholesterol, and diet can play a role in controlling each of these. Behavioral factors in CVD include smoking and a diet high in saturated fat and low in fiber and antioxidant vitamins. Psychosocial risks include persistently high levels of anxiety, low educational levels, low income, lack of social support, and loud, violent expressions of anger.

5. **What approaches allow people to lower their cardiovascular risks?**
   Both before and after a diagnosis of heart disease, people can use a variety of approaches to reduce their risks for CVD. Hypertension can be controlled by drugs, sodium restriction, and relaxation techniques. Cholesterol levels can be lowered through drugs and, to some extent, through diet. Lowering the ratio of total choles-

terol to HDL is probably a better idea. Both regular exercise and moderate consumption of alcohol can improve this ratio. Also, people can learn to modify loud, quick outbursts of anger by expressing their frustrations in a soft, slow manner or by using various relaxation techniques. Cardiac patients who receive social support, especially after a diagnosis of heart disease, can reduce their risk of a subsequent heart attack.

Suggested Readings

Cooper, K. H. (1994). *Dr. Kenneth H. Cooper's antioxidant revolution.* Nashville, TN: Nelson. In this very readable book, Kenneth Cooper, one of the early promoters of aerobic exercise for a healthy heart, discusses the value of antioxidants, including vitamin E.

Siegman, A. W. (1994). From Type A to hostility to anger: Reflections on the history of coronary-prone behavior. In A. W. Siegman & T. W. Smith (Eds.), *Anger, hostility, and the heart* (pp. 1–21). Hillsdale, NJ: Erlbaum. One of the leading advocates of the notion that anger is the toxic component of the Type A behavior pattern discusses the evolution of Type A to hostility to anger.

Stamler, J., Stamler, R., Neaton, J. D., Wentworth, D., Daviglus, M. L. Garside, D., Dyer, A. R., Liu, K., & Greenland, P. (1999). Low risk-factor profile and long-term cardiovascular and noncardiovascular mortality and life expectancy: Findings for 5 large cohorts of young adult and middle-aged men and women. *Journal of the American Medical Association, 282,* 2012–2018. This analysis represents the largest and most comprehensive study of cardiovascular risk factors and their effect on life expectancy. The authors projected an additional 6 to 10 years of life for low-risk people.

Voelker, R. (1998). A "family heirloom" turns 50. *Journal of the American Medical Association, 279,* 1241–1245. Rebecca Voelker's interview with William Castelli, who directed the famous Framingham Heart Study from 1965 to 1995, reveals an interesting history of this study. Castelli contends that epidemiologists still know only about one half of the risk factors for heart disease.

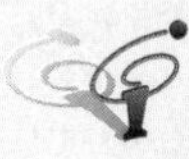

Search InfoTrac College Edition

Search these terms to learn more about topics in this chapter:

- Coronary heart disease and causes of
- Coronary heart disease and demographic aspects
- Stroke and demographic aspects
- Coronary heart disease and statistics
- Coronary heart disease and genetic aspects
- Coronary heart disease and world
- Heart disease and longitudinal study
- Heart function tests
- African Americans and heart disease
- Heart disease and women and risk
- Diet and heart disease
- Framingham study
- Blood cholesterol and heart disease risk
- Smoking and heart disease risk
- Social support and heart disease
- Type A behavior and heart disease
- Hostility and heart disease
- Heart disease prevention
- Cardiac rehabilitation

10

Behavioral Factors in Cancer

The Story of Victoria

CHAPTER OUTLINE

What Is Cancer?

The Changing Rates of Cancer Deaths

Behavioral Risk Factors for Cancer

Cancer Risk Factors beyond Personal Control

Personality As a Risk Factor for Cancer

Living with Cancer

QUESTIONS

This chapter focuses on six basic questions:

1. What is cancer?
2. Are cancer death rates increasing or decreasing?
3. What are the behavioral risk factors for cancer?
4. What are the environmental and inherent risk factors for cancer?
5. How do personality traits relate to cancer?
6. How can patients be helped in coping with cancer?

The Story of Victoria

Victoria was a 16-year-old high school junior when she was diagnosed with **non-Hodgkin's lymphoma**, cancer of the lymphatic system. She had noticed a lump on her head and knew of no reason for it. Her mother took Victoria to her pediatrician, who referred her to several specialists. One of these specialists was a dermatologist who took a **biopsy** and diagnosed lymphoma.

The dermatologist did not explain his reasoning or the procedures. Even when he told Victoria and her mother that the lump was lymphoma, he didn't really explain what it was or what she should expect. He did, however, refer her to an **oncologist**, a physician who specializes in the treatment of cancer. The oncologist conducted further tests and confirmed the diagnosis.

Victoria's parents were not pleased with her medical care and took her to a large research hospital that specializes in children's cancer. The hospital physicians repeated some of the testing and rapidly confirmed the diagnosis of lymphoma. The treatment Victoria received there was different—the staff was ready to explain any facet of the diagnosis and treatment, and they were also prepared to deal with her reaction to the diagnosis.

Victoria's first reaction was anger. Initially she was angry with everyone. Her doctors' understanding helped her to deal with her anger and to accept her diagnosis and treatment. For the first 3 months, treatment consisted of intensive chemotherapy, an experience she described as terrible. She lost 30 pounds, experienced muscle atrophy and coordination problems, and lost her hair, but her tumor started to shrink. After another 6 months of less intensive chemotherapy, she began to feel better.

Victoria's life was disrupted by her illness as well as by the treatment. In addition to the difficulties of traveling to the hospital to receive treatment and coping with its side effects, she was faced with changes in her life. Her friends became awkward around her and didn't know what to say. Victoria knew that they had never been faced with a life-threatening illness in someone their own age. "I didn't think it could happen to anyone I know," she said. She had been dating a young man for about 3 months when she was diagnosed, and she thought that her illness would end their relationship. She told him that if he couldn't handle it, she would understand. He said that he thought he could, and he did.

Victoria could not attend school during her treatment but received home schooling and graduated from high school with her class. She remembers that keeping up with schoolwork was not difficult but being alone was. Rather than going to school and being with her friends, she had to study at home by herself. She believes that the experience changed her, making her less sociable and less outgoing.

Victoria's lymphoma went into remission and has remained so for more than 15 years. Although her diagnosis and treatment were difficult and painful, she said that she always thought, "It could have been worse." She never believed she was going to die and never tried to live each day as though it was her last. She did, however, lose her feeling of invincibility.

In this chapter, we examine cancer, the second most frequent cause of death in the United States and many other industrialized countries. We look at the demographics and risk factors for cancer and then discuss behavioral changes that can help to alter risk factors. First, however, we define cancer and describe its biology.

What Is Cancer?

The first medical document to describe cancer was the *Ebers Papyrus*, written around 1500 B.C. That document did not give a detailed description of cancer, only a description of the swellings that accompany some tumors. Hippocrates gave the disorder the name *cancer*, and the Greek physician, Galen, first used the word *tumor*. These ancient physicians did not know much about cancer, however, because they did not have microscopes or use dissection, two procedures that greatly facilitated an understanding of cancer.

CHECK YOUR HEALTH RISKS

Check the items that apply to you.

- ☐ 1. Someone in my immediate family (a parent, sibling, aunt, uncle, grandparent) developed cancer before age 50.
- ☐ 2. I am African American.
- ☐ 3. I have never had a job where I was exposed to radiation or hazardous chemicals.
- ☐ 4. I never have been a cigarette smoker.
- ☐ 5. I am a former smoker who quit during the past 5 years.
- ☐ 6. I have used tobacco products other than cigarettes (such as chewing tobacco, a pipe, or cigars).
- ☐ 7. My diet is low in fat.
- ☐ 8. My diet includes lots of smoked, salt-cured, or pickled foods.
- ☐ 9. I rarely eat fruits or vegetables.
- ☐ 10. My diet is high in fiber.
- ☐ 11. I have light-colored skin, but I like to get at least one nice tan every year.
- ☐ 12. I have had more than 15 sexual partners during my life.
- ☐ 13. I have never had unprotected sex with a partner who was at high risk for HIV infection.
- ☐ 14. I am a woman over age 30 who has not given birth to a child.
- ☐ 15. I have at least two alcoholic drinks every day.
- ☐ 16. I exercise on a regular basis.

Each of these topics is either a known risk factor for some type of cancer or has the potential to protect against it. Items 3, 4, 7, 10, 13, and 16 describe situations that may offer some protection against cancer. If you checked none or only a few of these items and a large number of the remaining items, your risk for some type of cancer is higher than people who checked different items. Behaviors related to smoking and diet (Items 4–10) place you at a greater risk than other behaviors, such as Item 15 (alcohol) or Item 16 (lack of regular exercise).

Cancer is a group of diseases characterized by the presence of new cells that grow and spread beyond control. During the 19th century, the great physiologist, Johannes Muller, discovered that tumors, like other tissues, consisted of cells and were not formless collections of material. However, their growth seemed unrestrained by the mechanisms that control other body cells.

The finding that tumors consist of cells did not shed light on what causes their growth. During the 19th century, the leading theory of cancer was that a parasite or infectious agent caused the disorder, but researchers could find no such agent. Because of this failure, a mutation theory arose, holding that cancer originates because of a change in the cell, a mutation. The cell continues to grow and reproduce in its mutated form, and the result is a tumor.

Cancers is not unique to humans; all animals get cancers, as do plants. Indeed, any cell that is capable of division can be transformed into a cancer cell. In addition to the diverse *causes* of cancer, many different *types* exist. However, different cancers share certain characteristics, the most common of which is the presence of **neoplastic** tissue cells. Neoplastic cells are characterized by new and nearly unlimited growth that robs the host of nutrients and that yields no compensatory beneficial effects. All true cancers share this characteristic of neoplastic growth.

Neoplastic cells may be **benign** or **malignant**, although this distinction is not always easy to determine. Both types consist of altered cells that reproduce true to their altered type. However, benign and malignant neoplasms have some differences: benign growths tend to remain localized, whereas malignant tumors tend to spread and establish secondary colonies. The tendency for benign tumors to remain localized usually makes them less threatening than malignant tumors, but not all benign tumors are harmless. Malignant tumors are much more dangerous because they invade and destroy surrounding tissue and may also move or **metastasize** through blood or lymph and thus spread to other sites in the body.

The most dangerous characteristic of tumor cells is their autonomy—that is, their ability to grow without regard to the needs of other body cells and without being subject to the restraints of growth that govern other cells. This unrestrained tumor growth makes cancer capable of overwhelming its host, damaging other organs or physiological processes, or using nutrients necessary for body functions. The tumor takes priority, becoming like a parasite on its host.

Malignant growths can be divided into four main groups—carcinomas, sarcomas, leukemias, and lymphomas. **Carcinomas** are cancers of the epithelial tissue, cells that line the outer and inner surfaces of the body, such as skin, stomach lining, and mucous membranes. **Sarcomas** are cancers that arise from cells in connective tissue, such as bone, muscles, and cartilage. **Leukemias** are cancers that originate in the blood or blood-forming cells, such as stem cells in the bone marrow. Three types of cancers—carcinomas, sarcomas, and leukemias—account for over 95% of malignancies. Victoria's cancer, **lymphoma**, a cancer of the lymphatic system, was one of the rarer types of cancer.

Although some people may have a genetic predisposition to cancer, the disease itself is almost never inherited. Behavior and lifestyle are the primary contributors to cancer, and our concern is with those behaviors and lifestyles that have been identified as risk factors in the development of cancer.

The Changing Rates of Cancer Deaths

For the first time since records have been kept, the death rates from cancer in the United States has leveled off and even begun to decline. This trend ends a century-long steady increase in cancer deaths that peaked in 1993 when cancer mortality was more than three times higher than in 1900. Figure 10.1 shows the total cancer death rates in the United States from 1900 to 1999.

Why have cancer death rates dropped in recent years? At least two explanations are possible. First, the decline might be due to improved treatment that prolongs the life of cancer patients. The validity of this explanation can be tested by looking at the difference between cancer incidence and cancer deaths. If incidence remained the same or even increased while deaths declined, then better treatment would account for the drop in cancer deaths. However, the evidence does not support this hypothesis. A recent review from the National Cancer Institute (Howe et al., 2001) reported that both the incidence rate and the death rate for all cancers decreased an average of 1.1% per year between 1992 and 1998. This result suggests that better treatment regimens do not account for the recent decrease in cancer rates. Instead, people are developing cancer less often, and an explanation for that situation comes from changes in U.S. lifestyle. People are smoking much less and eating a more healthy diet than they did 40 years ago. Because smoking and diet account for about two thirds of all cancer deaths in the United States (American Cancer Society, 2002), improvements in these two areas should result in lower rates of cancer.

Although the incidence for all cancer combined declined 1.1% a year between 1992 and 1998, men profited from these changes more than women. New cases among European American men dropped 2.9% annually, whereas the incidence rate for African American men decreased 3.1% a year over this time period (Howe et al.,

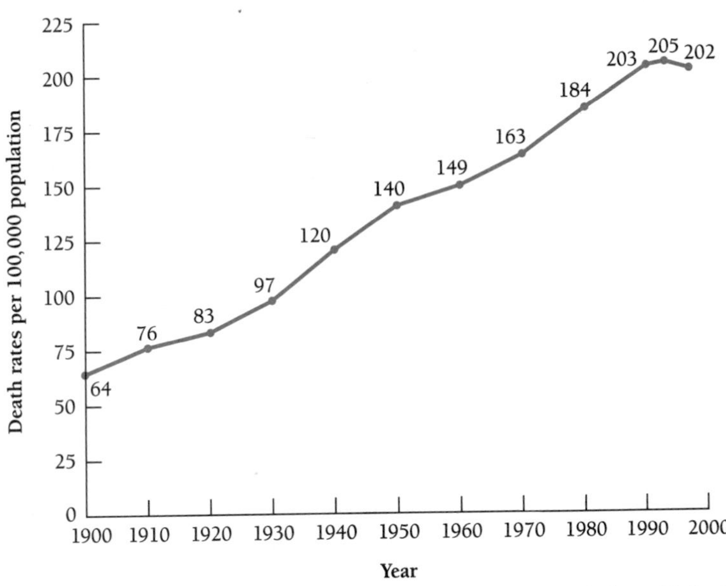

Figure 10.1 Death rates from cancer per 100,000 population, United States, 1900–1999.

Sources: Data from Historical Statistics of the United States: Colonial Times to 1990, Part 1 *(p. 68) by U.S. Bureau of the Census, 1975, Washington, DC: U.S. Government Printing Office;* Health, United States, 1998 *(p. 231) by USDHHS, 1998, Washington, DC: U.S. Government Printing Office; and the National Vital Statistics Systems,* Health, United States, 2001 *(p. 231), by National Center for Health Statistics, 2001, Hyattsville, MD: U.S. Government Printing Office.*

2001). The slight rise in incidence among women was mostly a result in an increase in new cases of breast cancer. The good news for women is that their mortality rate for all cancers combined declined by 0.8% per year between 1992 and 1998. Over this same time period, the mortality rate for men decreased by twice that level—1.6% per year.

Cancers with Decreasing Death Rates

Cancer of the lungs, breast, prostrate, and colon/rectum account for about half of all cancer deaths in the United States. and mortality rates for each of these sites are currently declining.

Lung cancer accounts for about 27% of all cancer deaths and about 13% of all cancer cases—figures that reveal the deadliness of lung cancer. Between 1992 and 1998, total lung cancer deaths in the United States declined 1.6% per year, but almost all of this decline was due to a decrease of 2.7% annually for men (Howe et al., 2001). Figure 10.2 shows that lung cancer mortality for women rose dramatically from 1965 to 1990, but since that time death rates have been almost level (Howe et al., 2001). Because cigarette smoking is the primary cause of lung cancer deaths among women, the current decline in women's smoking rates should eventually bring about a decrease in lung cancer mortality for women. Other than skin cancer, *breast cancer* has the highest incidence (but not death rate) of any cancer in the United States. Women account for about 99.2% of all new cases and men the remaining fraction of 1%. The incidence of breast cancer is increasing faster for women than any other cancer, suggesting that early detection through the use of mammography might be responsible for some of that increase, but another possible explanation is women's increasing

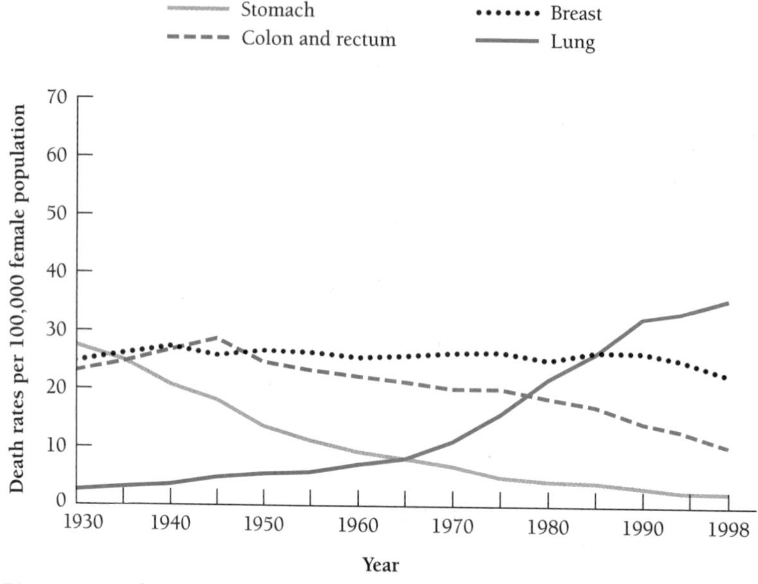

Figure 10.2 Cancer death rates for selected sites, men, United States, 1930–1998.

Sources: Data from Cancer Facts & Figures, 2002 *(p. 3) by American Cancer Society and* Factbook, *National Institutes of Health, 1993, p. 47. US Government Printing Office.*

obesity, a known risk factor for breast cancer (Howe at al., 2001). In the year 2002, the incidence of breast cancer among women was estimated to be more than twice as high as their incidence of lung cancer, but more women died of lung cancer (American Cancer Society, 2002). This suggests that people are much more likely to survive breast cancer than lung cancer.

Other than skin cancer, *prostate cancer* has the highest incidence of cancer among men in the United States, but again, it does not have the highest mortality rate; nearly twice as many men die each year from lung cancer as from prostate cancer. In 2002, the number of men diagnosed with prostate cancer was estimated to be nearly as high as the number of women diagnosed with breast cancer (American Cancer Society, 2002). Like breast cancer incidence, new cases of prostate cancer increased sharply during the 1980s when prostate-specific antigen (PSA) screening was first introduced. In more recent years, however, the number of new cases—about 15% of all cancer cases—has declined slightly (Howe et al., 2001). In the United States, African American men have much higher death rates from prostate cancer than European American men, but interestingly, these differences are not related to socioeconomic status and remain a mystery (Robbins, Whittemore & Thom, 2000). Also, large geographical differences exist for prostate cancer rates, a situation that may be due to regional differences in PSA screening.

Colorectal cancer is the second leading cause of cancer deaths in the United States and other developed countries, exceeded only by lung cancer. However, in the United States, both the incidence and the mortality rates of colorectal cancer are going down. Incidence and morality rates vary widely by ethnic background, with African Americans much more likely to be diagnosed with colorectal cancer than either Hispanic Americans or European Americans. For all groups combined, the incidence of colorectal cancer has declined 1.8% per year from 1992 to 1998, but the rate for African American women has remained about the same. Although incidence of colorectal cancer increased slightly until

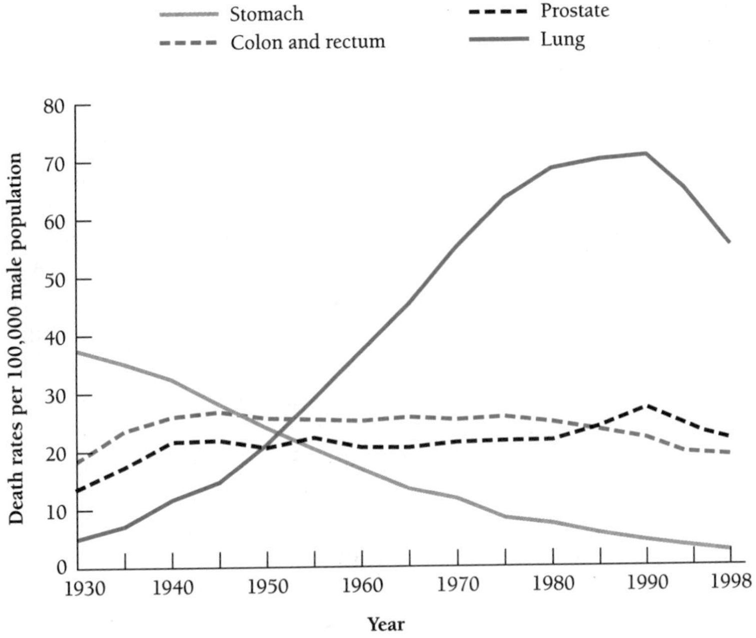

Figure 10.3 Cancer death rates for selected sites, men, United States, 1930–1998.

Sources: Data from Cancer Facts & Figures, 2002, *(p. 2) by American Cancer Society and* Factbook, *National Institutes of Health, 1993, p. 47, US Government Printing Office.*

about 1985, the mortality rate has been declining since about 1945 (see Figures 10.2 and 10.3).

Death rates from *stomach cancer* have dropped from being the leading cause of cancer deaths for both women and men to having a very low mortality rate. As we discuss later, modern refrigeration and fewer salt-cured foods probably account for most of the decrease in stomach cancer.

Cancers with Increasing Incidence and Mortality Rates

In general, incidence rates for the four leading cancers—lung, breast, prostate, and colorectal—are declining, especially for men. However, not all cancer rates are decreasing. Several cancers have recently increased (Howe et al., 2001).

Non-Hodgkin's lymphoma has the highest death rates among the cancers that are increasing. It accounts for 4% of the cases and 4.4% of deaths. Non-Hodgkin's lymphoma is one type of cancer found among AIDS patients (although, like our opening case study Victoria, most people with non-Hodgkin's lymphoma do not have AIDS). *Liver cancer*, like lung cancer, is quite lethal, with a death rate nearly twice as high as its incidence rate. *Melanoma*, a potentially fatal form of skin cancer, accounts for 1.4% of all cancer deaths in the United States. Other cancers with increasing incidence and mortality rates are cancer of the esophagus, some types of leukemia, cancer of the soft connective tissue, thyroid, small intestine, and vulva. These cancers combined account for 13% of all cancer cases and deaths in the United States.

In Summary

Cancer is a group of diseases characterized by the presence of neoplastic cells that grow and spread without control. These new cells may form benign tumors, which tend to remain localized, or malignant tumors, which may metastasize and spread to other organs.

After more than a century of rising mortality rates, cancer deaths are beginning to decline. This decrease is most evident from a look at the incidence and mortality of the four cancers that contribute to about half of all cancer deaths—lung, breast, prostate, and colorectal cancers. Since 1992, incidence and death rates among men for these four cancers have declined at a slow but steady pace, whereas comparable rates for women have risen very slightly. The leading cause of cancer deaths for both women and men continues to be lung cancer. The incidence of breast cancer among women and prostate cancer among men is much higher than the incidence of lung cancer, but lung cancer kills far more people in the United States than do either breast cancer or prostate cancer.

Behavioral Risk Factors for Cancer

Cancer results from an interaction of genetic, behavioral, and environmental conditions, most of which are still not clearly understood. However, researchers are making progress in understanding how genes and environment contribute to the development of cancer. For example, the BRCA 1 and BRCA 2 genes are involved in the development of breast and ovarian cancer. These genes protect against cancer by providing the code for a protective protein (Paull, Cortez, Bowers, Elledge, & Gellert, 2001). When a woman has a mutated form of BRCA 1, that mutation does not allow the development of that protective protein, and she is as much as seven times more likely to develop breast cancer than women with the healthy form of this gene. Mutations in BRCA 1 and BRCA 2 have also been implicated in the development of breast cancer in men and in pancreatic cancer in both women and men (Li, Cass, & Karlan, 2001). This gene does not create a certainty of developing cancer, but people with the mutation have an increased risk.

The form of breast cancer involving BRCA 1 and BRCA 2 are responsible for no more than 10% of breast cancer, and the other cancers associated with BRCA are even less common. Despite the widespread publicity about genetic causes of cancer, genetics plays a fairly minor role in the development of cancer; lifestyle factors are much more important (Vineis, Schulte, & McMichael, 2001).

As with cardiovascular diseases, however, a number of cancer risk factors have been identified. Recall that risk factors are not necessarily *causes* of a disease, but they do predict the likelihood of a person developing or dying from that disease. Most risk factors for cancer relate to personal behavior and lifestyle, especially smoking and diet. Other known behavioral risks include alcohol, physical inactivity, exposure to ultraviolet light, and sexual behavior.

Smoking

Cigarette smoking is the primary cause of preventable deaths in the United States, accounting for about 440,000 deaths per year; about 40% of these deaths are from lung cancer. More people die from smoking than from motor vehicle crashes, AIDS, alcohol, cocaine, heroin, homicide, and suicide—combined (USDHHS, 2000). The vast majority of smoking-related cancer deaths are from lung cancer, but smoking is also implicated in deaths from several other cancers, including leukemia and cancers of the breast, lip, oral cavity, pharynx, esophagus, pancreas, larynx, trachea, urinary bladder, and kidney (CDC, 2002).

What Is the Risk? Epidemiologists generally agree that sufficient research evidence exists for a causal relationship between cigarette smoking and lung cancer. Chapter 2 includes a review of that evidence and also explains how epidemiologists can infer causation from nonexperimental

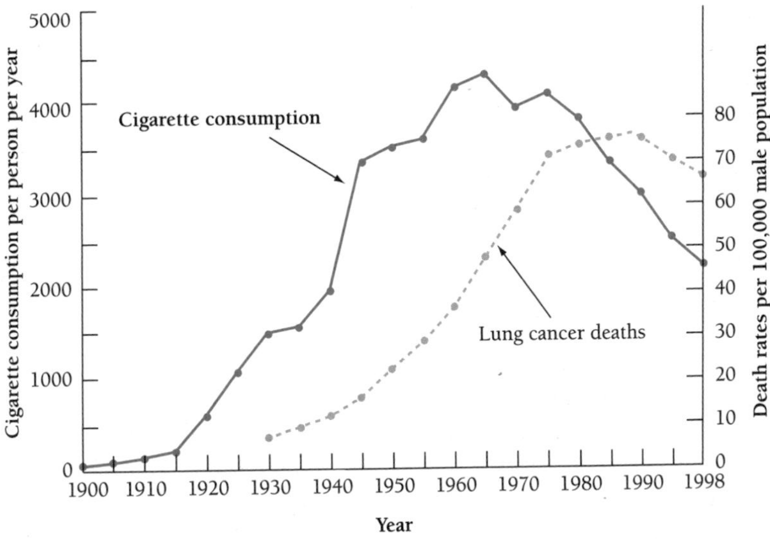

Figure 10.4. The parallel paths of cigarette consumption and lung cancer deaths among men, United States, 1900–1998.

Sources: "Surveillance for Selected Tobacco Use Behaviors—United States, 1900–1994" by G. A. Givovino et al., 1994, Morbidity and Mortality Weekly Report, 43, *No. SS-3, pp. 6–7;* Health, United States *by 2001, National Center for Health Statistics Hyattsville, MD: U.S. Government Printing Office;* Cancer Facts & Figures, 2002. *(p. 2) by American Cancer Society.*

studies. A strong case for a causal relationship between smoking and lung cancer can be seen by observing the way lung cancer rates track smoking rates. About 25 to 40 years after smoking rates began to increase for men, lung cancer rates started a steep rise; about 25 to 40 years after cigarette consumption decreased for men, lung cancer death rates for men began to drop (see Figure 10.4). The decline in smoking among women has been more gradual than among men, and their lung cancer mortality rates have also been slower to show a decline (see Figure 10.2).

Low-income men smoke more than high-income men, and they have a higher lung cancer mortality rate; low-income women smoke a little less than high-income women, and they have a slightly lower rate of lung cancer mortality (National Center for Health Statistics [NCHS] 2001). The dose-response relationship between cigarette smoking and lung cancer and the close tracking of smoking rates and lung cancer rates provide compelling evidence for a causal relationship between smoking behavior and the development of lung cancer.

How high is the risk for lung cancer among cigarette smokers? A very conservative estimate (Lubin, Richter, & Blot, 1984) placed the relative risk at 9.0, meaning that lung cancer was nine times higher among smokers than among nonsmokers. The risk that cigarette smokers have of dying of lung cancer is the strongest link between any behavior and a major cause of death. In Chapter 2, we saw that a relative risk of 1.3 can suggest causality and that a relative risk of 2.0 or greater is considered strong. Thus, cigarette smokers' relative risk in the vicinity of 9.0 for lung cancer clearly establishes smoking as a primary contributor to death from lung cancer—the leading cancer-related death for both men and women. This link is so well established that epidemiologists now have moved beyond conducting research in this area. Instead, they are more concerned with the risk to passive smokers—that is, people exposed to the smoke of others. (See Chapter 13 for a review of this research.)

Cigarette smoking also contributes to breast cancer. Women who smoke and women who live with a smoker have an elevated risk for both breast cancer incidence and breast cancer mortality, and the risk is dose related. One study (Calle, Miracle-McMahill, Thun, & Heath, 1994) found that women who smoked 40 or more cigarettes daily had a 75% increase in breast cancer, whereas those who smoked 10 to 19 cigarettes a day had only a 20% increase. Also, the number of years of smoking history was directly related to risk of breast cancer, as was early initiation of smoking. These findings present powerful evidence that smoking increases a woman's chances of dying of breast cancer.

In addition to smoking, such factors as polluted air, socioeconomic level, occupation, ethnic background, and building material in one's house have all been linked to lung cancer. Each of these has an additive or possibly a **synergistic effect** with smoking, so studies of different populations may yield quite different risk factor rates, depending on the combination of risks that cigarette smokers have in addition to their risk as a smoker.

What Is the Perceived Risk? Despite their heightened vulnerability to cancer, many smokers do not perceive that their behavior puts them at risk. They show what Neil Weinstein (1984) referred to as an *optimistic bias* concerning their chances of dying from cigarette-related causes. One study of high school students (Reppucci, Revenson, Aber, & Reppucci, 1991) found that, despite their knowledge of a strong relationship between smoking and lung cancer, these young smokers judged their chances of developing lung cancer as about average. Adult smokers, too, have an optimistic bias concerning their personal risks from smoking. Michael Schoenbaum (1997) found that nonsmokers, former smokers, and current light smokers, made fairly accurate guesses of their chances of living to age 75, but heavy smokers greatly overestimated their chances of living to that age. Possibly influenced by their optimistic bias, smokers are more likely than nonsmokers to say that smoking tastes good, smells good, is sociable, or is good for one's nerves (van Assema, Pieterse, Kok, Eriksen, & de Vries, 1993).

Is Smoking Ever Safe? Is smoking ever safe? Many people have taken up cigars and pipes in the belief that they are less hazardous than cigarettes (Rigotti, Lee, & Wechsler, 2000). Is this belief justified? Evidence suggests that cigars and pipes are safer than cigarettes, but each has a relatively high risk for lung cancer. One study (Lubin et al., 1984) found that the relative risk for cigarette-only smokers was 9.0, whereas the risks for cigar-only and pipe-only smokers were 2.9 and 2.5, respectively. Interestingly, when cigars or pipes were combined with cigarettes, the relative risk for lung cancer increased dramatically. Cigars and cigarettes combined yielded a 6.9 risk, whereas pipes and cigarettes raised the relative risk to 8.1, or nearly as high as cigarettes alone. Results from this research are clear: *Smoking any tobacco product is never safe.*

Diet

Another risk factor for cancer is an unhealthy diet. The American Cancer Society (2002) estimated that one third of all cancer deaths in the United States are a result of dietary choices, but other estimates (Simone, 1983) yield rates as high as 50%. Poor dietary practices are associated with cancers of the breast, stomach, uterus, endometrium, rectum, colon, kidneys, small intestine, pancreas, liver, ovary, bladder, prostate, mouth, pharynx, thyroid, and esophagus.

Which Foods May Promote Cancer? Some foods are suspected of being **carcinogenic**, that is, of causing cancer, and these may be either "natural" foods or foods with additives. Natural foods—those without added chemicals or preservatives—are not necessarily safer than those containing preservatives, and some may be less so. Also, the lack of preservatives can result in high levels of bacteria and fungi. Spoiled food is a risk factor in stomach cancer, and the sharp decline in this cancer (see Figures 10.2 and 10.3) is due in part to increased refrigeration during the last 75 years and to lower consumption of salt-cured foods, smoked foods, and foods stored at room temperature.

In Chapter 9, we saw that dietary fat is an established risk for cardiovascular disease, and a number of studies have shown that dietary fat is a risk for cancer. However, it is not as strong as risk for cancer as it is for cardiovascular disease. Much of the research on dietary fat and cancer has centered on breast cancer, but the results are inconsistent. Reports from the Nurses' Health Study show that neither eating a high-fat diet (Holmes et al., 1999) nor a history of being overweight (Huang et al., 1997) increases women's chances of breast cancer. However, weight *gain* after age 18 was positively associated with breast cancer after menopause, especially in women who never used hormone replacement therapy. Women in the Nurses' study may not be typical of all women in the United States, and a study of Italian women (Toniolo, Riboli, Protta, Charrel, & Coppa, 1989) showed that breast cancer patients had a slightly higher consumption of protein and nonvegetable fats (milk, high-fat cheese, and butter) compared with healthy women. Women who consumed half their calories as fat had breast cancer rates that were three times higher than average. Thus, the relationship between high-fat diet and breast cancer is not clear.

Colorectal cancer is the second leading cause of cancer deaths in the United States and other developed countries, exceeded only by lung cancer. Yet the cause of colorectal cancer deaths is not well known. Most research on colon and rectal cancers have turned to obesity and diet, but the results of this research have not been definitive. A study on a national sample of adult U.S. men (Ford, 1999) found a clear dose-response relationship between weight and incidence of colon cancer in men; that is, the more extra weight a man carried, the greater his chances of developing colon cancer. However, a report from the Framingham Study (Zhang et al., 2001) found no relationship between weight and rectal cancer and an *inverse* relationship between weight and colon cancer in postmenopausal women. Authors of this study hypothesized that the inverse relationship between weight and colon cancer may be the result of greater cumulative estrogen exposure.

Much of the evidence for diet and colorectal cancer has centered on the "Western" eating pattern, a diet that includes large amounts of processed meat, fast foods, refined grains and potatoes, sugar-laden foods, and few fruits and vegetables. One study (Slattery, Boucher, Caan, Potter, & Ma, 1998) reported that such a diet may contribute to colon cancer, but a later study (Terry, Hu, Hansen, & Wolk, 2001) found little evidence to support the hypothesis that the "Western" eating pattern makes a significant contribution to colorectal cancer deaths in women.

Researchers have also investigated the relationship between diet and lung and bladder cancers. For example, the Western Electric study (Shekelle, Rossof, & Stamler, 1991) found that men who consumed high levels of cholesterol had nearly twice the rate of lung cancer as men who were low consumers of cholesterol and that much of this added risk came from consumption of eggs. A recent meta-analysis (Steinmaus, Nuñez, & Smith, 2000) revealed that diets high in fat generally increase people's chances of bladder cancer.

Although the role of diet in the development of colorectal cancer is not clear, evidence suggests that some foods may increase one's risk for bladder and lung cancer. Even with these somewhat mixed results, it would seem prudent to adopt an eating pattern that includes a large supply of fruits and vegetables, fish, poultry, cereals, and whole grain bread.

Which Foods May Protect Against Cancer? If eating certain foods increases the risk for cancer, do other dietary measures offer protection? Which foods should people consume to reduce their risk for cancer? Research in this area has

WOULD YOU BELIEVE

Pizza May Prevent Cancer

Would you believe that pizza may prevent cancer? For pizza lovers everywhere, this indeed is good news. However, before you begin eating two or three pizzas a day, you should be aware of a few cautions. Pizza is not an entirely healthy food; the cancer-protective effects of pizza are limited to the tomato sauce that contains a specific nutrient—lycopene. Toppings such as ground meat, pepperoni, anchovies, and cheese are high in fat, and high-fat diets have many risks. In addition, the protective value is not large.

The lycopene in tomato sauce is a type of chemical that is inversely related to the development of cancer (Giovannucci, 1999). That is, people who eat more tomatoes, especially cooked tomatoes, are less likely to get cancer. Lycopene is not the only nutrient that protects against cancer. Some researchers (Freeman et al., 2000; Norrish et al., 2000) are beginning to find a number of specific nutrients that may have the ability to influence origin and development of cancer.

What are the pathways through which lycopene and other nutrients in food may protect against cancer? At the earliest stage of prevention, antioxidants can counteract carcinogens before they damage cells; the polyphenols in green tea as well as the lycopene in cooked tomatoes seem to work in this way (Cowley, 1998). After entering the body, carcinogens are converted from precursors into agents that damage DNA and produce malignancies. You can slow this process, however, by eating lots of vegetables, including tomato paste and garlic.

Another possibility for the preventive power of nutrients comes from the body's ability to destroy damaged or mutated cells; the omega-3 fatty acids found in flaxseed and fatty fish may have the ability to hinder tumor growth in this way. Not all fats are protective; the fat in corn and safflower oils are believed to promote tumor growth (Cowley, 1998). Therefore, a low-fat diet is a good general dietary strategy for lowering cancer risk. But, eating fish and flaxseed may help protect against cancer.

Tissues of reproductive organs are especially vulnerable to malignancies, and estrogen is a culprit for breast cancer in women. Soy products can diminish the estrogen risk, because soy contains a chemical that binds to estrogen receptors but is much weaker than estrogen, diminishing the effect. This substitution can be an advantage in slowing cell division and, thus, tumor growth. Countries in which soy is an important part of the diet have lower rates of both breast and prostate cancer than the United States (Cowley, 1998).

Another possible route for protection comes from nutrients that suppress tumor growth. Like other growing cells, malignancies depend on growth factors to establish and promote growth, and suppression of these factors can thwart cancer proliferation. A chemical in red grapes, carrots, rosemary, and turmeric has the ability to block blood vessel formation, thus preventing a tumor from establishing itself (Cowley, 1998). Eating these foods will not cure cancer, and most of the research on the preventive powers of nutrients has been carried out on rats. However, diet is a factor in the establishment and spread of cancer, so a cancer-healthy diet exists. This diet includes foods with specific nutrients that seem to offer protection against particular types of cancer—so have a slice of pizza.

focused both on types of foods that relate to lowered risks for cancer of different sites and on nutrients that may protect against the development or proliferation of cancer (see Would You Believe . . . ? box).

Deficiencies in vitamin A result in deterioration of the stomach's protective lining—a situation that has prompted several investigators to look for a possible association between cancer and low intake of vitamin A and **beta-carotene**, a form of vitamin A found abundantly in vegetables such as carrots and sweet potatoes. Beta-carotene has been promoted as a protector against several cancers. What is the evidence for this claim? In general, research has found no relationship between intake of beta-carotene and either bladder cancer (Steinmaus et al., 2000) or prostate cancer (Norrish, Jackson, Sharpe, & Skeaff, 2000) and only a weak protective effective of beta-carotene for breast cancer (Hunter et al., 1993) and lung cancer (Yong et al., 1997). These findings suggest that intake of beta-carotene-rich foods or dietary supplements probably provides some protection against breast and lung cancer.

Twenty-five years ago, Linus Pauling (1980) created much interest (and some controversy) with his claim that taking large doses of vitamin C (ascorbic acid) was an effective protector against cancer. Ascorbic acid acts as a nitrite scavenger and antioxidant, thus inhibiting the formation of **nitrosamine** carcinogens. For this reason, vitamin C does appear to have some *potential* to protect against cancer. Is this potential effect supported by the evidence? Epidemiological studies suggest that diets high in vitamin C provide moderate protection against lung cancer. For example, the First National Health and Nutrition Examination Survey (NHANES I) (Yong et al., 1997) found that adults in the top level of vitamin C consumption, compared with those in the bottom level, had only two thirds the incidence of lung cancer.

Selenium is an important trace element found in grain products and in meat from grain-fed animals. It enters the food chain through the soil, but not all soils throughout the world contain equal amounts of selenium. In excess, selenium is toxic, but in moderate amounts, it provides some protection against colon and prostate cancers. Foods with high levels of selenium protect against colon cancer in laboratory rats (Finley, Davis, & Feng, 2000), and selenium supplements have been reported to reduce prostate cancer by 66% (Tracey, 2001). These findings suggest that moderate levels of selenium provide some protection against colon and prostate cancers. Researchers (Knekt et al., 1997) have also looked at dietary flavinoids as a possible buffer against lung and other cancers. Flavinoids, which are products of plant metabolism, are effective antioxidants and, thus, have some potential to protect against cancer. Apples are an excellent source of flavinoids, but other good sources include onions, garlic, scallions, and leeks. High levels of dietary flavinoids are associated with decreased rates of lung cancer in men and women, independent of vitamin E, vitamin C, and beta-carotene.

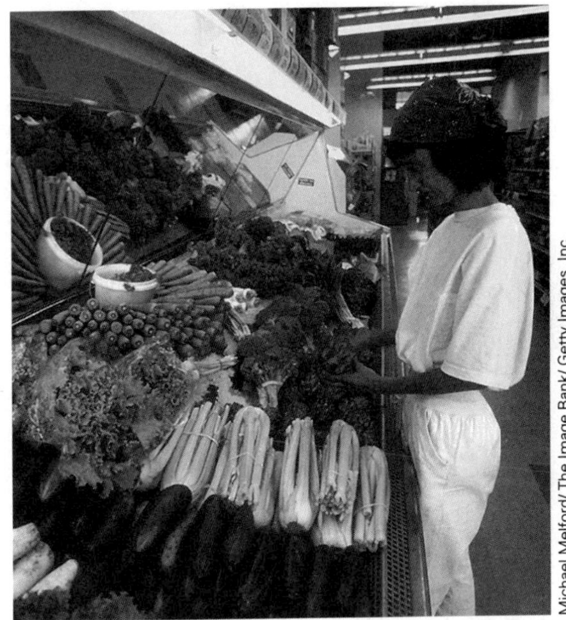
Michael Melford/ The Image Bank/ Getty Images, Inc.

A diet high in fruits and vegetables offers protection against both cancer and cardiovascular disease.

A high-fiber diet may provide some protection against colon and rectum cancers. Martha Slattery and her associates (Slattery et al., 1998) found that a "prudent" pattern of eating helps reduce one's risk of colon cancer. A "prudent" diet consists of all types of fruits and vegetables, some fish and poultry, but very little red meat, processed meat, or sugar-laden foods. This is the same study that found that a "Western" eating pattern—lots of red meat, processed meat, fast foods, refined grains, and sugar—was positively related to the development of colon cancer.

One of the most effective foods in the fight against bladder cancer—and certainty the least expensive—is water. Dominique Michaud and her colleagues (Michaud et al., 1999) found that people who drink lots of plain water or juices have a significantly reduced risk of bladder cancer compared with people who consume less water. These

TABLE 10.1 *Diet and Its Effects on Cancer*

Type of Food	Findings	Studies
A. High-fat diet	Does not cause breast cancer	Holmes et al., 1999
	Contributes to colon cancer	Slattery et al., 1998
	No relation to colorectal cancer	Terry et al., 2001
	May cause bladder cancer	Steinmaus et al., 2000
B. Very high consumption of milk, cheese, and butter	Triples chance of breast cancer	Toniolo et al., 1989
C. Being overweight	Increases chances of rectal cancer	Ford, 1999
	Reduces risk for colon cancer	Zhang et al., 2001
	Does not relate to rectal cancer	Zhang et al., 2001
D. High-cholesterol diet	Doubles chances for lung cancer	Shekelle et al., 1991
E. Beta-carotene	Does not reduce risk for bladder or prostate cancer	Steinmaus et al., 2000;
	Has a weak relationship to breast and lung cancers	Norrish et al., 2000; Hunter et al., 1993; Yong et al., 1997
F. Dietary vitamin A	Some protection against lung and stomach cancer	Yong et al., 1997
G. Dietary vitamin C	Reduces lung cancer by one third	Yong et al., 1997
H. Selenium	Offers some protection against colon and prostate cancer	Finley et al., 2000; Tracey, 2001
I. Vitamin E and C supplements	No added benefit in protecting against lung cancer	Yong et al., 1997
J. Beta-carotene supplements	Does no harm but offers no benefit for any cancers	Hennekens et al., 1996
K. Dietary flavinoids (apples, onions, etc.)	Reduce all cancer, but especially lung cancer	Knekt et al., 1997
L. Water and other fluids	Greatly reduce risk for bladder cancer	Michaud et al., 1999

researchers hypothesized that drinking large amounts of fluids would dilute the urine in the bladder and thus lower the concentration of potential carcinogens. These researchers followed a group of male health professionals for 10 years and found that men who drank 10 or more 8-ounce glasses of fluid every day had only half the risk of bladder cancer as men who consumed five or fewer glasses per day. They also found that every extra glass of fluids consumed decreased the risk of bladder cancer by 7%. These findings suggest that people should not pass a water cooler without taking a drink.

People who drink lots of water and eat four or five moderate servings of fruits and vegetables daily probably have no need to supplement their diet with additional amounts of selenium, beta-carotene, vitamin E, or vitamin C. Little evidence exists that adding vitamin supplements is an effective approach to further lowering of one's risk of cancer. For example, the NHANES I study (Yong et al., 1997) found that dietary consumption of vitamin E, vitamin C, and vitamin A all had some ability to reduce lung cancer in some people but found no added benefit in supplementing these vitamins. Also, a study of male physicians (Hennekens et al., 1996) used only beta-carotene supplements and found neither harm nor benefit; that is, beta-carotene supplements neither raised nor lowered these men's incidence of cancer (or cardiovascular disease). Table 10.1 summarizes some of the research on diet and cancer.

Alcohol

For cancers of all sites, alcohol is not as strong a risk factor as either smoking or imprudent diet. Nevertheless, alcohol has been implicated in cancers of the tongue, tonsils, esophagus, pancreas, breast, and liver. Pancreatic cancer has a special affinity to alcohol consumption, and some evidence ties alcohol consumption to liver cancer. The liver has primary responsibility for detoxifying alcohol. Therefore, persistent and excessive drinking often leads to cirrhosis of the liver, a degenerative disease that curtails the organ's effectiveness. Cancer is more likely to occur in cirrhotic livers than in healthy ones (Leevy, Gellene, & Ning, 1964), but alcohol abusers are likely to die of a variety of causes before liver cancer.

Does drinking alcohol cause breast cancer? Current evidence indicates that high levels of alcohol consumption are related to breast cancer, but the evidence for lower levels of drinking is still is not overwhelming. Keith Singletary and Susan Gapstur (2001) reviewed 33 recent studies on this question and found much variation in the strength of the association between alcohol and breast cancer. In general, women who consume three or more drinks per day have a moderate to strong risk for breast cancer, and women who consume as little as one to two drinks daily have some risk. The risk is not equal in all countries. Singletary and Gapstur estimated that in the United States, about 2% of breast cancer cases can be attributed to alcohol, but in Italy where alcohol intake is much higher, as much as 15% of breast cancer cases may be due to drinking. Alcohol has a synergistic effect with smoking, so people who both smoke and drink heavily have a relative risk for certain cancers exceeding that of the two independent risk factors added together. Research (Flanders & Rothman, 1982) has found a synergistic effect between alcohol and tobacco on cancer of the larynx. Exposure to both substances increases the risk for laryngeal cancer by about 50% more than would be expected if the effect were merely additive. These data suggest that people who both drink heavily and smoke could substantially reduce their chances of developing laryngeal cancer by giving up either smoking or drinking. Quitting both, of course, would reduce the risk still more.

Sedentary Lifestyle

A sedentary lifestyle seems to promote some types of cancer, whereas regular physical activity may provide some protection against breast cancer in women. Current evidence (Gilliland, Li, Baumgartner, Crumley, & Samet, 2001) suggests that both pre- and postmenopausal women who engage in rigorous physical activity have a lower risk for breast cancer than inactive women. Other studies (Bernstein, Henderson, Hanisch, Sullivan-Halley, & Ross, 1994; Thune, Brenn, Lund, & Gaard, 1997) suggest that women who begin a physical activity program when they are young and who continue to exercise 4 hours a week greatly reduce their risk for breast cancer.

Does physical activity decrease men's chances of prostate cancer, or does it elevate the risk? Evidence on this question suggests that either situation may occur, depending on the type of physical activity. For example, a case-control study (Le Marchand, Kolonel, & Yoshizawa, 1991) found that older men who had worked many years on jobs demanding strenuous activity had higher rates of prostate cancer than men who had spent most of their lives in sedentary or low-activity jobs. However, I-M Lee and colleagues (Lee, Paffenbarger, & Hsieh, 1992) measured all types of exercise, including leisure-time activities and found that physically active men had a much reduced rate of prostate cancer compared with men who exercised infrequently or not at all. Lee et al. hypothesized that physical activity may protect against prostate cancer because it moderates the production of testosterone, a hormone that seems to increase the risk of prostate cancer.

As for colon cancer, physical activity seems to offer some protection to both men and women. A review by David Batty and Inger Thune (2000) concluded that a dose-response relationship exists between physical activity and colon cancer for both women and men; that is, the higher the levels of physical activity, the lower the rate of colon cancer. In summary, these studies indicate that regular leisure-time physical activity probably protects against cancer of the breast, prostate, and colon. The potential risks and benefits of physical activity are discussed more fully in Chapter 16.

Ultraviolet Light

Exposure to ultraviolet light, particularly from the sun, has long been recognized as a cause of skin cancer, especially for light-skinned people (Levy, 1985). Yet, 25% of White adults in the United States sunbathe frequently, and one-fourth of those do not use sunscreens at the recommended levels (Koh et al., 1997). Both cumulative exposure and occasional severe sunburn seem to relate to subsequent risk of skin cancer. Since the mid-1970s, the incidence of skin cancer has risen dramatically, but because this form of cancer has a low mortality rate, it has only slightly affected total cancer mortality statistics. Not all skin cancers, however, are innocuous. One form, malignant melanoma, can be deadly. Malignant melanoma is especially prevalent among light-skinned people exposed to the sun.

Although skin cancer is associated with a behavioral risk (voluntary exposure to the sun over a long period of time), it also has a strong genetic component. Light-skinned, fair-haired, blue-eyed individuals, compared with dark-skinned people, are more likely to develop skin cancer, and much of their damage occurs with sun exposure during childhood. During the past 50 years, the relationship between melanoma mortality rates and geographic latitude has gradually decreased, so that residence in the southern part of the United Stales is no longer a risk factor for women and is a decreasing risk factor for men (Lee, 1997).

Even if geography ceases to be a risk for malignant melanoma, fair-skin people will remain vulnerable to this disease. These people should avoid prolonged and frequent exposure to the sun by taking protective measures, including using sunscreen lotions and wearing protective clothing while exposed to the sun. Presently, the people least likely to protect themselves against the harmful effects of the sun are young White men who have no history of skin cancer (Hall, May, Lew, Koh, & Nadel, 1997). Just because skin cancer is not in their history does not mean it is absent from their future.

Sexual Behavior

Some sexual behaviors also contribute to cancer deaths, especially cancers resulting from acquired immune deficiency syndrome (AIDS). Two common forms of AIDS-related cancers are Kaposi's sarcoma and non-Hodgkin's lymphoma. Kaposi's sarcoma is a malignancy characterized by soft, dark blue or purple nodules on the skin, often with large lesions. The lesions can be so small as to look like a rash but can grow to be large and disfiguring. Besides covering the skin, these lesions can spread to the lung, spleen, bladder, lymph nodes, mouth, and adrenal glands. Until the 1980s, this type of cancer was quite rare and was limited mostly to older men with a Mediterranean background. However, AIDS-related Kaposi's sarcoma occurs in every age group and in both men and women. But not all people with AIDS are equally susceptible to this disease; gay men with AIDS are much more likely to develop Kaposi's sarcoma than people who developed AIDS due to injection drug use or to heterosexual contact (Schulz, Boshoff, & Weiss, 1996).

Non-Hodgkin's lymphoma is characterized by rapidly growing tumors that are spread through the circulatory or lymphatic systems. Most people with non-Hodgkin's lymphoma, like Victoria our chapter-opening case study, do *not* have AIDS. Like Kaposi's sarcoma, non-Hodgkin's lymphoma can occur in AIDS patients of all ages and both genders. The greatest risk for AIDS-related cancers continues to be unprotected sex with an HIV-positive partner.

The presence of invasive cervical cancer has also become a basis for diagnosing AIDS (CDC, 1992), but the majority of cases of cervical cancer are unrelated to HIV infection. Cancer of the cervix accounts for only a small number of all cancer deaths among women in the United States, but some women are at greater risk than others.

Women in low socioeconomic groups, those who have had many sex partners, those whose first sexual intercourse experience occurred early in life, and those who have had early pregnancies are most vulnerable to cervical cancer.

Cervical cancer is related not only to the sexual behavior of women but also to the sex practices of their male partners. When men have multiple sex partners, specifically with women who have had many sex partners, their female sex partners are at an increased risk of cervical cancer.

Other sexual practices put both women and men at risk for cancer. For women, early age at first intercourse and a large number of sex partners are both strongly implicated in the development of cancer of the cervix, vagina, and ovary. However, some of the danger is offset by physiological changes in women's bodies resulting from pregnancy and childbirth that seem to protect against breast, ovarian, and endometrial cancers. These cancers are less common in women who have had children early in life compared with those who have had children later in life or who have no children (Levy, 1985). Having a first child later in the childbearing years does not confer the same protection as it does during early years.

For men, too, sexual practices can increase the risk of cancer, especially prostate cancer. Karin Rosenblatt and her associates (Rosenblatt, Wicklund, & Stanford, 2000) found a significant and positive relationship between prostate cancer and lifetime number of female sex partners (but not male sex partners), early age of first intercourse, and prior infection with gonorrhea. However, they found no risk for prostate cancer and lifetime frequency of sexual intercourse.

In Summary

Cigarette smoking and unwise dietary choices may account for as much as two thirds of cancer deaths in the United States. In addition, alcohol, an inactive lifestyle, ultraviolet light, and some sexual behaviors may contribute to cancer risk.

Cigarette smoking is the leading risk factor for lung cancer. Although not all cigarette smokers die of lung cancer and some nonsmokers develop this disease, clear evidence exists that smokers have a greatly increased chance of developing some form of cancer, particularly lung cancer. The more cigarettes per day people smoke and the more years they continue this practice, the more they are at risk. Cigars and pipes are safer than cigarettes, but no type of smoking is safe. Cancers of the mouth, pharynx, and esophagus have also been associated with cigars and pipes as well as with cigarettes.

Poor dietary habits, especially high-fat diets, are related to cancers of the digestive and excretory systems, breasts, and lungs. Women who consume half their calories in fat have an elevated chance of developing breast cancer, but the relationship between specific diets and various cancers is quite complex. Currently, no convincing evidence exists that proper diet can cure cancer or can offer a strong buffer against this disease.

Alcohol is probably only a weak risk factor for cancer. Nevertheless, it has a synergistic effect with cigarette smoking; when the two are combined, the total relative risk is much greater than the risks of the two factors added together. Lack of physical activity and exposure to ultraviolet light are additional risk factors for cancer. Also, certain sexual behaviors, such as number of lifetime sex partners, relate to both cervical and prostate cancer as well as to cancers associated with AIDS—Kaposi's sarcoma and non-Hodgkin's lymphoma.

Cancer Risk Factors beyond Personal Control

Most risk factors for cancer result from personal behavior, especially diet and smoking. However, some are largely beyond personal control, and these include both environmental and inherent risks.

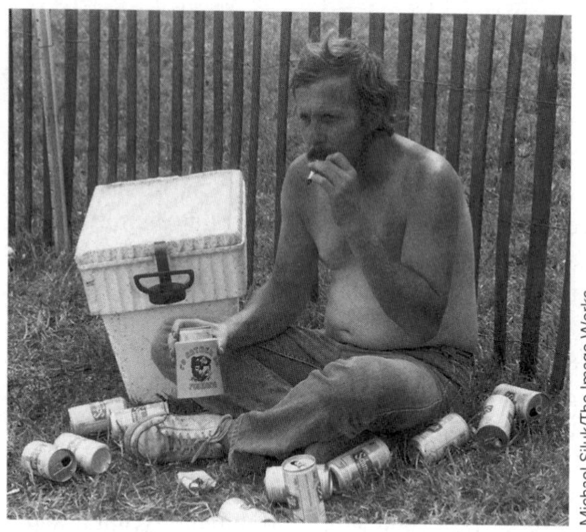
Michael Siluk/The Image Works

Risks from smoking, drinking, and sun exposure can have a synergistic effect, multiplying the chances of developing cancer.

Environmental Risk Factors for Cancer

Environmental cancer risk factors include such conditions as exposure to radiation, asbestos, pesticides, motor exhaust, and other chemicals and may also include living near a nuclear facility. In addition, arsenic, benzene, chromium, nickel, vinyl chloride, and various petroleum products are possible suspects in a number of cancers.

Longtime exposure to asbestos can produce risk for lung cancers, depending on the type of asbestos and the frequency and duration of exposure. A study in Sweden (Gustavsson et al., 2000) looked into the possible carcinogenic effects of asbestos as well as diesel exhaust, motor exhaust, metals, welding fumes, and other environmental conditions that some workers encounter on the job. They found that workers who were most exposed to environmental carcinogen had about a 9% additional chance of developing lung cancer compared with people who were not exposed to these conditions. A study of rubber workers exposed to asbestos (Straif et al., 2000) found slightly increased risks for lung and stomach cancer. However, other studies have found much stronger evidence for an association between asbestos exposure and lung cancer. For example, a study in Malaysia (Luce et al., 2000) found that women who worked with asbestos whitewash had more than four times as much lung cancer than other women. Men in this study had lower exposure to whitewash and no elevated risk for lung cancer. Also, a 25-year longitudinal study of asbestos workers in China (Yano, Wang, Wang, Wang, & Lan, 2001) reported that male asbestos workers, compared with other workers, had a relative risk of 6.6 for lung cancer and 4.3 for all cancers. These findings strongly suggest that long-time exposure to asbestos increase the risk for cancer deaths and especially lung cancer deaths.

Environmental exposure to radiation is also a risk for cancer, especially among nuclear plant workers. An early study from the National Dose Registry of Canada (Ashmore et al., 1998) measured radiation exposure in nuclear power workers and compared their death rates to expected death rates. Nuclear power plant workers with high lifetime accumulations of radiation had an increase in deaths not only from cancer but also from cardiovascular disease and from unintentional injuries. A later report from this Canadian group (Sont et al., 2001) yielded more specific results. This study found workers exposed to high levels of radiation had elevated risks for leukemia, cancers of the rectum, colon, testis, and lung. These results suggest that longtime cumulative exposure to high levels of radiation increases the risk of death from several cancers.

If working in a nuclear plant can elevate one's risk of cancer, can merely living near a nuclear plant increase the risk of environmental cancer? Presently, scientists have found no evidence that simply residing near a nuclear power plant elevates one's risk for cancer. A study (Jablon, Hrubec, & Boise, 1991) that investigated this question compared cancer mortality rates of people living in U.S. counties where nuclear facilities were located with the rates of people living in counties without such facilities. This large-scale study, which included more than 40 million peo-

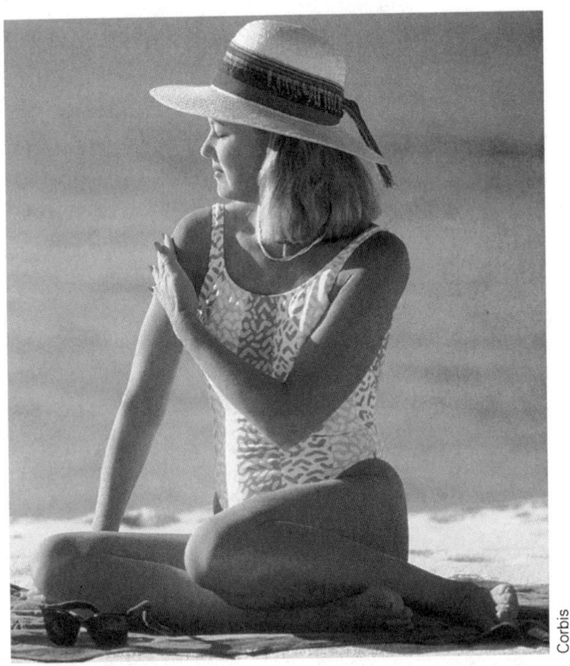

Protective clothing and sunscreen can decrease the risks associated with exposure to ultraviolet light.

ple covering a 35-year period, found no increased cancer mortality for people living near nuclear electrical generating plants.

Some people are concerned about the cancer risks of sleeping with an electric blanket or living near an electric power plant. Are these concerns justified? A report from the Nurses' Health Study (Laden et al., 2000) found no evidence that sleeping with electric blankets had any effect on breast cancer. Similarly, scientific research does not confirm the belief that living near electromagnetic power plants can cause cancer. Edward Campion (1997) conducted a review of 18 years of research on all cancer as well as specific cancers and concluded that no convincing evidence existed that power lines contribute to cancer or any other health hazard. Campion noted that small, poorly controlled early studies that had found a link between cancer and living near power lines generated stories in the popular media, causing many people to be needlessly concerned about power lines. These studies indicate that exposure to environmental conditions other than those encountered by working with air-born asbestos or working in a nuclear power plant presents little or no added risk for cancer.

Inherent Risk Factors for Cancer

Inherent risks for cancer include family history, ethnic background, and age. Although these risks are beyond personal control, people with inherent risk factors for cancer can reduce their risk through modifying their behavior, such as eating more fruits and vegetables and quitting smoking.

Family History Most research on family history as a risk for cancer has centered on breast cancer. Having a mother or sister with early breast cancer doubles or triples a woman's risk for this disease. The Nurses' Health Study (Colditz et al., 1993) observed women whose mothers had been diagnosed with breast cancer and compared their cancer rates to those of women whose mothers had no history of breast cancer. Women whose mothers had been diagnosed with breast cancer before age 40 were more than twice as likely to have breast cancer. Those who had a sister with breast cancer also had a twofold chance of developing this same disease, and having both a sister and a mother with breast cancer increased a woman's risk by about two and a half times. Similarly, a study of Mormon women in Utah (Slattery & Kerber, 1993) found that women with the strongest family history of cancer had three times the risk of breast cancer compared to those with the lowest risk. Looking at this issue from a different view, approximately one third of all women with breast cancer have a family history of the disease (Esplen et al., 1998).

Ethnic Background Compared with European Americans, African Americans have about a 40% to 50% greater incidence of and mortality from cancer. However, Hispanic Americans, Asian Americans, and Native Americans have lower rates than either African Americans or European Americans (NCHS, 2001). Reasons for these discrepancies appear to be due to behavioral and psychosocial factors rather than to biology. For example, although Asian Americans generally have lower total cancer death rates than European Americans, they have a much higher mortality rate for stomach cancer, which is strongly influenced by diet (Miller et al., 1996).

Minority status plays a greater role in survival of cancer than it does in incidence of this disease. For cancer sites with a high 5-year survival rate, the discrepancy between incidence and mortality widens with ethnic background. With breast cancer, for example, non-Hispanic White women have a higher incidence rate than African American women, but African American women have a higher mortality rate from cancer (Miller et al., 1996).

How does minority status contribute to cancer outcomes, that is, length of survival and quality of life? A comprehensive review of research on this question (Meyerowitz, Richardson, Hudson, & Leedham, 1998) showed that several variables contribute to different cancer outcomes among ethnic groups. These variables include socioeconomic status, knowledge about cancer and its treatment, and attitudes toward the disease. These factors can affect access to medical care as well as adherence to medical advice. Access and adherence, in turn, influence both survival time and quality of life. No direct link exists between ethnicity itself and cancer outcome; the association between ethnic background and cancer mortality stems from differences in access, adherence, knowledge and attitudes, and socioeconomic status.

Advancing Age The strongest risk factor for cancer—and many other diseases—is advancing age. The older people become, the greater their chances of developing and dying of cancer; that is, 80-year-old people are more likely than 50-year-old people to die of cancer. However, the percent of total deaths due to cancer is higher for 50-year-olds than for 80-year-olds. Figure 10.5 shows a steep increase in cancer mortality by age for both men and women, but especially for men.

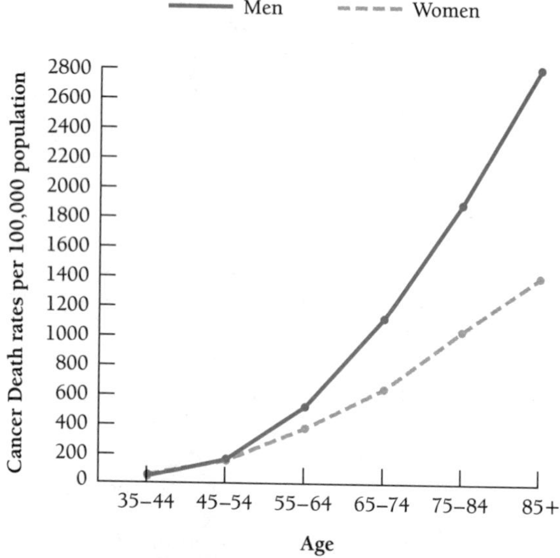

Figure 10.5. Cancer death rates by age and gender, per 100,000 of U.S population, 1999.

Source: Data from Health United States, 2001 *(p. 195) National Center for Health Statistics, 2001, Hyattsville, MD: U.S. Government Printing Office.*

In Summary

Inherent risks for cancer include family history, ethnic background, and advancing age. Although cancer is seldom inherited, family history and a genetic predisposition play a major role in its development. A woman who has a mother or sister with breast cancer has a two- to threefold chance of developing that disease. About one third of all women with breast cancer have a family history of the disease.

African Americans have a higher cancer incidence and higher death rates than European Americans, but people from other ethnic backgrounds have a lower incidence. These differences are not due to biology but to differences in socioeconomic status, knowledge about cancer, and attitudes toward the disease. Each of these is related to both the incidence of cancer and to 5-year survival with the disease.

The strongest risk factor for cancer—as well as many other diseases—is advancing age. The older one becomes, the greater that person's risk for cancer. Both men and women increase their risk for cancer as they get older, but men have an even greater increase than women.

Personality As a Risk for Cancer

Since the days of the Greek physician Galen (131–201 CE), people have speculated about the relationship between personality traits and certain diseases, including cancer. However, that speculation does not match the findings from scientific research. For example, Ina Schapiro and associates (Schapiro et al., 2001) found that neither extraversion nor neuroticism—as measured by the Eysenck Personality Inventory—were related to increased risks of cancer.

Although global personality traits, such as extraversion/introversion and neuroticism/emotional stability do not predict incidence or mortality of cancer, one specific personal trait—suppression of emotion—places people at an elevated risk for cancer. A much weaker psychological risk factor for cancer is clinical depression.

Suppression of Emotion

During the 1970s, evidence began to emerge showing that the suppression of emotion was an important risk factor for cancer. Steven Greer and Thomas Morris (1978) published one of the earliest prospective studies on the relationship between suppression of emotion and incidence of cancer. Participants in this study were women who had been admitted to a hospital for biopsy of a lump in the breast and who had anxiety about their test results. Greer and Morris placed the women into one of three groups: (1) those who suppressed emotion, (2) those who were extreme in their expression of feelings, and (3) those who were apparently normal in their emotional response. A 5-year follow-up revealed that the suppression or denial of anger was significantly related to increased chances of a later diagnosis of breast cancer. These findings led many other researchers to study the relationship between suppression of emotion and incidence of cancer.

A study with male patients at a Veterans Administration hospital (Dattore, Shontz, & Coyne, 1980) also found that suppression of emotion was related to later development of cancer. Ten years prior to diagnosis, these veterans had filled out the Minnesota Multiphasic Personality Inventory (MMPI), giving the researchers early information on their tendencies to suppress emotion. Men later diagnosed with cancer were more likely than other participants to have had a history of suppressing emotion.

A 30-year follow-up of medical school students (Shaffer, Graves, Swank, & Pearson, 1987) provided powerful evidence that suppression was a risk factor for cancer. These medical students had taken a series of psychological tests and questionnaires, which allowed researchers to assign them to groups such as "acting out" and suppression of emotion. Only 1% of physicians in the "acting out" group had developed cancer 30 years later. However, physicians who suppressed their emotions and who were characterized as loners were 16 times more likely to have developed cancer than physicians in the acting-out group. These results suggest that suppressing emotion and being a loner may be as great a risk for cancer as cigarette smoking.

Depression

A second personal characteristic that may place people at risk for cancer is clinical depression. Cancer patients are often depressed, but the evidence that depression causes cancer is neither clear nor strong.

One early study (Dattore et al., 1980) showed that cancer patients were more likely not only to suppress emotion but also to score high on the depression scale of the MMPI years before they developed cancer. Another study (Shekelle et al., 1981) showed that depressed men were at elevated risk for cancer 17 years later. A follow-up report on this study (Persky, Kempthrone-Rawson, & Shekelle, 1987) showed somewhat different results: depression was a risk factor for dying of cancer but not for developing it. These results suggest that depression may promote established cancers, but it probably does not initiate them. However, a later study (Zonderman, Costa, & McCrae, 1989) showed no significant relationship between depression and either cancer morbidity or mortality. Taken together, this body of research does not leave a clear picture of the relationship between depression and cancer. After reviewing this research, Spiegel and Kato (1996) concluded that there is little support for any relationship between depression and incidence of cancer and no evidence of a *causal* association.

In Summary

Of all possible personality traits that may cause cancer, only suppression of emotion is a strong risk. People who suppress or deny their feelings, particularly anger and hostility, have an increased risk for cancer. One study (Shaffer et al., 1987) showed that only about 1% of people who habitually "act out" in anger developed cancer. This same study found that people who suppress strong emotions were 16 times more likely to get cancer than were the people who "acted out." Evidence that depression may cause cancer is weak and inconsistent.

Living with Cancer

The American Cancer Society (2002) estimated that more than 1.28 million people in the United States would be diagnosed with cancer in 2002. Most of those people experienced feelings of fear, anxiety, and anger. Indeed, the diagnosis of cancer nearly always has a significant psychological impact on patients and their families. Psychologists have been involved in assisting patients cope with their emotional reactions to a cancer diagnosis, providing social support to patients and families, and helping patients prepare for the negative side effects of some cancer treatments.

Once people develop cancer, can they improve their chances of survival through nonmedical means? More precisely, do psychosocial factors such as a "fighting spirit," social support, or marital status play a role in length of survival of cancer patients? Is psychotherapy successful in prolonging the lives of cancer patients? What are the problems associated with cancer treatments?

Emotional Responses to a Diagnosis of Cancer

The same emotional factors that enhance the survival of heart disease patients may be precisely the wrong reactions for cancer patients. That is, the calm expression of emotion that seems to help cardiovascular patients cannot be recommended for cancer patients, who may lengthen their survival time by angrily fighting against their illness. One early study (Pettingale, Morris, Greer, & Haybittle, 1985) found that cancer patients who fight angrily against their diagnosis tended to live longer than those who calmly accept their fate. Interestingly, those cancer patients who were poorly adjusted to their illness outlived those who were more accepting of their cancer diagnosis. Specifically, the long-term survivors had higher levels of anxiety, depression, and guilt as well as stronger feelings of alienation. Patients who did not survive the first year were less hostile, better adjusted to their illness, and showed less anger and fewer feelings of discontentment. A review of later studies by Spiegel and Kato (1996) concluded that a "fighting spirit" tends to help cancer patients prolong their life, whereas a hopeless/helpless attitude and difficulty in expressing distress are related to a shorter survival time. Recall that Victoria, the 16-year-old who

BECOMING HEALTHIER

1. Know your family history for cancer. Although you cannot alter this risk factor, you can change modifiable behaviors that relate to cancer.
2. If you smoke, try to quit and keep trying. Most ex-smokers tried more than once to quit before they were successful. Also, do not switch to cigars or pipes. Remember, too, that smoking interacts with alcohol to create an even higher risk for cancer.
3. Keep a food diary for at least one week. (We also recommended this in Chapter 9). Note the amount of fat and the number of servings of fruits and vegetables you eat. Try to find a varied, colorful, low-fat, high-fiber diet that appeals to you. Imprudent eating relates to a number of cancers, including lung cancer.
4. If you are currently sedentary, take up some type of exercise program. Begin slowly at first and try to make it fun. (We have more recommendations for this at the end of Chapter 16.)
5. Practice expressing your emotions, especially anger and hostility, in a quiet, soft, and slow manner. Do not suppress your feelings; recognize them, but do not traumatize other people with a violent expression, although if you have been diagnosed with cancer, go ahead and vent your feelings.
6. If you are frequently depressed or if you have a hopeless/helpless attitude toward life, seek professional help. Qualified psychologists and counselors may be able to help you change your behavior and way of looking at things.

was diagnosed with lymphoma, initially felt angry with everyone. Perhaps that attitude was better than she imagined; more than 15 years later, she is still alive.

Another emotional response to a diagnosis of cancer is self-blame. Judith Glinder and Bruce Compas (1999) investigated the effects of two types of self-blame on women with recently diagnosed breast cancer. *Characterological self-blame* is a stable personality trait marked by a sense of helplessness and a tendency of people to blame themselves for who they are, whereas *behavioral self-blame* is directed at specific behaviors, such as blaming one's self for drinking too much or for not eating enough fruits and vegetables. Glinder and Compas found that both types of self-blame were related to increased symptoms of anxiety and depression immediately after a diagnosis of cancer. However, only characterological self-blame was able at diagnosis to predict breast cancer patients' distress 1 year later. Thus, characterological self-blame can have damaging effects on breast cancer patients for at least 1 year after diagnosis.

Social Support for Cancer Patients

How do social support and an extensive social network increase length of survival of cancer patients? Vicki Helgeson and her colleagues (Helgeson, Cohen, & Fritz, 1998) found that the support of spouses, family members, and friends can help cancer patients by increasing their access to information, strengthening a sense of personal control, fostering self-esteem, and boosting their feelings of optimism. However, some types of marital support may be ineffective. For example, Mariet Hagedoorn and colleagues (Hagedoorn et al., 2000) found that attempts by partners of cancer patients to protect their spouses from the reality of their illness were not helpful. Also, women with breast cancer who lacked adequate marital support profited more from peer-group support than from support of their partners, whereas women with strong support from their partners were actually harmed by peer-discussion support (Helgeson, Cohen, Schulz, & Yasko, 2000).

Nial Bolger and his colleagues (Bolger et al., 2000) found that "invisible" support may be the best kind. These researchers studied providing and receiving support in couples and concluded that support that one partner provides but the other partner does not notice was better at relieving stress than more obvious types of supportive interactions. Receiving support entails obligations, which may be especially troubling for people who are ill. Thus, partners who are supportive without being obvious provide many advantages to cancer patients.

Psychotherapy with Cancer Patients

In addition to a fighting spirit and marital status, certain types of psychotherapy may relate to survival time of cancer patients. The benefits of psychotherapy and counseling to alleviate stress and improve patients' emotional well-being are well established (Jacobsen & Hann, 1998), but the ability of psychological interventions to extend the life of cancer patients is less firmly established. David Spiegel and his colleagues (Spiegel, Kraemer, Bloom, & Gottheil, 1989) found that psychotherapy substantially increased the life of women with metastatic breast cancer. In this study, women who participated in weekly group therapy sessions in which they were free to express their fears and other negative emotions not only benefited emotionally but lived an average of 18 months longer than breast cancer patients who received only medical treatment.

Spiegel et al. expected that group therapy would contribute to improved psychosocial functioning, but they neither planned for nor expected greater survival time for the therapy group. However, a later study by Pamela Goodwin et al., (2001) found that, although group therapy reduced sensations of pain and increased psychological functioning, it did not increase survival time of women with metastatic breast cancer. Because the design of this study was nearly identical to that of Spiegel et al., the results need some interpretation. At least two explanations are possible. First, the differences between the Spiegel and the Goodwin studies may have been the result of the experience and skill of the therapists; and second, newer treatment programs since the Spiegel et al. study have resulted in increased survival rates for all breast cancer patients, whether or not they receive group therapy (Spiegel, 2001).

Problems Associated with Cancer Treatments

Currently, nearly all medical treatments for cancer have negative side effects that may add stress to the lives of cancer patients. These therapies include surgery, radiation, chemotherapy, hormonal treatment, and immunotherapy. The first three are the most common and also the most stressful.

Barbara Andersen (1998) reported that psychological interventions can effectively reduce distress and pain in patients undergoing treatment for cancer. Cancer patients who undergo surgery are likely to experience distress, rejection, and fears, and often receive less emotional support than other surgery patients. Postsurgery stress leads to lower levels of immunity, which may prolong rate of recovery and increase vulnerability to other disorders. Radiation and chemotherapy also have severe side effects. Many patients who receive radiation therapy anticipate their treatment with fear and anxiety, fearing the loss of hair, burns, nausea, vomiting, fatigue, and sterility. Most of these conditions do occur, so patients' fears are not unreasonable. However, patients are seldom adequately prepared for their radiation treatments, and thus their fears and anxieties may exaggerate the severity of these side effects.

Chemotherapy is also frequently accompanied by unpleasant side effects that precipitate stressful reactions in cancer patients. At least half those cancer patients treated with chemotherapy experience nausea, fatigue, depression, weight change, hair loss, sleep problems, and loss of appetite (Burish, Meyerowitz, Carey, & Morrow,

1987). Sexual problems are also common, regardless of the cancer site, and 70% of women interviewed 3 years after chemotherapy had decreased or no sexual interest.

Victoria described her chemotherapy treatments as "terrible." Some of the procedures were painful, and the side effects made Victoria feel helpless and out of control. During the course of her chemotherapy treatments, Victoria experienced nausea and vomiting. She lost her appetite and all interest in eating, so she lost 30 pounds. Her hair fell out, and she experienced a significant loss of coordination and a decreased ability to concentrate. Years later, she believes that she has still not regained her former ability to concentrate.

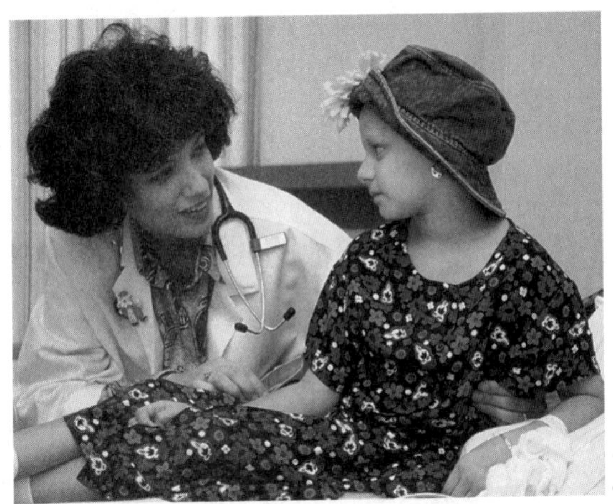
Corbis

Negative side effects of chemotherapy add to the stress of cancer patients.

In Summary

Once people have been diagnosed with cancer, they can affect their survival time by adopting a "fighting spirit," having strong emotional and social support, joining support groups, or attending group psychotherapy sessions. Poor adjustment and a nonacceptance of the cancer diagnosis may tend to prolong the lives of cancer patients. For several reasons, cancer patients who are married tend to live longer than those who are not. Therapy that allows the expression of negative emotions reduces sensations of pain and improves psychological functioning and may add time to the life of breast cancer patients. However, the evidence that psychotherapy can increase survival time is mixed. The standard medical treatments for cancer—surgery, chemotherapy, and radiation—all have negative side effects that often produce added stress. These side effects include changes in body image, loss of hair, nausea, fatigue, and sterility.

Answers

This chapter addressed six basic questions:

1. **What is cancer?**
   Cancer is a group of diseases characterized by the presence of new (neoplastic) cells that grow and spread beyond control. These cells may be either benign or malignant, and both types of neoplastic cells are dangerous. Malignant cells sometimes metastasize and spread through the blood or lymph to other organs of the body; thus malignancies are life threatening.

2. **Are cancer death rates increasing or decreasing?**
   Cancer is the second leading cause of death in the United States, accounting for about 20% of deaths. During the first 9 1/2 decades of the 20th century, cancer rates in the United States rose threefold, but since the mid-1990s, the death rates have begun to decline, especially for cancers of the lung, colon and rectum, breast,

and prostate—the four leading causes of cancer deaths in the United States. One important exception is the rise in lung cancer mortality among women, but women's death rates from lung cancer are beginning to level off and may soon begin to decline.

3. **What are the behavioral risk factors for cancer?**
As many as two thirds of all cancer deaths in the United States have been attributed to either smoking or unwise dietary choices. Smoking cigarettes raises the risk of lung cancer 9 times, but smoking also accounts for other cancer deaths. Cigars and pipes are less dangerous than cigarettes, but they each present a very high risk for cancer.
High-fat diets are related to cancer of several sites, whereas diets that include lots of fruits, vegetables, and grains seem to offer some protection against cancer. Alcohol is not as strong a risk for cancer as diet, but when combined with smoking, it sharply increases the risk. A sedentary lifestyle also presents a risk, especially for breast cancer, and exposure to ultraviolet light and sexual behaviors can increase the risks for various cancers.

4. **What are the inherent and environmental risk factors for cancer?**
The uncontrollable risk factors for cancer include age, family history, and ethnic background. Advancing age is the single most powerful mortality risk for cancer, but age is also the leading risk for death from cardiovascular and other diseases. Family history is a factor in many types of cancer, and women whose mothers or sisters had breast cancer have a two- to threefold risk for breast cancer. Ethnic background is also a factor; compared with European Americans, African Americans have a significantly higher rate of mortality from cancer, but other ethnic groups have lower rates. Environmental exposure to air-borne asbestos and radiation constitute significant risks for cancer, but the exposure is usually heavy and prolonged.

5. **What personality traits relate to cancer?**
Psychological risk factors for cancer are not as powerful as behavioral risks. Nevertheless, some personality traits may relate to cancer. Suppression of emotion, especially anger and hostility, greatly increases cancer risk. Research has also revealed a link between depression and cancer, but the effect is not strong.

6. **How can patients be helped in dealing with cancer?**
To help cancer patients cope with their illness, therapists can encourage them to develop a "fighting spirit" and to loudly express negative emotions rather than suppressing them. In addition, cancer patients usually benefit from social support from spouse, family, and support groups. Psychotherapy may increase survival time of cancer patients, but the evidence for this is mixed. Therapists can use relaxation methods to assist cancer patients in coping with some of the negative aspects of cancer treatments.

Suggested Readings

Dooley, J. F., & Betancourt, M. (2002). *Cancer breakthroughs: What you need to know about the latest cancer treatment options.* New York: Kensington. Clinical biochemist Joseph Dooley and science writer and cancer survivor Marian Betancourt teamed to examine the latest cancer treatments and to explain the physiological basis for these treatments in terms that are easy to understand. Thus, this book offers information about cancer and practical advice about seeking treatment.

Harvard Health Letter. (2002, August). How you can lower your cancer risk. *Harvard Health Letter, 27* (10). This article summarizes the research on lowering risks for cancer, including the usual suspects of smoking and unhealthy diet. In addition, these recommendations draw from recent research and make suggestions about other lifestyle factors.

Perera, F. P. (1997). Environment and cancer: Who are susceptible? *Science, 278,* 1068–1073. This article reviews the evidence linking environmental factors such as smoking, diet, and pollutants with cancer and the interaction of these environmental factors with individual differences arising from genetic factors, ethnic background, and gender. Thus, the article explores complex relationships that produce cancer.

Singletary, K. W., & Gapstur, S. M. (2001). Alcohol and breast cancer: A review of epidemiologic and experimental evidence and potential mechanisms. *Journal of the American Medical Association, 286,* 2143–2151. An up-to-date review of all recent studies on the effects of alcohol on breast cancer. The authors also hypothesize potential mechanisms responsible for the relationship of alcohol to breast cancer.

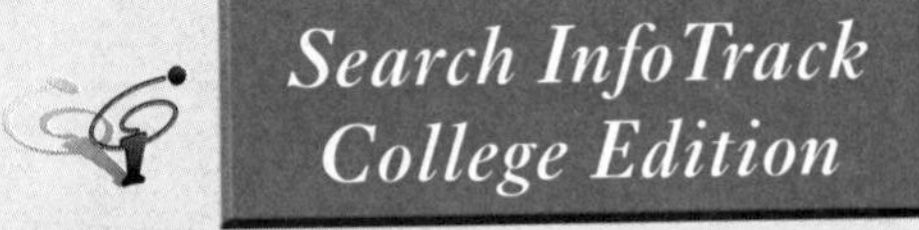

Search these terms to learn more about topics in this chapter:

Cancer and statistics and rates

Smoking and cancer and risk

Alcohol and cancer and risk

Oncogenes

Carcinogens and food

Cancer and environmental aspects

Cancer and stress and health

Social support and cancer patients

Depression and cancer cause

Cancer and diagnosis and distress

Psychotherapy and cancer

Cancer and support groups

11

Living with Chronic Illness

The Story of Brenda

CHAPTER OUTLINE

The Impact of Chronic Disease

Adjusting to Diabetes

The Impact of Asthma

Dealing with HIV and AIDS

Living with Alzheimer's Disease

QUESTIONS

This chapter focuses on five basic questions:

1. What is the impact of chronic illness?
2. What is involved in adjusting to diabetes?
3. How does asthma affect the lives of people with this disease?
4. How can HIV infection be managed?
5. What is the impact of Alzheimer's disease on patients and their families?

The Story of Brenda

Brenda was concerned about her mother, Sylvia, who seemed to be more and more forgetful. At first, Brenda attributed the lapses in Sylvia's memory to her age. She was 81 and entitled to be forgetful at times, but the times were becoming progressively more frequent and disturbing. One day when she was visiting her mother, Brenda noticed that the electric stove in the kitchen was still turned on to the highest setting. She turned it off without saying anything to Sylvia. Later that afternoon, Brenda asked her mother what she had fixed for dinner and was quite surprised when Sylvia replied that she had forgotten to eat. Could it be that Sylvia had turned on the stove and then forgotten to cook anything? The question bothered Brenda.

Several months later when Brenda was visiting her mother, Sylvia suddenly became angry and accused her daughter of throwing away her reading glasses. "You threw out my glasses," Sylvia shouted. "You don't want me to read the newspaper. What are you trying to do to me?" Brenda tried to assure her mother that she had not thrown out her glasses and that she wasn't trying to do anything to her, but Sylvia remained unconvinced.

As time passed, Sylvia's failing memory became even more disconcerting to Brenda. Sylvia often forgot to eat, to bathe, to comb her hair, or to feed her cat. Moreover, she repeatedly confused the names of her children, lost interest in reading and watching television, failed to understand directions, and had difficulty making herself understood.

Sylvia was aware of her loss of memory and would become angry with herself when she could not think of names for simple objects like the chair, the table, or the radio. Her memory for past events seemed to be largely unaffected. She frequently showed old photo albums to Brenda and told stories about the people in the pictures. However, she had little memory for what happened the day before or even the minute before. One day when Brenda was preparing to leave, she said to Sylvia, "I'm going home now, Mother. Do you understand?" Sylvia replied that she did, but when Brenda started for the door, Sylvia asked, "Where are you going?"

Brenda had two brothers and an older sister, but they lived in other cities, and the closest was more than 200 miles away. Brenda knew that she would be the one primarily responsible for her mother. She wondered whether her mother might have Alzheimer's disease, so she sought the opinion of Sylvia's physician. The doctor was unable to confirm a diagnosis and pointed out that no absolute diagnosis of Alzheimer's disease is possible while the patient is still living. Only by eliminating other possible causes of Sylvia's dementia, the doctor told Brenda, could he determine that Sylvia was likely to have Alzheimer's disease.

This chapter looks at the consequences of living with chronic illnesses, such as Alzheimer's disease, diabetes, asthma, and AIDS, but other chronic illnesses share many elements with these. The physiology of the diseases varies, but the emotional and physical adjustments, the disruption of family dynamics, the need for continued medical care, and the necessity for self-management also apply to such chronic diseases as arthritis, kidney disease, multiple sclerosis, head injury, and spinal cord injury.

The Impact of Chronic Disease

As Chapter 1 explained, the patterns of death and disease in the United States have changed during the past 100 years. Acute diseases such as pneumonia and influenza were once among the leading causes of death, but today such chronic illnesses as heart disease and cancer have replaced them on that list. Acute diseases do not last long; people either recover relatively quickly or die rapidly. Long-lasting, chronic diseases are now far more common in the United States than short-term, acute ones. Most of these chronic conditions are not severe or life threatening, but if fatal, they cause death only after a lengthy period of illness. The number of people affected presents a major problem for the medical profession and for health psychology because such conditions affect not only the person with the disease but friends and family members as well.

Serious illness poses a crisis in people's lives. For serious acute illness, the disease may be a crisis, but the danger passes quickly, requiring little adaptation. Chronic illness, on the other hand, presents a range of situations that require adaptation, including financial hardship, change in the way patients see themselves, and altered relationships with family members and friends.

Crisis theory (Moos & Schaefer, 1984) is one way to attempt to explain the impact of disruptions on established patterns of personal and social functioning. Crisis theory holds that individuals need to operate in a state of equilibrium and when this state is disrupted for any reason, including illness, people rely on previously successful ways of responding in an effort to restore balance. Crises occur when events are so unusual or major that habitual patterns of coping are inadequate, then people experience heightened feelings of anxiety, fear, and stress. Because people cannot tolerate a crisis state for very long, they adopt new ways of responding and attempt to "normalize" their lives (Knafl & Deatrick, 2002). Some of these new patterns of coping may lead to healthy adaptation, but others result in unhealthy adjustment and psychological deterioration. The crisis itself is neither healthy nor pathological. Rather, it is a turning point in a person's life, resulting in either a healthy adjustment to the precipitating event or a psychologically unhealthy adaptation. Crisis theory suggests that chronic illness would not inevitably bring about psychological distress.

Other models of responses to chronic illness have emphasized the context of chronic illness and the adjustment that sick people need to make (Livneh, 2001; Stanton, Collins, & Sworowski, 2001). These models focus on the person who is ill and the impact of chronic illness on the patient.

Impact on the Patient

All patients must cope with their illness, which includes dealing with the symptoms of the disease, the stresses of treatment, and living as normal a life as possible. This adjustment is not easy. When patients are forced to interact with the health care system, they tend to feel deprived not only of their sense of competence and mastery but also of their rights and privileges. That is, sick people begin to be treated as "nonpersons" and to experience loss of personal control and threats to self-esteem (Stanton et al., 2001). Being ill leads to feelings of vulnerability and loss of control over the future as well as changes in how others think of patients and how patients think of themselves. The longtime course of chronic diseases demands that chronically ill patients manage problems beyond those faced by patients with an acute disease.

Several studies have explored the impact of chronic illness on the lives of patients. Research that evaluated the functioning of a large group of patients with a variety of chronic illnesses (Stewart et al., 1989) found that patients with chronic illnesses showed worse social and physical functioning, poorer mental health, and greater pain than patients without chronic illnesses. Hypertension produced the lowest impact on functioning and gastrointestinal disorders and heart disease the highest. Patients with more than one chronic condition showed greater decrements in functioning than patients with only one chronic disease. Factors such as the time required for treatment of the condition, the symptoms, the amount of fatigue, and the degree to which the illness interfered with daily activities contribute to the intrusiveness of the illness, which is important in adjustment (Maes, Leventhal, & de Ridder, 1996). Thus, chronic diseases differ in their impact not only in severity but also in how much they disrupt patients' lives. Even serious diseases that have few symptoms and allow patients to function at near normal levels do not produce the adjustment problems caused by less serious but more intrusive diseases.

A major impact of chronic illness involves the changes that occur in how people think of themselves; that is, the diagnosis of a chronic disease changes self-perception. Diagnosis of a disease such as cancer or HIV changes people's lives, and they go through a process of understanding the meaning of their illness and integrating it into their lives and their perceptions of themselves.

Developing such an understanding is an important part of coping with chronic disease (Stanton et al., 2001). Chronic illness and treatment force many patients to reevaluate their lives, relationships, and body image. Contrary to what many healthy people believe, people with chronic diseases often find some positive aspect to their situation (Folkman & Moskowitz, 2000). Part of healthy adjustment is accepting the changes that disease brings, and in one study (Fife, 1994), the lives of all chronically ill patients changed after diagnosis, and all patients imagined that their lives would never be the same.

People with chronic diseases tend to adopt a number of coping strategies to deal with their illness, including attempts to focus on the positive aspect of the disease (Dunkel-Schetter, Feinstein, Taylor, & Falke, 1992). Besides focusing on the positive, the patients who experienced the least emotional distress tended to seek social support and to try to distance themselves emotionally from their illness. Those who experienced more emotional distress tended to cope by using strategies of cognitive or behavioral avoidance, such as wishing that the situation would go away or avoiding the situation by misusing drugs, alcohol, or food. People who used more problem-focused coping strategies were more successful than those who used avoidance-strategies (Stanton et al., 2001). In summary, people with chronic illnesses—like other stressed people—use a variety of coping strategies, but some strategies are more effective than others.

Like patients with acute diseases, those with chronic conditions must develop and maintain relationships with health care providers (Stanton et al., 2001), but the characteristics of these relationships differ. People with an acute illness usually believe in the power of modern medicine and are optimistic about cures. This attitude is shared by health care workers, creating a positive climate of trust and optimism. Conversely, people with a chronic illness may have a hopeless and even helpless attitude toward their condition, an attitude often reflected in their relationship with their physician. Health care providers too may feel less positive about those with chronic conditions (Turner & Kelly, 2000). These feelings can create a difficult climate for treatment, with patients questioning and resisting health care providers, and providers feeling frustrated and annoyed with patients who fail to follow treatment regimens and who do not get better.

Negative emotions are common among the chronically ill due to the uncertain course of chronic disease (Stanton et al., 2001), and physicians often feel less than adequately prepared to help patients deal with these emotional reactions (Turner & Kelly, 2000). Such deficits have led to two types of supplements: psychological interventions and support groups. For many chronic illnesses, health psychologists have created interventions that emphasize the management of emotions. Support groups have also addressed this need by providing emotional support to patients or family members who must confront an illness with little chance of a cure. These services supplement traditional health care and help chronically ill patients to maintain compliance with the prescribed regimen and sustain a working relationship with health care providers. A meta-analysis of studies dealing with the effectiveness of psychosocial interventions with cancer patients (Meyer & Mark, 1995) showed that a variety of behavioral, informational, and educational methods helped patients adjust emotionally and functionally to their symptoms and their treatment.

Sustaining personal relationships is another challenge for those who are ill (Stanton et al., 2001). When people become ill, their behavior often changes, and the relationships and the expectations of their friends and family members undergo significant shifts, even though social support is an important factor in maintaining health (Berkman & Syme, 1979; Wiley & Camacho, 1980). These changes are partly due to their role as sick people. However, people who are chronically ill do not fit the sick role as well as those who are acutely ill. Therefore, chronic illness can have a great impact on the families of the chronically ill.

Impact on the Family

Illness is a crisis not only for people who are ill but also for their families. As Sylvia's illness progressed, she became unable to live alone. She sometimes wandered about her neighborhood in the middle of the night, forgot to eat, set fires in her house to burn old letters, and behaved in other dangerous ways that made living alone an impossibility. Brenda realized that her mother needed constant care and vigilance, so she and her husband Bob decided to move Sylvia into their home. Sylvia resented this notion, claiming that nothing was wrong with her and that Brenda was trying to steal her money. With much rancor and bitterness all around, the move was made. Although Sylvia had previously spent a great deal of time in her daughter's house, this move confused and disoriented her. She couldn't find her personal belongings and had trouble understanding how to move from one room to another. She became increasingly angry with Brenda, her primary caregiver, and complained to Bob that "that woman (meaning Brenda) is mean to me." Paradoxically, Sylvia directed her fury almost exclusively at Brenda, the one person who spent so much time and effort caring for her. Brenda was unable to continue her law practice and yet care for her mother, so she gave up her practice to be with Sylvia 24 hours a day. Bob tried to relieve his wife whenever possible, but he too was a lawyer, and his income was important, so he worked longer hours to help make up for Brenda's loss of income. During the 3 years that Sylvia lived with Brenda and Bob, Brenda felt stressed and confined. Often she wondered who was the real victim of her mother's disease.

In adults like Sylvia, chronic illness may cause a redefinition of identity (Fife, 1994) and a change in relationships with others. Chronic illness in children also changes the lives not only of the patients but also of the entire family, as parents and siblings try to "normalize" family life while coping with therapy for the sick child (Knafl & Deatrick, 2002).

The relationship between married partners often undergoes changes when one of them develops a chronic illness. An analysis of coping responses in married couples with one partner undergoing kidney dialysis for renal failure (Palmer, Canzona, & Wai, 1984) showed that couples with flexible roles adapted better than those couples with fixed, inflexible roles. The treatment was not the major source of problems; rather, difficulties arose from a discrepancy between the patients' view of their problems and the partners' view of the patients' problems. These differing views contributed to feelings of being misunderstood and abandoned. Many couples became closer but not more satisfied with their relationship, because the closeness was a result of dependency and came at the price of sacrificing one partner for the other's needs.

An analysis of partner support (Bolger et al., 2000) indicated that "invisible" support was more effective in relieving stress than support that was obvious. This type of interaction may be easier to manage when a partner is not ill; a sick partner needs help, but being the obvious recipient of assistance makes that support stressful as well as helpful. Therefore, chronic illness presents difficulties even to well-intentioned, caring partners.

Chronically ill parents can also experience changes that produce problems in their relationships with their young children; these changes are most pronounced for children with a terminally ill parent (Christ et al., 1993). As part of the sick role, a parent may lose the authority to discipline a child, or a sick parent may be protected from children's misbehavior because of the illness. Children may avoid consulting a sick parent so as not to further burden the parent, leading to decreased closeness. Children may be even less comfortable than adults with sick people and may change their behavior toward their sick parent as a result. Children may fear or experience changes in family life, and their role in the family may change as a result of a parent's illness. Young children may even feel guilt for their parent's illness because they do not understand that their misbe-

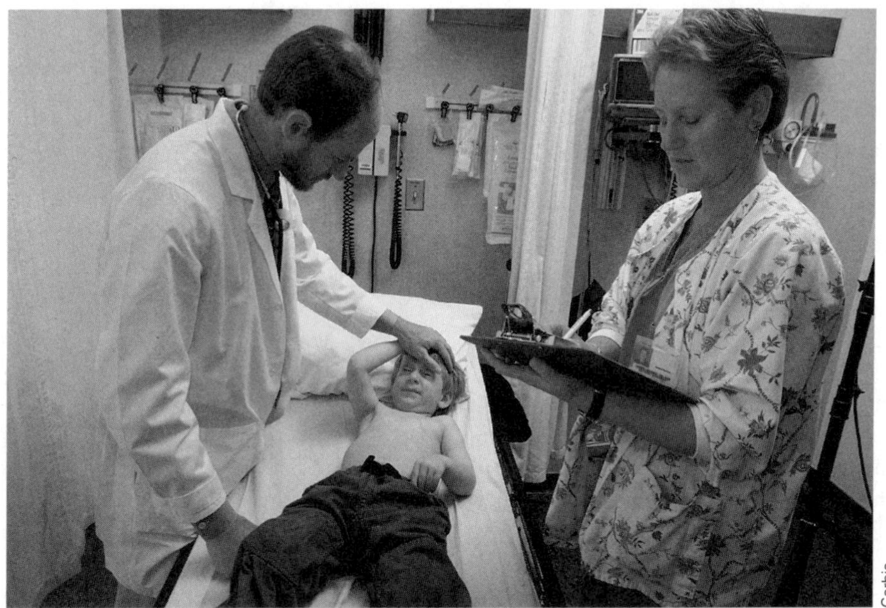

A chronically ill child can create financial and emotional problems within the family.

havior played no role in the development of the illness, and they may fear that their other parent will also get sick.

For adults, the changes that come with illness can alter their relationships and redefine their identity, but for children who are sick, illness can be an important factor in their identity formation. Although the rates of childhood diseases declined dramatically in the 20th century, a significant number of children still experience chronic diseases (Brace, Smith, McCauley, & Sherry, 2000). The majority of these illnesses are relatively minor, but many children experience severe chronic conditions such as cancer, asthma, rheumatoid arthritis, and diabetes, conditions that limit mobility and activity. For some children, these restrictions are very difficult, leading to isolation, depression, and distress, whereas other children cope more effectively (Melamed, Kaplan, & Fogel, 2001). Younger children have cognitive difficulties in conceptualizing the nature of their disease, and older children and adolescents may resent the restrictions that their disease imposes. Health care providers and parents can help these children make adjustments by offering alternative or modified activities.

Families of sick children face problems similar to couples: they must continue their relationships and manage the problems of caring for a sick child (Knafl & Deatrick, 2002). A child who is ill requires a great deal of emotional support, most of which is supplied by mothers. These efforts can leave mothers so drained that they have little emotional energy left for their husbands, which can leave husbands feeling abandoned, angry, and finally guilty over these feelings.

Added to these negative feelings are concerns over the financial demands of the illness and continuing concern for the sick child. Furthermore, a child's chronic illness can lead to sibling jealousy. Dependence in sick children can easily lead to overdependence, and they can learn to manipulate the family by becoming angry or depressed when they do not get their way. A child's illness, then, can disrupt family functioning at all levels, stressing each member's ability to cope.

Recommendations for families include trying to be flexible and establish a family routine that is as close to normal as they can manage (Knafl & Deatrick, 2002). One example of this would be to put the disease into the background and focus on the ways in which the sick child is similar to other children and other family members. Magnifying the ways that the disease makes the child different and focusing on the changes to family routine tend to lead to poorer adaptations. However, families should find ways to meet sick children's needs without reinforcing their anxiety and depression (Brace et al., 2000).

Families should find ways to express their negative emotions, such as anger and frustration over their situation. Families with sick children should also set aside time for themselves and not spend all their energy caring for the sick child. As a result of their own unmet emotional needs, many parents have joined support groups for families of children with chronic illnesses. These support groups can help families manage their emotions as well as receive information about their child's condition.

In Summary

Chronic illness affects not only the afflicted person but friends and family members as well. Unlike infectious diseases that last for a relatively short time, chronic illnesses such as heart disease, cancer, diabetes, asthma, AIDS, and Alzheimer's disease may persist for years.

Long-term chronic illnesses frequently bring about a crisis in people's lives, change the way patients see themselves, produce financial hardship, and disrupt family dynamics. Chronically ill patients have physiological, social, and emotional needs that are different from those of healthy people, and finding ways to satisfy these needs is part of the coping process. The social and emotional needs may be neglected by health care professionals who attend to the patient's physical needs. Health psychologists and support groups help provide for the emotional needs associated with chronic illness. Although some elements are common to all chronic diseases, special problems exist for people living with heart disease (see Chapter 9), cancer (see Chapter 10), diabetes, asthma, HIV, and Alzheimer's disease.

Adjusting to Diabetes

Dawn was diagnosed with **diabetes mellitus** when she was 4 years old. She has no clear memories of life without diabetes, and no facet of her life has been unaffected by the disease. She remembers being ostracized by other children during elementary school because they were afraid that playing with her would make them sick, too. She hid her condition during junior high and high school, but her attempts to fit in with her peers led her to neglect her diabetes regimen.

The Physiology of Diabetes

Before examining the psychological issues in the management of diabetes, let's look more closely at the physiology of the disorder. The **pancreas,** located below the stomach, produces different types of secretions. The **islet cells** of the pancreas produce several hormones, two of which, glucagon and insulin, are critically important in metabolism. **Glucagon** stimulates the release of glucose and, therefore, acts to elevate blood sugar levels. The action of **insulin** is the opposite. Insulin decreases the level of glucose in the blood by causing tissue cell membranes to open so glucose can enter the cells more freely. Disorders of the islet cells result in difficulties in sugar metabolism. Diabetes mellitus is a disorder caused by insulin deficiency. If the islet cells do not produce adequate insulin, sugar cannot be moved from the blood to the cells for use. Lack of insulin prevents the blood sugar level from being regulated by the body's control mechanisms. Excessive sugar accumulates in the blood and also appears in abnormally high levels in the urine. If unregulated or poorly regulated, diabetes may cause coma and death.

TABLE 11.1 *Characteristics of Type 1 and Type 2 Diabetes Mellitus*

Type 1	Type 2
Onset occurs before age 30	Onset may occur during childhood or adulthood
Patients are underweight	Patients are overweight
Patients experience frequent thirst and urination	Patients may or may not experience frequent thirst and urination
Affects equal numbers of men and women	Affects more women
Has no socioeconomic correlates	Affects more poor than middle-class people
Requires insulin injections	Requires no insulin injections
Carries risk of kidney damage	Carries risk of cardiovascular damage
Accounts for 10% of diabetics	Accounts for 90% of diabetics

The two types of diabetes mellitus are (1) insulin-dependent diabetes mellitus (IDDM), also known as Type 1 diabetes, and (2) noninsulin-dependent diabetes mellitus (NIDDM), also known as Type 2 diabetes. Type 1 diabetes is an autoimmune disease that occurs when the person's immune system attacks the insulin-making cells in the pancreas, destroying them (Roberts, 1998). This process usually occurs before age 30 and leaves the person without the capability to produce insulin and thus dependent on insulin injections.

Until a few years ago, Type 2 diabetes was called adult-onset diabetes because it typically developed in people past the age of 30. However, Type 2 diabetes has begun to appear among children and adolescents, accounting for at least 33% of diabetes cases among this age group (Ludwig & Ebbeling, 2001). This trend appears not only in the United States but also in developed countries throughout the world (Amschler, 2002). For both children and adults, Type 2 diabetes affects ethnic minorities disproportionately, and those who develop this disease are often overweight, sedentary, and poor. The characteristics of both types of diabetes are shown in Table 11.1.

Both types of diabetes require lifestyle changes in order for the person to adjust to the disease and to minimize health complications. Diabetes requires daily monitoring of blood sugar levels and relatively strict compliance to both medical and lifestyle regimens to regulate blood sugar.

In addition to the danger of coma, the inability to regulate blood sugar often causes diabetics to have other health problems. The administration of insulin can control the most severe symptoms of insulin deficiency but it does not cure the disorder. Nor do insulin injections mimic the normal production of insulin. Elevated levels of blood sugar seem to be involved in the development of (1) damage to the blood vessels, leaving diabetics prone to cardiovascular disease (diabetics are twice as likely as other people to have hypertension and to develop heart disease); (2) damage to the retina, leaving diabetics at risk for blindness (diabetics are 17 times as likely to go blind as nondiabetics); and (3) kidney diseases, leaving diabetics prone to renal failure. In addition, diabetics, compared with nondiabetics, have more than double the risk of cancer of the pancreas (Everhart & Wright, 1995). Dawn experienced damage to her retinas at age 17, and the laser surgery left her vision permanently impaired. She is not blind, as her doctors feared she would be, but she has no night vision, and she can focus only if given time. These visual impairments prevent her from qualifying for a driver's license, which makes her life different from most other young adults.

The Impact of Diabetes

The diagnosis of any chronic disease produces an impact on patients for two reasons: first, the emotional reaction to having a lifelong incurable disease, and second, the adjustments to lifestyle required by the disease. For diabetes that begins during childhood, both children and their parents must come to terms with the child's loss of health (Kovacs et al., 1990) and the management of the

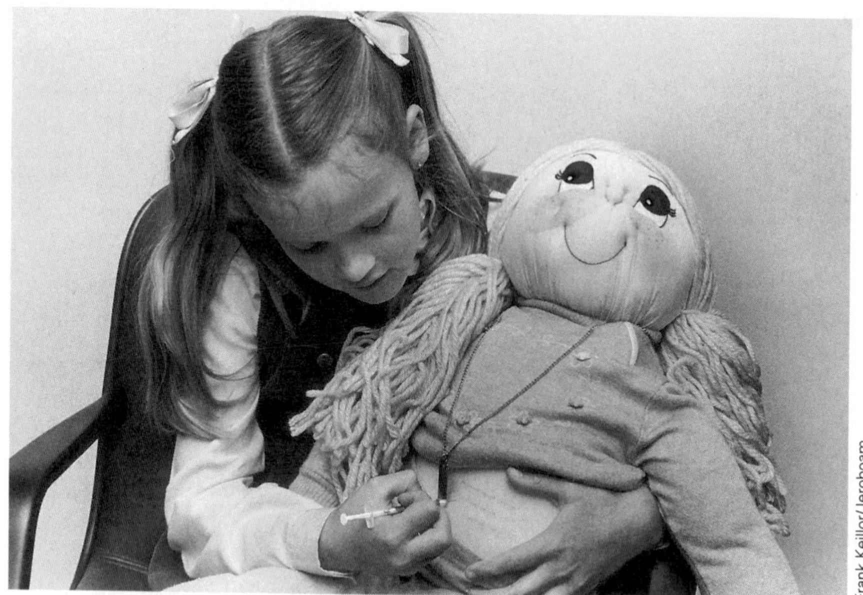

Learning to inject insulin is one of the skills that children with Type I diabetes must master.

disorder, which includes careful restrictions in diet, insulin injections, and recommendations for regular exercise. Dietary restrictions include careful scheduling of meals and snacks as well as adherence to a set of allowed and disallowed foods. Diabetics must test their blood sugar levels at least once (and possibly several times) per day, drawing a blood sample and using the testing equipment correctly. The results guide diabetics to appropriate levels of insulin injections. These injections are also a daily requirement and can be a source of fear and stress. Regular medical visits, which may frighten the children and create scheduling difficulties for the parents, are also part of the regimen.

Dawn did a poor job of taking care of herself when she was a teenager. She learned to give herself insulin injections when she was 6 years old, and her compliance with this aspect of her care has always been good. Eating was a problem. She never developed a taste for sweets, so avoiding them was not difficult, but she was always a finicky eater and did not like to eat three meals a day. She found skipping meals easy and saw it as a good strategy for losing weight. However, one diet put her in the hospital because of a very low blood sugar level.

Noninsulin-dependent (Type 2) diabetes often does not require insulin injections, but this type of diabetes does require lifestyle changes and oral medication. African Americans, Hispanic Americans, and Native Americans are at higher risk for Type 2 diabetes than are European Americans (NCHS, 2001), and being overweight is a risk for all groups. Indeed, gaining weight increases and losing weight decreases the risk for Type 2 diabetes (Colditz, 1995). Therefore, a frequent component of treatment is weight loss.

Type 2 diabetics must deal with dietary restrictions and attend to their schedule of oral medication. Diabetes often affects sexual functioning in both men and women, and diabetic women who become pregnant often have problem pregnancies. Type 2 diabetes is more likely to cause circulatory problems, leaving adult-onset diabetics prone to cardiovascular problems, which is their leading cause of death. Both women (Hu et al., 2001) and men (Lotufo et al., 2001) with Type 2 diabetes are at dramatically increased risk for death from all causes, but especially from cardiovascular disease.

Some diabetics deny the seriousness of their condition and ignore the need to restrict diet and take medication. Others acknowledge the seriousness of their problems but believe that the recommended regimen will be ineffective (Skinner, Hampson, & Fife-Schaw, 2002). Others become aggressive, and they either direct their aggression outward and refuse to comply with their treatment regimen or they turn their aggression inward and become depressed. Finally, many diabetics become dependent and rely on others to take care of them, thus taking no active part in their own care. All these reactions can interfere with the management of blood sugar levels and lead to serious health complications, including death.

Dawn was able to deny the seriousness of her condition until she experienced kidney failure at age 22. She was put on kidney dialysis and eventually received a kidney transplant. In the hospital, she became aware of the dangers of her disease in a way that she had never been before. Not only did she understand that she might die, but the possibility of nerve damage and amputation of a limb made her more vigilant about self-care. Now, she monitors her blood sugar at least three times a day, eats regularly, and gives herself appropriate insulin injections.

Health Psychology's Involvement with Diabetes

Health psychologists are involved in both researching and treating diabetes (Gonder-Frederick, Cox, & Ritterband, 2002). Research efforts have concentrated on the ways that diabetics understand and conceptualize their illness, the effect of stress on glucose metabolism, the dynamics of families with diabetic children, and the factors that influence patient compliance with medical regimens. Health psychologists orient their efforts toward improving adherence to medical regimens so diabetics can control their blood glucose levels and minimize health complications.

Stress has been hypothesized to play two roles in diabetes: as a possible cause of diabetes and as a factor in the regulation of blood sugar in diabetics (Wertlieb, Jacobson, & Hauser, 1990). The role of stress as a factor in blood glucose levels is clearer than any causal role stress may play in precipitating diabetes. For example, an active stressor such as solving math problems produced more effect on the blood glucose level of diabetics than did a passive stressor such as viewing a gory movie. Not all the diabetics showed blood glucose changes in response to stress, but more than half of them did. A longitudinal study (Goldston, Kovacs, Obrosky, & Iyengar, 1995) examined the role of stress in metabolic control for school-age children with Type 1 diabetes and found that the extent to which stressful negative events disrupted the children's life was a strong predictor of metabolic control. Dawn sees stressful negative events as major problems in her management of her condition. She has trouble staying on her regimen when she is having trouble with her boyfriend.

A study of people with Type 2 diabetes (Surwit et al., 2002) showed that adding a stress management component to diabetes education has a small but significant effect on blood sugar levels. Therefore, the impact of stress can be negative, but interventions to manage stress can be a worthwhile (and cost-effective) component for diabetes education programs.

Another line of research concerns diabetic patients' understanding of their illness and how their understanding affects their behavior. Both patients and health care workers assume that patients understand the disease and recognize the symptoms of high and low blood glucose levels. These assumptions are not always true. One study (Gonder-Frederick, Cox, Bobbitt, & Pennebaker, 1986) showed that 58% of the diabetics had inaccurate beliefs about high blood glucose levels and 42% had inaccurate beliefs about low levels. The beliefs erred in both directions: people with diabetes saw problems where none existed and overlooked others. The women in the study were more vigilant in both correctly and incorrectly perceiving symptoms, whereas the men were more likely to miss symptoms. These results suggest that education for diabetics does not succeed in teaching symptom perception and that diabetics have inaccurate beliefs about their condition.

Inaccurate beliefs can have a significant impact on self-care. In a study of the interrelationships among beliefs, personality characteristics, and self-care behavior among diabetics (Skinner et al., 2002), beliefs emerged as the most important component. The perceived effectiveness of the treatment regimen predicted all aspects of diabetes self-care. This finding emphasizes the importance of diabetes education in building adherence to the diet, exercise, and medication regimen that is necessary to control blood glucose levels.

Complete adherence to the medication and lifestyle regimen is rare (Cherner, 2001). As Chapter 4 explored, complexity makes adherence more difficult, and making lifestyle changes is more difficult than taking medication. Diabetics must do both and perform blood sugar testing several times a day. Poor adherence to the treatment regimen is of primary concern to psychologists involved in providing care for diabetics (Harris & Lustman, 1998; Johnson, Freund, Silverstein, Hansen, & Malone, 1990).

The role of health psychology in diabetes management is likely to expand, because behavioral components can add to the effectiveness of educational programs for diabetic patients. Education alone is not adequate in helping diabetics follow their regimen (Cherner, 2001). Because situational factors such as stress and social pressure to eat the wrong foods affect adherence, programs with a behavioral skills training component might be a valuable addition to diabetes management training. Problem-solving skills (Toobert & Glasgow, 1991) and feelings of control (Macrodimitris & Endler, 2001) improved diabetics' adherence to diet, exercise, and blood glucose testing.

Although behavior-based strategies can improve patients' control, Russell Glasgow and Richard Anderson (1999) argued that the approach to diabetes management needs to change from one that emphasizes patient compliance to an orientation that stresses responsibility and self-management. They urged health care professionals to make changes in their approach to dealing with patients, acknowledging that chronic illnesses are different from acute ones. People who are diabetic are totally responsible for their own care, and health care professionals should help them to do a good job.

In Summary

Diabetes mellitus is a chronic disease that results from failure of the islet cells of the pancreas to manufacture sufficient insulin, affecting blood glucose levels and producing effects in many organ systems. Type 1 diabetes is an autoimmune disease that typically appears during childhood; Type 2 diabetes also affects children but is more typical of people over age 30. Diabetics must maintain a strict regimen of diet, exercise, and insulin supplements to avoid the serious cardiovascular, neurological, and renal complications of the disorder.

As with other chronic diseases, a diagnosis of diabetes mellitus produces distress for both patients and their families. Health psychologists have studied the factors involved in adjusting to the disorder and those that affect compliance with the necessary lifestyle changes. Few people with diabetes adhere to all aspects of blood glucose testing, medication, diet, and exercise that minimize the risks of health complications. Skills and problem-solving training programs have shown some success in helping diabetics manage their disorder, but health care professionals need to find ways to encourage the development of responsibility and self-management in order to put diabetics in charge of their own health.

The Impact of Asthma

Sean Miller and his friends in Climb 4 Air reached the summit of Mt. Kilimanjaro coughing, wheezing, and having difficulty breathing (Asthma and Allergy Foundation of America, 2002). Their experience was not unusual for climbers or for the group they climbed to benefit: people with asthma. Since 1995, this group has climbed mountains around the world to benefit the Asthma and Allergy Foundation of America and to develop an understanding of the experience of difficulty in breathing. This experience is part of the lives of the millions of people with asthma.

The number of people with asthma grew throughout the 1980s and into the 1990s in the United States but began to decrease by the late 1990s (American Lung Association, 2002). About 10% of adults in the United States have asthma, but the rate is the highest for children and adolescents between 5 and 17 years old. The rates are higher for African Americans than for other ethnic groups. The death rate from asthma is not high, but it is the largest cause of disability among children and the leading cause of missed school days, making it a serious health problem in the United States.

The Disease of Asthma

Asthma is a chronic disease that causes constriction of the bronchial tubes, preventing air from passing freely. People experiencing an asthma attack will wheeze, cough, and have trouble breathing. They may die during such an attack, but at other times they are fine (Goff, 2000).

Asthma shares some features with chronic obstructive pulmonary disease (COPD) such as chronic bronchitis and emphysema, but asthma also differs in some ways (Jeffery, 2000). All of these conditions involve inflammation, but the extent of inflammation differs. The immune system activity also varies for these two types of conditions, but the most important difference is that people with COPD experience constant problems, whereas people with asthma may go for long periods of time without any problems in breathing.

The cause of asthma is not understood. Until recently, experts believed that asthma was an allergic reaction to substances in the environment, but several newer explanations involve more complex reactions of the immune system. One view holds that a genetic vulnerability makes some infants' immune systems respond with an allergic reaction to substances in the environment that other infants' immune systems encounter without problems. This *diathesis-stress model* is a variation on the traditional view that asthma is an allergic reaction triggered by environmental allergens. These allergens include an assortment of common substances such as tobacco smoke, household dust (along with dust mites), cockroaches, animal dander, and environmental pollutants. People with the vulnerability who are exposed to the substance to which they are sensitive develop asthma; those who are not exposed fail to develop asthma or show such mild symptoms that they are not diagnosed.

Another view is called the *hygiene hypothesis* and holds that asthma is a result of the *cleanliness* that has become common in modern societies (Shell, 2000). Infants have undeveloped immune systems and, in hygienic environments, they encounter too little bacteria and dirt, which leaves their immune systems underprepared to deal with these substances. Exposure leads to overresponsiveness, which produces an inflammation; this inflammation forms the basis for asthma.

Both of these views are consistent with some of the evidence about asthma. Support for the genetic vulnerability view is found in a study of the Hutterites, a religious group that immigrated to the United States from Europe in the 1870s (Shell, 2000). Symptoms of asthma are very uncommon among the Hutterites who nevertheless show high rates of the inflammation that characterizes asthma. The rural, farming lifestyle of these people puts them into contact with few of the triggers for asthma attacks, leaving these vulnerable individuals without serious symptoms. As the hygiene hypothesis suggests, this disease is more common in developed countries that emphasize cleanliness and a hygienic environment for infants. For example, asthma is less common in rural China than in the United States, Sweden, Australia, and New Zealand (Goff, 2000). However, in the United States asthma is more common in the urban inner city, and African Americans are more vulnerable than other ethnic groups.

Other risk factors for asthma include sedentary lifestyle and obesity (Goff, 2000). People take few deep breaths when they are sedentary, which may be the link between lack of exercise and asthma. In addition, staying inside puts people in situations with exposure to some of the allergens that provoke asthma attacks. The link between asthma and obesity is significant: obese people are 2 to 3 times more likely to have asthma than nonobese people (Goff, 2000). Although the factors related to the development of asthma are complex and not completely known, the triggers for attacks are better understood.

Triggers are substances or circumstances that cause the development of symptoms, provoking the narrowing of the airways that cause difficulty in breathing. The substances include allergens such as mold, pollen, dust and dust mites, cockroaches, and animal dander; infections of the respiratory tract; tobacco or wood smoke; irritants such as air pollutants, chemical sprays, or environmental pollution (Hwang, 1999). The circumstances include exercise and emotional reactions such as stress or fear. All of these substances and experiences may provoke an attack, but most people with asthma are sensitive to only a few. Identifying an individual's triggers is part of managing asthma.

Managing Asthma

Managing asthma shows some similarities (and similar problems) to managing diabetes. Both disorders require frequent contact with the health care system, can be life threatening, affect children and adolescents, impose restrictions on lifestyle, and pose substantial adherence problems (Bryant, 2001). People with diabetes may manage their blood sugar levels so that they have no symptoms, but even with careful management, people with asthma have attacks. The underlying inflammation of the bronchial tract is always present, but a person with asthma may go for weeks or months without an attack. Daily attention to symptoms and status improves the chances of avoiding attacks, and behaviors are critical.

Managing asthma requires a variety of medications as well as learning personal triggers and avoiding them (Goff, 2000). To decrease the chances of an attack, people with asthma must take medication, which is usually an anti-inflammatory corticosteroid. This type of drug decreases the respiratory inflammation that underlies asthma. These drugs require daily attention and have unpleasant side effects, such as weight gain and lack of energy. The schedule may be very complicated, and as Chapter 4 detailed, complexity decreases compliance with medical regimens. The side effects also contribute to problems in adherence. Thus, adherence to their preventive medication is a major problem for people with asthma, especially for children and adolescents (Shell, 2000).

When people with asthma have an attack, they have trouble breathing or cannot breathe. Gasping for breath, they either use a bronchodilater to inhale medication that relieves the symptoms or they go to a hospital emergency room for treatment (Shell, 2000). If used improperly, bronchodilaters produce a type of "high," and asthma experts believe that most people with asthma rely on bronchodilaters too much and on preventive medication too little.

Asthma attacks can cause respiratory failure, which may be fatal. Such an attack is a frightening experience and affects asthma patients' attitudes and behaviors (Greaves, Eiser, Seamark, & Halpin, 2002). Attacks tend to produce fear, and having frequent attacks increases fear and diminishes people's beliefs that they can control their asthma. Those who experienced a recent attack but low levels of fear showed a greater chance of needing emergency care. This finding suggests that low fear may be related to denying the seriousness of the disease and to poor attention to self-care, whereas high fear may lead to appropriate care. In addition, caregivers' attitudes about asthma affect children's hospitalization (Chen, Bloomberg, Fisher, & Strunk, 2003); those caregivers who were less bothered had children who were more frequently hospitalized. Therefore, the attitudes of both people with asthma and their caregivers affect behaviors that relate to attacks.

Boosting self-care and adherence to medication regimens are major goals for improving asthma care. One group of researchers (Guendelman, Meade, Benson, Chen, & Samuels, 2002) developed a novel approach to asthma education: an interactive computer with a Web link to a health care provider. They tested this system on a group of inner-city children and adolescents with asthma and found that these young participants used the system and improved their self-care. They experienced one of the major goals of care: their asthma interfered less with their daily activities. Therefore, behavioral interventions can help in developing strategies to help people with asthma take their medication and avoid situations that precipitate attacks.

In Summary

Asthma is a chronic disease that involves inflammation of the bronchial tubes, which leads to difficulties in breathing. Substances such as smoke or allergens and situations such as fear can trigger attacks that have symptoms of coughing, wheezing, and choking. The cause for the inflammation that underlies asthma remains unknown, but theories include a genetic component and an overreaction of the immune system that occurs in hygienic environments.

Asthma usually develops during childhood, and children and adolescents experience problems in coping with their disease. People with asthma need to take medication to decrease the chances of attacks and identify their triggers so as to avoid them. The complex schedule of medication and their unpleasant side effects contribute to adherence problems, and a major goal of treatment is to help people with asthma take the medication to prevent attacks rather than rely on inhaled medications to stop symptoms or use hospital emergency room assistance.

Dealing with HIV and AIDS

Glenn Burke had always wanted to play baseball, and he had enough skill to become a major league player. From 1976 to 1979, he was a gifted outfielder for the Los Angles Dodgers and Oakland Athletics and played for the Dodgers in the 1977 World Series. Burke's promising career was never fulfilled—not because he lacked ability but because players, managers, and general managers suspected that he was gay, and they made his life as a ballplayer miserable. Burke *was* gay, but he did not acknowledge his sexual orientation openly until 2 years after he left baseball. He was also an African American, and the combination of being gay and being African American probably cut short his baseball career. Prejudice in organized baseball in the late 1970s was so strong that the Dodgers offered to pay Burke for an expensive honeymoon—if only he would get married. After he was traded to the Oakland Athletics, Billy Martin, the controversial manager of the Athletics (as well as several other teams), told Burke, "I don't want no faggot on my team," and the team promptly refused to sign Burke to an extended contract.

After his baseball career came to a premature end, Burke continued to have difficulties. He spent some time in San Quentin prison and more time as a homeless person on the streets of San

Francisco. Eventually he contracted AIDS, but he fought hard against the disease and survived many months longer than doctors had predicted. After developing AIDS-related illnesses and losing nearly 100 pounds from his once-powerful athletic frame, he died in 1995 at the age of 42.

AIDS is a disorder in which the immune system loses its effectiveness, leaving the body defenseless against bacterial, viral, fungal, parasitic, cancerous, and other opportunistic diseases. Without the immune system, the body cannot protect itself against the many organisms that can invade it and cause damage. (For a more complete discussion of the immune system and its function, see Chapter 6.) The danger from AIDS comes from the opportunistic infections that start when the immune system no longer functions effectively. In this way, AIDS is similar to the immune deficiency in children who have been born without immune system organs and are susceptible to a variety of infections.

AIDS is the result of exposure to a contagious virus, the **human immunodeficiency virus (HIV).** Presently, two variants of the human immunodeficiency virus have been discovered; HIV-1, which causes most AIDS cases in the United States, and HIV-2, which is responsible for most AIDS cases in Africa, although some HIV-2 cases have appeared in the United States. The progression from HIV infection to AIDS varies, and a few HIV-infected people have remained free of AIDS symptoms for many years.

Incidence and Mortality Rates for HIV/AIDS

AIDS appears to be a relatively new disease, first recognized in 1981 and identified in 1983. Some scientists (Corbitt, Bailey, & Williams, 1990; Froland et al., 1988) believe that the disease dates at least to the 1950s, and isolated cases of AIDS in humans may be thousands of years old. The current HIV epidemic originated in African chimpanzees (Gao et al., 1999) and probably occurred because the chimpanzees were hunted for food. Although the virus is not deadly in these chimpanzees, it is for humans. During the 1980s, both the number of new cases and the number of deaths from AIDS increased rapidly until HIV infection became one of the 10 leading causes of death in the United States.

In the mid-1990s, death rates from AIDS declined sharply in the United States, but some other countries continue to experience an increasing rate of HIV infection and AIDS deaths (*Population Reports,* 2001). According to one estimate (Lamptey, 2002), AIDS is the deadliest plague in history. About 40 million people were infected by 2001; when those people die, HIV will surpass the number of people killed by the bubonic plague in the 14th century.

In 1992, the Centers for Disease Control and Prevention (CDC, 1992) revised its definition of HIV infection so that incidence figures from 1992 and subsequent years are not directly comparable to earlier figures. The number of cases in 1992 appears to rise sharply (see Figure 11.1), but this count includes the large backlog of people who, in previous years, would not have been classified as having AIDS. As Figure 11.1 shows, AIDS cases reported each year (incidence) began a steady decline after 1992.

Not only has incidence declined, but also mortality from this disease has dropped even more. From 1996 to 1998, the mortality rates for AIDS in the Unites States dropped by 47%, a decrease far greater than that of any other leading cause of death. Subsequent drops were not as dramatic, but both incidence and death rates continue to decline (CDC, 2001b). One reason the number of deaths from AIDS has declined is that HIV-infected individuals are living longer. People diagnosed with AIDS in 1984 had an average survival time of 11 months, whereas people diagnosed in 1995 lived an average of 46 additional months (Lee, Karon, Selik, Neal, & Fleming, 2001). This increased survival time is a result of more effective drug therapies, early detection, and lifestyle changes. Figure 11.1 shows the number of people living with AIDS (prevalence) continues to increase. Combinations of antiretroviral drugs have changed the course of HIV infection,

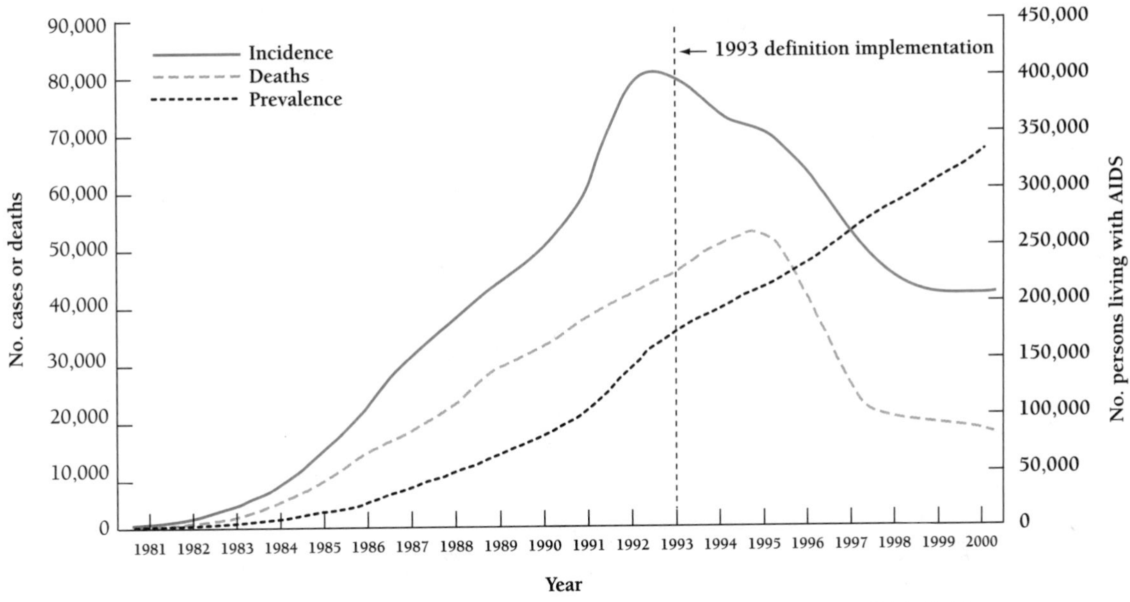

Figure 11.1 Incidence, prevalence, and deaths from AIDS cases by year, United States, 1981–2000.

Source: "Update, AIDS—United States, 2000," by R. M. Klevens & J. J. Neal, 2002, Morbidity and Mortality Weekly Report vol. 51, *no. 27, p. 593.*

slowing the progression of infection and prolonging lives (Schwarcz, Hsu, Vittinghoff, & Katz, 2000). In addition, giving up unhealthy habits such as smoking, drinking alcohol, and taking illicit drugs; becoming more vigilant about their health; and exercising more control over their treatment can help infected persons live longer and healthier lives (Folkman, 1993).

The HIV and AIDS Epidemics

In the United States and Europe, HIV infection was first associated with gay men, but an analysis of people infected with HIV reveals at least four distinct epidemics of the infection. These four epidemics exist around the world, but the proportion of people infected by each differs a great deal. For example, men who have sex with men accounted for many of the first U.S. cases of AIDS, but in Africa and Asia, heterosexual sex is the most common method of transmission. Male-male sexual contact is still the leading source of HIV infection in the United States, but this mode of transmission declined during the 1990s, and less than half of HIV transmissions are presently due to male-male sexual contact (CDC, 2001b).

A second epidemic affects injection drug users, with the percent of these cases remaining the same. A third epidemic includes transmission through heterosexual contact, and this number is increasing. A fourth epidemic occurs through transmission from women to their children during the birth process. This mode of transmission has decreased sharply with the advent of antiretroviral medication for pregnant women who are HIV positive.

Although incidence of HIV is declining for most modes of transmission, it is rising for male-female sexual contact, with women much more likely than men to be infected through this route. Of those cases for which transmission can be determined, heterosexual contact accounted for only about 2% to 3% of all HIV infections in 1985, but by 1999, male-female sexual contact accounted for 17% of all HIV infections (USBC, 2001).

In the United States and Europe, HIV infection affects men much more often than women

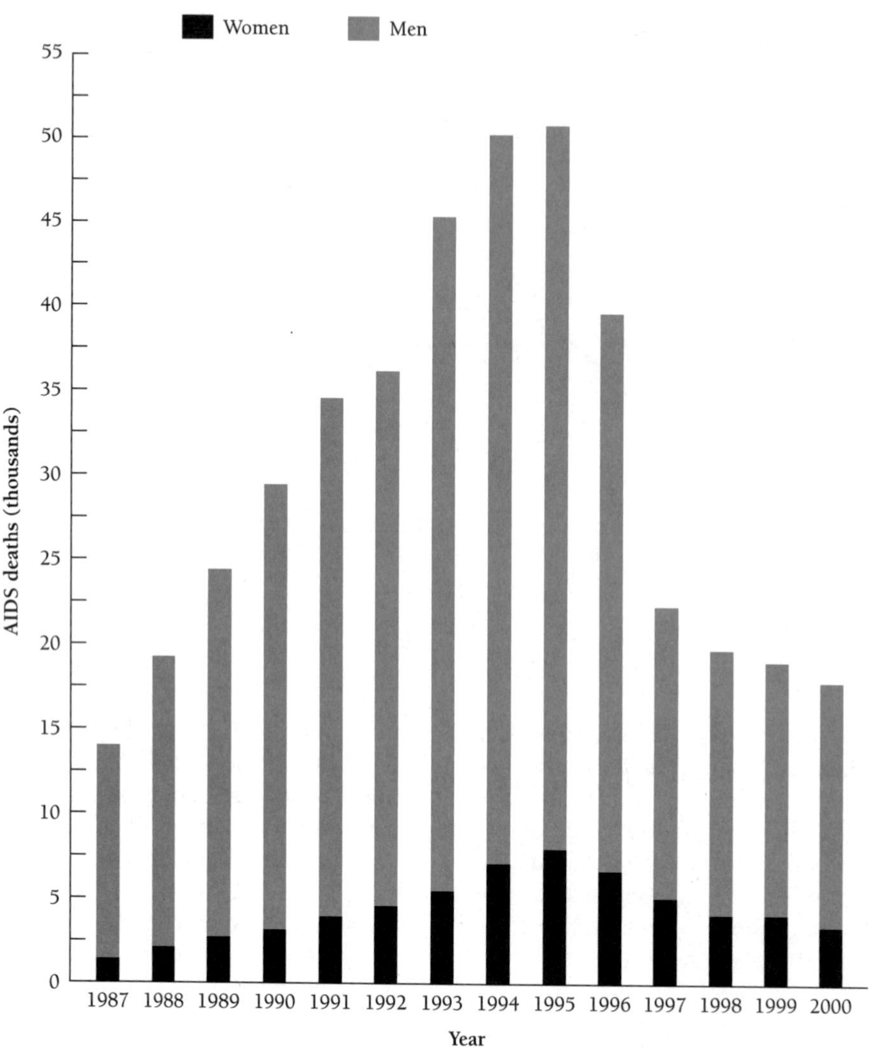

Figure 11.2 Deaths from AIDS by gender, United States, 1987–2000.

Sources: HIV/AIDS Surveillance Reports, 1989 (Table13), 1991 (Table 13), 1993 (Table 14), and 2001 (Mid-year report, Table 30). Centers for Disease Control and Prevention. Retrieved from the World Wide Web, July 31, 2002, www.cdc.gov/hiv/stats.htm

(see Figure 11.2). As of 1999, women accounted for slightly less than 20% of AIDS cases (USBC, 2001). Women are vulnerable to HIV infection primarily through two routes of transmission; heterosexual contact, which accounts for about half of all cases of AIDS in women, and injection drug use, which accounts for more than 40% of the cases. The third most frequent category is heterosexual contact with an injection drug user—a practice that makes classification difficult. However, women infected through this third mode have contracted the AIDS virus either through heterosexual contact or injection drug use, so these two methods of transmission currently are responsible for almost all AIDS cases among women (USBC, 2001). Worldwide, that situation

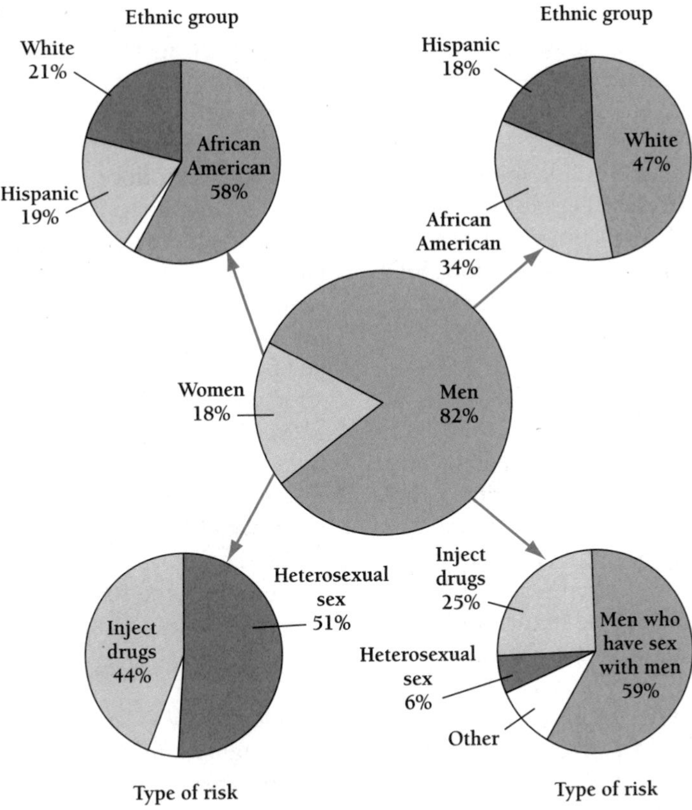

Figure 11.3 HIV infection for women and men, by ethnic group and type of risk.

Sources: Centers for Disease Control and Prevention, 2001, HIV Prevention Strategic Plan through 2005. *p. 12 and* HIV/AIDS Surveillance Report, vol. 13, *no 1, Tables 19 and 20.*

is different than in the United States: women account for 46% of the AIDS cases and half of the deaths, the majority of which are in sub-Saharan Africa (Matlin & Spence, 2001).

Minority ethnic groups in the United States have been affected disproportionately, especially by the epidemics affecting heterosexuals and injection drug users. In 1996, African Americans became the largest segment of the population with HIV, and by 1999, they accounted for 41% of HIV infections (CDC, 2001c). European Americans accounted for 38% of the cases, Hispanic Americans 20%, and Asian Americans less than 1%. The number of those infected through injection drug use has fallen, but heterosexual transmission has increased, especially among Hispanic and African American women. As of 1999, African American women made up 61% of women with HIV (Hader, Smith, Moore, & Holmberg, 2001). The trend toward declining rates of HIV infection has not occurred for minorities as rapidly as for European Americans. Figure 11.3 shows the percentages of men and women with different ethnic backgrounds infected with HIV.

Age is also a factor in HIV infection. The birth process is one mode of transmission, so some infants and children are HIV infected, but only about 1% of AIDS cases are younger than 13. Young adults are more likely to be infected than other age groups, largely due to their risky behaviors, lack of information about HIV, and lack of power to protect themselves (*Population Reports,* 2001). For these young adults, gender and ethnicity factors apply: most of the infected young adults are men, and ethnic minorities are disproportionately affected. People over age 50 are less likely to be infected than younger adults, but when infected, they tend to develop AIDS more rapidly and to get more opportunistic infections (CDC, 1998a).

Symptoms of HIV and AIDS

Typically, HIV progresses over a decade or more through four stages, but the length of time people spend at each stage varies. During the first stage of HIV infection, symptoms are not easily distinguishable from those of other diseases. Within a week or so of infection, people frequently experience fever, sore throat, skin rash, headache, and other mild symptoms (McCutchan, 1990). This relatively short first period of 1 to 8 weeks is typically followed by a latent period that may last as long as 10 years during which infected people are asymptomatic or experience only minimal symptoms. During the third stage, patients typically have a cluster of symptoms including swollen lymph nodes, fever, fatigue, night sweats, loss of appetite, loss of weight, persistent diarrhea, white spots in the mouth, and painful skin rash. During the final stage, the patients' CD4+ T-lymphocyte cell count drops to 200 or less per cubic millimeter of blood (healthy people have a CD4+ count of 1,000). As their immune system begins to lose its defensive capacities, patients become susceptible to various opportunistic infections involving the lungs, gastrointestinal tract, nervous system, liver, bones, and brain. Symptoms include greater weight loss, general fatigue, fever, shortness of breath, dry cough, purplish bumps on the skin, and AIDS-related dementia. At this point, HIV becomes AIDS, which is a fatal disease.

The supply of CD4+ T-lymphocytes is depleted, so the immune system no longer has a mechanism for fighting infections within cells. The diseases associated with AIDS are caused by a variety of agents, including viruses, bacteria, fungi, and parasites. The HIV virus damages or kills the part of the immune system that fights *viral* infections, leaving no way for the body to fight HIV. But HIV does not destroy the antibodies that the immune system has already manufactured, so the immune system response that occurs through antibodies circulating in the blood remains intact. Therefore, being HIV positive does not often cause a person, for example, to develop infections with the bacterium that causes strep throat or the virus that causes influenza. Most HIV-infected people have antibodies to fight against these common agents. Instead, HIV results in infection from otherwise rare organisms, which leads to such diseases as *Pneumocystis carinii* pneumonia, Kaposi's sarcoma, tuberculosis, and toxoplasmic encephalitis.

The Transmission of HIV

Although HIV is an infectious organism with a high fatality rate, the virus is not easily transmitted from person to person. The main routes of infection are from person to person during sex, from mother to child during pregnancy or birth, and from direct contact with blood or blood products (CDC, 2001b). Concentrations of HIV are especially high in the semen and blood of infected people. Therefore, contact with infected semen or blood is a risk. Other body fluids do not contain such a high concentration of HIV, making contact with saliva, urine, or tears much less of a risk. No evidence exists that any sort of casual contact spreads the infection. Eating with the same utensils or plates or drinking from the same cup as someone who is infected does not transmit HIV, nor does touching or even kissing someone who is infected. Insect bites do not spread the virus, and even being bitten by someone who is infected will not infect the person who is bitten.

People most at risk for HIV infection are those affected by causes of the four epidemics—male-male sexual contact, injection drug use, het-

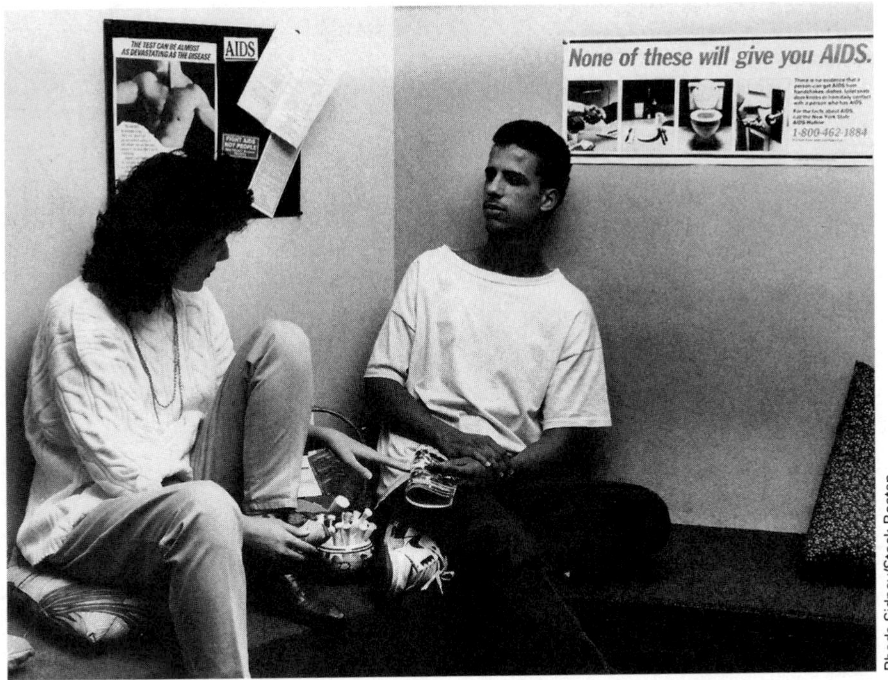

AIDS
None of these will give you AIDS.
1-800-462-1884
Rhoda Sidney/Stock Boston

Interventions to change risky behaviors are currently the most effective way to decrease the transmission of HIV.

erosexual contact, and transmission from mother to baby during birth. Each of the groups reflected by these four epidemics experiences somewhat different risks.

Male-Male Sexual Contact In the early years of AIDS, men who had sex with men made up the majority of AIDS cases. In recent years, HIV infection rates have decreased among gay and bisexual men, but this group still remains the largest risk group. Among gay and bisexual men, unprotected anal intercourse is an especially risky behavior, particularly for the receptive partner. Because the delicate lining of the rectum is often damaged during anal intercourse, the receptive person is at high risk if his partner is infected with HIV. The damaged rectum makes an excellent route for the virus to enter the body, and infected semen has a high concentration of HIV. Unprotected oral sex with an infected partner is also a risky practice because HIV can enter the body through any tiny cut or other lesion in the mouth.

Condom use has become common among older gay men, but many younger ones engage in unsafe sexual practices, especially after using alcohol or other drugs (LaBrie & Earleywine, 2000). Young men who have sex with other men are at increased risk if they also fail to use condoms, have 20 or more sex partners, or fail to take other precautions to avoid HIV infection (*AIDS Alert,* 2001). Unprotected sex has an attraction for some gay men, an attraction that can overcome knowledge of the risks posed by this behavior (Kelly & Kalichman, 1998). Risk-taking individuals may engage in a variety of dangerous behaviors, including unprotected sex. In addition, the use of intoxicants can cloud people's ability to make wise decisions about potentially dangerous sexual practices.

WOULD YOU BELIEVE

It's Not Safe to Stay in the Closet

Would you believe that gay men who conceal their sexual orientation experience greater health risks? These risks include a greater likelihood of engaging in risky sexual behaivors as well as a more rapid decline in health for those who are HIV positive.

Being "in the closet" or "out of the closet" is an important factor in the lives of gay men and lesbians. Concealment of sexual orientation allows gay men and lesbians to avoid the social censure that often accompanies being openly gay, and thus one might reason that being in the closet has advantages. It also requires misrepresentation and effort to maintain this facade, and in this sense, being in the closet may present problems. Research has confirmed the risks of being in the closet and the benefits of coming out.

A study of gay, lesbian, and bisexual young people (Rosario, Hunter, Maguen, Gwadz, & Smith, 2001) found that the coming out process involved changes in self-esteem and behavior. Those with negative attitudes about homosexuality were more likely to participate in unprotected sexual behavior. Those who were no longer "in the closet" had higher self-esteem and were less likely to engage in unprotected sexual activities. Therefore, coming out seems to lead to health advantages.

In a group of HIV-positive gay men, those who concealed their sexual orientation developed AIDS symptoms more rapidly and died earlier than those who were more open about their sexual orientation (Cole, Kemeny, Taylor, Visscher, & Fahey, 1996). Furthermore, the rapidity of progression was related to how strongly the men concealed their sexual orientation—the more "closeted," the faster HIV progressed. This progression was unrelated to demographic characteristics, health practices, or sexual behavior. Men who concealed their homosexuality most, compared with those who concealed least, experienced a 1.5- to 2-year faster progression of HIV. The magnitude of this difference was significant. Indeed, the difference was comparable to the effect of using versus not using some types of antiretroviral therapy!

In this study (Cole et al., 1996), few of the gay men were completely in the closet, but some were much more so than others. For example, some men were in the closet at work but not with their friends. These men needed to conceal a very relevant aspect of their lives for a large portion of the day. This type of inhibition might have some impact on health, thus affecting HIV progression (Cole et al., 1996).

Inhibiting significant factors about themselves might affect physiological mechanisms, including the immune system. This route is one possible explanation for the relationship between concealment and HIV progression. Others include reluctance to be identified as gay, which might also cause delays in seeking treatment for HIV infection. Such delays could, of course, affect the progression of the infection.

A complicating factor is sensitivity to social censure. Gay men who conceal their sexual orientation might do so to avoid the censure that often accompanies coming out of the closet. This rejection sensitivity is related to HIV progression (Cole, Kemeny, & Taylor, 1997). Indeed, the rejection-sensitive men who concealed their sexual orientation did not accelerate their HIV progression. Therefore, coming out is not equally advantageous for all gay men and may be an increased risk for those who are sensitive to social censure.

Injection Drug Use Another high-risk behavior is the sharing of unsterilized needles by injection drug users, a practice that allows the direct transmission of blood from one person to another. Injection drug use is the second most frequent source of HIV infection in the United States (USBC, 2001). Some injection drug users engage in this behavior in certain situations, for example, when intoxicated or when there is no immediate access to sterile drug equipment. Fortunately, evidence is beginning to indicate that incidence of HIV among injection drug users may be declining (Des Jarlais et al., 2000).

Transmission through injection drug use accounts for a greater percentage of infected African Americans and Hispanic Americans than European Americans (USBC, 2001). Also, a higher percentage of infected women than men are exposed to the virus through this route. Several behavioral factors are related to HIV infection for women who inject drugs, including the number of sex partners and whether or not they traded sex for money or drugs. Women are often vulnerable to infection if they are financially dependent on men; they may not be free to refuse sex, even if their partner is HIV positive and refuses to use a condom (*Population Reports,* 2001).

Heterosexual Contact Heterosexual contact is the leading source of HIV infection in Africa (*Population Reports,* 2001) and the fastest growing source in the United States (CDC, 2001b). African Americans and Hispanic Americans are disproportionately represented among those infected through heterosexual contact, and women from these two ethnic backgrounds are in greater danger than men from heterosexual contact.

This gender asymmetry comes from ease of transmission during sexual intercourse: male-to-female transmission is eight times more likely than female-to-male transmission (Padian, Shiboski, Glass, & Vittinghoff, 1997). Although men are susceptible to HIV through sexual contact with women, their risk is quite small. Despite women's greater likelihood of being infected through heterosexual sex, they tend to see their sexual partners as safer than do men (Crowell & Emmers-Sommers, 2001).

Trust and confidence of one's partner in a heterosexual relationship is not a good predictor of who later becomes HIV infected and who does not. One recent study (Crowell & Emmers-Sommers, 2001) asked HIV-infected women and men to look backward to assess their perceived risk prior to becoming infected and to compare those beliefs to their current beliefs. When HIV-positive individuals looked back at their sexual attitudes, beliefs, and behaviors they saw themselves as having a high level of trust in their partners and a low level of perceived risk for themselves. Moreover, their sexual attitudes and behaviors were no different from HIV-negative people. Thus, one reason why people engage in unprotected sex is because they see themselves as invulnerable to a very serious disease. Regular use of condoms may provide a high level of safety for heterosexual men and women, but many young heterosexual couples use condoms more as a means of preventing pregnancy than preventing HIV (Bird, Harvey, Beckman, & Johnson, 2000).

Transmission during the Birth Process Another group at risk for HIV infection includes children born to HIV-positive women. This transmission tends to occur during the birth process. Breastfeeding can also transmit the virus (*Population Reports,* 2001). Children infected with HIV during the birth process suffer a variety of developmental disabilities including intellectual and academic impairment, psychomotor dysfunction, and emotional and behavioral difficulties (Levenson & Mellins, 1992). In addition, many of these children are born to mothers who ingested drugs during pregnancy and are thus put at further risk for developmental difficulties.

Knowledge of HIV-positive status does not deter young women from becoming pregnant (Murphy, Mann, O'Keefe, & Rotherram-Borus, 1998). Between 15% and 30% of children born to HIV-positive women are infected, but this percentage can be cut to 8% or less if the pregnant woman receives prenatal treatment with antiretroviral drugs. Therefore, seeking prenatal care is critically important for HIV-positive women who become pregnant, and early prenatal care is responsible for much of the decline in this version of the epidemic (CDC, 2001b).

Psychologists' Role in the HIV Epidemic

From the beginning of the AIDS epidemic, psychologists have had an important role in combating the spread of infection (Kelly & Kalichman, 2002). During the early years of the epidemic, psychologists were involved in both primary and secondary prevention efforts. Primary prevention includes changing behavior to decrease HIV transmission. Secondary prevention includes helping people who are HIV positive to live with the infection, counseling people about being tested for HIV, helping patients deal with social and interpersonal aspects of the disease, and helping patients adhere to their complex treatment program. Much of the recent improvement in length of survival of HIV-infected patients rests with the effectiveness of drug treatments, and psychologists' knowledge concerning adherence to medical regimens is now relevant to managing HIV infection.

Encouraging Protective Measures Except for infants born to HIV-infected mothers, most people have some control in protecting themselves from the human immunodeficiency virus. Fortunately, HIV is not easily transmitted from person to person, making casual contact with infected persons a low risk. People can protect themselves against infection with HIV by changing those behaviors that are high risks for acquiring the infection—namely, having unprotected sexual contact or sharing needles with an infected person. The majority of people who are infected have become so in one of these two ways. Limiting the number of sex partners, using condoms, and avoiding shared needles are three behaviors that will protect the largest number of people from HIV infection.

However, other protective measures may be applicable for some people. Health care workers who participate in surgery, emergency care, or other procedures that bring them into contact with blood should be careful to prevent infected blood from entering their body through an open wound. For example, dentists and dental hygienists now wear protective gloves, and health care workers are taught to adhere to a set of standard protective measures.

The tendency to base judgment on appearances can be dangerous when it comes to HIV infection. Because HIV infection typically has a long incubation period without symptoms, people can be contagious and still appear healthy. Choosing sex partners based on the appearance of health can be very risky.

Most people in the United States do not perceive that they are at risk for HIV infection, and they are correct (Holtzman, Bland, Lansky, & Mack, 2001). That is, most adults do not engage in behaviors that are HIV risks. Those who do are more likely to engage in protective behaviors. This appropriate caution does not apply to everyone; many people continue to engage in high-risk behaviors. Younger men who have sex with men, African Americans, and Hispanic Americans are at higher risk, yet prevention efforts have been less successful with these groups (CDC, 2001c). Developing interventions that will affect these vulnerable groups is a priority.

Taking a cautionary lesson from the worldwide epidemic, authorities understand that containing the heterosexual transmission of HIV is an important goal. Changing sexual behavior is a difficult process that occurs within a complex personal and cultural context. Nevertheless, in New York City during the 1990s, cases of HIV infection decreased drastically among men who have sex with men and among injection drug users (CDC, 2001c). This recent research strongly suggests that prevention for all risk groups can be effective.

Helping People with HIV Infection People who believe they may be infected with HIV, as well as those who know that they are, can benefit from various psychological interventions. People with high-risk behaviors may have difficulty deciding whether to be tested for HIV, and psychologists can provide both information and support for these people. A significant minority of gay and bisexual men, injection drug users, and a larger proportion of heterosexual men and women with multiple partners and inconsistent use of condoms have never been tested for HIV. Indeed, an estimated 70% of people who are HIV positive have not been tested and thus do not know their HIV status (CDC, 2001c). Because HIV infection has a long incubation period, at-risk heterosexual men and women may contaminate others for years before they learn they have HIV.

The decision to be tested for HIV has both benefits and costs. The benefit, of course, is that people can find out their serostatus; if it is positive, they can begin treatment that will prolong their lives. Another potentially positive benefit of early testing is the reduction or elimination of behaviors that place others at risk. Many, but not all, gay and bisexual men reduce risky sexual behaviors, and most inform their primary partner of the results of testing. However, some research (Ickovics et al., 1998) indicated that women's sexual behavior tends not to change as a result of HIV testing.

What are the psychological costs of receiving an HIV-positive test result? People learning of a positive result typically react with increased anxiety, depression, anger, and distress, whereas people with existing psychiatric problems often react to a positive HIV test result with severe psychopathology, which may lead to a decrease in quality of life (Holmes, Bix, Meritz, Turner, & Hutelmyer, 1997). Therefore, trained therapists are needed to help people cope with their diagnosis. Coping processes can affect the amount of distress experienced by those who learn they are HIV positive, and psychological interventions can reduce their distress. Avoidance coping, such as denying reality or clinging to illusory hope, is associated with high levels of psychological distress and with lower levels of CD4 cells (Mulder, van Griensven, Sandfort, de Vroome, & Antoni, 1999). Active coping, including problem solving and seeking social support, is related to better adjustment.

Finding meaning and positive experience is important for people who are HIV positive. Research (Folkman & Moskowitz, 2000) showed that people with AIDS and their caregivers succeeded in working toward creating positive experiences in their lives, with over 99% able to recall a positive experience. For AIDS patients struggling with depression and negative feelings, cognitive behavioral stress management interventions have been successful in boosting adaptive coping and increasing social support (Lutgendorf et al., 1998), indicating that psychological interventions have a place in HIV management.

Psychologists can also help HIV patients adhere to the complex medical regimens designed to control HIV infection (Kelly & Kalichman, 2002). A combination of drug treatments became common in 1996 after its effectiveness became apparent. Patients typically take at least three different antiretroviral medications; they often take other drugs to combat side effects of the antiretroviral drugs as well as drugs to fight opportunistic infections. These regimens can include as many as a dozen drugs, all of which must be timed precisely. When patients do not follow the schedule, the effectiveness diminishes. Psychologists can help patients adhere to this schedule as well as facilitate their self-management skills.

In Summary

Acquired immune deficiency syndrome (AIDS) is the result of the depletion of the immune system after infection with the human immunodeficiency virus (HIV). When the immune system fails to defend the body, a number of diseases may develop, including bacterial, viral, fungal, and parasitic infections that are uncommon in people who have functioning immune systems.

The modes of transmission of HIV are behavioral, with receptive anal intercourse and the sharing of needles for intravenous drug injection the two behaviors that have spread the infection to the most people in the United States. Unprotected heterosexual contact with an infected partner accounts for an increasing proportion of people with HIV, the majority of whom are African American or Hispanic American women. The number of babies infected with HIV decreased because antiretroviral drug therapies sharply decrease transmission from an infected mother during the birth process.

Psychologists use a variety of interventions to help patients reduce high-risk behaviors, to cope with their illness, to manage their symptoms, and to adhere to the complex drug regimens that improve survival. In addition, psychologists have provided counseling services for those seeking to be tested and for those whose tests reveal infection. These programs not only encourage protective behaviors but also emphasize the role of positive health in combating AIDS.

Living with Alzheimer's Disease

Alzheimer's disease, a degenerative disease of the brain, is a major source of impairment among older people, affecting nearly half the people over 85 in the United States (Plaud, Mosley, & Moberg, 1998). Medical researchers identified the brain abnormalities that underlie Alzheimer's disease in the late 19th century. In 1907, a German physician, Alois Alzheimer, reported on the relationship between autopsy findings of neurological abnormalities and psychiatric symptoms before death. Shortly after his report, other researchers began to call the disorder Alzheimer's disease.

The disease can be diagnosed definitively only through autopsy, but Alzheimer's patients show behavioral symptoms of cognitive impairment and memory loss that may lead to a provisional diagnosis. In addition, brain imaging techniques have some ability to reveal the underlying degeneration (Pinsky, Burke, & Bird, 2001). During autopsy, a microscopic examination of the brain of those with Alzheimer's disease reveals "plaques" and tangles of nerve fibers in the cerebral cortex and hippocampus. These tangles of nerve fibers are the physical basis for Alzheimer's disease.

The underlying mechanisms in the development of the disease are not yet completely understood, but research has identified two different forms of the disease: an early-onset version that occurs before age 60 and a late-onset version that occurs after age 65. The early-onset type is quite rare, representing less than 1% of all Alzheimer's patients (Mayeux & Schupf, 1995). Early-onset Alzheimer's seems to be due to a genetic defect, and at least three different genes have been implicated on chromosomes 1, 14, and 21 (Daly, 1998).

The late-onset type, which has symptoms similar to the early-onset type, may occur with or without a family history of the disease (Pinsky et al., 2001). The risk for developing this version of the disease is related to apolipoprotein ϵ, a protein involved in cholesterol metabolism (Tang et al., 1998). One form of apolipoprotein, the $\epsilon 4$ form, increases the risk for developing the tangles of neurons that are characteristic of Alzheimer's disease by about three times (Farrer et al., 1998), but the $\epsilon 2$ form may offer some protection. The genetic contribution is not straightforward: African Americans experience increased risk, even with the same genetic risk (Green et al., 2002).

In addition to the genetic contribution, environmental and experiential factors contribute to the risk and interact with the genetics of Alzheimer's disease. For example, Type 2 diabetes increases the risk for Alzheimer's disease, but the combination of apolipoprotein and diabetes raises the risk by over five times (Peila, Rodriguez, & Launer, 2002). Mild brain trauma also contributes to the progress of the disease (Uryu et al., 2002); that is, repeated head injuries speed the plaque deposits that underlie the disease. Aluminum concentrations in drinking water are another risk, but silica in drinking water decreased risk (Rondeau, Commenges, Jacqmin-Gadda, & Dartigues, 2000).

Research into risk factors for Alzheimer's disease has also revealed some protective factors. Low levels of alcohol consumption cut the risk in half (Ruitenberg et al., 2002). Nonsteroidal anti-inflammatory drugs (NSAIDs) also appear to cut the risk. In an epidemiological study (In'tVeld et al., 2001), people who took NSAIDs such as ibuprophen for two years or longer showed a sharply decreased risk for Alzheimer's disease. The presence of the amino acid homocysteine raises the risk for both heart disease and Alzheimer's disease. Taking folic acid reduces the risk for heart disease and may do so for Alzheimer's disease as well (Seshadri et al., 2002). In addition, cognitive activity decreases the risk. People whose jobs demand a high level of cognitive processing are less likely to develop Alzheimer's disease than others with less cognitively demanding jobs (Wilson et al., 2002). Therefore, a combination of genetic and environmental factors contributes to the development of Alzheimer's disease, but other factors may offer protection.

The biggest risk factor for Alzheimer's disease is age; the incidence of Alzheimer's disease rises sharply with advancing age. One study (Evans et al., 1989) found that only 3% of the people between ages 65 and 74 demonstrate symptoms of the disease; 19% of people between ages 75 and 84 manifest symptoms; and 47% of people over age 85 show symptoms of Alzheimer's disease. The increase does not continue, however, and people who have not developed symptoms of Alzheimer's disease by their mid-80s are less likely to do so than people in their 70s (Ritchie & Kildea, 1995). The high number of people over 85 years old who have symptoms of probable Alzheimer's disease presents a pessimistic picture for the aging population in developed countries, where Alzheimer's is likely to become a large public health problem (Brookmeyer, Gray, & Kawas, 1998).

Because the symptoms of Alzheimer's include a number of behavior problems that are also symptoms of psychiatric disorders, the disease can be difficult to diagnose. These symptoms include memory loss, language problems, agitation and irritability, sleep disorders, suspiciousness and paranoia, incontinence, and sexual disorders (Plaud et al., 1998). These behavioral symptoms can be the source of much distress to patients as well as to their caregivers. The most common psychiatric problem among Alzheimer's patients is depression, with as many as 20% of patients exhibiting symptoms of clinical depression and an additional 30% to 50% suffering from depressed mood (Mulsant, Pollock, Nebes, Hoch, & Reynolds, 1997). Depression is especially common among people in the early phases of the disease and in early-onset Alzheimer's. Those people who retain much awareness of their problems find their deterioration distressing and respond with a feeling of helplessness and depression.

The memory loss that characterizes Alzheimer's patients may first appear in the form of small, ordinary failures of memory, which represents the early stages of the disease (Morris et al., 2001). This memory loss progresses to the point that Alzheimer's patients fail to recognize family members and forget how to perform even routine self-care (Rabins, 1989). In the early phases of the disease, patients are usually aware of their memory failures, making this symptom even more distressing. For example, former newspaper publisher Thomas DeBaggio chronicled his life after diagnosis of early-onset Alzheimer's disease in the book, *Losing My Mind* (2002). His book is filled with anger and loss as he felt himself losing abilities that were always easy for him. His vocabulary slipped away, and he found writing increasingly difficult. His ability was unusual, but his losses were typical of people with Alzheimer's disease.

Patients with Alzheimer's disease often exhibit symptoms of agitation, irritability, and even violence. Sylvia, the case that began this chapter, was no exception. A gentle, even passive woman during the first 80 years of her life, she frequently became aggressive and threatening as her disease progressed. She accused Brenda of mistreating her and on one occasion cut up all her old photos of Brenda. In some cases, Sylvia's explosive agitation was related to her memory failure. Sometimes, she would have an outburst of anger while getting dressed because she had forgotten how to complete the task and had become confused and frustrated. At other times, she would become angry because her daily routine had been disrupted and she was uncertain about how she should behave.

The common symptoms of paranoia and suspiciousness may also relate to cognitive impairments. Alzheimer's patients may forget where they have put belongings, and because they cannot find their possessions, accuse others of taking them. However, suspicious and accusatory behaviors are not limited to misplaced belongings. Like many Alzheimer's patients, Sylvia concentrated her suspicions and accusations on her primary caregiver, leading Brenda to become resentful and emotionally distressed.

Although difficulties in staying asleep are common among older adults, Alzheimer's patients have even more severe problems than their peers. As a result, these patients tend to wander at all times of the day and night (Rabins, 1989). This behavior can disturb those who sleep in the same house and provide opportunities for the patients to injure themselves. After Brenda and Bob moved Sylvia into their house, this problem became so serious that they were required to retain a "sitter" to watch Sylvia at night. The sitter was instructed to gently lead Sylvia back to her bedroom whenever she roamed around at night.

Incontinence and sexual disorders are acutely distressing problems to both the patients and their caregivers. Incontinence is very common in patients with advanced cases of Alzheimer's disease. In the year before she died, Sylvia lost all control over her bowel movements. Even more distressing to Brenda, she seemed also to have lost her awareness of normal excretory functions and showed no appreciation for her daughter's extra work in cleaning her. A pattern of behavioral symptoms, such as Sylvia's, is strong indication of Alzheimer's disease and the only means of diagnosis before autopsy.

Helping the Patient

Several drugs that may prevent or reverse the symptoms or underlying disease processes are in development (Martindale, 2002), but presently, no cure for Alzheimer's disease exists. Incurability and untreatability are two different things, and the physical symptoms and other accompanying disorders of Alzheimer's disease can be treated, but not cured. Treatment approaches include drugs for delaying the progression of cognitive deficits, neuroleptic drugs for reducing agitation and aggression, and the use of music and pets to relax Alzheimer's patients. At best, these techniques slow the progress of the disease by months or even a few years but do not cure it (Rabins, 1996).

In addition to these interventions, several researchers have advocated behavioral approaches in treating Alzheimer's patients. An analysis of the antecedents of patients' problem behaviors allows modification of the environment of Alzheimer's patients so they can adjust better to their lives (Plaud et al., 1998; Reese, 2002). By identifying the events that precede problem behaviors, family members can eliminate or reduce those events and thus perhaps decrease patients' undesirable behaviors. Changes include alterations in the environment and in the patient's behaviors. For example, patients with awareness of their memory loss can learn to write notes as a way of keeping track of the important things in their lives. For those who get lost in their own homes, labeling the doors can be helpful.

Although none of these treatments can cure Alzheimer's disease, most will help control undesirable behaviors and alleviate some of the distressing symptoms of the disease. Any treatment that can delay symptoms of Alzheimer's disease can make significant differences in the number of cases and in the costs of management (Brookmeyer et al., 1998). In the early phases of Alzheimer's disease, both patients and their families are distressed by its symptoms, but as the patients worsen and lose awareness, the stress of Alzheimer's becomes more severe for the family.

Helping the Family

As with other chronic illnesses, Alzheimer's disease affects not only patients but also their families. For Alzheimer's disease, however, the symptoms of the illness are particularly distressing to the families (Cohler, Groves, Borden, & Lazarus, 1989). The memory impairments are disturbing, because patients may fail to recognize their spouses and children. Cognitive impairments lead to changes in personality, and the one affected no longer seems like the same person. The suspiciousness that Alzheimer's patients frequently manifest can lead to accusations that hurt family members, and Alzheimer's patients who are violent upset normal family functioning. Families tend to find dangerous or embarrassing behaviors especially distressing (Barrett, Ford, Stewart, & Haley, 1994). In addition to this emotional burden, the problems of taking care of an Alzheimer's patient greatly disrupt family routine.

For instance, arguments between Brenda and Bob increased during the time Sylvia lived with them. Brenda neglected her own appearance, became absorbed in her caregiving duties, and lost interest in sexual relations with Bob. Before Sylvia's illness, Brenda and Bob shared interests in the law, movies, books, and traveling. Although she could have arranged to do so, during the 3 years her mother lived with them, Brenda never took a vacation or even went to a movie.

In the United States, the caregiver role is occupied mostly by women (Cancian & Oliker, 2000), and an unmarried woman has the greatest likelihood of becoming the primary caretaker for Alzheimer's patients (Modesti & Tryon, 1994). The National Long-term Care Survey (Stone, Cafferata, & Sangl, 1987) showed that family caregivers are usually the patients' wives or daughters. For Alzheimer's patients with spouses who are able to provide care, the caregiving falls to the spouse, but men often receive more help than women in care giving, and women provide the assistance.

In some ways, Brenda was more fortunate than the typical caregiver. Bob's income was sufficient, and Brenda suspended her career to care for her mother. Brenda could have continued with her law practice and hired a full-time nurse, but she felt that she should be the one to provide care. Brenda's feelings were typical of caregivers for Alzheimer's patients (Cancian & Oliker, 2000).

Caregivers experiencing the stress and strain of their role exhibit a number of symptoms of their own distress, including fatigue, frustration, helplessness, grief, shame, embarrassment, anger, and depression (Soukup, 1996). Anger is a common problem with Alzheimer's caregivers. Spouses become angry and frightened when they realize that they are faced with years of a deteriorating relationship. Caregivers who are adult children are often sandwiched between helping an Alzheimer's parent and taking care of children, and this strain can lead to anger, fatigue, depression, and loss of sleep (Soukup, 1996).

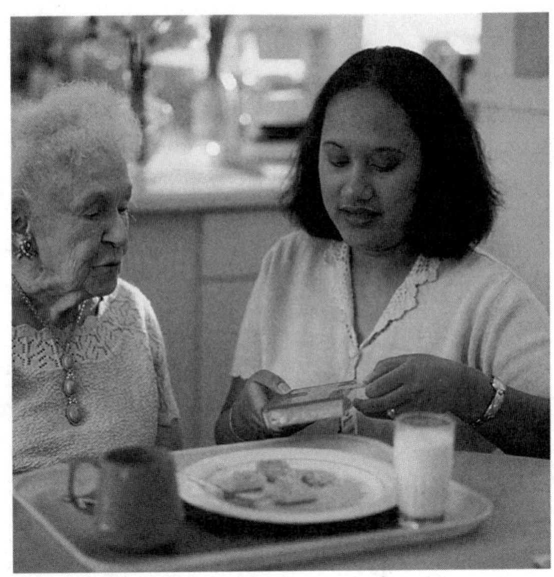
PhotoDisc

Caring for an Alzheimer's patient can produce high levels of stress, making caregivers vulnerable to illness.

The chronic stress of caregiving makes these individuals of interest to psychoneuroimmunologists, who have studied how this chronic stress affects the immune system (Cacioppo et al., 1998; Kiecolt-Glaser, 1999). Janice Kiecolt-Glaser and her colleagues have studied Alzheimer's caregivers and found that these caregivers experience poorer physical and psychological health and poorer immunological function compared to people of similar age who were not caregivers. Also, the level of impairment of the Alzheimer's patient is directly related to the level of distress in the caregiver

BECOMING HEALTHIER

1. If you have a chronic illness, understand your condition, form a cooperative relationship with health care professionals, but take charge of its management yourself. You are the person most affected by your condition.
2. If you are the primary caregiver to someone who is chronically ill, don't ignore your own health—both physical and psychological. Regularly schedule some time for yourself.
3. If you have Type 1 diabetes, don't try to hide your illness from your friends. Although you have a chronic disease, you can live a long and productive life, but you must adhere faithfully to a lifelong regimen that includes diet, insulin injection, and regular exercise. If you live with someone with diabetes, offer social and emotional support, and encourage that person to stick with required health practices.
4. Know your blood sugar level. Type 2 diabetes can develop at any age, and this disorder may have few symptoms.
5. If you have asthma, try to minimize attacks and use of dilators. Concentrate on taking preventive medication and knowing your triggers to avoid attacks.
6. Protect yourself against HIV infection. The most common mode of transmission is sexual, and condoms make sex safer.
7. If you are the primary caregiver to someone with HIV or AIDS, seek social and emotional support through groups specifically convened to offer such support. The white pages of your telephone book lists numbers to call for information.
8. If you are a caregiver to someone with Alzheimer's disease, take regular breaks. (You have friends who can assume caregiver duties for short periods.) Look for an Alzheimer's support group in your community and attend meetings as frequently as possible.

(Robinson-Whelen et al., 2001), that is, the more impaired the patient, the more distressed the caregiver. Furthermore, their distress does not decrease when their caregiving is ended. Therefore, caregiving imposes severe burdens, extending even after the death of the Alzheimer's patient.

Cognitive-behavioral therapies can help caregivers manage their negative emotions (Plaud et al., 1998). In addition, support groups can help people who care for Alzheimer's patients. Participation in a group that encourages an open, honest sharing of feelings, including negative feelings, can provide support that families may not be able to give. This additional support may be needed because of the strain imposed on the family and friends of the patient, people who would otherwise be the main sources of support. Support groups can also be sources of information about caring for the patients and about community resources that provide respite care.

Alzheimer's caregivers frequently experience feelings of loss for the relationship that they once shared with the patient. This sense of loss may be similar to bereavement, only the person is still alive (Kiecolt-Glaser, 1999). To cope with her distress, Brenda joined a support group but attended meetings only irregularly. The other caregivers at these meetings often talked about their feelings of loss, and Brenda could identify with those feelings. During her times alone, she found herself reminiscing more and more about her childhood and the pleasant times she enjoyed with her mother. She knew that Sylvia would never regain the loving person that marked her earlier life. The woman Brenda once knew no longer lived in her mother's body, and she grieved over her loss.

In Summary

Alzheimer's disease is a progressive, degenerative disease of the brain that affects cognitive functioning, especially memory. Other symptoms include language problems, agitation and irritability, paranoia and suspiciousness, sleep disorders, depression, incontinence, and sexual problems. These symptoms are also indicative of some psychiatric disorders and make Alzheimer's disease distressing to both patients and caretakers.

Increasing age is a risk factor for Alzheimer's disease, with nearly half the people over 85 exhibiting symptoms. Both genetics and environment seem to play a role in the development of the disease, and early-onset and late-onset varieties exist.

Drug treatments intended to slow the progress of the disease have limited effectiveness, but active research may soon be more successful in formulating a treatment. At this point, treatment is largely oriented toward slowing the progress of the disease, managing the negative symptoms, and helping family caregivers cope with the stress. Management of symptoms can include changing the environment to make care less difficult. Treatment may also be desirable for those who provide care to Alzheimer's patients, because a high percentage of these caregivers experience stress and stress-related problems, depression being the most common. Individual therapy or increased social support from an Alzheimer's support group can help the caregivers and families of Alzheimer's patients cope with the stress of providing care.

Answers

This chapter addressed five basic questions:

1. **What is the impact of chronic illness?**
   Unlike acute diseases, chronic illnesses can persist for years and affect not only the afflicted person but friends and family members as well. Long-term chronic illnesses frequently bring about a crisis in people's lives, change the way people see themselves, produce financial hardship, and disrupt family dynamics. Support groups and programs designed by health psychologists help people cope with the emotional problems associated with chronic illness, problems that traditional medical care often overlooks.

2. **What is involved in adjusting to diabetes?**
   Diabetes, both insulin-dependent (Type 1) and noninsulin-dependent (Type 2), requires changes in lifestyle, including monitoring and adherence to a treatment regimen. Treatments include insulin injections for Type 1 diabetics and adherence to careful dietary restrictions, scheduling of meals, avoidance of certain foods, regular medical visits, and routine exercise for all diabetics. Health psychologists are involved in helping diabetics learn self-care to control the dangerous effects of their condition.

3. **How does asthma affect the lives of people with this disease?**
   Inflammation of the bronchial tubes is the underlying basis for asthma. Combined with this inflammation, triggering stimuli or events cause bronchial constriction that produces difficulty in breathing. Asthma is not often fatal, but it is the leading cause of disability among children. The origin of this process is not understood, but medication can control the inflammation and decrease the risk of attacks. People with asthma are faced with a complex medication regimen that they must follow, and they may also need to avoid exertion, which can be a difficult restriction

for children. People with asthma must develop ways to care for themselves to minimize the chances of attacks.

4. **How can HIV infection be managed?**
Infection with the human immunodeficiency virus (HIV) depletes the immune system, leaving the body vulnerable to acquired immune deficiency syndrome (AIDS) and a variety of opportunistic infections. Four different populations in the United States have been affected by HIV epidemics; (1) men who have sex with men, (2) injection drug users, (3) heterosexuals, and (4) children born to HIV-positive mothers. Psychologists are involved in the HIV epidemic by encouraging protective behaviors, counseling infected people to help them cope with living with a chronic disease, and helping patients adhere to complex medical regimens that have changed HIV infection to a manageable chronic disease.

5. **What is the impact of Alzheimer's disease on patients and their families?**
Alzheimer's disease is a brain disease that produces memory loss, language problems, agitation and irritability, sleep disorders, suspiciousness, wandering, incontinence, and loss of ability to perform routine care. Alzheimer's disease has a genetic risk, but this risk combines with environmental risks to produce the most common variety of the disease. Age is the main risk, with the prevalence doubling for every decade after age 65. Medical treatments are being developed, but the main management strategies consist of interventions to allow patients longer periods of functioning and counseling and support groups for family members, who frequently experience more stress than the patient.

Suggested Readings

Amschler, D. H. (2002). The alarming increase of Type 2 diabetes in children. *Journal of School Health, 72,* 39–41. This article reviews the increase of Type 2 diabetes among children and covers the risks for this type of diabetes for all ages and the challenges of controlling the disease.

DeBaggio, T. (2002). *Losing my mind: An intimate look at life with Alzheimer's.* New York: Free Press. When former newspaper writer Thomas DeBaggio began to recognize symptoms of Alzheimer's disease at age 57, he decided to write about his experience of "losing his mind." The result is a moving account of Alzheimer's disease from an insider's point of view.

Kelly, J. A., & Kalichman, S. C. (2002). Behavioral research in HIV/AIDS primary and secondary prevention: Recent advances and future directions. *Journal of Consulting and Clinical Psychology, 70,* 626–639. Jeffrey Kelly and Seth Kalichman review the changed and changing field of HIV research and treatment, focusing on the advances and the evidence about prevention. This article not only discusses prevention efforts in the general population but considers prevention for people who are HIV positive and for populations who are difficult to reach, such as those who are homeless.

Shell, E. R. (2000, May). Does civilization cause asthma? *Atlantic Monthly, 285,* 90–92, 94, 96–98, 100. This article reviews the provocative notion that the cleanliness of modern society may underlie the increased frequency of asthma as well as considers the challenges of treatment in the lives of affected children and young adults.

Stanton, A. L., Collins, C. A., & Sworowski, L. A. (2001). Adjustment to chronic illness: Theory and research. In A. Baum, T. A. Revenson, & J. E. Singer (Eds.), *Handbook of health psychology* (pp. 387–403). Mahwah, NJ: Erlbaum. This article takes a biopsychosocial view of adjustment to chronic illness, adopting the point of view that coping with chronic illness has important environmental and personal influences.

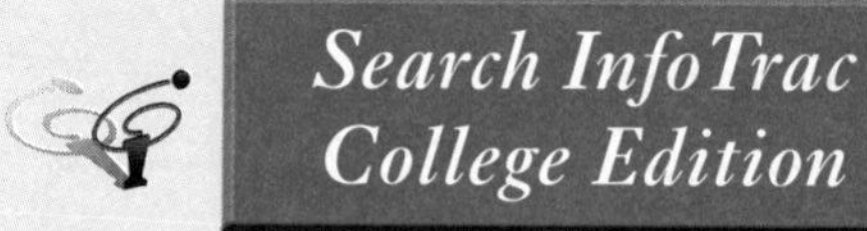

Search these terms to learn more about topics in this chapter:

Chronic illness and adaptation

Impact and chronic illness

Family and chronic illness

Children and chronic illness

Diabetes and statistics

Diabetes susceptibility and genetic aspects

Diabetes and adherence

Diabetes in youth

Diabetes in children

Diabetes in adults

Health psychology and diabetes

Asthma and causes of

Asthma and cleanliness

Asthma and statistics

Asthma and demographic aspects

Asthma and management

Asthma and self-management

HIV and statistics

HIV and demographic aspects and ethnic

HIV and transmission and modes

HIV and prevention and behavior

HIV and coping

Alzheimer and apolipoprotein

Alzheimer and protective

Alzheimer and progression

Alzheimer and drug treatment

Alzheimer and caregiver

12

Preventing Injuries

The Story of James

CHAPTER OUTLINE

Unintentional Injuries

Strategies for Reducing Unintentional Injuries

Intentional Injuries

Strategies to Reduce Intentional Injuries

QUESTIONS

This chapter focuses on six basic questions:

1. How can adults make children's worlds safer?
2. What can young people do to reduce their chances of unintentional injuries?
3. What unintentional injuries are most likely to affect adults?
4. What are some of the strategies for reducing unintentional injuries?
5. What are the major types and the impact of intentional injuries?
6. How can intentional injuries be reduced?

The Story of James

James, a European American college student, acknowledges that he took many safety risks in his 23 years and feels lucky that he was not injured seriously. James grew up in a small Southern town where drinking alcohol was a primary recreation for him and his friends, and many of his risks involved alcohol, motor vehicles, firearms, or some combination of the three. When he was in high school, James and his friends drank heavily on weekends. A group of them played a game that involved one member of the group riding on the top of the cab of James's truck in order to shoot whatever came into the headlights. The person who was shooting was strapped to the top of the cab to prevent him from falling, but some falls did occur. One resulted in a broken leg, so the group decided to stop playing that game.

James continued to take risks, including driving after he had been drinking. He says that he had a drinking problem during high school but that he never hesitated to drive. His drinking habits changed when he started college; he drinks much less but continues to drive after drinking. Although he knows the risks, he doesn't believe that these risks apply to him because he changes his driving behavior after he has been drinking; that is, he avoids busy streets and drives more slowly. He has had one crash while he was driving drunk, but that crash resulted in only a minor injury. James has not experienced any major injury despite his many risks.

James likes guns and owns both handguns and hunting rifles. Indeed, he carries a firearm in his truck and has done so ever since high school. He knows the risks involved with guns, and he is more cautious with firearms than he is with driving after drinking. He knows the proper safety procedures for handling guns and insists that his friends observe these procedures. He acknowledges that drinking makes people less safety conscious and slows their reflexes, but he still feels that he is careful with firearms. However, James knows that having a gun in his truck can be a risk—once a friend became angry with another person and wanted to get the gun from James's truck to shoot that person. James talked his friend out of it, but the incident made James aware that having a gun might be a danger even if he was not going to use the firearm himself.

Although James has taken a great many risks, he sees those risks more clearly now than during the gun incident. He now considers himself very lucky to have experienced only minor injuries, but he believes that the precautions he has taken after drinking and his training in firearm safety have contributed to his escape from injury. He has taken more than his share of chances, but his beliefs concerning precautions are similar to those of many people. His belief that he will escape the negative consequences of risky behavior fits into the framework of **optimistic bias** (Weinstein, 1980), in which one believes that negative events will happen to others more often than to oneself. Most people take some type of precaution to avoid injury or crime victimization. Unfortunately, most people also put themselves at risk in some ways, and, like James, they may not acknowledge it.

Just as healthy behaviors tend to cluster together, so too do unhealthy habits. When young children begin to engage in one risky behavior, it increases their chances of engaging in a multitude of such behaviors. If children 11 years old and younger begin to smoke, they are also more likely than other children to use cocaine, alcohol, and other drugs, go skating without a helmet, refuse to use a seatbelt, and engage in violent behavior (DuRant, Smith, Kreiter, & Krowchuk, 1999). These same children are also likely to carry a gun or other weapon, rank low in school, have an older age for their grade in school, be a European American boy, and come from a single-parent household.

Before 1970, psychologists, like nearly everyone else, referred to unintentional injuries as *accidents,* a term with connotations of chance, fate, or inevitability. During the 1970s and 1980s, physician William Haddon, Jr. (Haddon, 1970, 1972, 1980) began to change the way psychologists and many others looked at these injuries. Rather than viewing them simply as a consequence of unavoidable human error, health psychologists now see unintentional injuries as resulting from a complex of conditions, including individual behaviors, dangerous environmental conditions, and lack of tough legislation and enforcement. Health psychologists are concerned with each of these three areas in unintentional injuries at the various developmental stages.

CHECK YOUR SAFETY RISKS

Check the items that apply to you.

If you do not have a young child in your home, go to Item 7.

- ☐ 1. Children in my home always wear helmets when they ride a bicycle or use a skateboard.
- ☐ 2. In my home, cleaning materials, chemicals, or poisons are stored in an unlocked cabinet under the sink.
- ☐ 3. In my home, a child under the age of 2 sleeps in the top bunk of a bunk bed.
- ☐ 4. In my home, a child under the age of 2 is never left unattended in a highchair.
- ☐ 5. Children in my home sometimes go swimming without an adult supervisor.
- ☐ 6. I never allow young children to ride in the front seat of a car.
- ☐ 7. I keep a loaded gun in my home.
- ☐ 8. I always use a seatbelt when driving or riding in a motor vehicle.
- ☐ 9. I sometimes drive after having more than two drinks.
- ☐ 10. I sometimes ride with someone who has been drinking.
- ☐ 11. I sometimes ride a bicycle or motorcycle without a helmet.
- ☐ 12. I usually ride my bicycle on the right side of the road, in the same direction as automobile traffic.
- ☐ 13. I sometimes smoke in bed.
- ☐ 14. While swimming I have sometimes dived into a body of water without knowing exactly what was in the water.
- ☐ 15. I sometimes ride a bicycle after drinking alcohol.
- ☐ 16. I sometimes play sports after drinking alcohol.

If you answered "yes" to items 1, 4, 6, 8, and 12 and "no" to each of the other items, you have a generally safe lifestyle. Although potential harm cannot be avoided completely, most safety rules do not greatly restrict one's freedom or limit one's enjoyment of leisure-time activities.

Unintentional Injuries

Unintentional injuries are the fourth leading cause of death in the United States, accounted for more than 97,000, or about 4% of all, deaths in the year 2000 (NCHS, 2001). Fatalities from unintentional injuries dropped sharply from 1965 to 1985, but as Figure 12.1 shows, the *rate* of decline has leveled off since 1985.

Unintentional injuries remain the leading cause of death in the United States for all groups up to age 35 and account for more than 40% of all deaths among young people 15 to 24 years of age (USBC, 2001). Age of victim has an interesting relationship with death from unintentional injuries in the United States. The safest age is 5 to 14 years, with fewer than 10 children per 100,000 dying from unintentional injuries. Figure 12.2 shows this relationship and also the large jump in deaths rates for people between ages 15 to 24 years. Adolescents and young adults continue to have the highest rate of deaths from unintentional injuries until age 65, after which the rate skyrockets to nearly 100 per 100,000 population. Gender also relates to unintentional injury deaths—men are more than twice as likely as women to die from this cause (USBC, 2001).

The primary cause of death from unintentional injuries is motor vehicle crashes, which account for almost half of all unintentional deaths. Figure 12.1 shows a continuous decline in deaths from motor vehicle injuries from 1965 to 1998. In addition to this drop in the rate of deaths, the *total number* of deaths from motor vehicle crashes steadily dropped from almost 55,000 in 1970 to less than 42,000 in 1998

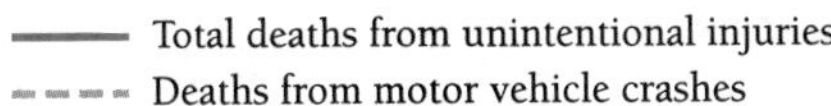

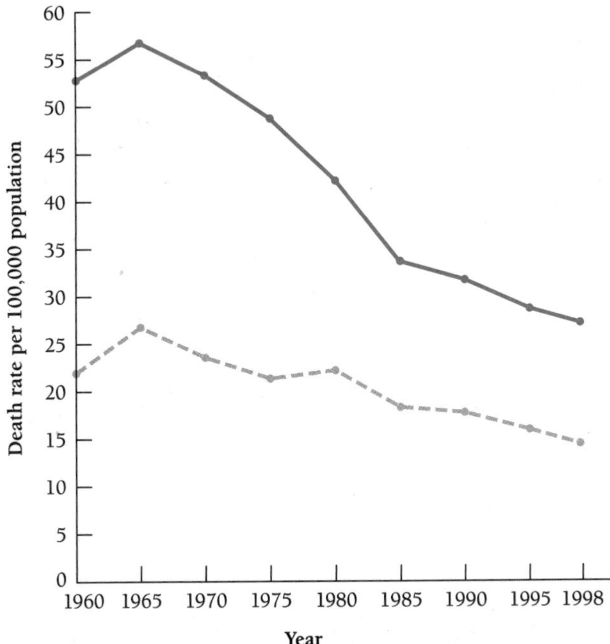

Figure 12.1 Deaths from unintentional injuries (total and motor vehicle related) per 100,000 population, United States, 1960–1998.

Source: Data from Statistical Abstracts of the United States, *1973, (p. 61); 1988, (p. 77); 2001 (p. 79) by U.S. Bureau of the Census, Washington D.C.: U.S. Government Printing Office.*

(USBC, 2001). This decline in the total number of deaths from motor vehicles crashes is remarkable in view of large increases in the number of drivers and the number of miles driven. The use of seatbelts and airbags, better built cars, safer roads, and stiffer penalties for driving while intoxicated have each contributed to this decline.

Because about half the deaths from unintentional injuries are due to motor vehicle crashes, the pattern of these deaths closely parallels those of all unintentional injuries. A comparison of Figure 12.2 and Figure 12.3 shows this profile; that is, up to age 15, relatively few children die from motor vehicle crashes or from other unintentional injuries. As childhood turns into adolescence, however, death from both categories rise dramatically, reaching a peak during adolescence and young adulthood and then declining gradually until age 65, after which time deaths from all unintentional injuries as well as motor vehicle crashes both rise sharply.

In addition to the large number of fatalities from unintentional injuries, even larger numbers of people suffer nonfatal injuries every year. Nonfatal injuries are responsible for increased health care costs, lost work and school days, disability, and pain. Clearly, violent death and injury are major health problems in the United States, and health scientists have been involved in strategies to reduce their number (Collins et al., 2002; Saldana & Peterson, 1997).

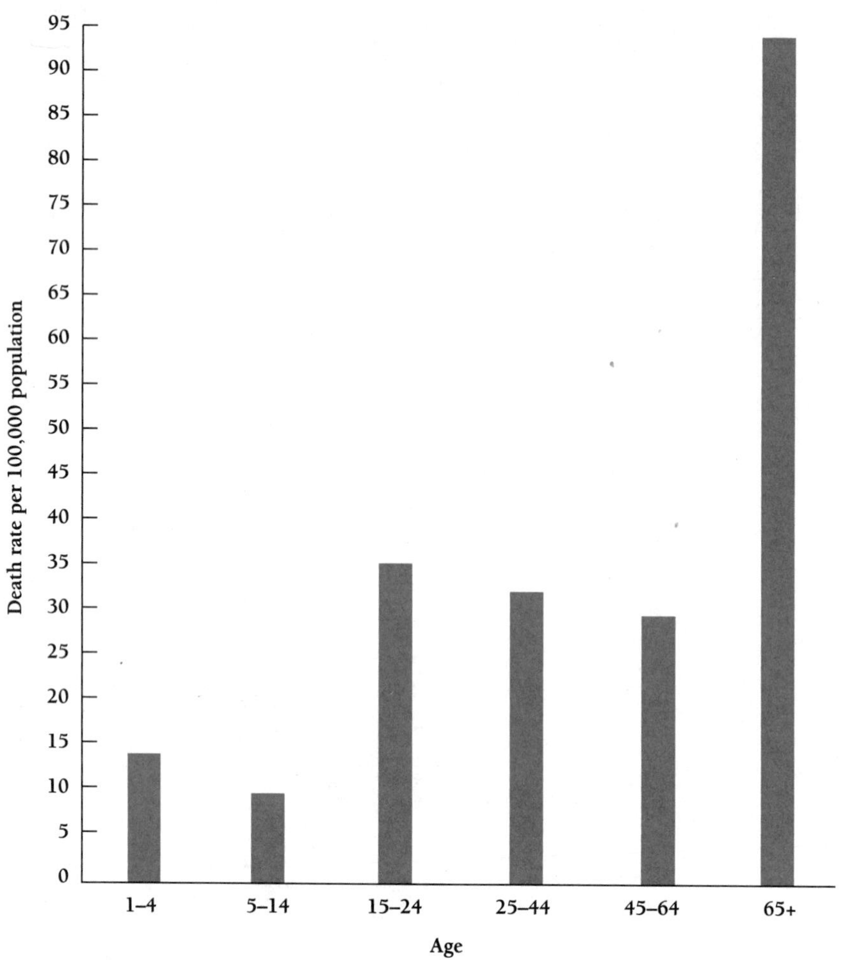

Figure 12.2 Deaths from unintentional injuries by age, per 100,000 of U.S. population, 1998.

Source: Data from Statistical Abstracts of the United States, *2001 (121st ed.) (p. 82) by U.S. Bureau of the Census, 2001, Washington, D.C.: U.S. Government Printing Office.*

Although all age groups are vulnerable to unintentional injuries, the pattern of death and injury varies with different developmental stages.

Childhood

Unintentional injuries are the leading cause of death for children in the United States, accounting for about 40% of all deaths among children under age 15 (NCHS, 2001). However, because children of this age have a relatively low death rate, the number of young children killed unintentionally is much lower than it is for adolescents or older people (see Figure 12.2).

Unintentional injuries to children are often caused by the unsafe acts of adults or an environment made unsafe by adults. The most frequent fatal injuries are from motor vehicle crashes, the major cause of unintentional injuries at every age. Motor vehicle crashes account for about one third of all unintentional injury deaths of children 1 to 4 years of age, and for children 5 to 14, more

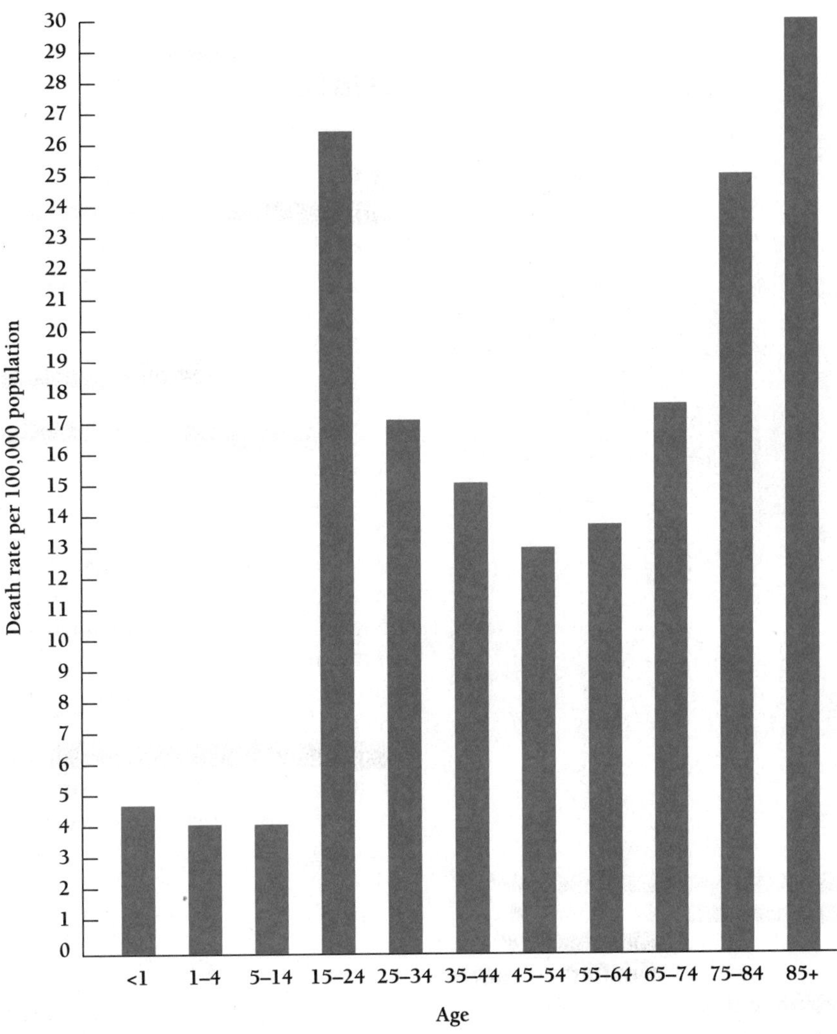

Figure 12.3 Death rates from motor vehicle injuries by age per 100,000 U.S. population, 1999.

Source: Data from National Center for Health Statistics (2001). Health, United States, 2001. *(p. 210). Hyattsville, MD: U.S. Government Printing Office.*

than half the deaths from unintentional injuries are due to motor vehicle crashes. The majority of automobile-related injuries to children under age 5 result from an adult's failure to properly restrain an infant or toddler in the back seat of a car (Saldana & Peterson, 1997). Unfortunately, several infants and young children in the front seat of a car have been killed or seriously injured by the deployment of passenger-side airbags, but nearly all these injuries could have been avoided by properly restraining children in the *back* seat (National Highway Traffic Safety Administration, 1993–1996). Alcohol is involved in about 20% of motor vehicle-related deaths of children as pedestrians, bicyclists, or passengers, but like most alcohol-related causes of deaths, this percentage is declining (Margolis, Foss, & Tolbert, 2000).

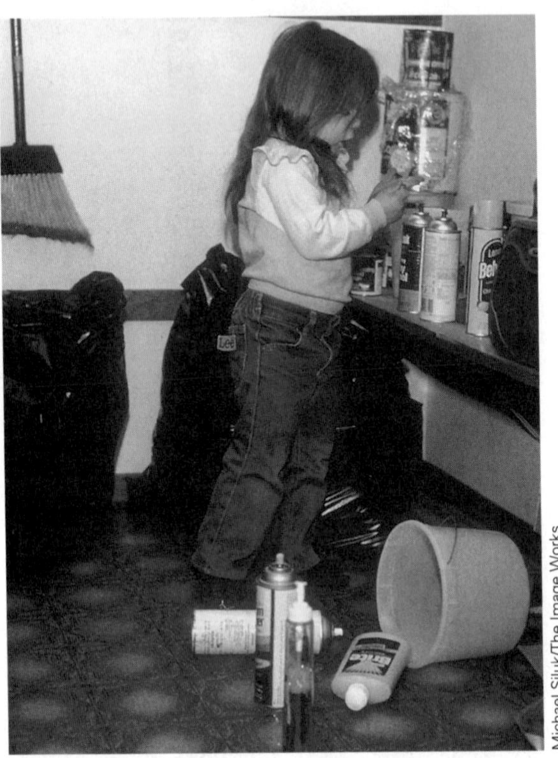
Michael Siluk/The Image Works

Homes include a number of safety hazards for young children.

Drownings are the second leading cause of children's death from unintentional injuries, and not all drownings occur in a swimming pool. For children under the age of 5, bathtubs and large buckets filled with water are potentially deadly containers. For older children, swimming pools are the most common place for drownings, and warm weather states such as California, Arizona, and Florida have more than their share of swimming pool drownings (Saldana & Peterson, 1997).

Children are also killed and injured by burns, most of which result from house fires. Many house fires are due to adults' smoking, but children are often the victims. Children under the age of 5 have an increased risk of death from residential fires, and the younger the child, the greater the risk. As with most childhood injuries, burns are much more common among boys than girls (Saldana & Peterson, 1997).

Other causes of childhood unintentional injuries include falls, suffocations, poisonings, and bicycle mishaps. Falls contribute significantly to childhood unintentional injuries. Children under age 4 can be severely injured or killed by falling from relatively short distances, such as from a bunk bed, a swing, or an open window. Suffocation is the second leading cause of death from unintentional injuries for children under the age of 1 year and is the fourth leading causes of death among children 1 to 4 years old (Saldana & Peterson, 1997). Poisoning deaths have decreased for young children in recent years, largely because of the increased use of child-resistant containers. Nevertheless, thousands of children become ill each year from exposure to dangerous chemicals. Finally, unintentional bicycle injuries result in more visits to emergency rooms than any other injuries. Bicycle injuries are related to both age and gender; the number of deaths and injuries increase up to early adolescence, with boys between the ages of 10 and 14 having the highest rates (Saldana & Peterson, 1997). The majority of bicycle fatalities are due to head injuries, and many of these could have been prevented by the proper use of bicycle helmets. (We discuss use of helmets later in the section on prevention of injuries.)

Youth

The passage from childhood to adolescence in the United States carries with it a greatly increased risk of death from unintentional injuries, especially those resulting from automobile crashes. Figure 12.3 shows that death rates from motor vehicle injuries increased sixfold as individuals moved from childhood to adolescence and young adulthood. The primary reason for this jump, of course, is that young people are beginning to drive and also to ride with other neophyte drivers. Like James, adolescents are also likely to drive after drinking alcohol or to ride with someone who has been drinking. Moreover, nearly half the teenager deaths from motor vehicle crashes occur during the nighttime hours and more than half take place on weekends (Lescohier & Gal-

TABLE 12.1 *Percentage of High School Students Who Participated in Behaviors that Contribute to Unintentional Injuries, by Gender and Ethnicity—United States,* Youth Risk Behavior Survey, *2001*

Ethnic Group	Rarely or never used seatbelts	Rarely or never used motorcycle helmets	Rarely or never used bicycle helmets	Rode with a driver who had been drinking	Drove after drinking alcohol
White	14%	34%	84%	30%	15%
Female	10	26	81	29	11
Male	18	37	86	30	19
Black	16	45	91	28	8
Female	12	32	90	24	3
Male	18	51	91	31	13
Hispanic	15	55	89	38	13
Female	11	51	87	39	11
Male	18	58	91	37	16
Total	14	37	85	31	13
Female	10	30	83	30	10
Male	18	41	86	32	17

Source: Data from Youth Risk Behavior Surveillance—United States, 2001, by J. A. Grunbaum et al., 2002, *Morbidity and Mortality Weekly Report, 51,* No. SS-4 (pp. 23, 25).

lagher, 1996). In addition, teenagers are the age group least likely to use seatbelts (Saldana & Peterson, 1997).

Because they are a leading killer of young people, injuries are responsible for more lost years of life than any other source. For example, each death through heart disease equals 13 lost years, and each cancer-related death accounts for 16 lost years of life, but each death due to unintentional injury subtracts an average of 35 years from life expectancy (USBC, 2001). Just as older people can reduce their risk of heart disease and cancer by changing their behavior, young people can decrease their risk of unintentional injuries and add to their life expectancy by altering their behavior. Most deaths among high school students are the result of behaviors that contribute to either unintentional or intentional injuries.

The behaviors that lead to unintentional injuries include not using seatbelts, not using bicycle and motorcycle helmets, driving after drinking, and riding with a driver who has been drinking. Jo Anne Grunbaum, Laura Kann, and their associates (Grunbaum et al., 2002) reported that one in seven students in grades 9 to 12 rarely or never used seatbelts while riding in a car or truck driven by someone else and that male students were less likely than female students to use seatbelts. Of students who had ridden a motorcycle during the past year, more than one third rarely or never wore a motorcycle helmet. Grunbaum et al. also found that five out of six students who had ridden a bicycle rarely or never used a helmet. Nearly one third of students nationwide had ridden at least once during the past month with a driver who had been drinking. Although these figures suggest that high school students in the United States engage in many unsafe behaviors, a comparison with 1997 and 1999 data (Kann et al., 1998, 2000) shows a slight trend toward safer behaviors, especially among African American and European American youth.

Some gender and ethnic differences appear in frequency of behaviors contributing to unintentional injuries (Grunbaum et al., 2002), but there were more similarities than differences among the various groups. Table 12.1 shows that high school boys were less likely to use seatbelts than high school girls and much more likely to drive after drinking. African American students were somewhat more reluctant than European American youth to wear helmets and more likely to have ridden with a driver who had been drinking. Nevertheless, different ethnic groups are quite similar in risk-taking behaviors. For example, a very high percentage of high school students in all three ethnic groups rarely or never wore bicycle helmets. This survey revealed that young people, regardless of gender or ethnicity, are willing to engage in a variety of risky behaviors.

Automobile crashes are by far the leading cause of fatal and nonfatal injuries among adolescents and young adults. For young people 15 to 24, about three fourths of fatalities from unintentional injuries are due to motor vehicle crashes. Alcohol has been identified in nearly half the motor vehicle deaths involving teenagers, despite more severe penalties for drunken driving. At the same blood alcohol level, teenager drivers are much more likely than adult drivers to have fatal automobile crashes. As we saw earlier, a significant number of high school students rarely or never use seatbelts (Grunbaum et al., 2002), but disdaining use of seatbelts is not the only dangerous decision young drivers make. The combination of drinking while driving at night and with friends who are not wearing a seatbelt can be a deadly one (Cvijanovich, Cook, Mann, & Dean, 2001). People 15 to 44 years of age not only have a high rate of death from motor vehicle crashes, but they also have the highest number of alcohol-impaired driving episodes (Liu et al., 1997). Alcohol's major contribution to motor vehicle injuries and fatalities among young people comes from three sources: greater risk-taking behavior, fatigue, and impaired psychomotor functioning (Vervialle, Le Breton, Taillard, & Home, 2001).

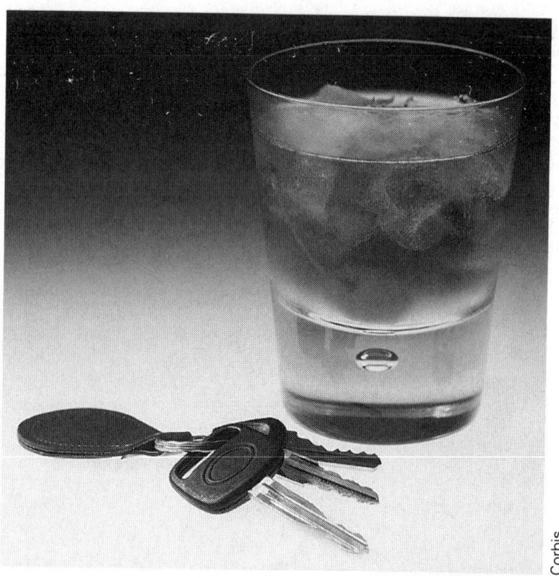

Corbis

Alcohol is a significant contributor to motor vehicle crashes.

During the past 2 decades, the number of bicycle trips more than doubled in the United States, and with that increase came a greater number of injuries, many of which involved alcohol. Indeed, for adolescents and young adults, alcohol is involved in nearly as high a percentage of bicycle-associated fatal injuries as it is in automobile fatalities. One study (Li, Baker, Smialek, & Soderstrom, 2001) found that almost one fourth of fatally injured bicyclists 15 years old or older tested positive for alcohol, and nearly one tenth were legally intoxicated. Compared with bicyclists who had not been drinking, those who were legally drunk were more than 20 times more likely to have had a fatality or serious injury. Also, only 5% of intoxicated riders wore a helmet, whereas 35% of sober riders wore a helmet at the time of the accident.

A case-control study in Finland (Olkkonen & Honkanen, 1990), where bicycling is an important mode of transportation, showed that intoxicated bicyclists had a more than tenfold risk of accidental injury compared with bicyclists who had not been drinking. This study also revealed that bicycle injuries were more likely to result from falling than from collisions. In other words, drunken bicycle riders seem to need neither another vehicle nor a fixed object (other than the road) to injure themselves.

Besides alcohol, failure to use bicycle helmets is an important contributor to unintentional injuries. Nevertheless, as Table 12.1 shows, more than 80% of high school students rarely or never wear helmets while riding a bicycle (Grunbaum et al., 2002).

Alcohol, which is involved in about 40% of drowning deaths, is a dangerous companion to water in at least two ways; it impairs judgment and it reduces dexterity. Death rates from drowning increase through late childhood and early adolescence, reaching a peak at age 18. Gender and ethnicity play a role in drowning deaths; young men are 10 times more likely than young women to die from drowning, and African American youth are three times more likely to drown than European American youth (Lescohier & Gallagher, 1996). James and his friends often went swimming after they had been drinking, and he remembers jumping into water of unknown depth while he was drunk. The next day, he realized how dangerous his behavior was, but drinking and the social situation contributed to his risky behavior.

Gunshot wounds are another source of death and injury for young people. In the United States, most deaths from gunshot wounds are intentional—people aim to shoot others or themselves. Nevertheless, a sizable number of deaths from firearms are unintentional. In the United States, one third of all households with young children have some sort of firearm, and in those homes, one fifth of the guns are kept loaded and unlocked (Berns, 2000). The availability of firearms in the United States results in nearly 500 deaths per year from unintentional gunshot wounds, and most of these deaths are of young people between ages 10 and 19 (Lescohier & Gallagher, 1996). Regardless of intention, firearms are the second leading cause of deaths in every age category from 10 to young adulthood (Berns, 2000). For youths 15 to 19 years old, more than half the unintentional fatalities from firearms were either hunting related or the result of playing with a gun (Lescohier & Gallagher, 1996). Neither James nor any of his friends experienced a firearms injury, and James believes that his awareness of the dangers and his caution when handling guns contributed to this outcome.

Although falls, bicycle mishaps, drowning, and gunshot wounds are responsible for most non-motor vehicle fatalities among young people, sport-related injuries account for far more emergency room visits and more hospitalizations than any other category of unintentional injury. Sports injuries are seldom fatal, but each year an estimated 3 million people seek emergency room treatment because of a sports injury, and nearly all these people are teenagers or young adults (Hambidge, Davidson, Gonzales, Steiner, 2002). As with other unintentional injuries, boys have more than twice the number of sports-related injuries than girls, and that ratio moves to about 3 to 1 for older adolescents.

Adulthood

Whereas the passage from childhood to youth is marked by a vast increase in unintentional fatal injuries, the transition from youth to adulthood brings about little change in a person's risk. As people advance from adolescence and young adulthood to mature adulthood, they have a somewhat smaller overall risk of total unintentional fatalities as well as motor vehicle fatalities (see Figures 12.2 and 12.3). As noted earlier, deaths from motor vehicle crashes have declined during the past 25 years, despite the addition of many more drivers and considerably more miles driven.

Besides improved roads, safer cars, and harsher penalties for drinking under the influence of alcohol, the use of seatbelts and airbags has brought down the number of motor vehicle fatalities. Passenger-side airbags have saved the lives of many adults in frontal and other crashes (Braver, Ferguson, Greene, & Lund, 1997). The use of seatbelts and airbags not only lowers one's chance of death, but it also lessens one's chances of serious injury, for both the driver and passenger. One recent study (Mouzakes et al., 2001) found that a combination of seatbelts and airbags reduced the risk of severe facial injuries by 90% and that seatbelts alone were somewhat more effective than airbags alone in reducing facial injuries.

Compared with younger and middle-aged adults, older adults have higher mortality rates from both total unintentional injuries and from

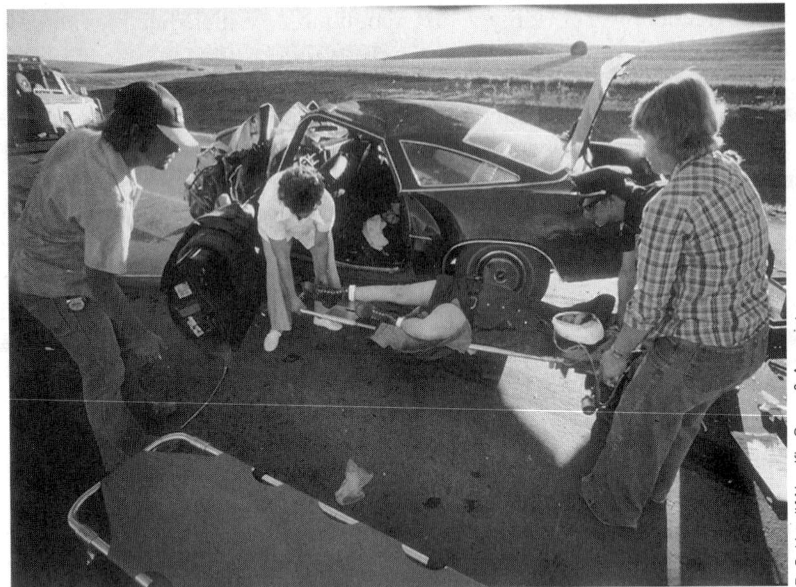

R. S. Uzzell/Woodfin Camp & Associates

Automobile crashes continue to be the leading cause of both fatal and nonfatal injuries in the United States.

motor vehicle injuries. Figure 12.3 shows that people over age 85, compared with those 45 to 64, have double the rate of unintentional fatalities from car crashes. People 85 and older drive only about one third as many miles as do younger adults, but after age 85, the number of fatal crashes per mile rises sharply, thus negating the reduction in total miles driven by older people (Dellinger, Langlois, & Li, 2002). For reasons not yet clear, older drivers who consume alcohol are more likely to be killed or seriously injured than younger individuals who drink while driving (Khattak, Pawlovich, Souleyrette, & Hallmark, 2002).

In addition to automobile crashes, older people die from many of the same unintentional injuries that kill children, especially falls and fires. Children under the age of 5 have an increased risk of death from residential fires, but older people have an even greater risk. After the age of 65, the death rate from residential fires rises sharply as people age. Older people are at an increased risk from residential fires for two possible reasons—infirmity, which can make escape more difficult, and diminished cognitive functioning, which can lead to cooking devices left unattended or improperly used (McGwin, 2000). In addition to falls and fires, older people often die from complications of medical procedures and misuse of legal drugs and medicines.

In contrast to children and older people, who suffer most of their unintentional injuries at home, young and middle-aged adults are most often injured in the workplace. Both gender and ethnic background influence the frequency of workplace injuries. African Americans and men of all ethnic backgrounds are at a higher risk than European Americans and women, largely because they have more hazardous jobs. An examination of all occupation-related deaths over a 15-year period (Loomis & Richardson, 1998) revealed that African Americans had a 36% greater risk of fatal unintentional job-related injuries than European Americans. In this analysis, African American men had the greatest risk followed by European American men, African American women, and European American women. If African Americans and European Americans worked at the same jobs, the gap in occupation-related deaths would almost disappear. The gap, however, would not completely vanish, and African American men would still have a slightly higher mortality rate than European American men, a difference that is difficult to explain (Loomis & Richardson, 1998).

Hazardous industries such as construction, transportation, manufacturing, and agriculture place workers in dangerous conditions, but work conditions are not the only contributor to unintentional injuries on the job; attitudes toward safety also affect injury risk (Cohen & Colligan, 1997). The attitudes of both workers and managers are important in creating a workplace atmosphere that can increase or decrease the risk for injuries. When managers place workers under time pressure to perform hazardous tasks, safety precautions become a lower priority, thereby increasing the chances of injury. Workers contribute to unsafe behaviors when they maintain the attitude that safety practices are for "wimps" and impinge on their freedom to do their job. These attitudes create a climate of disdain for safety measures that increases risk.

Even when danger is acknowledged, managers often believe that safety is the workers' (and not the manager's) responsibility (Eakin, 1997). This belief leads managers to provide safety equipment or procedures but not to provide training or to ensure enforcement of procedures for its use. When injuries occur, such managers blame their employees. Workers who are aware of hazards may not take appropriate precautions because they believe that the hazards are part of the work or that safety procedures are too much trouble. This attitude is consistent with the view that "accidents happen" and are beyond personal control.

In Summary

Unintentional injuries are the fourth leading cause of death in the United States and the leading cause of death among young people. About half of all fatal unintentional injuries are due to motor vehicle crashes—the leading cause of unintentional injuries for all age ranges.

Children under the age of 15 have the lowest death rates from unintentional injuries. Besides motor vehicle crashes, children die from drownings, fires, falls, suffocation, poisoning, and bicycle injuries. For young adults, motor vehicle crashes account for more than four out of five unintentional deaths. The other deaths are largely from falls, bicycle mishaps, drowning, and gunshot wounds. Alcohol is a major contributor to many unintentional injuries among adolescents and young adults. The most common sources of unintentional injuries to adolescents and young adults are sports, but sports-related injuries have a very low mortality rate.

For adults, motor vehicle crashes account for a very high proportion of deaths from unintentional injuries. Older adults have the highest death rate from unintentional injuries and tend to die from motor vehicle crashes, falls, fires, and complications following medical procedures. In all age groups, African American adults have a higher mortality rate from unintentional injuries than European American adults. Much, but not all, of the difference for adults is a result of African Americans working in more hazardous jobs. Many unintentional injuries on the job are a consequence of both managers and workers underestimating the potential hazards of the workplace.

Strategies for Reducing Unintentional Injuries

Death rates from unintentional injuries have been going down, and much of this decline is due to interventions aimed at (1) changing individual behaviors, (2) changing the environment, or (3) changing the law.

Changing the Individual's Behavior

Changing an individual's behavior is one component of a comprehensive program to reduce unintentional injuries. Most of the emphasis on reducing unintentional injuries through changes in the individual's behavior has centered on home safety, workplace safety, motor vehicle safety, and bicycle safety. In all four areas, however, individually oriented interventions have been, at best, only moderately successful.

Strategies to Prevent Home Injuries Psychologist Lizette Peterson and her colleagues (Peterson, DiLillo, Lewis, & Sher, 2002; Peterson & Tremblay, 1999; Saldana & Peterson, 1997) have been concerned with reducing injuries to children, especially those that occur in the home. The most effective interventions to reduce children's injuries are directed at parents. Peterson and Brenda Schick (1993) trained both children and their mothers in setting rules of safe behavior. Using a behavior analysis approach suggested by B. F. Skinner (1953), Peterson and Schick examined minor unintentional injuries experienced by second grade children with respect to the injuries' antecedents, the event itself, and the consequences of the event. Using this analysis as a guide, Peterson and Schick developed categories of rules for injury prevention. Their analysis revealed that most of the injuries could have been avoided if children had followed such basic rules as "Don't walk backwards," "Don't run with anything in your mouth," or "Don't touch, taste, or smell medicines or cleaners." This strategy holds some promise of reducing unintentional injuries to children, provided parents are willing and able to implement such a program. Later, a research project (Heck, Collins, & Peterson, 2001) applied the same behavioral principles to train school age children to adopt behaviors that reduced dangerous behaviors on playground equipment.

Injuries from falls in the home are a serious threat to the health of both infants and many older persons, but strategies to change individual behavior have not been a very effective means of reducing these unintentional injuries. A recent study compared the effectiveness of two programs: (1) safety counseling plus parents' visit to a safety center and (2) these two interventions plus a home safety visit by a community health worker (Gielen et al., 2002). The results indicated that families who visited a children's safety center gained additional information about safety, but this additional information did not result in fewer injuries to the infants whose parents had visited the safety center. Similarly, a study of older members of the Kaiser Permanente health maintenance organization found that a comprehensive program emphasizing home safety, exercise, and risky behaviors reduced the number of falls by only 7% (Hornbrook et al., 1994). Moreover, this study reported that the participants' chances of avoiding falls serious enough to require medical treatment were not significantly improved by the intervention. Results from these studies suggest that interventions aimed at changing behavior of individuals are not, by themselves, sufficient to reduce unintentional injuries in the home.

Strategies to Prevent Workplace Injuries During the 20th century, deaths from workplace injuries declined by more than 90%, a remarkable achievement brought about largely by safer environments (CDC, 1999b). Building safer workplace environments has been a collective endeavor, including efforts by individual workers, unions, employers, and governmental agencies, such as the National Safety Council, the Occupational Safety and Health Administration (OSHA), and the National Institute for Occupational Safety and Health (NIOSH).

Changing the environment is generally a more effective way to prevent workplace injuries than changing individual behavior. Nevertheless, modifying individual behaviors can play an important role in providing a safer workplace. Environmental changes often rely on workers' behavior. For example, protective clothing does not protect when it remains on the rack; ventilation systems do not work unless activated; alarms that have been disconnected to eliminate their annoying noise fail to alert workers of dangers.

Training workers and enforcing safety procedures can reduce workplace injuries by changing individual behavior. Workers cannot behave safely without knowledge and skills that allow them to recognize and avoid dangers on the job (Cohen & Colligan, 1997). Therefore, worker education is one strategy to prevent workplace injuries, and this approach shows some success. Unfortunately, even workers who know what is safe do not always behave accordingly. Pressure to complete tasks and a workplace climate that disdains safety can prevent even knowledgeable and well-trained workers from adhering to safety procedures. Training alone is not sufficient. Developing a workplace climate that values safety is a more important step in creating safer workplaces (Eakin, 1997).

Like any other skill, safety techniques are most effective when workers receive feedback about their performance (Cohen & Colligan, 1997). Many safety training procedures involve only a single training session. One session can provide information and training that prompts behavior changes, but these changes may disappear as workers revert to older behavior patterns. Feedback can help sustain the changes by providing reminders and monitoring new behaviors. The addition of incentives for desirable performance can be even more effective. That is, when principles of behavior modification are applied to safety behaviors, those behaviors increase in frequency.

Strategies to Prevent Motor Vehicle Injuries

Much of the decline in motor vehicle deaths is due to safer cars, better roads, and stricter laws against drunken driving. Two strategies aimed at changing individual behavior center around reducing driver drowsiness and using the designated driver program.

Driving while drowsy, independent of driving while intoxicated, is a risk for both fatal and nonfatal injuries. One team of investigators (Cummings, Koepsell, Moffat, & Rivara, 2001) studied a variety of conditions related to drowsiness. After analyzing data from drivers who had crashed and those who had not, the researchers suggested several behaviors that could reduce motor vehicle crashes. The suggested behaviors included stopping driving when first feeling sleepy, using highway rest stops, drinking coffee, turning on the radio, getting at least 12 hours of sleep during the 48 hours prior to the trip, and on long trips, sharing driving with another person. Most of these strategies seem obvious, but when combined with specific advice, they can significantly reduce drowsy driver's chances of a crash.

Alcohol is an even stronger risk factor for vehicle crashes than drowsiness. One strategy for reducing alcohol-related traffic injuries is the designated driver approach, whereby one person is supposed to abstain from alcohol and be responsible for driving and the overall safety of others in the party. Although this concept has been part of the social norm for a number of years, little evidence exists as to its effectiveness in reducing traffic-related injuries. One study of college students found that 40% of designated drivers did not drink while serving in that capacity (DeJong & Winsten, 1999), but other research indicated that more than 90% of designated drivers drank at least some alcohol (Barr & MacKinnon, 1998). Some observers (DeJong & Wallack, 1992) have argued that powerful economic interests (bars, restaurants, and the alcohol industry) are behind the designated driver concept and that these programs may encourage some underage adolescents to binge drink.

Strategies to Prevent Bicycle-Related Injuries

Fatal and nonfatal bicycle injuries are an important health problem in the United States, with nearly 600,000 bicyclists a year being injured badly enough to require medical attention and nearly 700 dying of various injuries from riding a bicycle. About one third of the injuries and two thirds of the fatalities could have been prevented if the rider had been wearing a protective helmet (Schulman, Sacks, & Provenzano, 2002). Regardless of a bicyclist's age or type of helmet worn, use of a helmet can significantly reduce the number of head injuries, brain injuries, and severe brain injuries, especially in collisions with motor vehicles (Thompson,

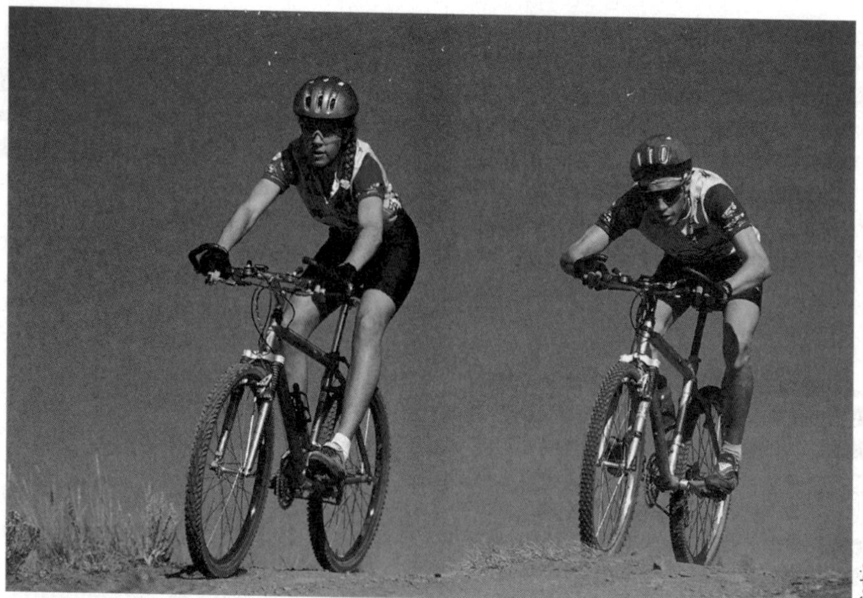

Corbis

Strategies to increase helmet use are effective in reducing bicycle injuries.

Rivara, & Thompson, 1996). Unfortunately, however, 86% of high school students seldom or never wear helmets while riding bicycles (Grunbaum et al., 2002). This situation suggests that more effective interventions are needed to help prevent bicycle-related injuries.

How can use of bicycle helmets be improved? Medical personnel have identified a number of possible barriers to the widespread use of helmets, including high costs, parental lack of interest, inconvenience, discomfort, poor fit, misconceptions about the risk of cycling, lack of knowledge about the effectiveness of a helmet, and negative attitudes of peers concerning the appearance of bicycle helmets, that is, the "nerd" factor (Berg & Westerling, 2001; Thompson & Rivara, 2001). Interventions to increase helmet use must overcome most or all of these barriers. The theory of reasoned action and the theory of planned behavior (see Chapter 3) both suggest that behavior follows intentions, and intentions are, in part, shaped by subjective norms. Thus, if children believe that their peers regard bicycle helmets as fashionable (the social norm), they are more likely to wear them.

Does research support this theoretical position? One study (Frank, Bouman, Cain, & Watts, 1992) indicated that changes in beliefs regarding the seriousness of injuries can lead to changes in safety-oriented behaviors. Additional evidence supports the notion that changes in attitudes and beliefs can alter behavior. For example, a team of Canadian investigators (Farley, Haddad, & Brown, 1996) used a variety of strategies in two similar communities to increase bicycle helmet use among children 5 to 12 years old. In the experimental community, the children were exposed to educational activities designed to change attitudes and beliefs regarding helmet use, discount coupons to purchase helmets, and reinforcement for wearing helmets. Children in the control community received no specific intervention. Children in cities that received the intervention increased bicycle helmet use from a very low rate of 1.3% to 33% after 4 years. During this same time, children in the control cities also increased their use of helmets but only to a level less than half that of children in the exposed cities.

Thus, theory and research have combined to provide effective strategies for increasing helmet use. However, the problem of implementing these tactics on an individual basis remains a huge hurdle to the regular use of bicycle helmets. As with other unintentional injury topics, changing the environment or enacting and enforcing legislation may be more efficient means of reducing fatal and nonfatal injuries.

Changing the Environment

A second strategy for reducing unintentional injuries is to make changes in the environment. Such an approach includes building safer cars and roads, manufacturing better bicycle and motorcycle helmets, and making the home and workplace safer. Although some of the changes may require new legislation, others have been and can be made without changing laws. For example, no law mandates that smoke alarms be placed in every residence. Yet state and local health departments, aided by mass advertising, information campaigns, and giveaway programs have placed smoke alarms in nearly all of U.S. households (CDC, 1998b); the presence of these alarms has cut residential fire-related deaths by 89% in one large investigation (Towner, Dowswell, & Jarvis, 2001). Also, people's demand for safer cars was an incentive for automobile manufacturers to build cars with seatbelts and airbags long before legislation mandated passive restraints. Similar environmental changes can be effective means of reducing unintentional injuries.

An example of modifying the environment was reported by one research team (Paul, Sanson-Fisher, Redman, & Carter, 1994) that trained volunteers to go into the homes of people with young children and check for unsafe conditions. More than three of every four homes had multiple safety hazards, but after residents became aware of these hazards, they made significant reductions in the number of dangerous environmental conditions. A more comprehensive approach (Davidson et al., 1994) targeted major hazards of 5- to 16-year-old children's environment. This program, conducted in Harlem and called the Safe Kids/Healthy Neighborhoods Injury Prevention Program, included such environmental interventions as (1) renovating playgrounds; (2) involving children and adolescents in safe, supervised activities, such as dance, art, sports, and carpentry; (3) conducting injury and violence prevention classes; and (4) providing bicycle helmets and other safety equipment. In a comparison of injuries during and after the intervention and injuries from the preceding years, the targeted age group cut their number of injuries nearly in half, thus indicating that a comprehensive program to alter specific environmental conditions can successfully reduce the rate of injury.

However, when people must make a major effort or a substantial financial commitment toward a safer environment, multifaceted community interventions are less successful. A comprehensive injury prevention program in an African American community in Philadelphia (Schwarz, Grisso, Miles, Holmes, & Sutton, 1993) consisted of (1) making simple modifications in the home such as providing smoke detectors, water thermometers, night lights, poison prevention supplies, and emergency telephone numbers; (2) inspecting the home to inform residents of hazards and ways to eliminate or reduce them; and (3) educating residents about specific injury prevention practices. After 12 months, residents in the intervention homes had more knowledge of injury prevention and had more safety supplies available than did residents in the control homes. However, the investigators found no difference between the intervention group and the control group in home hazards that required a major effort to correct. These results suggest that lack of money and lack of control over one's environment lead to an inability to comply with many injury-prevention strategies that call for changes in one's environment.

Changing the Law

In general, legal interventions that require safety have been more effective than either individual interventions or environmental manipulations

(Zador & Ciccone, 1993). Children now live in a safer environment because of laws that require protective action or prohibit the manufacture of hazardous products that can kill or injure children.

Many of the laws passed during the past 40 years have been designed to protect children, and the decreasing rate of children's deaths from unintentional injuries closely parallels the passage of safety legislation. During the 1960s and 1970s, many children suffocated inside abandoned refrigerators because there was no way to open the door from the inside. Since passage of the Refrigerator Safety Act, which banned products that could not be opened from the inside, children's' deaths from asphyxiation have been nearly eliminated (Durlak, 1997).

Similarly, the Poison Prevention Packaging Act of 1970, which mandated that dangerous household substances such as aspirin, paint solvent, and prescription drugs be sold in special packaging, has cut the number of children's deaths from poisoning to one fourth the previous rate. Laws banning cribs that could strangle infants and clothes that could easily catch fire have saved the lives of many children (Peterson & Gable, 1997). Child access prevention laws that hold adults criminally liable for unsafe storage of guns that lead to children being killed or injured is associated with a significant reduction of children's deaths from firearms (Webster & Starnes, 2000).

Children are injured and die from motor vehicle crashes more often than from any other cause, and legislation has been aimed at preventing children's deaths. In the United States, all 50 states and all territories have laws that mandate protection of children in motor vehicles (National Safe Kids Campaign, 1997). These laws vary in their requirements and enforcement, but the existence of laws increases the use of restraints, which in turn decreases the rate of injury and death to children riding in vehicles.

Laws mandating the use of bicycle helmets have been effective in preventing head injuries. Unfortunately, most state laws do not mandate helmet use after age 15 (Thompson & Rivara, 2001), and adolescents are likely to disdain the use of helmets (Grunbaum et al., 2002). A study in Florida (Kanny, Schieber, Pryor, & Kresnow, 2001) sought to determine the effectiveness of laws requiring helmet use. The researchers compared rate of helmet use in the 60 counties that had enacted laws requiring children under the age of 16 to wear a helmet with three counties that had no such laws. In general, children in the counties with helmet laws were more than twice as likely as those in the other counties to wear a helmet while riding a bicycle. More specifically, all ethnic groups reached at least 60% compliance in the counties mandating helmet use. In addition, both boys and girls increased compliance by at least 50%. These studies suggest that laws can increase injury-prevention behaviors among children and adolescents.

Laws have also decreased unintentional injuries in adults. In 1970, the Occupational Safety and Health Administration (OSHA) was founded to prevent injury and illness among U.S. workers (OSHA, 1998). This regulatory administration is part of the U.S. Department of Labor and employs inspectors to ensure compliance with workplace safety regulations, and its staff helps employers to develop safety and health programs. OSHA recognizes businesses that have excellent safety programs, and these businesses serve as models for others. The substantial decreases in workplace unintentional death and injury during the past 70 years (CDC, 1999b) point to the effectiveness of such an approach to increasing safety.

Laws that require seatbelt use have also had a positive impact on the rate of injuries and deaths from automobile crashes (National Highway Traffic Safety Administration [NHTSA], 1998), increasing use to over 60%. Another legal intervention that has improved vehicle safety is the requirement that new vehicles be equipped with driver and passenger airbags, which went into effect for cars with model year 1998 and for trucks for model year 1999. Airbags decrease fatalities by about one third but pose hazards for adults who are not properly seated or are not belted into their seats correctly (Braver et al., 1997). In ad-

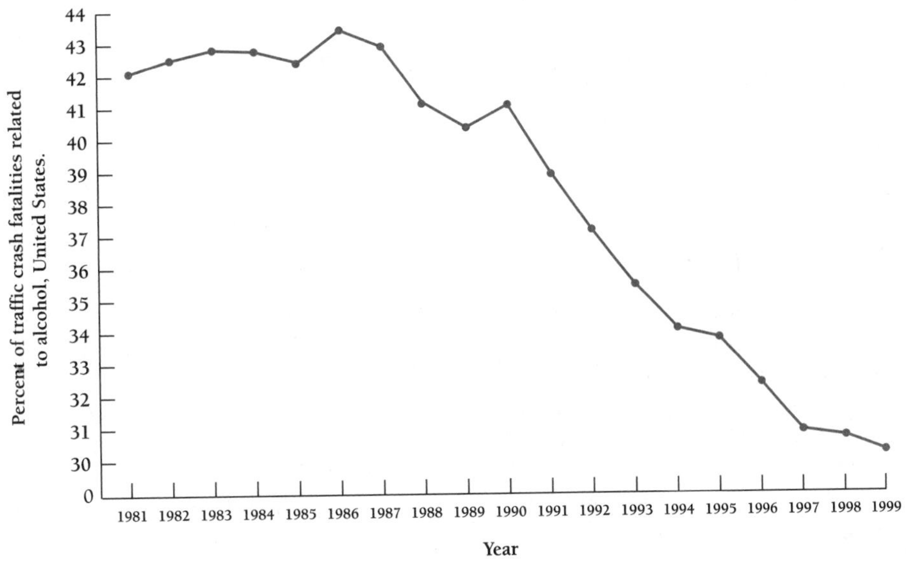

Figure 12.4 Percent of traffic crash fatalities involving alcohol, United States, 1981–1999.

Source: Data from Trends in alcohol-related fatal traffic crashes, United States, 1977–99, by H. Yi, C. D. Williams, & M. C. Dufour, 2001, Alcohol Epidemiologic Data System. Surveillance Report #56. *Rockville, MD: National Institute on Alcohol Abuse and Alcoholism, (December 2001).*

dition, airbags are a risk for children riding in the front seat, leading to the recommendation that children younger than 12 should not ride in the front seat of a vehicle. Despite these risks, airbags significantly decrease the risk to drivers and adult passengers during crashes, and the laws and regulations mandating their inclusion have been effective in decreasing risk.

Increasing the legal drinking age to 21 has led to a decline in alcohol-related motor vehicle injuries (Hingson, Heeren, Jamanka, & Howland, 2000). A survey of young drivers both before and after their state passed a law lowering the legal blood alcohol limit (Wagenaar, O'Malley, & LaFond, 2001) revealed a substantial reduction in driving after drinking. Also, harsher penalties for DWI seem to have lowered the rate of alcohol-related traffic crash fatalities. Figure 12.4 shows that since 1990, the percent of traffic crash fatalities in which alcohol was involved dropped steadily after several years of little change (Yi, Williams, & Dufour, 2001). Such evidence does not prove the effectiveness of legal interventions, but it does suggest that raising the drinking age and strictly reinforcing laws prohibiting drinking and driving may be two of several factors lowering the percent of traffic fatalities involving alcohol.

A combination of interventions aimed at the individual, the environment, and the law (including severe penalties for noncompliance) offers the most promise in preventing all types of unintentional injuries.

In Summary

Interventions for reducing unintentional injuries can be aimed at changing the individual's behavior, changing the environment, or changing legislation. Change in individual behavior is a goal of strategies to prevent home injuries, workplace injuries, motor vehicle injuries, and bicycle-related injuries.

Programs to prevent home injuries frequently target children and older people, but most of these programs have not been very successful. Changing worker behavior is not the preferred strategy for creating safer workplaces, but some interventions have prompted workers to use safety equipment and to follow safe procedures. Strategies, such as having a designated driver, that attempt to reduce motor vehicle fatalities by emphasizing individual behavior have been only marginally successful. Also, individualized approaches to increasing bicycle helmet use are not very effective, but when the cost of helmets goes down and their social acceptance goes up, adults and children are more likely to buy and use them.

Strategies to alter the environment are generally more successful than those that attempt change through individual interventions. Environmental changes include building safer cars and roads, making the home and neighborhood safer, and providing safer equipment for workers.

Laws, too, can have an impact on reducing unintentional injuries. Laws requiring child protection in motor vehicles, childproof medicine containers, flame-retardant clothing, refrigerators that open from the inside, the use of automobile seatbelts and bicycle helmets, and raising the legal drinking age have saved many lives and prevented thousands of serious injuries.

Intentional Injuries

Unintentional injuries are the leading cause of death for people in the United States below age 35, but intentional injuries are also among the leading causes of death for this age group. Both suicide and homicide are among the top 10 leading causes of death for children and youth, and many young people suffer nonfatal injuries as a result of the violent acts of others. Violence is a more common cause of injury and death in the United States than in other industrialized nations (Acierno, Resnick, & Kilpatrick, 1997), with violent crimes occurring at a rate of about 8 per 1,000 people. The settings for violence and its effects differ over the lifespan.

Childhood

Childhood is a period during which mortality rates are low. Children between ages 5 and 9 years have the lowest death rate for any age group (National Center for Injury Prevention and Control, 1998), but younger and older children are somewhat more vulnerable. Their risks are the highest for unintentional injuries, but children are also in danger from intentional violence, most often at the hands of their parents (U.S. Department of Health and Human Services [USDHHS] Administration on Children, Youth, and Families, 2001). Child maltreatment is by no means a recent phenomenon (ten Bensel, Rheinberger, & Radbill, 1997), but the identification of child battering as a social problem and its definition as a crime did not occur on a national level until the 1960s. Treating infants with skull and long bone fractures led pediatricians and radiologists to recognize that these injuries were caused by beatings. Evidence began to accumulate that such beatings were common and a major source of injury for infants and children.

Injuries at different ages during childhood have varying consequences, but such injuries have some consequences for all children (Kempe, 1997). One common result of intentional injuries is that abused children may be vigilant and feel threatened in a variety of situations—the world becomes a dangerous place. Abused children also tend to be fearful about rejection, abandonment, and additional abuse. Mistrust and poor self-esteem are problems common to abused persons of all ages. Problems in the nurturing relationship lead abused children to be thwarted in their attempts to seek nurturance. These children often grow to adulthood displaying aggressive behaviors, lacking the ability to adequately express emotions, and having inadequate cognitive and problem-solving skills.

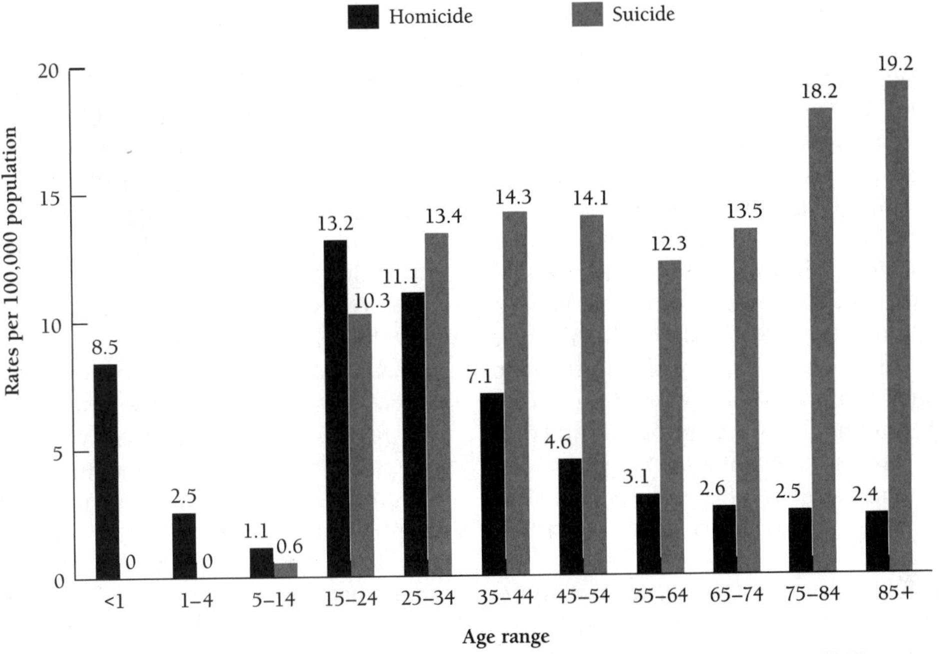

Figure 12.5 Homicide and suicide rates over the lifespan (per 100,000 population), 1999.

Source: Data from Health, United States, 2001, *(pp. 214, 217) National Center for Health Statistics, 2001, Hyattsville, MD: U.S. Government Printing Office.*

Infancy is a time during which children are particularly vulnerable and during which children are most likely to suffer from violence. Abuse is the leading cause of death for infants after the prenatal period, making the first year of life the most dangerous single year during childhood (USDHHS Administration on Children, Youth, and Families, 2001). Figure 12.5 shows the death rate for homicide at all ages, including infants' heightened vulnerability. Children injured during infancy are at risk for permanent damage to their nervous systems, which can lead to cognitive and developmental problems (Kempe, 1997).

Adults who abuse children were almost always abused themselves, but not all people who were abused during childhood become abusers. Many have experiences that compensate for the abuse, forming relationships that allow them to feel valued and safe in some ways and grow up to become good parents. However, children who do not form such relationships are at high risk to become abusers themselves.

Abuse can prevent children from accomplishing some of the developmental tasks of young childhood (Kempe, 1997), including forming attachments to others (usually parents), seeing themselves as separate individuals, and developing physical, cognitive, and language skills. Abuse during early childhood can impede the development of these tasks and impair children's ability to get along with their age-mates and to do well in school.

School-age children and adolescents who are abused may exhibit symptoms of psychopathology or behavior disorders (Dube et al., 2001). Physical abuse may continue during middle childhood, but it is not as likely to be initiated at this age as is sexual abuse. Girls between ages 10 and 13 are particularly vulnerable to sexual abuse, but boys are also victims (USDHHS Administration on Children, Youth, and Families,

2001). Biological fathers are much more likely than mothers to be perpetrators, but stepfathers and boyfriends are also frequent perpetrators, along with other male family members and adults in positions of trust.

Children are also exposed to violence in their communities, and children in poor urban neighborhoods are particularly vulnerable (Buka, Stichick, Birdthistle, & Earls, 2001). The dramatic increase in youth violence that began during the late 1980s affected children, who were often witnesses to violence in their communities and schools. Surveys of inner-city children reveal that between one fourth and one half have witnessed shootings, muggings, or stabbings, and as many as 30% reported that they have been mugged or threatened with a weapon.

Older children and adolescents are even more likely to be witnesses and victims of such violence. In many cases, those who witness violence are acquainted with both the victims and the assailants, making the experience more traumatic. Children exposed to violence can develop post-traumatic stress disorder (PTSD) and other stress-related and anxiety problems.

Youth

Violence is a more pervasive problem for adolescents and young adults than for children, and adolescents are substantially more likely than adults to be victims of violence (Hashima & Finkelhor, 1999). Unlike children, adolescents are frequent perpetrators of both minor and serious violence. In a survey of high school students (Grunbaum et al., 2002), about 43% of boys and 24% of girls had been in a physical fight during the previous 12 months; 4% of all students were injured in a fight. In addition to homicide, suicide is ranked among the leading causes of death beginning with 10-year-olds. Figure 12.5 shows the dramatic increase in both homicide and suicide beginning at age 15.

Neither homicide nor suicide rates reveal the full picture of violence: between 100 and 400 assaults occur for each homicide (Garbarino & Kostelny, 1997), and up to 20 suicide attempts exist for each suicide death (U.S. Department of Health and Human Services, 2001). A survey of high school students (Grunbaum et al., 2002) found that 24% of girls and 14% of boys had seriously considered attempting suicide, and nearly 8% of all students had made at least one attempt at suicide. The types and settings for youth violence are varied, and some young people are at much higher risk than others.

Being young and living in the United States are two conditions that place many people at risk for violence. Compared with other age groups and other countries, young people who live in the United States have an increased risk of intentional injury or death (Garbarino & Kostelny, 1997). In addition, economic factors, ethnic background, and gender all influence risks for being involved in violence either as a perpetrator or as a victim. Poor mental health, drug use, and problems at school are associated with violent behavior (Ellickson, Saner, & McGuigan, 1997). Poverty is a risk factor, and living in a poor neighborhood is often synonymous with living in a high-crime neighborhood (Greenberg & Schneider, 1994). Poverty tends to be associated with ethnic minority status in the United States, putting ethnic minority youth at increased risk (but also elevating the risk for all people living in these neighborhoods). Young men are more likely to be both perpetrators and victims of physical violence than young women. Those factors combine to put young African American men at particularly high risk for homicide.

Young African American men are much more likely to die from homicide than any other segment of U.S. society, including young European American men and African Americans in other age groups. For example, the death rate from homicide by firearms is about five times higher among male African Americans ages 15 to 24 than it is for male European Americans of the same age (NCHS, 2001). For all age groups, African Americans are nearly seven times more

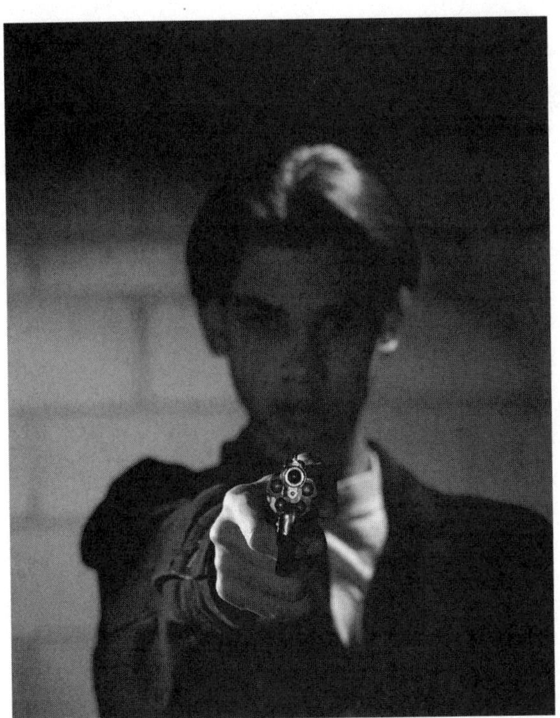

Access to guns is a significant factor in the deadliness of violence among youth.

likely to be victims of murder than European Americans. Figure 12.6 contrasts the homicide rates by ethnicity and gender of victims from 1980 to 1999. Note the sharp decrease in homicide for both genders and both ethnic groups in recent years after a peak in the early 1990s. Despite widespread publicity about growing violence, homicide rates are actually decreasing, but the rates for young African American men—despite their recent decline—continue to be much higher than for other groups.

Gender is also a factor in assaults. Young men are more likely to be both targets and perpetrators, but the methods of injury differ. Young men are more likely be shot, whereas young women are more likely to be stabbed, with injuries tending to occur in their homes (Moskowitz, Griffith, DiScala, & Sege, 2001). Young women are at higher risk for sexual assault (Heise, Ellsberg, & Gottemoeller, 1999). Between half and two thirds of all sexual assaults occur before the victims reach age 18, making late childhood and adolescence a vulnerable time. Unfortunately, those who have been victimized are at increased risk for future incidents. Ethnicity is also a factor, with non-Hispanic European American women at higher risk than Hispanic American or African American women. The official reports of rape do not capture the magnitude of the problem, because a large majority of victims of sexual assault do not report the incident to police and are thus not counted in the official crime statistics. When they are forced to have sex, men are even less likely than women to report to authorities. Perhaps as few as 16% of sexual assaults are reported to police, but about half of all rape victims experience either minor or serious physical injury as a result of the sexual assault. In addition to physical injury, assault and rape increase the risk for mental health problems that are related to suicide (Koss & Kilpatrick, 2001).

Access to weapons contributes to the increased deadliness of violence among adolescents versus children. In 2001, about 29% of high school boys and 6% of girls reported that they had carried a gun, knife, or club during the 30 days preceding the survey (Grunbaum et al., 2002), but this represents a drop from 1993, when 34% of high school boys and 9% of high school girls reported carrying a weapon to school (Kann et al., 1995). In high-violence neighborhoods, the percentages are higher. Nearly half of inner-city 7th- and 8th-grade boys in one survey (Webster, Gainer, & Champion, 1993) carried knives and one fourth carried guns. Among 7th- and 8th-grade girls, 37% carried a knife. Although adolescents report that they believe their schools are dangerous and they are in need of self-protection, these junior high school students carried guns more for aggressive purposes than for defensive reasons. Indeed, students in elementary and middle school who owned guns were likely to do so in order to gain respect, frighten, and bully others (Cunningham, Henggeler, Limber, Melton, & Nation, 2000).

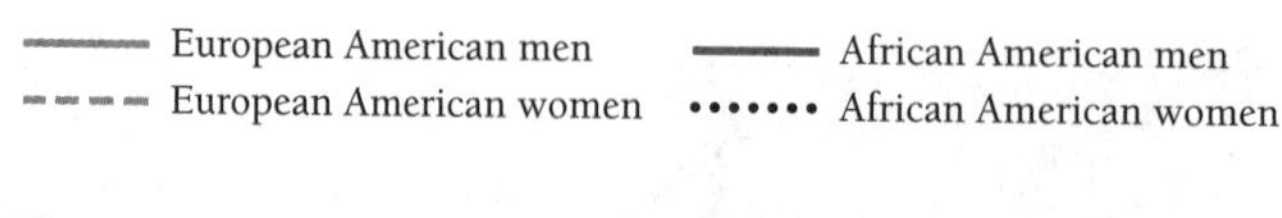

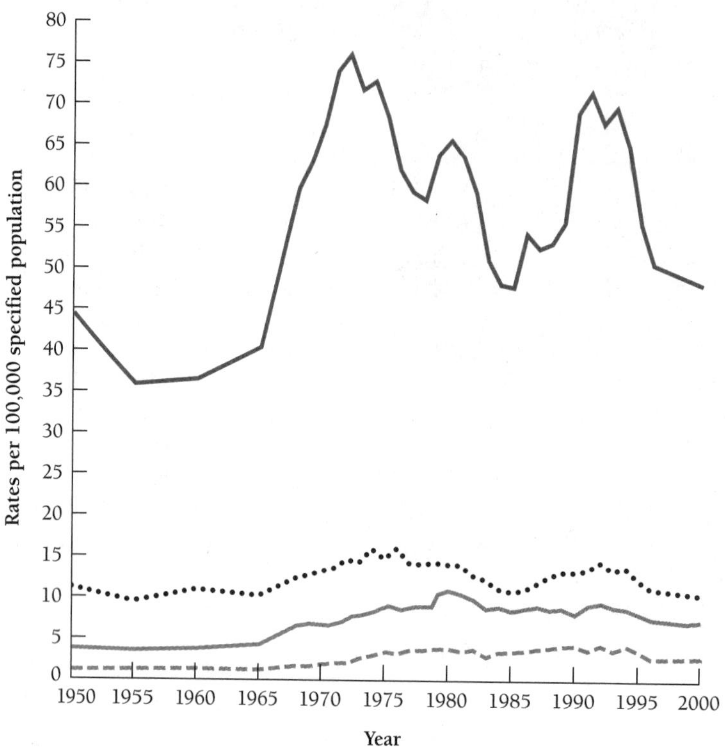

Figure 12.6 Homicide rates in the United States by ethnicity and gender of victim, 1950–1999 (rates per 100,000 of specified population).

Source: Data from Health, United States 2001, *(p. 214) National Center for Health Statistics, 2001, Hyattsville, MD: U.S. Government Printing Office.*

Easy access to firearms is a factor in homicide and suicide among young people: firearms are used in a majority of homicides and suicides among youth (O'Donnell, 1995). Federal laws prohibit gun sales to adolescents, but they have access to firearms through family and friends as well as through theft. Young people with behavior problems are more likely than other adolescents to carry a gun (Cunningham et al., 2000), and over three fourths of young people with guns are involved in gangs, drugs, or other illegal activities. About 30% of adolescents with guns have used them to shoot at someone.

Weapon-related violence received a great deal of publicity due to a series of shootings in U.S. public schools beginning in 1997 (Witkin, Tharp, Schrof, Toch, & Scattarella, 1998). The children who committed these shootings gained access to a variety of guns, which are more plentiful than in years past. With easy access to guns, adolescents who are troubled and angry can fantasize about revenge, and the publicity over each shooting made this action attractive to others, promoting additional shootings. The school shootings brought publicity, but school violence has been a topic of concern to educators for years. Bringing weapons to school has been one focus of this concern, but fights without weapons have been the most common type of school violence during recent years (National

Education Association, 1998). The publicity generated by the shootings has given a boost to strategies to reduce school violence.

The increased access to weapons has not only led to an increase in homicide and assault-related injuries among teenagers, but it has also contributed to suicide attempts among young people (Resnick et al., 1997). The risk factors for suicide attempts among youth are similar to risk factors for other age groups—easy access to weapons, alcohol and drugs, feelings of isolation, lack of social support, and low self-esteem. Also, junior high and high school students who lack a sense of being connected to family or school are at significantly increased risk for suicide attempts. In young people, estrangement from family and trouble in romantic relationships can lead to the feelings of isolation that are related to suicide attempts (Lester, 1994). Being gay or bisexual also increases the suicide risk for young men (Remafedi, French, Story, Resnick, & Blum, 1998). Because youth suicide produces so many years of lost life, many prevention strategies are aimed at this age group (USDHHS, 2001).

Adulthood

Intentional violence is also a cause of injury and death for adults, but the context of this violence shows some differences from violence in youth. As Figure 12.5 shows, suicide becomes a more common cause of death than homicide beginning at age 25; the number of suicides increases and homicides decreases. Violence in the streets and workplace has an impact on adults, but homes are more dangerous (Carden, 1994). Domestic violence is a major cause of injury and death, and partner violence and elder abuse are the two varieties of domestic abuse that affect adults. In addition, intentional injuries occur in the workplace as well as on the streets and in homes. Therefore, adulthood is a period during which intentional violence continues to be a source of death and injury.

The same social and economic factors that influence violence in youth apply to adults as well. Income level, ethnicity, and gender relate to risk of victimization. These factors converge in inner-city neighborhoods, putting poor African American men at increased risk for street violence. Men are more likely than women to be murder victims for all income levels, ages, and ethnicities (NCHS, 2001), but adults over age 25 are much less likely than those between 15 and 24 to be victims. Street violence becomes less of a risk for adults, but violence at home remains a major problem.

The scope of worldwide domestic violence is beginning to become clear (Heise et al., 1999). In some societies, a majority of women report violence at the hands of male family members. Many societies include cultural values that allow this abuse to occur, and women have little recourse and sometimes few options. Similar to women in the United States, abused women around the world report that they are dependent on the men who abuse them and have no economic resources that would allow them to leave the abusive relationship. Beginning in the 1990s, international organizations such as the United Nations emphasized these problems and organized efforts to combat them.

Early publicity on domestic violence focused on husbands who physically abused their wives, but research soon appeared indicating that women also initiate partner violence. In a representative sample of young adults in New Zealand (Magdol et al., 1997), women were more likely to be perpetrators of violent acts than men, although serious violence was unusual for either. For severe domestic violence, men were more common perpetrators than women. This finding is consistent with other research (Hale-Carlsson et al., 1996; Kurz, 1997) showing that women are more likely to be injured as a result of partner abuse.

Michael Johnson (1995) argued that domestic violence can be divided into two types. He called one type common couple violence, which fits into the pattern of conflicts in which an argument escalates into a fight. The physical violence can be minor, but when it becomes serious, women are

WOULD YOU BELIEVE

Cholesterol Level Is Related to Violent Death

Would you believe that having a low cholesterol level may *increase* your chance of violent death, including suicide? Since the 1980s, evidence has been accumulating that, despite the positive relationship between cholesterol levels and incidence of coronary artery disease, low cholesterol does not lower all-cause mortality. Curiously, there seems to be a U-shaped relationship between total cholesterol and death from all causes, with both high and low levels of cholesterol associated with higher death rates. For example, two early studies (Holme, 1990; Iso et al. 1989) indicated that men with either very high or very low total cholesterol levels had a much higher death rate than men with cholesterol levels between 180 and 220.

The possibility that violent deaths account for the difference was confirmed by two meta-analyses (Cummings & Psaty, 1994; Muldoon, Manuck, & Matthews, 1992), which revealed that men with low levels of cholesterol had significantly higher rates of deaths from violence or suicide. But why should low cholesterol be related to violent death? Researchers looking for the underlying connection discovered a link between low cholesterol and depression in men over 70 (Morgan, Palinkas, Barrett-Connor, & Wingard, 1993). Depression was about three times higher for men with cholesterol below 160 than for those with higher cholesterol.

Most of the earlier studies demonstrating a link between lower cholesterol and violent death involved participants on a low-fat diet who may have been experiencing the unpleasantness of such a diet. Could this deprivation have made them irritable and thus aggressive? Existing evidence does not support this hypothesis. A study of psychiatric patients (Mufti, Balon, & Arfken, 1998) found that the strong relationship between low cholesterol levels and violent behavior could not be accounted for by cholesterol-lowering medication, alcohol use, or diet. However, research with animals by Jay Kaplan and his associates (Kaplan, Fontenot, Manuck, & Muldoon, 1996) found that monkeys on a cholesterol-lowering diet behaved more aggressively than those on a high-fat diet, suggesting that a low-fat diet may be at least partially responsible for aggressive and violent behavior.

The frequently observed relationship between low cholesterol and violent death has led many authorities to rethink the standard recommendation to lower cholesterol. If gains from decreased heart disease deaths are offset by increased deaths from other causes (including violent deaths), should people stop trying to lower their cholesterol?

If deciding whether or not you should continue efforts to lower your total cholesterol, you should be aware of several points. First, the studies we have discussed included people with very low total cholesterol, below 140 or even lower. Second, a recent meta-analysis of the effectiveness of drug interventions to lower total cholesterol found no significant increase in non-illness mortality as cholesterol dropped (Muldoon, Manuck, Mendelsohn, Kaplan, & Belle, 2001). So, if you are taking a drug to lower your cholesterol to the average range, you should continue to do so. Third, recall evidence from Chapter 9 that total cholesterol levels are not as important as the ratio of total cholesterol to high-density lipoprotein (HLD). Our best advice is to maintain a cholesterol level between about 170 and 200, with a ratio of total cholesterol to HLD of about 4.5 to 1 or lower.

more likely than men to be injured. Johnson termed the other type of domestic violence *patriarchal terrorism,* which describes a situation in which a man dominates his family by using physical force as well as other control strategies. This pattern of domestic violence is an extension of male dominance in families and results in injury and death to both women and children. This description is consistent with that of partner violence in many societies (Heise et al., 1999). In summary, women are more likely than men to be homicide victims as a result of domestic violence and more likely to be injured or killed by an intimate partner than by a stranger.

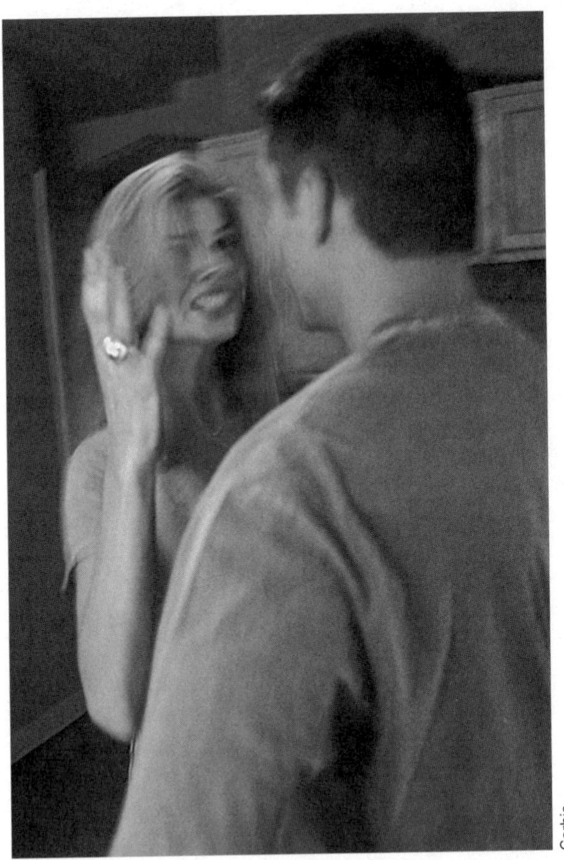
Corbis

Domestic disagreements can escalate into domestic abuse.

Availability of weapons is also a factor in domestic violence and suicide. Having a loaded gun in the house is a way to turn an argument into a homicide. Because shooting is one of the most effective methods of killing oneself, having a gun also increases the odds that a suicide attempt will be completed. Thus, having a gun in the house increases the risk of both homicide and suicide. Other factors that relate to suicide are a history of mental illness and living alone (Bailey et al., 1997).

Domestic violence can spill out into the workplace. A number of homicides have occurred when angry spouses entered a workplace and attacked or killed their partners as well as others who happened to be present (Solomon, 1998). Other workplace violence incidents involve angry employees or former employees who threaten, harm, or kill supervisors or coworkers. These two types of violence may be related, and perpetrators of domestic violence are at increased risk for workplace violence as well (Brownell, 1996). Workplace violence does not come "out of nowhere," and both corporate policy and workers' behavior can be predictors of violent outbursts. For example, a failure to set limits on harassment and intimidation or insensitive discipline and terminations can lead to employee violence. In addition, a failure to take the possibility of violence seriously can endanger managers and human resources personnel (Caudron, 1998).

The gender difference in risk for violence applies to suicide: men are more likely to commit suicide than women, especially at younger ages. In addition, suicide rates vary a great deal among countries (Ruzicka, 1995). For example, Hungary has the highest rate and Greece the lowest. In most developed countries, suicide rates increased during the past 15 years. The United States has a suicide rate in the lower half of the distribution of countries, similar to the rates in Canada and Japan. In the United States, variation occurs among ethnic groups, and European Americans have the highest suicide rates, followed by Native Americans (NCHS, 2001). African Americans, Hispanic Americans, and Asian Americans commit suicide only about half as often, and some Native American tribes have much lower rates than others do.

Alcohol is connected to suicide and suicide attempts in people of nearly every age and ethnic background (USDHHS, 2001). This connection may come through alcohol's disinhibiting effects; some people may decide to kill themselves while sober and then use alcohol as an anesthetic. However, an inability to control alcohol consumption is related to one's chances of attempting suicide, and people diagnosed with alcoholism are at increased risk for suicide. People with drinking problems are often also depressed; feelings of despair and hopelessness lead some people to both abuse alcohol and to attempt suicide.

Suicide also varies with age. Youth suicide has gained a great deal of publicity, but adults are even more likely to commit suicide. Suicides among older adults account for a lower percentage of their deaths but only because older people have higher rates of death from other causes. Figure 12.5 shows that suicide rates are higher for middle-aged adults than for youth and even higher among older people. Indeed, individuals over age 85 have the highest suicide rate of any age category.

Older people are also at risk for violence from others, which can come from family caregivers in the home or from professional caregivers in institutions. Elder abuse includes physical, psychological, sexual, or financial abuse or neglect of older people (Chalk & King, 1998). This type of domestic violence is less common than child abuse or partner violence but still constitutes a substantial problem.

Being in need of care puts older people at risk for emotional, physical, and possibly financial dependence on others, who may be abusive or neglectful. Risk factors for elder abuse include functional impairment and cognitive disability as well as age and economic dependence (National Center on Elder Abuse, 1998). Caring for elders who are poor or who are functionally or cognitively impaired places burdens on caregivers that may be overwhelming. Thus, factors that make caregiving more stressful increase the risk for abuse. In addition, lack of awareness of the specific needs of older people can contribute to neglect.

Elder abuse is a significant risk for older people, affecting over half a million people per year in the United States (National Center on Elder Abuse, 1998). Like other types of domestic violence, elder abuse can be difficult to diagnose because the abused person depends on the abuser and may be reluctant to complain to authorities. In addition, physicians may not be alert to the possibility of abuse or reluctant to intervene.

In Summary

Intentional violence is a problem that affects people throughout the lifespan. For children, homicide is one of the leading causes of death, and violence is a major source of injury. This violence can come from abuse by parents and from exposure to community violence. Abuse not only causes injury but also can prevent children from accomplishing developmental tasks such as forming close relationships and learning problem-solving skills. In addition to physical abuse, children are at risk for sexual abuse, with girls at higher risk than boys.

Young people are the perpetrators as well as victims of violence. Several types of violence affect youth, including community violence, school violence, sexual assault, homicide, and suicide. Young men are at higher risk than young women for all types of violence except sexual assault. In addition to gender, several risk factors combine to put young African American men living in inner-city neighborhoods at a sharply increased risk for assault and homicide in both their communities and their schools. Availability of firearms is one factor that relates to the deadliness of violence. Several well-publicized school shootings highlighted the easy availability of guns for youth, but school violence was a problem years before these incidents brought the problem to public attention. Access to firearms also relates to suicide risk for youth.

Adults are also in jeopardy from violence. Two types of domestic violence—partner abuse and elder abuse—affect adults. In addition, adults experience violence in their communities and workplaces. People in intimate relationships behave violently toward each other, but women are the targets of the most severe attacks and suffer more injuries than men from partner abuse. The availability of firearms can turn partner abuse into homicide. Community violence rates are lower for adults than for adolescents, but suicide rates increase with increasing age. Elder abuse can occur in the form of physical, emotional, or financial abuse or neglect of older people. Thus, all age groups are at risk for various types of intentional violence.

Strategies to Reduce Intentional Injuries

Strategies for reducing intentional injuries include interventions aimed at changing individual behavior, the environment, and the law. The interventions tend to be aimed at specific problems, and some strategies for reducing intentional injuries combine changes in individual behavior, the environment, and the law. Indeed, changes in all three will be necessary to make substantial progress in reducing intentional injuries. Joyce Osofsky (1997) contended that individual efforts to reduce various types of violence must be supplemented by a national campaign in the media to "change the image of violence from one that is acceptable, even admired, to something disdained and considered unacceptable" (p. 326). Such a strategy would go beyond any of the three approaches to changing public opinion. Enactments of this strategy have begun and include presidential proclamation about domestic violence and child abuse, community programs to raise awareness of domestic and family violence, and school-based programs to decrease sexual abuse, interpersonal conflicts, and bullying.

Domestic Violence

Three types of domestic violence—child abuse, partner violence, and elder abuse—have been targets of interventions. However, child abuse prevention differs from partner violence interventions, and both differ from programs aimed at elder abuse. One overarching problem with all domestic abuse programs is the sparseness of evaluations for their effectiveness. According to the report of a special committee assembled to evaluate domestic violence interventions (Chalk & King, 1998), services are fragmented by jurisdiction and specialty, and evaluations for effectiveness are not routine. Therefore, many programs with intuitive appeal may not have supporting evidence for their effectiveness, and without evidence for effectiveness, some professionals are unwilling to implement programs. However, information about evaluations is beginning to collect, and these findings suggest that interventions can be effective.

Child Abuse Programs Interventions for child abuse are aimed at both parents and children. The programs for parents include programs to help parents do a better job (and thus prevent abuse) as well as legal interventions to restrain violence or to remove the child from an abusive environment. Other programs are intended to minimize the harm that violence has done to children who have been abused. In addition, legal strategies focus on compulsory reporting of suspected child abuse to remove children from abusive environments before more harm can occur.

Some programs have targeted high-risk parents, attempting to prevent initial incidents of abuse (Chalk & King, 1998; Eckenrode et al., 2000). Factors that contribute to risk include poverty, young age, and a history of abuse, either as a victim or as a perpetrator. Programs may consist of parent support in the form of education or support groups, home visits, and mental health counseling. All of these approaches take the form of changing the individual behavior of abusive or potentially abusive parents. Follow-up evaluation has demonstrated that these interventions are beneficial for the mother-child relationship and for these children's early development.

Preserving the family by changing dysfunctional family interactions has been the goal of many social service interventions. The goal may not be realistic unless interventions are long term (Chalk & King, 1998), and programs with additional follow-up indicate more success than those without continued attention. In some cases, children may be safer in another setting than in a preserved yet still abusive family. However, placing an abused child in foster care or a group home may not be sufficient, because the experience of violence has already produced damage. Children placed in alternative living environments need services to help them recover from the violence that prompted their placement.

Whereas interventions to decrease child abuse focus on parents' behavior, sexual abuse prevention is aimed at changing children's behavior. The goal of these programs, which are often school based, is to change the individual behavior of children so that they avoid sexual abuse (Davis & Gidycz, 2000). These programs provide information to children on how to behave in potentially abusive situations. Children are taught to flee from people or situations in which a person tries to touch them sexually and to tell about such attempts. Evaluations for these programs indicate that they increase knowledge, and a survey of college women who had participated in "good touch–bad touch" school sexual abuse programs (Gibson & Leittenberg, 2000) reported substantially lower levels of sexual abuse (8%) than women who had not (14%). Therefore, programs that train children about abuse may be effective in increasing knowledge, and more important, in decreasing sexual abuse.

Changes in the law have made reporting of child abuse mandatory for health care and education professionals. The rationale is that, by requiring physicians, psychologists, nurses, counselors, and teachers to report suspicious cases, children can be protected from escalating violence. Physicians must overcome many barriers to question their patients about abuse and, thus, often do not learn enough to report, which makes these mandatory reporting laws ineffective (Gerbert et al., 2000). In addition, these laws may have unexpected and negative consequences for children, forcing the disintegration of families (Landsberg & Wattam, 2001).

In summary, the interventions aimed at changing parents' behavior and teaching children to avoid and report sexual abuse have some effect. Changing the environment is not a strategy used to prevent child abuse, and changing the law has been very effective in decreasing risks of violence to children.

Partner Abuse Interventions The ideal strategy to prevent partner abuse would be to change social values so that violence is not an acceptable way to resolve conflicts and to allow women the power and resources to leave violent relationships (Jewkes, 2002). That level of social change is beginning to happen in many societies around the world, but others retain values that allow husbands to behave violently toward their wives.

Strategies for reducing partner abuse focus on caring for victims and preventing additional incidents. These strategies fall into two groups: social services and legal interventions. The majority of social services programs are shelters to which abused women can escape (Chalk & King, 1998), although some inventive approaches exist. For example, the Donate a Phone program asks people to donate wireless phones to victims of domestic violence so that they can call for help in case of repeated attack ("Cell Phones," 2000). Shelters offer a range of services such as counseling, job training, legal advice, and housing assistance, making evaluation of these programs difficult. A community-based advocacy program for women with abusive partners has demonstrated positive effects that persist over time (Bybee & Sullivan, 2002). This program was designed to help women find and use community resources and increase their level of social support to protect them against violent partners. Women who participated in this program experienced an improved quality of life and a decreased risk of partner violence two years later.

Legal interventions are also intended to decrease partner violence. Legal strategies include protective orders to keep batterers away from their partners, mandatory arrest and prosecution, and legal reporting requirements. Protective orders can be good short-term solutions to partner abuse, but studies that evaluate their effectiveness are lacking (Chalk & King, 1998), and protective orders are typically part of a legal response that involves arrest and prosecution.

Incidents of partner violence prompt mandatory arrest in some states and many jurisdictions; this strategy is the most common legal intervention (Mills, 1998). Mandatory arrest and prosecution laws or policies appeared as a result of pressure on police departments that had responded to domestic violence with too little concern and had held the view that these incidents were not important instances of violent crime. Some evidence suggests that mandatory arrest deters further violence, but the policy can also create unwanted effects and possibly even increase violence in some cases (Mills, 1998). Mandatory prosecution has not been studied as extensively, but one study (Davis, Smith, & Nickles, 1998) found that mandatory prosecution was no more effective than mandatory arrest in deterring additional domestic violence.

Legal reporting requirements are not very effective in reducing partner violence, because those responsible for reporting are reluctant do so. Less than 15% of physicians questioned female assault victims about partner abuse, and few women who sought emergency room services for physical assault were referred for additional services (Acierno et al., 1997). In addition, physicians did not want to question women about domestic abuse because such inquiries would be personal and distressing and would make physicians responsible for taking additional action. This attitude is a barrier to identifying and decreasing partner abuse (Gerbert et al., 2000).

The acceptance of violence as a way of resolving conflicts is another barrier. Nearly 3 million married couples do some type of violence to each other each year (Sorenson, Upchurch, & Shen, 1996). Furthermore, many people find such behavior acceptable, at least under some circumstances. A survey of American couples (Straus, Gelles, & Steinmetz, 1980) found that 25% of wives and over 30% of husbands considered violence an acceptable way to resolve some disputes. This attitude is a major barrier to reducing partner violence.

Reducing Elder Abuse Programs for reducing elder abuse are less common and less frequently evaluated than other types of domestic abuse programs (Chalk & King, 1998). In many ways, efforts to reduce elder abuse parallel approaches to decrease child abuse; both concentrate on protecting individuals who cannot protect themselves, and both use social and legal interventions.

All states in the United States have some protective services oriented toward elder people (Chalk & King, 1998). Such services investigate cases of suspected abuse or neglect combined with case management that include medical, educational, and legal services. These services may help either older people or their caregivers. For example, caregivers for Alzheimer's disease patients are one such targeted group, and support groups and respite care can help caregivers cope with the stress of providing care for older patients with dementia. Services to older people include assistance with the things that would allow them to live independently and care for themselves. Such programs remain largely unevaluated.

Legal interventions include mandatory or voluntary reporting laws in most states in the United States, protective orders, arrest and prosecution, legal counseling, and appointment of guardians (Chalk & King, 1998). Those who abuse the elderly are less likely to be prosecuted than child abusers (Young, 2000), and social and legal service workers typically seek a resolution to a problem situation that allows for the care of the older person.

Creating Safer Workplaces

Although unintentional injuries are common in the workplace, three types of intentional workplace violence pose hazards. One type is violent crime; assault and homicide at work is the most common source of workplace violence. Another type is an extension of partner abuse and occurs when domestic disputes are carried into the workplace. The third occurs when angry employees or former employees come into the workplace and retaliate against supervisors and coworkers.

BECOMING SAFER

1. If you have young children in your home, you can make their lives safer by adopting a few basic rules and following these rules consistently.
2. Always properly buckle your seatbelt when riding in a motor vehicle.
3. Never ride a bicycle, motorcycle, or skateboard without a helmet.
4. Don't drive after drinking even a small amount.
5. Never ride with a driver who has been drinking.
6. Don't keep a loaded firearm in your residence or clean a firearm unless you are certain that it is not loaded.
7. Don't ride a bicycle, play sports, or work with machinery after you have been drinking.
8. Follow safety rules at work even if your coworkers ignore them.
9. Do not endorse violence as a way to deal with problems with children, in relationships, or in school.
10. Find ways to manage conflict that do not involve violence, and provide models for child of ways to settle conflicts constructively.
11. If you are a victim of violence, get out of the situation and seek help so that you can recover psychologically as well as physically.
12. If you feel tempted to injure someone in your care, join a support group that will provide strategies for coping with this stressful situation.
13. Learn to recognize the warning signs of suicide, both in yourself and others, and seek help.

Efforts to decrease workplace violence have concentrated on robbery and other violent crimes perpetrated by those who come into a workplace (Loomis, Marshall, Wolf, Runyan, & Butts, 2002). Strategies such as bright external lighting, forbidding working alone at night, and keeping doors locked decreases the chances of worksite homicide from robbers; however, these same strategies do not combat violence from other employees or from workers' partners.

The dramatic cases of a former employee or employee's partner entering a workplace with a gun represent only a small part of the workplace violence. Unhappy employees or former employees create conflicts and do damage that diminishes productivity, creates workplace tension, and adds to health care costs. The same risks occur when domestic violence spills over into the workplace.

The realization that domestic violence has workplace implications led Polaroid Corporation to start a women's group for battered employees (Solomon, 1998). The group helped women get out of their abusive situations and put the company in a position to respond to threats to workers by employees or former employees. The Polaroid Corporation's attention to domestic violence was unusual for a large business, but attention to potentially violent employees has become a part of modern corporations, which recognize that unhappy employees and former employees can be serious threats. An increasing number of companies have developed policies and procedures to deal with violent situations.

Current recommendations (Barrett, Riggar, & Flowers, 1997) include a variety of strategies to prevent workplace violence. Identifying employees who may be violent is difficult, but preemployment screenings can identify those with a history of harassing or violent behavior. Businesses should complete a risk assessment that includes an examination of the physical work environment as well as workplace climate for situations that promote risk. The physical environment can provide opportunities for intruders to hide or can allow easy access to employees, both of which can increase risk of violent attacks. Managers and supervisors who allow hostile interactions of others or initiate such interactions create a hostile working environment, which increases risks of frustrated, angry employees within their organization. Supervisors who are authoritarian and insensitive in handling discipline or layoffs increase the possibility for violence among former employees. Employers with effective harassment and grievance processes are less likely to have problems than those without such policies and procedures.

Companies should formulate a plan for dealing with dangerous employees, develop a reasonable grievance procedure to defuse employee anger, safeguard against dismissed employees, and protect potential targets such as supervisors, managers, and human resources personnel. Sending clear messages to employees about the unacceptability of threats concerning violence is another precaution. This last recommendation is consistent with discouraging violence in all aspects of society.

Legal regulations have also been aimed at workplace violence. The Occupational Safety and Health Administration (1996) issued guidelines for prevention of violence in the workplace for workers in health care and social service settings. These regulations encourage employers to develop violence prevention plans for their employees. Included in the regulations are components requiring worksite analysis, safety and health training, management commitment to safer workplaces, and control of hazards. Therefore, workplace violence prevention has been attempted through changes in individual behavior, altering the environment, and enacting laws to control workplace violence.

Reducing Community and School Violence

Violence in the community and the school affect young people in two ways—as victims and as perpetrators. Changing the behavior of a large segment of the population seems an overwhelming task, but violence of all types decreased in the late 1990s in the United States (USBC, 2001). These decreases are probably not due to any program efforts, but many programs have targeted community and school violence. These programs have taken each of the three approaches—changing individual behavior, the environment, and the law.

Programs that attempt to change individual behavior take a variety of approaches. For example, the American Psychological Association teamed with Music Television (MTV) in a program, brochure, and Web site called "Warning Signs" (APA, 1999). These messages are aimed at youth and help young people analyze and deal with conflict in nonviolent ways. Programs aimed at alcohol and drug use can also decrease violence because use of these substances often increases aggression. However, programs aimed specifically at youth include conflict resolution programs, mentoring, and psychological and peer counseling.

Conflict resolution programs often appear as part of the school curriculum and teach problem-solving skills as well as violence prevention. One such program is the Teaching Students to be Peacemakers program (Johnson & Johnson, 2002). This program acknowledges the benefits as well as the dangers of conflict and tries to help students find the benefits. Students learn negotiation and mediation skills during a sequence of exercises as well as participate in booster sessions to maintain their skills. Evaluation has revealed that this program not only decreases violence but also helps youth think of conflict in different ways. Other school programs are oriented toward decreasing bullying (Bullock, 2002). Long considered an inevitable part of childhood, bullying has now been identified as generating violence and a poor learning environment. By sensitizing teachers to its negative effects and providing family support, bullying can be decreased.

The strategy of providing mentors who furnish positive role models may also be effective in combating violence (Murray, Guerra, & Williams,

1997). Programs such as Big Brothers/Big Sisters provide children with adult mentors who form nurturing relationships with the children. This type of mentoring program can have positive effects in decreasing the use of violence to solve interpersonal problems, but programs that provide experiences that help young people prepare for, obtain, and keep jobs are more successful.

Job training and access to jobs can be part of a successful strategy for reducing violence by changing the environment (Stiffman, Earls, Dore, Cunningham, & Farber, 1996). In some communities, the most attractive employment options involve illegal activities, and offering meaningful alternatives can be a powerful deterrent to crime. Other community changes include recreational programs, such as midnight basketball, and street monitoring, such as Neighborhood Watch.

Altering the environment can also help to decrease school violence (National Education Association, 1998). In addition to attempting to change children's behavior, alterations in building arrangement can eliminate opportunities for fights. Wooded areas on or near campuses can give intruders the opportunity to approach unobserved, and secluded wings or classrooms give students chances to begin fights without being interrupted. Some schools have hired consultants to perform safety "audits" in which dangerous features of the school environment are located and changed.

Changing the law is another strategy designed to reduce youth violence in schools and communities. Legal approaches include removing violent youth from communities, restricting access to weapons, and arrest and incarceration. Residential treatment programs for violent youth are not a new approach, but the latest version is the "boot camp" in which young offenders are placed in military-type programs. Unfortunately, these programs have not demonstrated a great deal of effectiveness, and youth who participate have a high rate of committing additional crimes (Stiffman et al., 1996).

Restricting weapons is an important component of reducing community and school violence, and this approach has shown more promise of decreasing violence than residential programs or incarceration (Stiffman et al., 1996). A growing belief that access to firearms posed a serious threat to school safety led the U.S. government to pass a public law in 1994 that mandated a "zero tolerance" policy toward weapons in schools (Pipho, 1998). The goal of this legislation was to decrease the number of guns in schools, and the law included several mandated penalties for bringing guns or explosives into school. Although case-by-case exceptions are allowed under the law, expulsion for one year is the required penalty for most weapons violations. Strategies to restrict firearms access have been effective in decreasing injuries and deaths (Cole & Flanagin, 1999), so perhaps these laws will decrease the danger in schools and in communities.

Cutting Suicide Rates

In 1999, the U.S. Surgeon General called for the development of a national strategy to prevent suicide, which resulted in a comprehensive plan that includes many levels of prevention (USDHHS, 2001). This strategy has taken the approach of suicide as a public health problem that needs to be controlled. The plan emphasizes identifying risk factors, then developing, implementing, and evaluating interventions.

The national strategy includes all three approaches to intervention, but many of its goals are oriented toward changing the environment. This program aims to change societal attitudes toward disorders such as depression, which elevate the risk for suicide, and toward seeking mental health care, which decreases risk. Goals also include making the means of suicide less available, such as limiting access to guns and drugs. Individual behavior is also addressed. Those individuals who are at risk will be targets for special interventions as will family and friends of suicide victims.

The national strategy to prevent suicide (USDHHS, 2001) includes plans for rigorous evaluation of the effectiveness of interventions, but it also relies on research concerning effective suicide prevention efforts. Existing research offers some suggestions about effective interventions.

One intervention that is not very effective is the telephone hot line service that allows suicidal people to call suicide prevention centers and talk to trained volunteers. A meta-analysis of studies over a 70-year period indicated that traditional hot line services had little or no effect on the rate of suicide for people who call (Dew, Bromet, Brent, & Greenhouse, 1987).

The sharp increase in suicide among adolescents during the 1980s led to the development of school-based programs. These suicide prevention programs often include training faculty to identify warning signs, forming mental health teams for counseling at-risk students, and developing written formal suicide policies (King, 2001). Other components of school-based interventions include training parents to identify problems in their children. Teaching students to identify and report problems to responsible adults seems like the ideal approach, but students have proven reluctant to consult adults when they or their friends show the warning signs of suicide (USDHHS, 2001). Decreasing this reluctance is a goal, but providing a peer referral network is an alternative (King, 2001).

An evaluation of a school program (Kalafat & Elias, 1994) found that students who had taken part in the intervention classes gained more knowledge about suicidal peers and had more favorable attitudes toward helping troubled schoolmates than did the controls. Assessing long-term benefits of suicide prevention programs is difficult, but some evidence indicates that school-based programs can be effective. One study (Kalafat, 1997) found a county with a suicide prevention program had a lower suicide rate than the state average. No causal conclusions can be drawn from these results, but the differences suggest that a widely implemented school-based program can be effective.

Another suicide reduction strategy is limiting access to the means to commit suicide, including drugs and firearms (Cohen, Spirito, & Brown, 1996). Use of firearms to commit suicide has increased, and a majority of completed suicides involves firearms. For young people, suicide is often an impulsive action, and access to a gun makes the chances of death more likely. Restricting access to firearms, especially loaded guns, can be beneficial. Training or mandating parents to take precautions with their firearms as well as other strategies to limit access may be helpful. Restricting access to drugs can also make suicide more difficult. Limiting the number of pills per prescription for sedatives reduced the number of suicides in Australia (Cohen et al., 1996).

Therefore, some existing suicide prevention programs have demonstrated positive effects, and the national strategy to prevent suicide has the development of such programs among its goals. Changes in societal attitudes and environment, laws, and individual behavior will be necessary to cut suicide rates.

In Summary

Violence prevention strategies can work through changing individual behavior, the environment, or the law. In addition, a societal change in the acceptability of violence is necessary to decrease violence on many levels. Domestic violence interventions are aimed at decreasing child, partner, and elder abuse through all three strategies. Reducing parental violence can have long-term benefits for reducing societal violence because abused children can grow into people who do violence to others. Some commonalties exist among interventions for all types of domestic violence, including help for stressed caregivers, alternative living arrangements for the abused, and laws that mandate arrest and prosecution. Evaluations of the effectiveness of interventions for domestic violence are sparse, but some indicate that programs can decrease child and spouse abuse.

Reducing workplace violence may include strategies to reduce domestic violence because partner abuse may occur in a workplace, endangering the partner as well as other employees and even customers. Other violence reduction strategies are aimed at preventing crime in the workplace and keeping angry employees or former employees from committing violence in the workplace.

Community and school violence are more difficult to reduce than domestic or workplace violence, but violent crimes decreased during the late 1990s. Conflict resolution programs in schools can help students deal with others in nonviolent ways, and mentoring and jobs programs are among the more successful approaches. Reducing access to firearms can also decrease community and school violence.

Suicide and suicide prevention are the focus of a national initiative. This plan includes goals of changing attitudes about suicide and prevention so as to allow people with mental disorders to receive appropriate care that decreases suicide risk. People at increased risk are targeted for special intervention, and reducing access to the means of suicide is also a goal.

Answers

This chapter addressed six basic questions:

1. **How can adults make children's worlds safer?**
   Adults can make children's worlds safer by following several basic, nonrestrictive rules: (1) Don't allow children under the age of 5 to ride in the front seat of a motor vehicle. Restrain young children in the back seat; (2) Supervise young children while they are taking a bath, sitting in a highchair, or using a knife or scissors; (3) Don't store chemicals, cleaning supplies, or poisons in areas assessable to children; (4) Don't permit children to swim without adult supervision.
2. **What can young people do to reduce their chances of unintentional injuries?**
   Young people can reduce their chances of unintentional injuries by following several basic rules: (1) Use seatbelts while driving or riding in a motor vehicle; (2) Don't drive after drinking or ride with someone who has been drinking; (3) Never ride a bicycle or use a skateboard without a helmet; (4) Don't ride a bicycle or participate in sports after you have been drinking; (5) Don't play with or clean a firearm that has some possibility of being loaded.
3. **What unintentional injuries are most likely to affect adults?**
   The leading unintentional injury to adults is motor vehicle crashes, but seatbelts and airbags can help many people survive these crashes. Alcohol is involved in nearly half of motor vehicle fatalities among adults, but it is also a factor in many other unintentional injuries. Many adults are injured or killed in the workplace, with men being far more vulnerable than women, and African Americans somewhat more vulnerable than European Americans.
4. **What are some of the strategies for reducing unintentional injuries?**
   Strategies for reducing unintentional injuries can be divided into three areas of focus—those aimed at (1) changing the individual's behavior, (2) changing the environment, and (3) changing the law. Attempts to change individual behavior through education, lectures, or advice are not very effective. Changing the environment is somewhat more effective than attempts to change an individual's behavior. Examples of changing the environment include building

safer cars and roads and making changes in the home and neighborhood. Laws that mandate use of seatbelts and the manufacture of flame-retardant children's clothes, childproof medicine containers, and refrigerators that open from the inside have reduced unintentional injuries to adults and children.

5. **What are the major types and the impact of intentional injuries?**
Intentional violence is a problem that affects people throughout the lifespan, but children and youth are more frequent targets of assault and homicide than middle-aged or older people. Child abuse can have life-long effects for victims, creating a cycle of violence that produces violent adolescents and adults. Youth violence extends to perpetration as well as victimization, and youth are involved in community violence, school violence, sexual assault, homicide, and suicide. Young African American men are at a particularly high risk. Adults are also in jeopardy from violence. Two types of domestic violence—partner abuse and elder abuse—affect adults. In addition, adults experience violence in their communities and workplaces as well as suicide.

6. **How can intentional injuries be reduced?**
Violence prevention strategies can work through changing individual behavior, the environment, or the law. In addition, a societal change in the acceptability of violence is necessary to decrease intentional violence. Domestic violence interventions are aimed at decreasing child, partner, and elder abuse through all three strategies by providing support for stressed caregivers, alternative living arrangement for the abused, and legal requirements for arrest and prosecution of offenders. Reducing workplace violence includes strategies to reduce crime in the workplace, domestic violence that spills over into the workplace, and angry employees or former employees. Conflict resolution programs in schools can help students deal with others in nonviolent ways, creating mentoring experiences and jobs in the community can help at-risk individuals, and reducing access to firearms can also decrease community and school violence. Strategies to prevent suicide have become a national priority, with an emphasis on prevention and research into effective preventive strategies. Increasing access to mental health services, decreasing the stigma of seeking help, and reducing access to the means of suicide can prevent impulsive suicide attempts.

Suggested Readings

Jewkes, R. (2002). Intimate partner violence: Causes and prevention. *Lancet, 359,* 1423–1429. Rachel Jewkes discusses the social underpinnings, risk factors, and dynamics of intimate partner violence and presents a multifaceted program to address these issues.

Johnson, D. W., & Johnson, R. T. (2002). Teaching students to resolve their own and their schoolmates' conflicts. *Counseling and Human Development, 34,* 1–11. David Johnson and Roger Johnson present the view that conflict can be a positive factor in schools if teachers and students know how to resolve the inevitable conflicts that arise. They discuss many strategies to handle school conflict, including negotiation and mediation.

Saldana, L., & Peterson, L. (1997). Preventing injury in children: The need for parental involvement. In T. S. Watson & F. M. Gresham (Eds.), pp. 221–238. *Handbook of child behavior therapy.* New York: Plenum Press. Psychologists Lisa Saldana and Lizette Peterson discuss the variety of unintentional injuries to children and offer strategies for reducing these injuries.

Williams, A. F., & Lund, A. K. (1992). Injury control: What psychologists can contribute. *American Psychologist, 47,* 1036–1039. This brief article provides some background to the injury control field and discusses the role of psychologists in injury reduction.

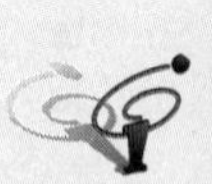

Search InfoTrac College Edition

Search these terms to learn more about topics in this chapter:

Injuries and seatbelts
Unintentional injuries and children
Alcohol and unintentional injury
Safety and corporate culture
Bicycle helmet use
Violence and United States and statistics
Child abuse and health effects
Witnessing and violence and children
Violence and demographic aspects
Violence and cholesterol
Intimate partner violence
Domestic violence and statistics
Workplace violence and statistics
Elder abuse
Domestic violence and prevention
Child abuse prevention
Elder abuse and prevention
Community violence and prevention
School violence and prevention
Suicide prevention

13

Smoking Tobacco

The Story of Lisa

CHAPTER OUTLINE

QUESTIONS

This chapter focuses on five basic questions:

1. How does smoking affect the respiratory system?
2. Who chooses to smoke and why?
3. What are the health consequences of tobacco use?
4. How can smoking rates be reduced?
5. What are the effects of quitting?

The Story of Lisa

Lisa, a 31-year-old African American office manager, has been smoking for 9 years. Neither of her parents smoked, and as a teenager, Lisa was never tempted to try smoking. After working in an office for about 3 years, one day Lisa had a particularly unpleasant argument with a coworker in another office. When she returned to her desk, Lisa was still angry. She asked her friend, Karen, for a cigarette. Lisa smoked just one that day, but about 10 days later, after another altercation with the same coworker, she stormed back to her office and almost demanded a cigarette from Karen. Again, she smoked just one, but the next morning she stopped at a convenience store and bought a pack of cigarettes. At first, she smoked just two a day—one at work and one in the evening.

Gradually, Lisa increased her rate of smoking. After about a year, she was up to a pack a day, a number that she maintains at present. Interestingly, she has never purchased cigarettes by the carton, reasoning that quitting would be easier if she did not have several unused packs around her apartment. Twice Lisa has made serious attempts to stop smoking. The first time was about 3 years ago when she tried the nicotine patch. That procedure was partially successful—she quit for 4 months. When she began smoking again, she returned almost immediately to one pack a day. About a year later, she tried for a second time to quit—this time on her own. Once again, she was partly successful, but she refrained from cigarettes for only 3 weeks.

Why did she go back to smoking after wanting to quit and succeeding at doing so? Lisa says that one day she got angry with her boss, and she knew if she didn't do something to occupy her hands and mouth, she might do or say something she would later regret.

When Lisa first began smoking, people were permitted to smoke in her building. When the building became smoke free, Lisa would step outside to smoke, or she would smoke while running errands between one building and another. The prohibition against smoking in her building neither reduced nor increased the number of cigarettes Lisa smokes at work.

Lisa believes that she is at greater risk for cancer than other people because she had cancer when she was 12 years old. Lisa's attitude of vulnerability is therefore different from that of most smokers who think that smoking is generally unhealthy but who nevertheless believe that other smokers are at greater risk for cancer and heart disease than they are. This chapter summarizes the level of those risks, the risks for other tobacco products, the nonlethal hazards of smoking, the dangers of passive smoking (environmental tobacco smoke), the prevalence of smoking in the United States, the reasons why people smoke, and some methods of preventing and reducing smoking. First, however, we briefly review the effects of smoking on the respiratory system, the body system most immediately affected by smoking.

Smoking and the Respiratory System

Through respiration, oxygen is taken into the body and carbon dioxide is expelled. This process draws air deep into the lungs, and with the air can come other particles that may damage the lungs. Smoking routinely introduces a variety of particles into the lungs, and several diseases are associated with smoking.

Functioning of the Respiratory System

The exchange of oxygen and carbon dioxide occurs deep in the lungs. To get air into the lungs, the **diaphragm** and the muscles between the ribs (intercostal muscles) contract, increasing the volume within the chest. As the space inside the chest increases, the pressure within the chest falls below atmospheric pressure, and air is forced into the lungs by that pressure.

CHECK YOUR HEALTH RISKS

Check the items that apply to you.

- ☐ 1. I have not smoked more than 100 cigarettes in my life.
- ☐ 2. I have probably smoked between 100 and 200 cigarettes in my life, but I have not smoked at all in more than 5 years and have no desire to do so.
- ☐ 3. I currently smoke more than 10 cigarettes a day.
- ☐ 4. I currently smoke more than two packs of cigarettes a day.
- ☐ 5. I am a smoker who believes that the health risks of smoking have been exaggerated.
- ☐ 6. I am a smoker who believes that smoking is probably harmful, but I plan to stop smoking before those effects can harm me.
- ☐ 7. I don't smoke cigarettes, but I do smoke a least one cigar a day.
- ☐ 8. I don't smoke cigarettes, but I do smoke my pipe at least once a day.
- ☐ 9. I smoke cigars because I believe that they carry a very low risk for heart disease and cancer.
- ☐ 10. I smoke a pipe because I believe that pipe smoking is not very harmful.
- ☐ 11. I live with someone who is a heavy smoker.
- ☐ 12. I use smokeless tobacco (chewing tobacco) on a daily basis.

Except for the first two statements, each of these items represents a health risk from tobacco products, which account for about 440,000 deaths a year in the United States, mostly from heart disease, cancer, and chronic obstructive pulmonary disease. Count your check marks for the last 10 items to evaluate your risks. As you read this chapter, you will see that some of these items are more risky than others.

Figure 13.1 traces the flow of air into the lungs. The nasal passages, pharynx, larynx, trachea, bronchi, and bronchioles conduct air into the lungs. These passages have little ability to absorb oxygen, but in the process of inhalation, the air is warmed, humidified, and cleansed. Millions of **alveoli,** located at the ends of the bronchioles, are the site of oxygen and carbon dioxide exchange. Each tiny alveolus in the lungs is like a bubble, giving the lungs a spongy appearance. The alveoli have thin walls (only one cell in thickness) that allow the easy exchange of gases.

Air rich in oxygen is drawn into the lungs and reaches the alveoli. Blood that has circulated through the body travels back to the heart and then back to the lungs. This blood has a high carbon dioxide content and a low oxygen content. In the lungs, the blood circulates to the capillaries that surround each alveolus, where an exchange of carbon dioxide and oxygen occurs based on differences in diffusion pressures. The blood, now oxygen rich, travels back to the heart and is pumped out to all areas of the body.

During exhalation, the diaphragm and the muscles between the ribs relax. The air in the alveoli is compressed, and the increased pressure forces the air out of the lungs by the same route through which it entered. The expelled air contains a great deal of carbon dioxide and little oxygen. Not all air leaves the lungs during exhalation, and each breath mixes new air with air that remains in the lungs.

Air is an excellent medium for the introduction of foreign matter into the body. Airborne particles potentially move into the lungs with every breath. Protective mechanisms in the respiratory

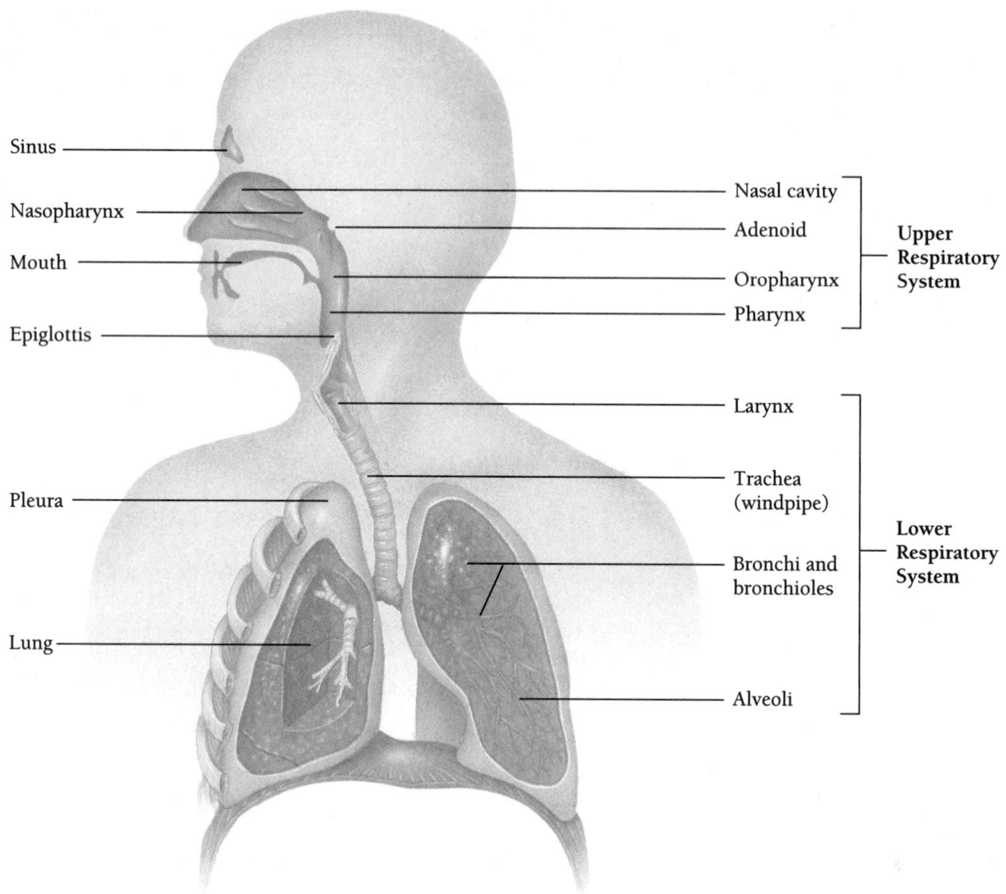

Figure 13.1 Respiratory system.

Source: Introduction to Microbiology *(p. 525) by J. L. Ingraham & C. A. Ingraham, 1995, Belmont, CA: Wadsworth. Copyright 1995 by Wadsworth Publishing Company. Reprinted by permission.*

system, such as sneezing and coughing, expel some of the dangerous particles. Noxious stimulation in the nasal passages may activate the sneeze reflex, whereas stimulation in the lower respiratory system promotes the cough reflex.

Another protective mechanism in the respiratory system is called the **mucociliary escalator.** Diffusion of gases requires a moist environment, and the respiratory system is kept moist by its mucous membrane lining. In the nasal cavity, pharynx, and bronchi, the lining of the respiratory system contains **cilia,** tiny hairlike structures. The cilia and mucous membranes form the mucociliary escalator. Mucus is secreted in the respiratory system, and the beating of the cilia moves the mucus toward the pharynx, where it is usually swallowed or coughed out. This transport mechanism cleanses the system of inhaled particles, providing an important defense against dangerous particles.

Several respiratory disorders are of interest to health psychologists. All kinds of smoke, as well as other types of air pollution, increase mucus secretion in the respiratory system but decrease the activity of the cilia, thus decreasing the efficiency of the mucociliary escalator. As mucus builds up, people cough to get rid of the mucus, but coughing may also irritate the bronchial walls. Irritation and infection of the bronchial walls may damage the cilia and destroy tissue in the bronchi. The formation of scar tissue in the bronchi, irritation or

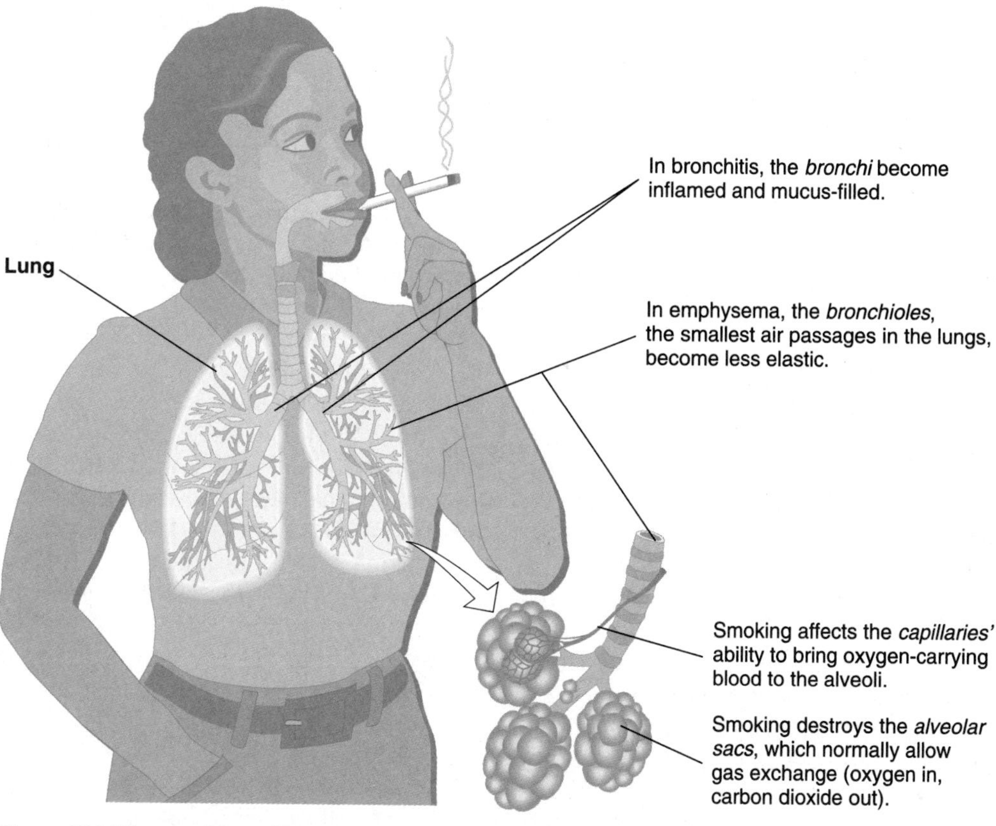

Figure 13.2 How smoking affects the lungs.

Source: An Invitation to Health *(7th ed. p. 493) by D. Hales, 1997, Belmont, CA: Brooks/Cole. Copyright 1997 by Brooks/Cole Publishing Company. Reprinted by permission.*

infection of bronchial tissue, and coughing are characteristics of **bronchitis,** one of several chronic obstructive pulmonary diseases that are the third leading cause of death in the United States.

Acute bronchitis is caused by infection and usually responds quickly to antibiotics. When the irritation persists and the mechanism underlying the illness continues, it can become a chronic problem and thus one of the chronic obstructive pulmonary diseases. Cigarette smoke is the major cause of chronic bronchitis, but environmental air pollution and occupational hazards may also underlie chronic bronchitis.

Another chronic obstructive pulmonary disease is **emphysema,** a disorder that develops when scar tissue and mucus obstruct the respiratory passages, bronchi lose their elasticity and collapse, and air is trapped in the alveoli. The trapped air breaks down the alveolar walls, and the remaining alveoli become enlarged. Both damaged and enlarged alveoli have reduced surface area for the exchange of oxygen and carbon dioxide. Damage also obstructs blood flow to the undamaged alveoli, and so the respiratory system becomes restricted. The loss of efficiency in the respiratory system means that respiration delivers a limited amount of oxygen. People with emphysema usually cannot exercise strenuously, and even normal breathing can become impossible for them.

Chronic bronchitis, emphysema, and lung cancer are all diseases of the respiratory system associated with the inhalation of irritating, damaging particles. Figure 13.2 shows how smoke can damage the lungs, producing bronchitis and emphysema. Cigarette smoking is of particular interest to health psychologists because it is a voluntary behavior that can be avoided, whereas air pollution and occupational hazards are social problems not under direct personal control. Thus, smoking is the target for much negative publicity and for interventions for change. But what specifically makes inhaled smoke dangerous?

What Components in Smoke Are Dangerous?

The processed tobacco in cigarettes contains at least 2,550 compounds, and burning increases the number to over 4,000 (USDHHS, 1989). But which of these components in cigarette smoke might be dangerous? Nicotine is the pharmacological agent that underlies addiction to cigarette smoking (Kluger, 1996), but is nicotine the main culprit responsible for the adverse health effects of smoking? Can nicotine cause coronary heart disease, cancer, bronchitis, and emphysema? What does this drug do in the body?

Nicotine is a stimulant drug, an "upper." It affects both the central and the peripheral nervous systems. Certain central nervous system receptor sites are specific for nicotine; that is, the brain responds to nicotine, as it does to many drugs. But smoking is a particularly effective means of delivering drugs to the brain. Nicotine, for example, can be found in the brain 7 seconds after having been ingested by smoking—twice as fast as via intravenous injection. The half-life of nicotine, the time it takes to lose half its strength, is 30 to 40 minutes. Addicted smokers rarely go more than this length of time between "fixes."

When nicotine is delivered to the brain, catecholamines, neurotransmitters that include epinephrine and norephinephrine, are released. These substances act as stimulants, increasing cortical arousal, which can be measured by an electroencephalograph (EEG). In addition, smoking releases beta-endorphins, and the pleasurable effects of smoking may be due to the release of these opiates produced by the body. Nicotine also increases the metabolic level, which explains the tendency for smokers to be thinner than nonsmokers (Perkins, Epstein, Marks, Stiller, & Jacob, 1989).

The term *tars* describes the water-soluble residue of tobacco smoke condensate, which is known to contain a number of compounds identified or suspected as **carcinogens**—that is, agents that may cause cancer. Mortality from smoking-related diseases decreases with decreasing tar yields (Tang et al., 1995), but the problem in evaluating the role of tars in cigarette smoke is that tars and nicotine vary together in commercially available cigarettes. Some cigarettes are high in both, although the trend is toward cigarettes that are relatively low in both. Currently, no commercially available cigarettes are low in tars and high in nicotine, even though such a product might have advantages. For low-nicotine cigarettes, smokers increase their smoking rate (Maron & Fortmann, 1987) and inhale more deeply (Herning, Jones, Bachman, & Mines, 1981), exposing themselves to more of the dangerous tars. Thus, there may be few health advantages to low-yield cigarettes.

Several other by-products of tobacco smoke are suspected of being health risks. **Acrolein** and **formaldehyde** belong to a class of irritating compounds called **aldehydes.** Formaldehyde, a demonstrated carcinogen, disrupts tissue proteins and causes cell damage. **Nitric oxide** and **hydrocyanic acid** are gases generated in smoking tobacco that affect oxygen metabolism and, thus, could be dangerous.

In Summary

The respiratory system allows oxygen to be taken into the lungs, where an exchange with carbon dioxide occurs at the level of the alveoli. Along with air, other particles can enter the lungs; some of these particles can be harmful. Cigarette smoke can cause damage to the lungs, and smokers are prone to bronchitis, an inflammation of the bronchi. Cigarette smoke contributes heavily to the development of chronic obstructive pulmonary diseases, such as chronic bronchitis and emphysema.

Several chemicals, either within the tobacco itself or produced as a by-product of smoking, can cause organic damage. Although nicotine in large doses is extremely toxic, its precise harmful effects on the average smoker are difficult to assess. This difficulty exists because the level of nicotine in commercial cigarettes varies with the level of tars, another class of potentially hazardous substances. Thus, determining what specific components of smoke connect to which sources of illness and death is difficult.

A Brief History of Tobacco Use

When Christopher Columbus and other early European explorers arrived in the Western hemisphere, they found that the Native Americans had a custom considered odd by European standards: the natives carried rolls of dried leaves, which they set afire, and then they "drank" the smoke. The leaves were, of course, tobacco. Those early European sailors tried smoking, liked it, and soon became quite dependent on it. Although Columbus disapproved of his sailors using tobacco, he quickly recognized that "it was not within their power to refrain from indulging in the habit" (Kluger, 1996, p. 9). Within a century, smoking and the cultivation of tobacco spread around the world, and no country where people have learned to use tobacco has ever successfully barred the habit (Brecher, 1972).

Smoking was a habit that grew rapidly in popularity among Europeans, but it was not without its detractors. Elizabethan England adopted the use of tobacco, although Elizabeth I disapproved, as did her successor, James I. Another prominent Elizabethan, Sir Francis Bacon, spoke against tobacco and the hold it exerted over its users. Many objections to tobacco were of a similar nature—namely, that people who became addicted to it often spent money on it even though they could not afford to purchase it. Because of its scarcity, tobacco was expensive: in London in 1610, it sold for an equal weight of silver.

In 1633, the Turkish Sultan Murad IV decreed the death penalty for subjects who were caught smoking. He then conducted "sting" operations on the streets of his empire and beheaded those vulnerable people who were seduced to use tobacco (Kluger, 1996). From the early Romanoff Empire in Russia to 17th-century Japan, the penalties for tobacco use were also severe. Still the habit spread. In the Spanish colonies, smoking by priests during Mass became so prevalent that the Catholic Church forbade it. In 1642 and again in 1650, tobacco was the subject of two formal papal bulls, but in 1725, Pope Benedict XIII annulled all edicts against tobacco—he liked to use snuff, that is, ground tobacco.

Over the centuries, tobacco has been used in a variety of forms, including snuff, pipes, cigars, and cigarettes. Cigarettes (shredded tobacco rolled in paper) were not popular until the 20th century, although some soldiers smoked them during the U.S. Civil War. However, cigarette smoking was not widespread during the last half of the 19th century because many men considered it rather effeminate. Ironically, cigarette smoking was not socially acceptable for women either, and few women smoked during this period. Cigarette smoking became more popular during the 1880s when ready-made cigarettes came on the market. Gradually, people came to prefer factory-made cigarettes to those they had to roll themselves.

The widespread adoption of cigarette smoking was aided in 1913 by the development of the "blended" cigarette, a mixture of the air-cured Burley and Turkish varieties of tobacco mixed with flue-cured Virginia tobacco. This blend provided a cigarette with a pleasing flavor and aroma that was also easy to inhale. Cigarette smoking became increasingly popular during World War I, and during the 1920s, the age of the "flapper," cigarette smoking started to gain popularity among women.

From the time of Columbus until mid-19th century, tobacco did not lack enemies, but no one had tried to ban it for scientific or medical reasons. Historically, the assault on tobacco had come from people who damned it on moral, social, xenophobic, or economic grounds (Kluger, 1996). The tobacco industry continued to grow despite (or perhaps because of) the fact that many in authority had condemned the use of tobacco for one or more of these reasons. It was not until the mid-1960s that the scientific evidence on the dangerous consequences of smoking became widely recognized.

During the 1940s and 1950s, it was not uncommon for physicians to smoke and to recommend the practice to their patients as a method of relaxation and stress reduction. Tobacco companies, of course, used a variety of techniques to increase smoking rates. Besides multiple advertising approaches, they provided free cigarettes to soldiers during World War II and continued to give away free samples after the war. At that time, only a few people suspected that smoking might have negative health consequences, so the choice to smoke was a common one.

Sixty years after tobacco companies convinced people that cigarette smoking was chic, sexy and stylish, their approach to advertising continues to pay dividends (see the Would You Believe . . . ? box).

Choosing to Smoke

Unlike many health hazards, smoking is a voluntary behavior, making any negative consequences avoidable. In the recent history of the United States, the choice to smoke has become less and less common. Several different factors relate to the individual choice to smoke or not.

Who Smokes and Who Does Not?

Smokers differ from nonsmokers in gender, ethnicity, personal beliefs and behaviors, and educational level. In addition, changes have occurred over time, with the percentage of smokers decreasing since the 1960s. Currently, fewer than 25% of the adults in the United States are classified as smokers (NCHS, 2001). This percentage represents more than 47 million smokers, but it also means that more than three of every four adults in the United States are nonsmokers. In general terms, approximately one fourth of the adult population are cigarette smokers, one fourth are former smokers, and one half have never smoked. Figure 13.3 shows trends in smoking rates since 1965 when almost 45% of adults in the United States smoked and only about 14% were former smokers (CDC, 2001e).

In 1964, the U.S. Surgeon General issued a report spelling out the adverse effects of smoking on health (U.S. Public Health Service [USPHS], 1964). Beginning in 1967, each package of cigarettes had to carry a warning of the potential danger of smoking, and in 1970, cigarette advertising was banned from television. Coincidental with these warnings, smoking rates have declined in the United States. The highest rate of per capita cigarette consumption in the United States was in 1966, or 2 years after the first Surgeon General's report on the dangers of smoking. Figure 13.4 shows a significant decrease in the per capita consumption of cigarettes in the United States since 1968 and offers more evidence that the Surgeon General's report had some effect of reducing smoking in the United States. Figure 13.4 also shows historical events that may have increased or decreased the per capita consumption of cigarettes. The 49% price increase in cigarettes from December 1997 to December 1999 may help accentuate the decline in cigarette use.

At one time, gender was a good predictor of smoking. In 1965, for instance, more than half of all adult men in the United States were smokers, but only about a third of adult women smoked. Since that time, both men and women have begun to smoke less, and the rate of smoking for men declined more sharply until about 1985. Since that time, the difference between male and female smokers has remained at about

WOULD YOU BELIEVE

Tobacco Sales Are Doing Fine

Would you believe that tobacco companies continue to prosper, despite a decrease in smoking among people in the United States? Although U.S. tobacco companies seem to have lost some major legal battles, their future financial health appears much stronger than the future physical health of their regular customers.

Two relatively recent trends give the tobacco industry reason for optimism. First, their promotion of cigarettes to adolescents may be paying dividends. John Pierce and his associates (Pierce, Choi, Gilpin, Farkas, & Berry, 1998) surveyed adolescents who had no susceptibility to smoking when first interviewed. After 3 years, more than half these young people could name a favorite cigarette advertisement, and having a favorite commercial was a good predictor of who would begin smoking. Pierce et al. estimated that 34% of experimentation with cigarettes was due to advertising, a figure that would translate to more than 700,000 new smokers each year, or a quarter of a million more than the number of people who die each year of smoking-related causes.

A second reason for optimism in the tobacco industry lies in the expanding markets in Africa, Eastern Europe, and Asia. Richard Kluger (1996) has remarked that in these areas, smoking is regarded as a sign of being up-to-date, "an emblem of advancement, fashion, savoir faire, and adventure as projected in images beamed and plastered everywhere by its makers" (p. xii). To Kluger, the situation is ironic in that "the more evidence accumulated by science on the ravaging effects of tobacco, the more lucrative the business has become and the wider the margin of profit" (p. xii). In Kluger's interesting and informative book, *Ashes to Ashes,* he notes that many governments in emerging nations have, themselves, become addicted to cigarettes because of the taxes they receive from cigarette sales.

The nations of the former Soviet Union present an alluring potential market to American and British tobacco companies. Although the people in the former Soviet bloc have been longtime smokers, their consumption had traditionally been limited to inferior-tasting cigarettes manufactured in outmoded domestic factories that could not keep up with a growing demand. Despite a shortage of creature comforts, the people of the former Soviet Union continued their strong appetite for tobacco products.

Into this potentially lucrative market rode the Marlboro man, dispatched by his parent, Philip Morris. This prominent American tobacco company proceeded to renovate old factories, build new ones, and spend a total of $1.5 billion during the first 4 years after the Soviet breakup (Kluger, 1996). Their investment, of course, has reaped dividends. Thanks to the former Soviet countries and other eastern European nations, Philip Morris's international sales have increased by 10% a year, easily compensating for any erosion of the U.S. market (Kluger, 1996).

As appealing as the countries of eastern Europe appear, China presents an even larger prize to Western tobacco companies. The number of current smokers in China is not precisely known, but Kluger (1996) estimated the number at 300 million—about one quarter of the population and about 30% of the world's smoking population. However, unlike governments of the former communist countries of eastern Europe, the Chinese government has been more reluctant to open its doors to foreign tobacco and has actively sought to reduce smoking among its people by restricting cigarette advertising and putting health warnings on cigarette packs. Undaunted, Philip Morris has taken a patient course of action. It has sponsored a national soccer league, presented U.S. style television shows, and displayed other forms of advertising, even "though the average Chinese couldn't get near the product" (Kluger, 1996, p. 721). Only time will tell if these tactics will be successful, but given the history of tobacco companies, it seems safe to predict that these efforts will eventually pay off.

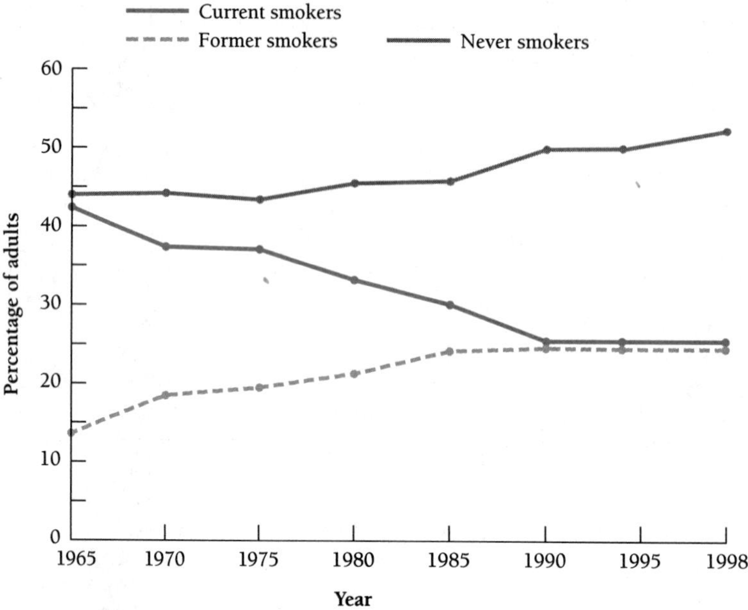

Figure 13.3 Percentage of never smokers, current smokers, and former smokers among adults, United States, 1965–1998.

Source: Centers for Disease Control and Prevention (CDC), 2001, Tobacco information and prevention source (TIPS). http://www.cdc.gov/tobacco/research_data/adults_prev/tab_3.htm.

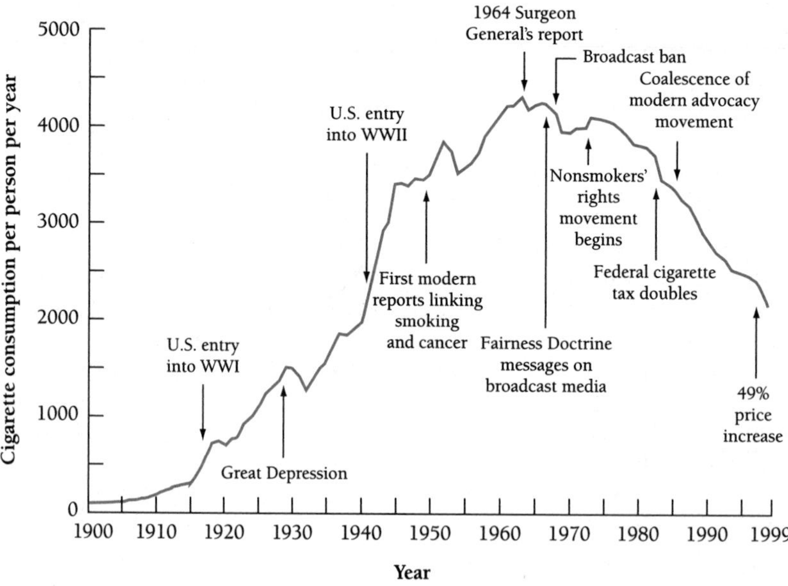

Figure 13.4 Cigarette consumption per person 18 and over, United States, 1900–1999.

Sources: "Surveillance for selected tobacco use behaviors—United States, 1900–1994" by G. A. Givovino et al., 1994, Morbidity and Mortality Weekly Report, 43, *No. SS-3, pp. 6–7, and National Center for Health Statistics, 2001,* Health, United States 2001. *Hyattsville, MD: U.S. Government Printing Office.*

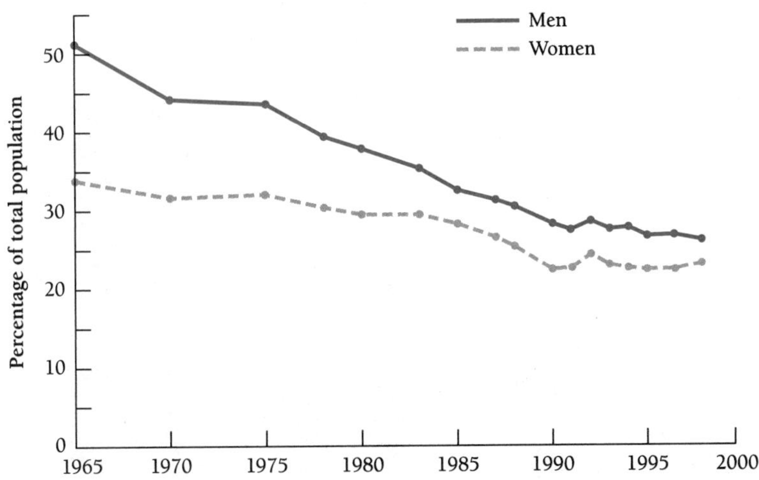

Figure 13.5 Percentages of adult male and female cigarette smokers, United States, 1965–1998.

Source: National Center for Health Statistics, 2001, Health, United States, 2001. *Hyattsville, MD. U.S. Government Printing Office.*

4%. Figure 13.5 shows these trends. Note that the 25-year steady decline in smoking rates for both men and women appears to have partly leveled off during the 1990s. However, this appearance is somewhat artificial because in 1994, the National Center for Health Statistics (1994) changed its definition of current smoker to include people who smoke only "some days" or have smoked at least 100 lifetime cigarettes, thus including more people as smokers.

The change in definition of smoker was also partly responsible for an apparent *increase* in smoking among adolescents for the years 1992 to 1996. However, since 1996, smoking rates among adolescents have begun to *decline.* Figure 13.6 shows this apparent increase in adolescents' smoking from 1991 to 1996, but it also shows a substantial decrease in their smoking for the years 1995 to 2001. Figure 13.6 also reveals that high school is the time when many adolescents begin to smoke. Only 12% of eighth graders are smokers, whereas nearly 30% of 12th graders meet the definition of smoker. The decrease in teenage smoking for the period 1996 to 2001 is the largest for any age group during that same time period. However, because adolescent smoking rates fluctuate more than other age groups, they may not be accurate predictors of future smoking trends.

In 1965, gender was the factor most strongly associated with smoking, but as seen in Figure 13.5, the rates of smoking for women and men are now quite similar. Currently, the best predictor of smoking is educational level: the more years people attend school, the less likely they are to smoke. Moreover, the *rate* of decline has been steeper for college graduates than for high school dropouts. Figure 13.7 shows not only the inverse relationship between smoking and education but also the steeper decline for college graduates. Socioeconomic level is also related to amount of cigarette smoking. For adults, more than 33% of people below the poverty line are smokers whereas only 23% of those at or above the poverty line meet the definition of smoker (CDC, 2001a). Socioeconomic level is the best predictor of smoking for young adults, ages 18 to 24. More than 75% of young men and more than 60% of young women in low socioeconomic homes are current smokers (Winkleby, Robinson, Sundquist, & Kraemer, 1999).

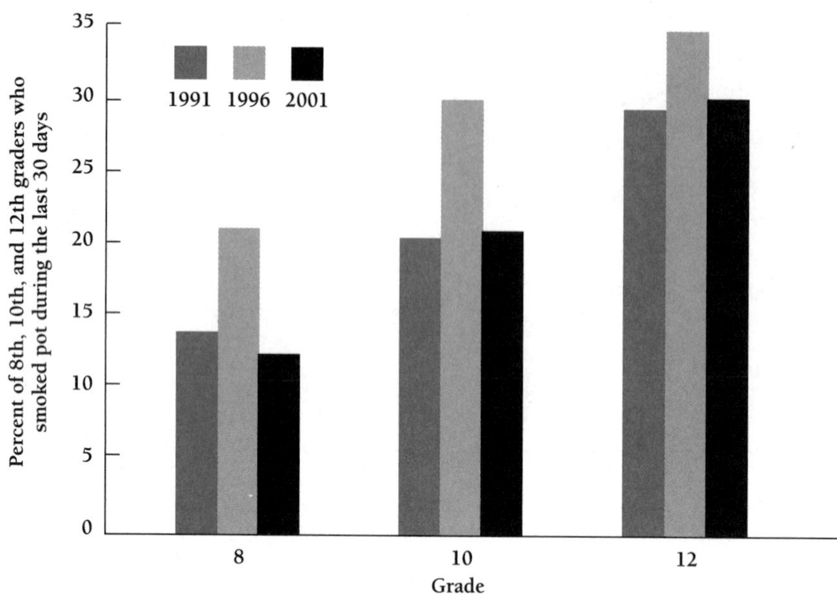

Figure 13.6 Percentage of smokers, past 30 days, grades 8, 10, and 12, for the years 1991, 1996 and 2001.

Source: Cigarette smoking among American teens declines sharply in 2001, *by L. D. Johnston, P. M. O'Malley, & J. G. Bachman, 2001, Ann Arbor, MI: University of Michigan News and Information Services. [online]. Retrieved from the World Wide Web, May 13, 2002. Available: www.monitoringthefuture.org.*

Why Do People Smoke?

Despite widespread publicity linking cigarette smoking to a variety of health problems, millions of people continue to smoke. That fact is puzzling because many smokers themselves acknowledge the potential dangers of their habit, and some even overestimate the dangers, especially of developing lung cancer (Jamieson & Romer, 2001). The question of why people smoke can be divided into two separate ones. Why do people begin to smoke and why do they continue? Answers to the first question are difficult because most young people are aware of the hazards of smoking. The best answer to the second question seems to be that different people smoke for different reasons, and the same person may smoke for different reasons in different situations.

Why Do People Start Smoking? Most young people are aware of the hazards of smoking (Jamieson & Romer, 2001), yet perhaps as many as 700,000 of them begin smoking each year (Pierce et al., 1998). Many of these young people have an optimistic bias, believing that these dangers do not apply to them. In addition to this optimistic bias, researchers have examined at least four explanations for why people begin smoking after becoming aware of the dangers of this practice: social pressure, genetics, advertising, and weight control. Most research on these hypotheses has centered on social pressure.

Social Pressure Many teenagers are sensitive to social pressure and may start smoking if they have friends who smoke (Mittelmark et al., 1987). Teenagers often are encouraged to smoke and to continue to smoke by peers who offer them cigarettes (Ary & Biglan, 1988). Also, young adolescents often cite "image" as an important reason for smoking (Stanton, Mahalski, McGee, & Silva, 1993).

Moreover, movies can be a source of social pressure. An analysis of smoking in movies (Es-

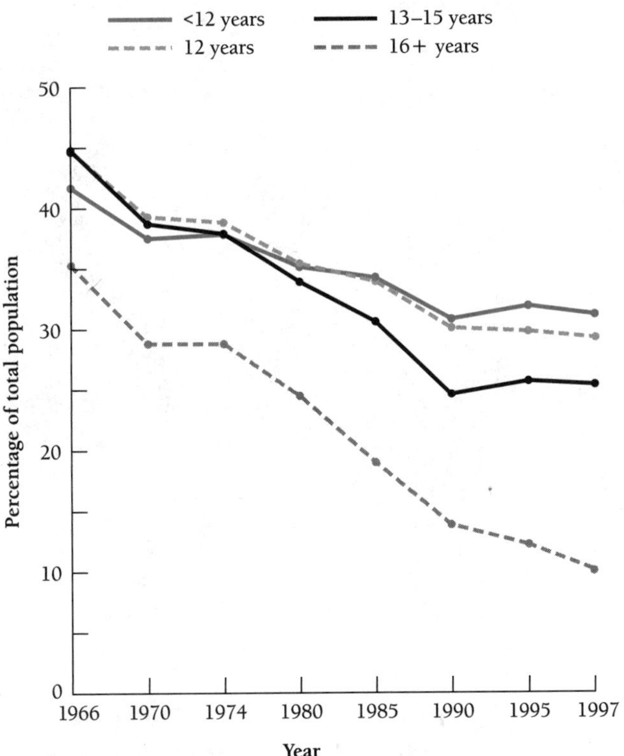

Figure 13.7 Smoking rates by number of years of education, United States, 1966–1997.

Sources: "Percentage of adults who were current, former, or never smokers, + overall and by race, Hispanic origin, age, and education, National Health Interview Surveys, selected years—United States, 1965–1994." Tobacco Information and Prevention Source, www.cdc.gov/tobacco; and "Cigarette smoking among adults—United States, 1999," by Centers for Disease Control and Prevention, 2001, Mortality and Mortality Weekly Report, vol. 50, *pp. 869, 873.*

camilla, Cradock, & Kawachi, 2000) revealed that female actors were as likely to smoke in PG/-PG-13 movies as in R-rated movies, whereas male actors were 2.5 times as likely to smoke in an R-rated movie. This same analysis showed that movies aimed at adolescent audiences contained more positive messages about cigarette smoking than did R-rated movies.

Social pressure affects different adolescent groups differently. In an early study (Mosbach & Leventhal, 1988), junior high school students identified four distinct peer groups with varying acceptance of smoking. The "dirtballs" were boys who smoked, used other drugs, were poor students, and had other personal or school-related problems. The "hotshots" were mainly girls who were popular and successful students, and the "jocks" were mainly boys who were interested in organized sports. The last group, the "regulars," was students who did not belong to any of these groups and were typical students. The "dirtballs" and the "hotshots" made up only 15% of their sample but accounted for 56% of the smokers. The attitudes and attractions of smoking differed in the two groups. The "dirtballs" were typically smokers before they entered junior high school and were attracted to one another and the behavior of the group because of the satisfaction of

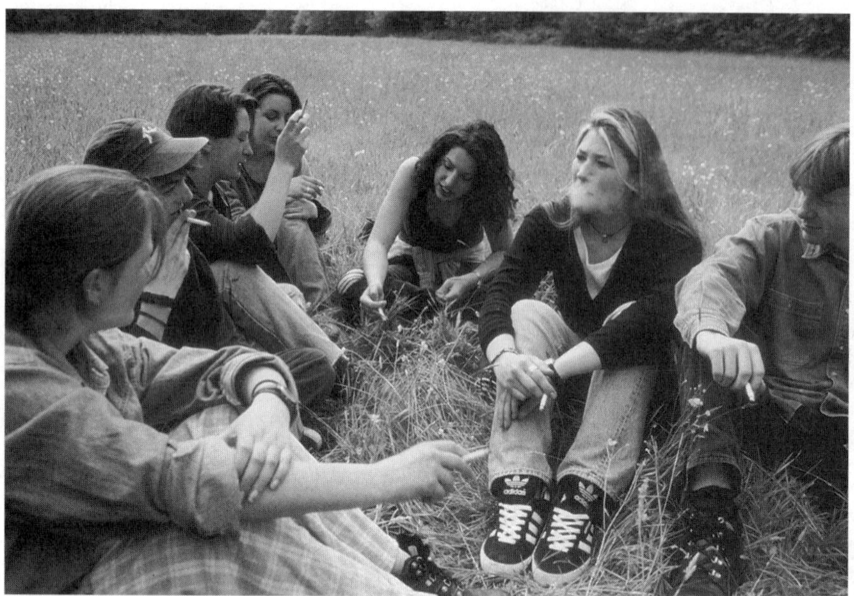

Acceptance into a social group can be a powerful source of reinforcement for adolescents, increasing the pressure to begin smoking.

excitement and danger. The "hotshots," on the other hand, experimented with smoking during junior high school because of peer pressure and a need for acceptance and excitement. Unlike the "dirtballs," who were unconcerned with the dangers of smoking, these girls were worried about smoking's hazards. This study explored the complexities of peer pressure in the initiation and maintenance of smoking in young adolescents.

Genetics The first evidence that smoking has some genetic component appeared in the 1950s from studies on twins (Pomerleau & Kardia, 1999). These studies indicated that identical twins tended to be more similar in their choice to smoke or not than did fraternal twins. More recent research has implicated a specific gene and a mechanism that is capable of explaining a genetic relationship in smoking. This research has concentrated on the SLC6A3 gene, which has several versions. People who have the SLC6A3–9 version are less likely to begin smoking before age 16 and less likely to smoke than people who have other variations of this gene (Lerman et al., 1999).

The SLC6A3–9 gene is involved with transport of the neurotransmitter dopamine, which is important in the brain's reward system. Part of nicotine's reinforcing properties is mediated through dopamine (Sabol et al., 1999). Thus, people who have the SLC6A3–9 gene may have some protection against nicotine addiction because they do not experience the same level of reward from smoking as others do. The personality factor of novelty seeking may be a link between the gene and smoking. (Sabol et al., 1999). People with the SLC6A3–9 version of the gene have lower levels of novelty seeking than others, which may translate into a lower need to smoke; people who are high in novelty seeking are more likely to smoke and less likely to quit than those who are lower in this trait. However, the effects of this gene are not large; the genetic difference accounts for only around 2% of the variance in novelty seeking and in smoking. Therefore, this specific gene is not a "no smoking" gene, but genes have some influence on smoking through their action on neurotransmitters.

Advertising In addition to social pressure, advertising and marketing are related to teenagers' initiation of smoking. During the late 1990s, tobacco companies argued that their marketing campaigns were directed at influencing people to switch brands and not aimed at getting young people to begin smoking. A study by Lois Biener and Michael Siegel (2000), however, repudiated these arguments. Biener and Siegel established a baseline of adolescents who had smoked no more than one cigarette during their lifetime. After 4 years, they interviewed these participants and found that young people who owned a tobacco promotional item and who could name a brand whose advertisements attracted their attention were nearly three times more likely to smoke. Biener and Siegel concluded that cigarette advertisements are not simply designed to get people to change brands but to influence adolescents to begin smoking.

If prosmoking advertising is effective, can antismoking advertising be effective as well? Siegel and Biener (2000) also studied this question and found that antismoking media campaigns are effective with young adolescents, aged 12 to 13; that is, young adolescents exposed to antismoking ads were only about half as likely as other young adolescents to progress to smoking. However, antismoking advertisements had no effect on 14- to 15-year-old adolescents, who progressed to smoking at the same rate as adolescents who were not exposed to the ads.

Weight Control Many young girls and some young boys begin smoking because they believe it will help them control their weight. A survey of mostly European American, upper middle class students in grades 7 to 10 (French, Perry, Leon, & Fulkerson, 1994) found that weight concerns were related to smoking initiation for girls but not for boys. Girls were most likely to begin smoking if they had two or more eating disorder symptoms, a history of attempts at weight loss, a fear of weight gain, or a strong wish to be thin. Girls who reported any one of these behaviors or concerns were about twice as likely as other girls to be current smokers.

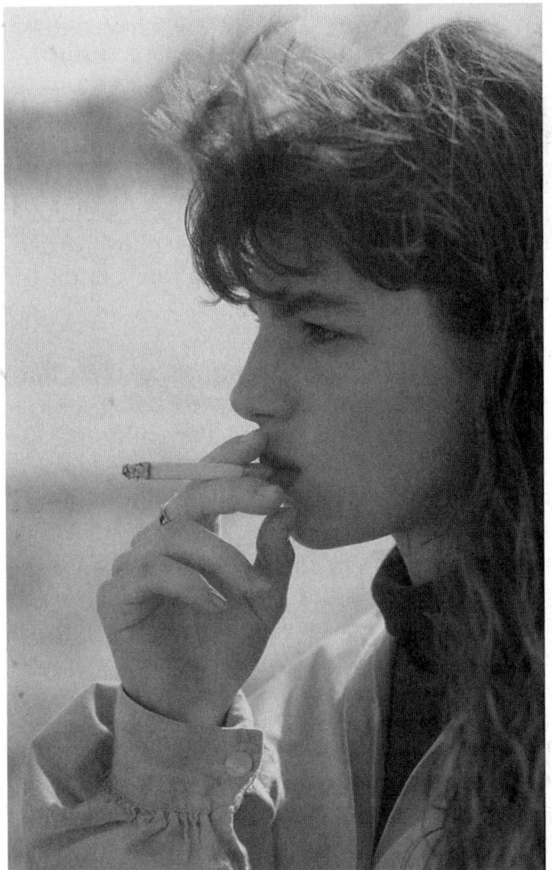

Corbis

Fear of weight gain motivates many young people to begin smoking.

A later study (Tomeo, Field, Berkey, Colditz & Frazier, 1999) found that both girls and boys sometimes initiate smoking because they see this behavior as a means of weight control. Participants were 9- to 14-year-old children of nurses in the Nurses Health Study II. About 9% of these children were smokers and another 6% were contemplating smoking. Both boys and girls who were unhappy with their weight were more likely than other children to consider smoking, and this tendency was stronger in girls. Boys who had experimented with cigarettes and who were dissatisfied with their appearance tended to exercise to control weight, whereas girls who were unhappy with their bodies turned to purging and daily dieting to supplement smoking as a means of weight control.

Why Do People Continue to Smoke? Research into why people smoke suggests that no single explanation is satisfactory and that different people probably smoke for different reasons, including being addicted to nicotine, receiving positive and negative reinforcement, having an optimistic bias, and fearing weight gain.

Addicted Once people begin to smoke, they quickly become dependent on the habit. The Centers for Disease Control and Prevention (CDC, 1994) surveyed smokers 10 to 22 years old and found that nearly two thirds of those who had smoked at least 100 cigarettes during their lifetime reported that "It's really hard to quit," but only a small number of those who had smoked fewer than 100 lifetime cigarettes gave this response. In addition, nearly 90% of participants who smoked more than 15 cigarettes a day found quitting to be very hard. These results suggest that people will become dependent on smoking and have great difficulty quitting once they have smoked about 100 cigarettes or have increased their cigarette consumption to more than 15 per day.

When addicted smokers are restricted to low-nicotine cigarettes, they will smoke more cigarettes to compensate for the scarcity of nicotine they are receiving. Stanley Schachter (1980) supplied heavy, long-duration smokers with cigarettes that alternately, over several weeks, were high or low in nicotine. The cigarettes all looked the same, and the smokers did not know how much nicotine they would be ingesting. On the average, the participants smoked 25% more low-nicotine than high-nicotine cigarettes. Schachter also noted that smokers took more puffs from low-nicotine cigarettes than from ones high in nicotine. Both experiments indicated that smokers are able to regulate the amount of nicotine they ingest, even when that amount is not directly related to the number of cigarettes smoked.

Addicted smokers are not only aware of smoking but are also keenly conscious of the fact that they are *not* smoking. They usually know how long it has been since their last cigarette and how long it will be before their next one. Addicted smokers are those who never leave home or office without first checking their supply of cigarettes. They often keep several extra packs available in case of emergency.

These smokers will go to extremes to ingest nicotine. Howard Leventhal and Nancy Avis (1976) drastically altered the taste of cigarettes by dipping them in vinegar and allowing them to dry, a process that drastically altered the taste of the cigarettes. Although people who smoked for relaxation or pleasure had little interest in the adulterated cigarettes, addicted smokers consumed as many of the bad-tasting cigarettes as regular ones, suggesting that nicotine addiction is one reason why some people continue to smoke.

Nicotine addiction, however, does not explain why some people are light smokers and others smoke heavily. If nicotine were the only reason for smoking, then other modes of nicotine delivery should substitute fully for smoking. Evidence, however, indicates that other delivery methods are not entirely satisfactory to smokers. Experiments with administering nicotine through the nicotine patch (Kenford et al., 1994), intravenously (Lucchesi, Schuster, & Emley, 1967), and with nicotine chewing gum (Hughes, Gust, Keenan, Fenwick, & Healey, 1989) indicate that, although smokers may decrease smoking when nicotine is available through other modes, they still find it difficult to stop smoking. Although nicotine may play a role in the reason people continue to smoke, this research indicates that something other than nicotine is involved.

Positive and Negative Reinforcement A second reason why people continue to smoke is that they receive either positive or negative reinforcement, or both. Behaviors are positively reinforced when they are followed immediately by a pleasant or pleasurable event. Positive reinforcers strengthen the smoking habit by providing smokers with a variety of positive reinforcers, including pleasure from the smell of tobacco smoke, feelings of relaxation, and satisfaction of manual needs.

Negative reinforcement may also account for why some people continue to smoke. Behaviors are negatively reinforced when they are followed immediately by the removal of or lessening of an unpleasant condition. After smokers become addicted, they must continue to smoke to avoid the aversive effects of withdrawal; that is, when addicted smokers begin to feel tense, anxious, or depressed after not smoking for some period of time, they can remove these unpleasant symptoms by smoking another cigarette. Some research on smokers' trying to quit (Brown, Kahler, Zvolensky, Lejuez, & Ransey, 2001) has found that the higher the smokers' level of anxiety, the more likely they are to relapse; that is, highly anxious smokers have much more trouble quitting smoking than do less anxious smokers. Avoiding unpleasant withdrawal symptoms is a powerful motivation for some people to continue to smoke.

Optimistic Bias In addition to addiction and reinforcement, many people continue to smoke because they have an **optimistic bias** that leads them to believe that they personally have a lower risk of disease and death than do other smokers (Weinstein, 1980). For example, when asked about their chances of living to be 75 years old, people who had never smoked and those who were former and light smokers estimated fairly accurately (Schoenbaum, 1997). Heavy smokers, on the other hand, greatly overestimated their chances of living to age 75. Some research (Ayanian & Cleary, 1999) has found that an optimistic bias extends to specific diseases, such as heart disease and cancer. In this study, more than 60% of heavy smokers failed to acknowledge their increased risk for heart disease and more than 50% failed to accept their heightened risk for cancer.

Neil Weinstein (2001) reviewed research on smokers' recognition of their vulnerability to harm and found strong support for the hypothesis that smokers tend to have an optimistic bias. In these studies, most smokers underestimated the dangers of smoking, but some actually overestimated the dangers. Nevertheless, whether smokers underestimated or overestimated the actual dangers of smoking, they failed to apply those dangers to themselves; that is, these studies found that smokers retain an optimistic bias concerning their vulnerability to harm.

Fear of Weight Gain Adolescents are not the only age group using cigarette smoking as a means of weight control. Adults, too, often continue to smoke from fear of weight gain. In a later section, we examine the validity of those concerns, but here we look at the magnitude of weight gain fears.

Concern about weight gain extends to a wide range of smokers. Pregnant women often experience conflict between their awareness of the potential harm to their fetus and their desire to keep from gaining too much weight (Pomerleau, Brouwer, & Jones, 2000). Both African American and European American women express some fears about gain weight. African American women who are smokers tend to have a higher acceptable weight than their European American counterparts (Pomerleau, Zucker, Brouwer, Pomerleau, & Stewart, 2001). Also, African American women, compared with European American women, are more resistant to quitting smoking if they believe that quitting will result in weight gain.

In addition to ethnic background, age is a predictor of weight concern. Young adults are more likely than older ones to use cigarette smoking as a means of weight control. Christina Wee and colleagues (Wee, Rigotti, Davis, & Phillips, 2001) looked at adults trying to lose weight and found that weight-conscious people 30 years old and younger were more likely than other young people to be current smokers, whereas older adults trying to control weight were no more likely than other older adults to be current smokers. These studies suggest that a diverse group of smokers have some concerns about gaining weight if they stopped smoking.

In Summary

The rate of smoking in the United States has slowly declined since the mid-1960s, especially among men. Presently, about 20% of adult women and 24% of adult men in the United States meet the definition of smoker. Ethnic background is a factor in smoking for both adolescents and adults, with Native Americans having the highest smoking rate, followed by African American, European Americans, Hispanic Americans, and Asian Americans. Currently, educational level is a better predictor of smoking status than gender, with more highly educated people smoking at a much lower rate than those with less education.

Reasons for smoking can be divided into questions concerning why people begin to smoke and why they continue to smoke. Most smokers begin as teenagers, at a time when peer pressure is especially strong. Young people recognize the dangers of smoking but they smoke anyway as part of a risk-taking, rebellious style of life. The question about why people continue is a difficult one because people smoke for a variety of reasons. Nearly every smoker in the United States is familiar with the potential dangers of smoking, but many do not relate those hazards to themselves; that is, their knowledge of the dangers of smoking is attenuated by an optimistic bias. In addition, for many people, smoking reduces stress, anxiety, and depression and is therefore negatively reinforcing. Also, some people smoke because they are addicted to the nicotine in tobacco products, and others smoke because they are concerned about weight gain.

Health Consequences of Tobacco Use

Cigarette smoking is the single deadliest behavior in the history of the United States, and it is the largest preventable cause of death and disability. Tobacco use is responsible for more than 440,000 deaths yearly in the United States, or more than 1,200 deaths a day (CDC, 2002). Until the mid-1990s, the largest number of these deaths was from cardiovascular disease. More recently, however, smoking deaths from cardiovascular disease have begun to decline, whereas those from cancer have increased—at least for women. As a result, smoking-attributable cancer deaths now exceed smoking-attributable cardiovascular deaths. Chronic obstructive pulmonary disease—the third leading cause of deaths in the United States—is also the third leading smoking-related cause of death.

In addition to these three causes of smoking deaths, as many as 1,000 people die each year from fires begun by cigarettes (CDC, 2002). Smoking cigarettes while drinking alcohol produces a number of fatal and nonfatal burns every year, but smoking by itself contributed more to those fires than drinking by itself (Ballard, Koepsell, & Rivara, 1992). Along with killing themselves, smokers contribute to the deaths of 1,700 infants a year by forcing them to breathe environmental tobacco smoke (CDC, 2002).

What Is the Evidence?

Is the evidence for the negative health consequences of tobacco merely correlational or has a causal link been established? Although experimental studies are lacking, sufficient evidence from descriptive investigations have firmly established a cause-and-effect relationship between cigarette smoking and several deadly diseases, namely lung cancer, heart disease, and chronic obstructive pulmonary disease. As we saw in Chapter 2, scientists can attribute causation from descriptive studies provided seven criteria are met. They can assume a cause and effect when (1) a dose-response relationship exists between smoking and the likelihood of developing a disease; (2) the incidence of the disease drops for people who quit smoking; (3) smoking precedes the disease; (4) plausible biological explanations exist for the link between smoking and disease; (5) a vast number of studies have consistently found an association between smoking and disease; (6) the strength of this association has been substantial, with some of the highest relative risks in all of health and medicine; and (7) the evidence for a causal relationship between smoking and disease is based on well-designed rigorous studies. As noted in Chapter 2, scientists have found evidence to support each of these seven criteria, thus offering strong evidence that smoking causes both lung cancer and heart disease. This chapter briefly summarizes some of that evidence and also provides support for a link between cigarette smoking and chronic obstructive pulmonary disease.

Evidence for the harmful effects of tobacco use began to emerge as early as the 1930s, and by the 1950s, the relationship between cigarette smoking and lung cancer, coronary heart disease, and emphysema was well established (Kluger, 1996). Despite this confirmation, many scientists and health professionals were still smoking during the 1950s and early 1960s, and they tended to exhibit an optimistic bias with regard to their own risk. But as a consequence of that bias, a full 10 years were lost in the fight against this deadly behavior.

The causal relationship between cigarette smoking and disease in Western nations is now so solidly established that many scientists have turned their research efforts toward the health effects of smoking in China. Results of their studies indicate that Chinese smokers have a risk of dying from lung cancer, heart disease, and chronic obstructive pulmonary disease that is quite similar to the risk for U.S. smokers (Chen, Xu, Collins, Li, & Peto, 1997). At their present rate of smoking, an estimated 2 million Chinese will die of smoking-related causes each year (Chen et al., 1997).

In the United States and other Western nations, most current research on smoking explores other smoking-related issues, for example, the effects of environmental tobacco smoke and the association between cigarette smoking and such nonlethal disorders as cognitive dysfunction, visual problems, accelerated aging, and male impotence. We look at this research later, but first we present data on the relationship between smoking and the three leading causes of death in the United States—cancer, cardiovascular disease, and chronic obstructive pulmonary disease.

Smoking and Cancer Cancer is the second leading cause of death in the United States, and smoking plays a role in the development of several cancers, especially lung cancer. Although smoking may also be responsible for deaths from cancers of the lip, pharynx, esophagus, pancreas, larynx, trachea, urinary bladder, and kidney (CDC, 2002), about 80% of smoking-related cancer deaths are from lung cancer. Stated differently, of the 150,000 people who die each year from smoking-related cancers, 120,000 of them die from lung cancer (CDC, 2002). Both female and male smokers have an extremely high relative risk of about 9.0 for lung cancer (Lubin, Blot et al., 1984). This risk is the strongest link established to date between any behavior and a major cause of death.

From 1950 to 1989, lung cancer deaths rose sharply, a trend that lagged about 20 to 25 years behind the rapid rise in cigarette consumption. During the mid 1960s, cigarette consumption began to drop sharply, and then about 25 to 30 years later, lung cancer deaths among men began to decline. Figure 10.4 (see Chapter 10) shows the close tracking of men's deaths from lung cancer and the rise and fall of cigarette consumption in the United States. This is strong circumstantial evidence for a causal link between smoking and lung cancer.

Could other factors, including environmental pollutants, have been responsible for the rapid rise in lung cancer deaths before 1990? Evidence from a prospective study (Thun, Day-Lally, Calle, Flanders, & Heath, 1995) strongly suggested that neither pollution nor any other nonsmoking factor was responsible for the increase in lung cancer deaths from 1959 to 1988. Another piece of evidence against smoking is data showing that lung cancer deaths for smokers rose significantly during this period, whereas lung cancer deaths among nonsmokers remained about the same (USDHHS, 1990), indicating that indoor/outdoor pollution, radon, and other suspected carcinogens had little or no effect on lung cancer mortality. These results, along with those from earlier epidemiological studies, strongly suggest that cigarette smoking is the primary contributor to lung cancer deaths.

Smoking and Cardiovascular Disease Cardiovascular disease (including both heart disease and stroke) is the leading cause of death in the United States and the second largest cause of tobacco-related deaths. Nearly 150,000 people die of smoking-related cardiovascular disease in the United States every year (CDC, 2002).

What is the level of risk for cardiovascular disease among people who smoke? In general, research suggests that the relative risk is about 2.0 (CDC, 1993), which means that people who smoke cigarettes are twice as likely to die of cardiovascular disease than people who do not smoke. The risk is slightly higher for men than for women, but both male and female smokers have a significantly increased chance of both fatal and nonfatal heart attack and stroke (Colditz et al., 1988).

What biological mechanism might explain the association between smoking and cardiovascular disease? Some evidence suggests that cigarette smoking increases the progression of atherosclerosis by as much as 50% during a 3-year period (Howard et al., 1998), speeding the formation of plaque within the arteries. In addition, nicotine itself may contribute to heart disease. This drug, which is the principal pharmacological agent in tobacco, has a stimulant effect on the nervous system, activating the sympathetic division of the peripheral nervous system. Under nicotine stimulation, heart rate, blood pressure, and cardiac output increase, but skin temperature decreases and blood vessels constrict. This combination of increased heart rate and constricted blood vessels places increased strain on the cardiovascular system and, thus, may elevate smokers' risk of coronary heart disease.

Smoking and Chronic Obstructive Pulmonary Disease Chronic obstructive pulmonary disease (COPD) is the third leading cause of death in the United States, and the third leading cause of tobacco-related deaths (CDC, 2002). Chronic obstructive pulmonary disease includes a number of respiratory and lung diseases; the two most deadly are chronic bronchitis and emphysema. Since 1950, mortality rates from COPD have increased faster than for any other major cause of death except HIV infection. By the beginning of the 21st century, deaths from COPD had risen to nearly 100,000 a year, and the death rate shot up 40% in the previous two decades (CDC, 2002).

Chronic obstructive pulmonary disease is relatively rare among nonsmokers. Only 4% of male nonsmokers and 5% of female nonsmokers receive a diagnosis of COPD, and a small of amount of this is due to passive smoking, mostly from a spouse who smokes (Whitemore, Perlin, & DiCiccio, 1995).

In summary, the three leading causes of death in the United States are also the three principal smoking-related causes of death. The U.S. Public Health Service has estimated that about half of all cigarette smokers eventually die from their habit (USDHHS, 1995).

Other Effects of Smoking

In addition to cancer, cardiovascular disease, and chronic obstructive pulmonary disease, a number of other problems have been linked to smoking. For example, smoking has an interactive effect with depression; that is, smokers have more than their share of depressive symptoms and depressed people do more than their share of smoking (Jung & Irwin, 1999; Windle & Windle, 2001). Also, people with various diagnoses of mental illness are about twice as likely as other people to be smokers (Lasser et al., 2000). In addition, smoking is related to diseases of the mouth, including periodontal disease (Ismail, Burt, & Eklund, 1983), to multiple sclerosis (Hernán, Olek, & Ascherio, 2001), and to diminished physical strength, poorer balance, and impaired neuromuscular performance (Nelson, Nevitt, Scott, Stone, & Cummings, 1994). Smokers are also more likely than nonsmokers to commit suicide (Miller, Hemenway, & Rimm, 2000), to develop the common cold (Cohen, Tyrrell, Russell, Jarvis, & Smith, 1993), to experience problems with cognitive functioning (Launer, Feskens, Kalmjin, & Kromhout, 1996), and to experience accelerated facial wrinkling, making them appear older than nonsmokers of their age (Ernster et al., 1995: Grady & Ernster, 1992). Smokers are more likely to suffer from two age-related problems: hearing loss (Cruickshanks et al., 1998) and macular degeneration, a serious visual impairment (Christen, Glynn, Manson, Ajani, & Buring, 1997; Klein, Klein, & Moss, 1998).

Female smokers have about twice the chance of developing ovarian cysts (Holt et al., 1994), and women who smoke at least one pack of cigarettes a day have a deficit in bone density sufficient to increase the risk of bone fractures (Hopper & Seeman, 1994). In addition, pregnant women who smoke double their chances of delivering a stillborn infant, and they also double their risk of having an infant die during the first year of life (Wisborg, Kesmodel, Henriksen, Olsen, & Secher, 2001). Also, adolescent girls and boys who smoke five or more cigarettes daily have slower growth of lung function than adolescents who do not smoke (Gold et al., 1996). Finally, male smokers may receive a double dose of undesirable effects from cigarettes. Smoking not only may make them older and less attractive in appearance (Ernster et al., 1995), but it also increases their chances of becoming sexually impotent (Mannino, Klevens, & Flanders, 1994).

The negative effects are not limited to individual smokers. Society, too, pays a price. The Centers for Disease Control and Prevention (CDC, 2002) estimated that smoking-related illnesses and economic losses cost the people of the United States $157 billion annually. These costs, of course, are not limited to smokers—they affect everyone who pays health insurance premiums and everyone who pays for lost worker productivity. Smokers obviously cannot legitimately argue that their smoking habit affects only themselves. They may pay $3.00 for a pack of cigarettes, but the cost to society is an additional $7.18 per pack (CDC, 2002).

Cigar and Pipe Smoking

Are cigar and pipe smoking as hazardous as cigarette smoking? The tobacco used in pipes and cigars differs somewhat from the tobacco used to make cigarettes, but pipe and cigar tobacco is similarly carcinogenic. The risk to pipe and cigar smokers, however, is not as elevated as it is for cigarette smokers because pipe and cigar smokers do not inhale as much smoke as cigarette smokers do.

As noted earlier, one study (Lubin, Richter, & Blot, 1984) found that the relative risk for people who smoked only cigarettes was about 9.0, indicating that cigarette smokers were nine times more likely than nonsmokers to die from lung cancer. In comparison, people who smoked only cigars had a risk of 2.9, and those who smoked only pipes had a 2.5 elevation in their risk for lung cancer. However, the combination of cigars or pipes with cigarettes dramatically increased the relative risk for lung cancer. The combination of cigars and cigarettes yielded a rate of 6.9, whereas the combination of pipes and cigarettes raised the relative risk to 8.1, a rate nearly as high as for cigarettes alone (Lubin, Richter, et al., 1984). These researchers found no elevation in risk for lung cancer for either cigar or pipe smokers who never inhaled. Cigar and pipe smoking may be less hazardous than cigarettes, but they are not safe.

The recent popularity of cigar smoking has led to renewed research interest in this form of nicotine delivery. As a result, evidence has revealed a dose-response relationship between cigar smoking and cardiovascular disease, chronic obstructive pulmonary disease, and several kinds of cancer (Irbarren, Tekawa, Sidney, & Friedman, 1999). In addition, heavy cigar smokers who inhale have the same risk for death as that of cigarette smoking (Baker et al., 2000), but those who do not inhale have about the same risk for diseases as passive smokers (Jacobs, Thun, & Appicella, 1999).

Passive Smoking

Many nonsmokers find the smoke of others to be a nuisance and even irritating to their eyes and nose. But is **passive smoking,** also known as **environmental tobacco smoke (ETS)** or secondhand smoke, harmful to the health of nonsmokers? In the 1980s, some evidence began to accrue that passive smoking might be a health hazard. Specifically, passive smoking has been linked to lung cancer, breast cancer, heart disease, and a variety of respiratory problems in children.

Passive Smoking and Lung Cancer The effect of passive smoking on lung cancer is difficult to determine because of the amount and duration of exposure. In general, the more smoke people are exposed to and the longer the exposure, the higher the risk for lung cancer. Exposure from a spouse (Fontham et al., 1994) or from coworkers (Kabat, Stellman, & Wynder, 1995) provides a slightly elevated risk, but the higher the level of exposure, the greater the risk. People exposed to environmental smoke during childhood have no elevated risk for lung cancer, and those exposed to their spouse's smoke have only a slight risk. However, people with a very high exposure to ETS in the workplace and in vehicles of transportation double their risk for lung cancer (Kreuzer, Krauss, Kreienbrock, Jóckel, & Wichmann, 2000).

Although evidence suggests that passive smoking may contribute to some additional risk for lung cancer, relative risks should be interpreted with reference to the prevalence of the disease within the comparison group—in this case, nonsmokers who are not exposed to cigarette smoke. Because lung cancer in this comparison group is quite rare, an elevated risk of 20% or 30% for nonsmokers exposed to environmental tobacco smoke does not add a great number of nonsmokers to the lung cancer mortality rates.

Passive Smoking and Breast Cancer Some early research seemed to implicate passive smoking as a risk in breast cancer, but most of the earlier studies were retrospective, based on relatively small sample sizes, and relied on smoking reports from the women exposed to environmental tobacco smoke.

However, a more recent and better controlled study from the American Cancer Society (Wartenberg at al., 2000) showed that women are not at increased risk from their smoking husbands. This investigation, which avoided most of the problems of earlier studies, found that women married to smokers for 30 years or more showed no greater number of deaths than women married to nonsmokers, regardless of the husband's level of smoking. These results are in contrast to some previous studies, but they are more compelling because they are based on a prospective design that used large numbers of exposed women and relied on smoking reports from both the wives and the husbands.

Passive Smoking and Cardiovascular Disease Although the effect of environmental tobacco smoke on breast cancer is nearly negligible, its effects on cardiovascular disease are substantial. A meta-analysis of studies (He, Vupputuri, et al., 1999) showed that the excess risk of heart disease for passive smokers is about 25%, or about the same as the relative risk for lung cancer, and a little less than the risk for stroke (You, Thrift, McNeil, Davis, & Donnan, 1999). However, even this small elevated risk for heart disease translates into thousands of deaths each year from passive smoking. This apparent discrepancy is explained by the huge number of smoke-free people in the comparison group. That is, many more people in the United States die from cardiovascular disease than from lung cancer, so that if the two diseases have the same excess mortality rate, many more people will die from CVD than from lung cancer. Thus, of the 30,000 to 60,000 people who die from ETS per year in the United States, about 75% of the deaths are from heart disease (Werner & Pearson, 1998). Although environmental tobacco smoke kills thousands of people each year, the risk from passive smoking is only about one tenth the risk from active smoking.

Passive Smoking and the Health of Children Infants are possibly the people at greatest risk from environmental tobacco smoke, and much of that risk is for death (CDC, 2002). Infants whose mother smoke have an increased chance for dying of sudden infant death syndrome (SIDS), and the more cigarettes that mothers smoke, the greater their infants' risk for sudden death (MacDorman, Cnattingius, Hoffman, Kramer, & Haglund, 1997).

Among the nonlethal problems faced by infants of parents who smoke are a greater incidence of bronchitis and pneumonia (USDHHS, 1990), an increased risk of asthma and lower respiratory tract illnesses (Larsson, Frisk, Hallstrom, Kiviloog, & Lundback, 2001), low birth weight (Ahluwalia, Grummer-Strawn, & Scanlon, 1997) and childhood cancers (John, Savitz, & Sandler, 1991). In general, the negative effects of environmental tobacco smoke diminish as children pass the age of 2 years (Wu, 1990), but school-age children exposed to passive smoking have more than their share of wheezing, more missed school days, and weaker lung function volume (Mannino, Moorman, Kingsley, Rose, & Repace, 2001).

In summary, passive smoking is a health risk for lung cancer, cardiovascular disease, and many health problems of children. In general, the greater the exposure, the greater the risk.

Smokeless Tobacco

Smokeless tobacco includes snuff and chewing tobacco, forms of tobacco that were more popular during the 19th century than at present. Currently, Hispanic American and European American male adolescents use smokeless tobacco more than any other segment of the U.S. population (Johnson et al., 2002). Who are these young male users of smokeless tobacco? In addition to gender and ethnic background, the people most likely to use smokeless tobacco are those who also smoke cigarettes, have low self-esteem, have parents who smoke, and participate in organized sports (Lewis, Harrell, Deng, & Bradley, 1999; Tomar & Giovino, 1998). The finding that users of smokeless tobacco are more likely than nonusers to participate in organized sports is an interesting one; professional athletes may be models for this behavior, or the ploy of marketing smokeless tobacco at sporting events may be successful. Young men—the segment of the population most likely to use smokeless tobacco—nearly all believe that smokeless tobacco can cause cancer, but this belief has almost no effect on their use of the product (Tomar & Giovino, 1998).

Health risks of smokeless tobacco include cancer of the oral cavity, periodontal disease, and heart disease. Also, people who use smokeless tobacco have a twofold risk for high cholesterol (Tucker, 1989) and 35- to 54-year-old men who use smokeless tobacco have more than a twofold risk of dying from cardiovascular disease (Bolinder, Alfredsson, England, & de Faire, 1994). The risks of smokeless tobacco are probably not as great as those of cigarette smoking; nevertheless, chewing tobacco has significant health hazards.

In Summary

The health consequences to tobacco use are multiple and serious. Smoking is the number one cause of preventable mortality in the United States, causing more than 440,000 deaths a year, mostly from cancer, cardiovascular disease, and chronic obstructive pulmonary disease. But smoking also carries a risk for nonfatal diseases and disorders such periodontal disease, loss of physical strength and bone density, respiratory disorders, cognitive dysfunction, facial wrinkling, sexual impotence, hearing loss, and macular degeneration.

Many nonsmokers are bothered by the smoking of others, and they also have an excess risk of respiratory disease from passive smoking. Research suggests that environmental tobacco smoke does not contribute substantially to death from lung cancer, but it may be responsible for several thousand deaths a year from cardiovascular disease.

Like cigars and pipes, smokeless tobacco is probably somewhat safer than cigarette smoking, but no use of tobacco is safe. Teenagers who use smokeless tobacco tend to believe that this form of tobacco is much safer than cigarette smoking, but the use of smokeless tobacco is associated with increased rates of oral cancer and periodontal disease and may be related to coronary heart disease.

Interventions for Reducing Smoking Rates

Interventions designed to reduce smoking rates can be divided into those that deter people (usually adolescents) from beginning and those that encourage current smokers to stop.

Deterring Smoking

Information alone is not an effective way to change behavior. Nearly every teenager in the United States knows that smoking is dangerous to health, yet almost one third of all 12th graders are smokers (Johnston et al., 2001). By the time adolescents are 14 years old, they pay little attention to health warnings, making such warnings ineffective as a means of deterring smoking (Siegel & Biener, 2000). In addition, smoking prevention programs that use lectures, posters, pamphlets, articles in school newspapers, and so forth are almost universally ineffective in preventing young people from starting to smoke (Cecil, Evans, & Stanley, 1996).

Psychological procedures aimed at buffering young adolescents against the social pressures to smoke have been more effective than educational programs. These techniques, usually called "inoculation" programs, are based on the same psychological concepts as the stress inoculation programs discussed in Chapter 8. Inoculation programs typically expose adolescents to social pressures to smoke, but they also arm them with techniques to refuse offers of cigarettes. Such programs are based on the notion that young adolescents can be inoculated against pressures emanating from parents, older siblings, and peers who model smoking behavior as well as from the media (including tobacco advertisements) that encourage cigarette smoking. This social pressure is analogous to a disease, and the therapy program is comparable to inoculation because it intervenes with small amounts of the disease rather than trying to cure an established disorder.

Smoking inoculation programs often call for young adolescents to view films in which teenage models are shown encountering and then resisting social pressure to smoke. After some initial success (Evans et al., 1981; Evans, Smith, & Raines, 1984), a follow-up study (Flay et al., 1989) found no differences in smoking rates of children who had received the inoculation intervention and those who had received the regular health education program.

However, when buffering techniques are combined with an intensive communitywide antismoking campaign, long-term positive results are possible. Seventh-grade students living in communities that had adopted intensive antismoking programs also experienced a psychological intervention that included training in resisting social pressure to smoke (Vartianen, Paavola, McAlister, & Puska, 1998). Comparison students received no intervention and lived in communities with no unusual media campaigns. After 15 years—well into young adulthood—both male and female participants who had received interventions were smoking at significantly lower rates than those in the control communities, suggesting that this combination can produce long-term gains.

Quitting Smoking

A second method of reducing smoking rates is for current smokers to quit. Although quitting smoking is not easy, millions of Americans have done so during the past 40 years. Currently, there are nearly as many former smokers in the United States as there are smokers—slightly less than one fourth of the adult population are in each category, or about 45 million people (CDC, 2001e). Figure 13.3 indicates that the decline in smoking rates is due not merely to fewer people starting to smoke but in large part to increased cessation rates.

Nevertheless, quitting smoking is usually difficult, in part because long-term smokers refuse to believe reports of the hazardous effects of smoking. For example, research (Chapman, Wong, & Smith, 1993) has found that many smokers believe that no strong evidence exists linking smoking and cancer, that most lung cancer is caused by things other than smoking, and that smoking fewer than 20 cigarettes per day is safe. Furthermore, this same study found that current smokers failed to believe that smokers have more than their share of heart disease, stroke, bronchitis, poor circulation, coughing, and breathlessness.

Also, an optimistic bias may contribute to the difficulty of quitting smoking. Former smokers who quit but then relapse tend to decrease their perception of smoking's dangers; that is, their bias tends to track their smoking status (Gibbons, Eggleston, & Benthin, 1997). Interestingly, relapsers with high self-esteem tend to rationalize that smoking is not all that bad. This finding suggests that high self-esteem may contribute to a strong belief of invincibility, making quitting quite difficult for these smokers.

Another factor contributing to the difficulty of quitting smoking is its addictive qualities. Most people who both smoke and drink alcohol consider smoking to be the more difficult habit to break. People seeking treatment for alcohol or drug dependence who also smoked were asked which would be most difficult to quit—their problem substance or tobacco (Kozlowski et al., 1989). A majority of these people reported that cigarettes would be more difficult to quit.

Despite the difficulties of quitting, many smokers have quit on their own, and others have found assistance through nicotine replacement therapy, psychological interventions, and communitywide antismoking campaigns.

Quitting without Therapy Most people who have quit smoking have done so on their own, without the aid of formal cessation programs. In order to understand this process, Stanley Schachter (1982) surveyed two populations: the psychology department at Columbia University and the resident population of Amaganset, New York. Schachter found a success rate of over 60% for both groups, with an average abstinence length of more than 7 years. Surprisingly, nearly a third of the heavy smokers who quit said they had no problems in quitting. Schachter interpreted the high success rate, even for heavy smokers, as evidence that quitting may be easier than the clinic evaluations indicate. He suggested that people who attend clinic programs are those who have, for the most part, failed in attempts to quit on their own. In addition, he hypothesized that the clinic success rates of 20% to 30% represent success for each program, with those who fail in one program going on to another, in which they may also have about a 20% to 30% chance for success. Schachter's data suggest that those who try to quit on their own largely succeed and never attend a clinic. Thus, people who attend clinics are an atypical group, self-selected on the basis of previous failure. These people, therefore, do not represent the general population of smokers, and failure rates based on clinic populations may be too high.

Using Nicotine Replacement Therapy People who have not been able to quit on their own often seek help from outside sources, including nicotine replacement therapy. The two most common nicotine replacement therapies are the nicotine patch and nicotine gum. Both work by providing nicotine-addicted smokers with a substitute for the nicotine they formerly obtained by smoking cigarettes. Nicotine patches, which resemble large bandages, work by releasing a small, continuous dose of nicotine into the body's system. People move from larger dose to smaller dose patches until they are no longer dependent on nicotine. With nicotine gum, ex-smokers receive small amounts of nicotine through chewing—a behavior that may guard against the unwanted weight gain that often follows smoking cessation. Presently, both the patch and nicotine gum are available without a physician's prescription, but the over-the-counter status has not increased the use of nicotine replacement and has actually lowered the use among African Americans (Thorndike, Biener, & Rigotti, 2002).

In 1996, the Agency for Health Care Policy and Research (AHCPR) suggested guidelines to clinicians, smoking cessation specialists, and health care administrators, insurers, and purchasers. Both a full report (Fiore et al., 1996) and a summary (Smoking Cessation Clinical Practice Guideline Panel and Staff, 1996) provide comprehensive information on the effectiveness of nicotine replacement therapy. After reviewing the evidence, the AHCPR identified only the nicotine patch and nicotine gum as effective pharmacological aids in smoking cessation. Moreover, the panel suggested that one or the other of these forms of nicotine replacement should be offered in any cessation program.

How effective are these nicotine replacement therapies? A review of previous research on this question (Tsoh et al., 1997) reported that the nicotine patch produced 22% success versus 9% for a placebo patch, whereas nicotine gum was slightly less effective—about 17–18% versus about 11% for a placebo. Later research (Thorndike et al., 2002) found basically the same results.

Although the effectiveness of the patch and the gum are similar, the AHCPR (Fiore et al., 1996) recommended the patch over the gum because compliance problems are fewer. On the other hand, the gum seems to have an advantage in helping control the weight gained by many ex-smokers. However, research reviewed by the panel found that nicotine gum provides only temporary help in controlling weight. Ex-smokers using the gum maintain weight better than those using the patch, but once they stop using the gum, they gain about as much as if they had never used it (Fiore et al., 1996).

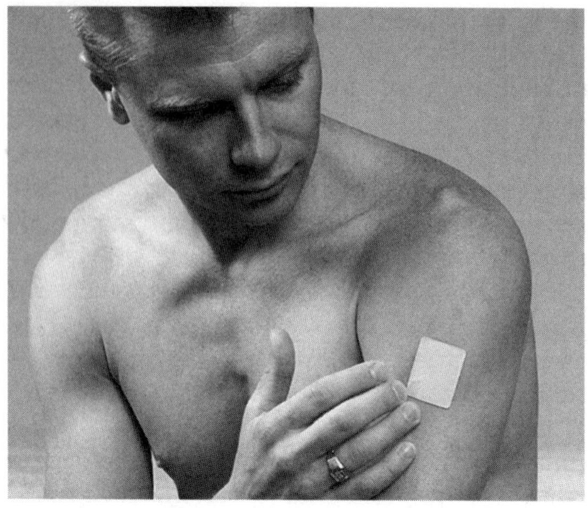
Corbis

Nicotine patches in a multimodal program can be effective in helping people quit smoking.

Neither the nicotine patch nor nicotine gum is without potential side effects. The AHCPR panel cautioned against the use of either by pregnant women, unless the beneficial effects of quitting clearly outweigh the potential risk of nicotine replacement. Also, people with recently diagnosed heart attack should not use the patch or the gum. In addition, the patch causes mild skin reactions in nearly half of the users, and the gum can cause mouth soreness, hiccups, and jaw ache. Other possible side effects of nicotine replacement methods include nausea, light headedness, and sleep disturbances (Tsoh et al., 1997).

In summary, nicotine replacement therapy is more effective than a placebo, but nicotine replacement alone will help less than 20% of smokers quit (Wetter et al., 1998). The effectiveness of both the nicotine patch and nicotine gum is enhanced when combined with various psychological approaches to smoking cessation.

Receiving a Psychological Intervention Psychological approaches aimed at smoking cessation typically include a combination of strategies, such as behavior modification, cognitive behavioral approaches, contracts made by smoker and therapist in which the smoker agrees to stop smoking, group therapy, social support, relaxation training, stress management, "booster" sessions to prevent relapse, and other treatment approaches (Niaura, & Abrams, 2002).

Most psychologists working with smoking cessation problems begin with some implicit or explicit theory, such as one or more of the models we discussed in Chapter 3. For example, they may use the stages of change model of James Prochaska (Prochaska et al., 1994) to assess a smoker's readiness to give up smoking. Smokers at the *precontemplation* stage have no intention to quit and, therefore, are not yet good candidates for psychological interventions. When smokers are at this level, some therapists will provide information about the hazards of smoking with the assumption that this strategy will help smokers move to the next *(contemplation)* stage, a point at which they are aware of the problem and may consider quitting sometime in the future. Although such a procedure agrees with common sense, some research (Quinlan & McCaul, 2000) has found that skipping a step, going from precontemplation to *preparation* for quitting, is more effective than moving only to the next step.

One psychological technique recommended by the AHCPR panel members is practitioner support. Their review found a 15% cessation rate for programs with strong provider support, compared with only a 9% success rate for those with no ongoing contact. Supportive practitioners are in a position to increase smokers' *self-efficacy,* that is, their belief that they can execute the behaviors necessary to stop smoking. One method of enhancing a smoker's self-efficacy is verbal persuasion. A therapist can explain that millions of people have successfully stopped smoking. Indeed, half of all living U.S. citizens who have ever smoked have quit. Self-help booklets and television segments aimed at increasing readiness to quit can also boost self-efficacy, which in turn can further enhance readiness to quit (Warnecke et al., 2001). However, information communicated through verbal persuasion has only a limited influence on self-efficacy. The strongest source of self-efficacy is previous successful performance. Thus, the therapist may be able to point to earlier successes in quitting, even if the smoker had quit for only a short time. If smokers can quit once, they can quit again.

A related approach is to encourage smokers to inform family and friends of their intentions to quit, a technique designed to give them a larger base of social support. Smokers also can be taught that changes in their environment can reduce cues to smoke; smokers can throw away their cigarettes, avoid places and events where others are smoking, and reduce consumption of alcohol, tea, colas, or other drinks associated with smoking. They can be taught that stress, arguments, and negative mood are associated with desire to light up a cigarette. These stressful situations cannot be entirely avoided, but smokers can learn other cognitive and behavioral strategies to distract attention from smoking. Therapists can train smokers to use such relaxation techniques as deep breathing, visual imagery, progressive muscle relaxation, and self-hypnosis. (We discussed these and other forms of stress management in Chapter 8.) Smokers effectively trained in stress-coping skills are more likely to quit than those who have not learned these techniques (Burling, Burling, & Latini, 2001; Fiore et al., 1996).

Both individual and group counseling can be successful in helping people to quit smoking. Psychologists, physicians, and nurses can be effective providers, but effectiveness is positively related to the amount of contact between client and therapist. The increased costs of intensive interventions are offset by their improved effectiveness. Programs that include more sessions tend to be more effective than programs with fewer sessions, but increases beyond about seven sessions merely increases costs, not effectiveness. The most effective programs include both a counseling component and a nicotine replacement component. These elements are both effective, and the combination of the two improves outcomes (Wetter et al., 1998).

Participating in a Community Campaign Many people stop smoking as a result of their participation in a communitywide health campaign. Such health campaigns are not new, dating back to Cotton Mather more than 2 centuries before anyone suspected the dangers of cigarette smoking. Mather used pamphlets and oratory to persuade the people of Boston to accept smallpox inoculations (Faden, 1987). Today, several hundred large community programs exist throughout the world (Secker-Walker et al., 2000). Such campaigns are typically sponsored by governmental agencies or by large corporations as an intervention designed to improve the health of large numbers of people.

The percentage of people who change behavior as a result of a health campaign is usually quite small, but if the message reaches millions of people, then thousands of lives may be saved. In 1989, the state of California enacted a cigarette surtax in order to fund an antismoking campaign (Fichtenberg & Glantz, 2000). This aggressive program not only reduced the number of smokers, but also saved an estimated 33,300 lives from heart disease between 1989 and 1997. An earlier intervention in Vermont and New Hampshire (Secker-Walker et al., 2000) was both less aggressive and less effective than the campaign in California. In the New England study, researchers used random-digit dialing to contact female smokers and to encourage them to quit. The quit rate was higher in the two intervention counties than in two matched comparison counties—24% versus 21% after 4 years. This difference may seem small, but it represents hundreds of women giving up cigarettes who might not otherwise quit smoking.

Community campaigns are frequently limited to a workplace community. Deborah Hennrikus and colleagues (Hennrikus et al., 2002) offered monetary incentives along with telephone counseling to smokers at various worksites in Minneapolis and St Paul, Minnesota. Workers were given $10 for participating in a smoking cessation program and $20 for completing three fourths of the program. In addition, workers who remained smoke free could register for a chance at a $500 drawing. These incentives doubled the number of smokers who signed up for the cessation program. However, they were not sufficient to produce a significant difference in cessation rates for workers who received a monetary incentive and those who did not. The authors concluded that a monetary incentive might not be an effective addition to a smoking cessation program that also included telephone counseling.

Who Quits and Who Does Not?

Who is successful at quitting and who is not? Investigators have examined several factors that may answer this question, including gender, age, educational level, quitting other drugs, and weight concern, which we discuss in a later section.

Are men more likely than women to quit smoking? Because men have had higher quit rates than women over the past 40 years, many observers assumed that women have more difficulty quitting than men. Although some evidence exists to support this idea (Vastag, 2001), the reason may be that female smokers who try to quit have more obstacles to overcome. Some research (Bjornson et al., 1995) suggests that gender differences could be explained by baseline differences. That is, at the beginning of the study, women are *less* likely to (1) be married, (2) have made a previous quit attempt, (3) have made longer quit attempts, and (4) be heavy smokers. Also, women were *more* likely to live with other smokers. Regardless of gender, each of these factors is associated with poorer quit rates. In other words, women generally have more obstacles to hurdle in trying to quit smoking.

Although women often have lower quit rates than men, the evidence for this is somewhat complex (Fortmann & Killen, 1994). First, women are more likely to volunteer to participate in such programs, but their motivation may simply be to go to therapy to support a friend. Second, once women express a genuine interest in quitting, they are as likely as men to quit. Third, although women have more difficulty during the first 24 hours, after that time they have the same quit rates as men. In summary, women may be more willing to make quit attempts, and may be less successful during the first

24 hours, but they are equal to men in avoiding relapse once they have quit.

Another factor relating to quitting is age. In general, younger smokers, especially those who smoke at a high level, are more likely to continue smoking than older smokers who smoke at a low level (Nordstrom et al., 2000).

A supportive social network may also help people quit smoking. Cessation programs are more effective in maintaining abstinence when spouses of participants are trained to offer support to the partner who is trying to quit. In contrast, having a greater than average number of smokers in one's social network may be a hindrance to initiating a cessation program (Klonoff & Landrine, 1999). Similarly, pregnant women who smoke are more likely to quit if their partners are nonsmokers or if they receive support from their partners (McBride et al., 1998).

Do difficulties in quitting smoking explain the inverse relationship between educational level and rate of smoking; that is, does educational level relate to quitting? Recent research (Droomers, Schrijvers, & Mackenbach, 2002) suggests an affirmative answer. This longitudinal study of Dutch participants found that people with low educational levels at baseline were more than twice as likely to remain smokers. More important, smokers with lower levels of education (1) begin smoking earlier, (2) have higher scores of neuroticism (anxiety, depression, guilt, and low self-esteem), (3) have lower scores on emotional support, and (4) have low levels of perceived personal control. These factors, rather than knowledge of the hazards of smoking, may be important reasons why lower educational level is associated with higher smoking rates.

Finally, do smokers who abuse alcohol and other drugs find it harder to give up cigarettes? Clinical psychologists have long recognized the strong relationship between smoking and drinking, but until recently there has been little research on how quitting one substance affects quitting the other. Some evidence now suggests that problem drinkers who are able to stop drinking are also able to quit smoking (Breslau, Peterson, Schultz, Andreski, & Chilcoat, 1996). Similarly, cognitive behavioral programs designed to help homeless veterans stop smoking contained the same elements that enabled these men to stop using alcohol and other drugs (Burling et al., 2001). This finding indicates that many people can stop two addictive behaviors simultaneously.

Relapse Prevention

The problem of relapse is not unique to smoking. Relapse rates are quite similar among people who have quit smoking, given up alcohol, and stopped using heroin (Hunt, Barnett, & Branch, 1971). The high rate of relapse after smoking cessation treatment prompted G. Alan Marlatt and Judith Gordon (1980) to examine the relapse process itself. For many people who have been successful in quitting, one cigarette precipitates a full relapse, complete with feelings of total failure. Marlatt and Gordon termed this phenomenon the *abstinence violation effect*. They incorporated strategies into their treatment to cope with patients' despair when they violate their intention to remain abstinent. By training patients that one "slip" does not constitute relapse, Marlatt and Gordon buffer them against a full relapse. Slips are common even among people who will eventually quit. One fourth of successful self-quitters slip at one time or another (Hughes et al., 1992). Thus, a single slip should not discourage people from continuing their effort to stop smoking.

Self-quitters have very high relapse rates. One study (Hughes et al., 1992) found that two thirds of smokers who quit on their own had relapsed after only 2 days and 92% had resumed smoking after 6 months. In formal smoking cessation programs that include relapse prevention, failure rates are not quite so high—about 70 to 80%.

The AHCPR guidelines (Fiore et al., 1996) suggest several procedures for preventing relapse and strongly recommend they be incorporated into all cessation programs. First, therapists should review reasons for relapse, such as fear of weight gain, unpleasant withdrawal symptoms, negative mood or depression, and lack of social support for cessation. Once these factors have been identified, therapists can work to reduce or

BECOMING HEALTHIER

1. If you do not smoke, don't start. College students are still susceptible to the pressure to smoke if their friends are smokers. The easiest way to be a nonsmoker is to stay a nonsmoker.
2. If you smoke, don't fool yourself into believing that the risks of smoking do not apply to you. Examine your own optimistic biases regarding smoking. Do not imagine that smoking low-tar and low-nicotine cigarettes makes smoking safe. Research indicates that these cigarettes are about as risky as any others.
3. If you smoke, quit. Even if you feel that quitting will be difficult, make an attempt to quit. If your first attempt is not successful, try again. Research indicates that people who keep trying are very likely to succeed.
4. If you have tried to quit on your own and have failed, look for a program to help you. Remember that not all programs are equally successful. Research indicates that the most effective programs combine some psychological techniques with nicotine replacement therapy.
5. The best cessation programs allow for some individual tailoring to meet personal needs. Try different techniques until you find one that works for you.
6. If you are trying to quit smoking, find a supportive network of friends and acquaintances to help you stop and to boost your motivation to quit. Avoid people who try to sabotage your attempts to quit, and be cautious in going to places or engaging in activities that have a high association with smoking.
7. Cigar smoking has undergone a resurgence in popularity. Cigar and pipe smoking are not as dangerous as cigarette smoking, but remember that no level of smoking is safe.
8. No level of tobacco exposure is safe. Exposure to environmental tobacco smoke is not nearly as dangerous as smoking, but it is not safe either. Smokeless tobacco use carries a number of health risks.
9. If you smoke, do not expose others to your smoke. Young children are especially vulnerable, and smoking parents can minimize the risks of respiratory disease in their children by keeping smoke away from their children.

eliminate them. For example, for smokers who fear gaining weight, the practitioner can inform them that the health benefits of quitting smoking are far greater than any health problems that might accompany weight gain. For smokers who are depressed, the therapist can provide individual or group counseling. For those suffering prolonged withdrawal symptoms, the therapist can recommend nicotine replacement therapy. For smokers needing more social support, the intervention can include making follow-up telephone calls and enlisting encouragement from the ex-smoker's family and friends. Research with some of these techniques (Brandon, Collins, Juliano, & Lazev, 2000) suggests that people who have given up smoking can remain abstinent if they receive repeated mailings of relapse prevention booklets. After 12 months, only 12% of ex-smokers who received the mail intervention returned to smoking, compared with 35% of ex-smokers who did not receive the periodic mailings. However, having access to a telephone hotline did not effectively prevent relapse. No intervention keeps every former smoker abstinent, and relapse remains a problem even in programs designed to cope with it.

In Summary

Smoking rates can be reduced either by prevention or by quitting. One approach to preventing young people from starting is the "inoculation" method, in which teenagers are given information to buffer them against the persuasive arguments of peers and media. These behavioral interventions—which include peer influence, training in refusal skills, and practice at making decisions—have had some success in deterring young people from smoking.

How can people quit smoking? Because giving up nicotine may result in withdrawal symptoms, many successful cessation programs include nicotine replacement in the form of a nicotine patch or nicotine gum. Both are more effective than a placebo, but without counseling, neither can claim high success rates. A second approach to quitting is psychological counseling, which usually includes assertiveness training, enhanced self-efficacy, relaxation training, social support, and stress management. An approach to reducing smoking rates involves large-scale community programs, which usually include antitobacco mass media campaigns. If even a small percentage of people exposed to such campaigns stops smoking, this can translate into thousands of people giving up tobacco. By combining nicotine replacement with psychological interventions, quit rates become higher—perhaps as high as 30%. In addition, millions of people have stopped smoking on their own. Men are more likely to be successful at quitting than women, perhaps because women face more barriers when they try to quit. Many people are able to quit for 6 months to 1 year, but the problem of relapse remains serious. Programs aimed at this relapse problem can be successful, but cessation programs need to address the issue of relapse.

Effects of Quitting

When smokers quit, they experience a number of effects, almost all of which are positive. However, one possible negative effect is the weight gain.

Quitting and Weight Gain

We have seen that many smokers fear weight gain if they give up smoking. Are such concerns justified? Several factors need to be examined when considering the health benefits of quitting smoking and adding weight.

First, middle-aged people will probably gain some weight whether they are smokers, have quit smoking, or have never smoked (Pirie, Murray, & Luepker, 1991).

Second, the weight gain is quite modest for most people who have stopped smoking. Peggy O'Hara and colleagues (1998) studied weight gain of former smokers and found that after 1 year, the average gain for women was a little more than 11 pounds and after 5 years, it was about 7.5 pounds. For men, the average weight gain after 1 year was a little less than 11 pounds and after 5 years, it was about 6 pounds.

Third, although most people who quit smoking experience only modest weight gain, some individuals gain large amounts of weight. O'Hara et al. (1998) found that 19% of women and 7% of men who quit smoking gained 20% or more of their baseline weight and that most of that gain occurred during the first year.

Fourth, although women are generally more concerned about weight gain than are men, their total weight gain after smoking cessation is about the same as that of men (Nides et al., 1994). However, because women are generally not as heavy as men at baseline, their *percentage* of weight gain is typically more than that of men.

Fifth, weight gain following smoking cessation can be temporary, and for female ex-smokers, both body mass index and body weight tend to decrease with years of smoking cessation (Chen, Horne, & Dosman, 1993). Former smokers are heaviest about 2 years after quitting, after which time their weight matches that of those who have never smoked.

Sixth, physical activity for ex-smokers can curtail weight gain in most people. Research from the Nurses Health Study (Kawachi, Troist, Robnitzky, Coakley, & Colditz, 1996) revealed that women who increased their level of exercise after quitting smoking gained less weight than women who quit but did not become more physically active. Similarly, a study with men (Froom et al., 1999) found that those who stopped smoking had a slight increase in body mass index, but men who were active in sports gained less than the sedentary ex-smokers.

Seventh, cognitive behavioral therapy can be successful in helping women to quit smoking and to reduce their concerns about weight gain without encouraging them to adopt an unhealthy diet (Perkins et al., 2001).

These findings suggest that the overall health of smokers is enhanced by quitting smoking. Smokers should be more concerned about the risks from smoking than from weight because the benefits of quitting smoking far outweigh the benefits of eating a low-fat diet—at least in terms of life expectancy (Grover, Gray-Donald, Joseph, Abrahamowicz, & Coupal, 1994). For the average male and female smokers who are free of heart disease, eating a diet of no more than 10% of calories from saturated fat would extend their lives somewhere between three days and three months. However, quitting smoking would add three or four years to life expectancy. The extra weight gained by former smokers—men and women—does not negate the health benefits of smoking cessation. Quitting smoking is much more beneficial to health than maintaining lower weight.

Health Benefits of Quitting

Can longtime cigarette smokers improve their health and add years to their life by quitting? One estimate suggests that the average reduction in life expectancy for smokers is 5 to 8 years, depending on the amount of smoking (Fielding, 1985). Can smokers regain some of their life expectancy by quitting? How long must ex-smokers remain abstinent before they reverse the detrimental effects of smoking?

The 1990 report of the Surgeon General summarized studies indicating that former light smokers (fewer than 20 cigarettes a day) who were able to abstain for 16 years had about the same rate of mortality as people who had never smoked (USDHHS, 1990). This encouraging finding was true for both women and men . Figure 13.8 shows that, after more than 15 years of abstinence, women who were either light or heavy smokers returned to the same risk for death as women who had never smoked. For women who were heavy smokers, the benefits of quitting were substantial, especially after the 3rd year of abstinence. Women who were light smokers seemed to have benefited almost immediately from quitting, and by the 16th year of abstinence, they had the same mortality rate as women who had never smoked. So Lisa, the smoker described in the introduction to this chapter who smokes 20 cigarettes or fewer a day, could eventually reduce her risk of death to a level about equal to what it would have been if she had never smoked.

Figure 13.9 shows that men who are current heavy smokers have a risk of death about 2.5 times greater than those who have never smoked. But those who quit show a steady reduction in mortality rate after the first year of abstinence if they have not already developed some smoking-related condition. After 16 years without smoking, men reduce their mortality risk to about half that of current smokers and only slightly more than that of nonsmokers. Men who were formerly light smokers do even better after 16 years of abstinence; they have about the same relative risk as men who have never smoked. For those with cancer, heart disease, or stroke, the benefits of quitting do not show up until after 3 years of abstinence, perhaps because many sick people quit in the years immediately before they die.

Longtime smokers who quit reduce their chances of dying from heart disease much more than they lower their risk of death from lung cancer. Several studies show that cigarette smokers who quit can eventually reduce their risk of cardiovascular disease to that of a nonsmoker, but their risk of cancer, especially lung cancer, remains elevated. For example, men who quit smoking for 30 years had only a very slightly

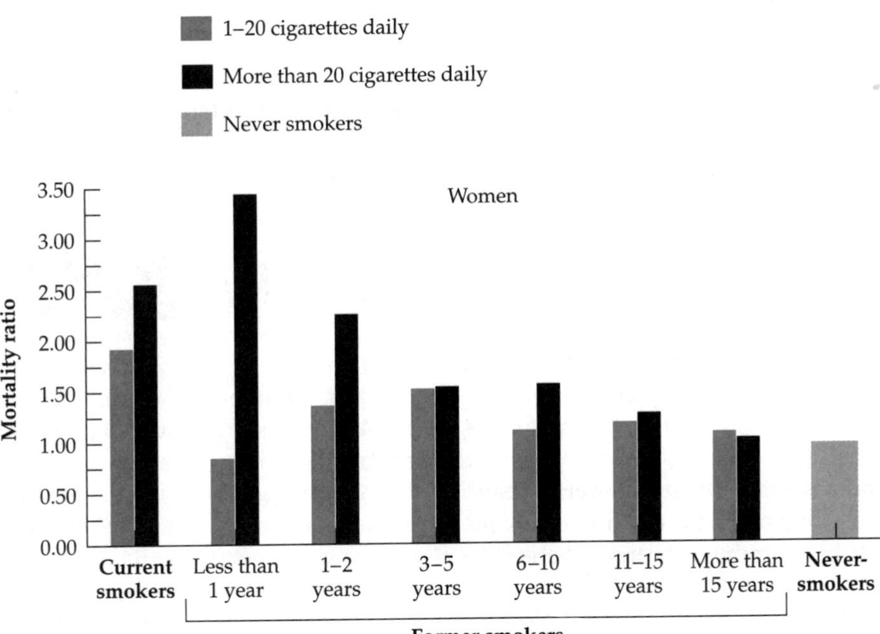

Figure 13.8 Overall mortality ratios for current and former female smokers compared with never smokers, by duration of abstinence.

Source: The Health Benefits of Smoking Cessation: A Report of the Surgeon General *(p. 78) by U.S. Department of Health and Human Services, 1990, (DHHS Publication No. CDC 90–8416), Washington, DC: U.S. Government Printing Office.*

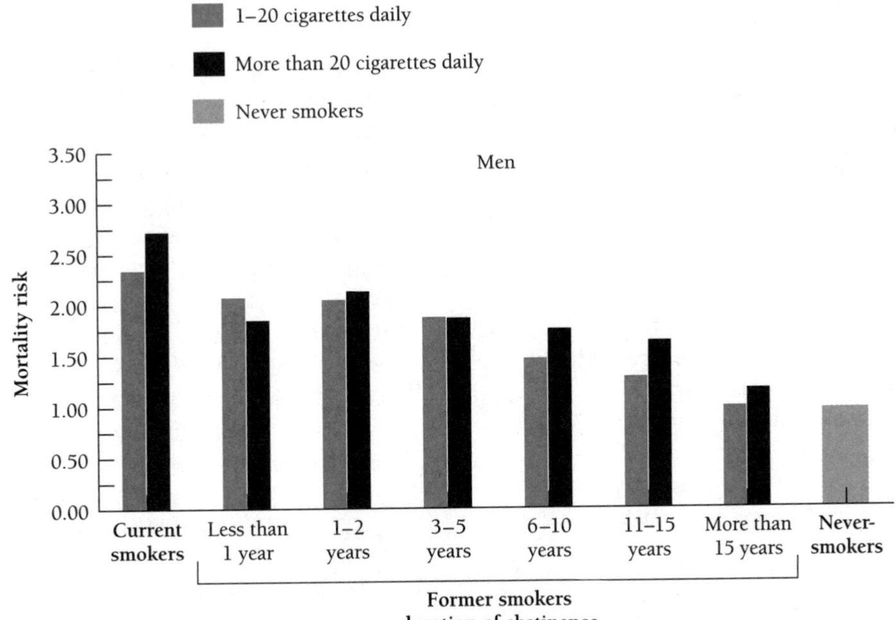

Figure 13.9 Overall mortality ratios for current and former male smokers compared with never smokers, by duration of abstinence.

Source: The Health Benefits of Smoking Cessation: A Report of the Surgeon General *(p. 78) by U.S. Department of Health and Human Services, 1990, (DHHS Publication No. CDC 90–8416), Washington, DC: U.S. Government Printing Office.*

elevated risk of coronary heart disease, but these same men had nearly a threefold risk for lung cancer (Ben-Shlomo et al., 1994). However, this increased risk of lung cancer for former smokers was less than one fourth the risk of men who continued smoking. Thus, men who quit smoking for 30 years reduce their risk of both cardiovascular disease and lung cancer, but their risk for lung cancer remains substantially higher than that of men who have never smoked. Women also reduce their risks by quitting. The excess risk of stroke disappears in middle-aged women who stop smoking, regardless of the number of cigarettes they had smoked, the age at which they had started, or the presence of other stroke risk factors (Kawachi et al., 1993).

These studies suggest that by quitting smoking, both male and female smokers can reduce their risk of cardiovascular disease to that of nonsmokers, although they may never completely erase their elevated risk of lung cancer. Thus, never starting to smoke is healthier than quitting, but quitting, though seldom easy, can pay off.

In Summary

Many smokers fear that if they stop smoking, they will gain weight, but the evidence shows that the average weight gain for most men and women is relatively modest—about 9 to 11 pounds. Even excessive weight gain is far less risky than continuing to smoke. On a more positive note, stopping smoking improves health and extends life expectancy. Some evidence suggests that after smokers have quit for 16 years, their all-cause mortality rate may return to that of nonsmokers, although they may continue to have an excess risk for lung cancer mortality.

Answers

This chapter addressed five basic questions.

1. How does smoking affect the respiratory system?

The respiratory system allows for the intake of oxygen and the elimination of carbon dioxide. Cigarette smoke drawn into the lungs eventually damages the lungs, and chronic bronchitis and emphysema are two chronic pulmonary diseases related to smoking. Tobacco contains several thousand compounds, including nicotine, and smoke exposes smokers to tars and other compounds that contribute to heart disease and cancer.

2. Who chooses to smoke and why?

Slightly less than one fourth of all U.S. adults smoke, about one fourth are former smokers, and a little more than one half have never smoked. Slightly more men than women smoke, but gender is not as important as educational level as a predictor of smoking—higher education is associated with lower smoking rates. Most smokers start as adolescents, and one motivation is that smoking is part of a risk-taking, rebellious style that is attractive to some adolescents. No conclusive answer exists for why people continue to smoke, but the nicotine plays a role, especially for some smokers. Other smokers list relaxation and stress reduction as reasons to continue.

3. What are the health consequences of tobacco use?

Smoking is the number one cause of preventable death in the United States, causing about 440,000 deaths a year, mostly from cancer, cardiovascular disease, and chronic obstructive pulmonary disease. Smoking also carries a risk of nonfatal diseases and disorders such as periodontal disease, loss of physical strength and bone density, respiratory disorders, cognitive dysfunction, facial wrinkling, sexual impotence, and macular degeneration. Passive smoking does not contribute substantially to death from lung cancer, but environmental tobacco smoke raises young children's risk of respiratory disease and even death. Adults exposed to environmental tobacco smoke have an elevated risk of death from cardiovascular disease. Smokeless tobacco is probably somewhat safer than cigarette smoking, but the use of smokeless tobacco is associated with increased rates of oral cancer and periodontal disease and may be related to coronary heart disease.

4. **How can smoking rates be reduced?**
   One way to reduce smoking rates is to prevent people from starting. One such program is the "inoculation" method in which teenagers are given information to buffer them against the persuasive arguments of peers and media. Most people who quit do so on their own without any formal cessation program, but relapse is a problem for these smokers. Nicotine replacement in the form of a nicotine patch or nicotine gum can be a useful component in smoking cessation, but use of nicotine replacement alone is not a very successful approach. Psychological counseling that includes enhanced self-efficacy, relaxation, and assertiveness training can be effective in helping people quit. Mass media campaigns that reach thousands or even millions of smokers are successful in helping some smokers quit.

5. **What are the effects of quitting?**
   Many smokers fear weight gain upon quitting, and a modest gain (9 to 11 pounds) is common. Nevertheless, gaining weight is not as hazardous to a person's health as continuing to smoke. Quitting improves health and extends life, but returning to the risk level of nonsmokers for cardiovascular mortality can take 16 years or longer, and most ex-smokers will retain some elevated risk for lung cancer.

Suggested Readings

Jamieson, P., & Romer, D. (2001). What do young people think they know about the risks of smoking? In P. Slovic (Ed.), *Smoking: Risk, perception & policy* (pp 51–63). Twin Oaks, CA: Sage. In this chapter, Patrick Jamieson and Daniel Romer review research on a variety of topics about young people's knowledge of the risks of smoking. In some areas, the beliefs of young people were reasonably accurate, but in other areas, their beliefs did not agree with the research. In general, however, these youth did not adequately understand the dangers of smoking.

Kluger, R. (1996). *Ashes to ashes; America's hundred-year cigarette war, the public health and the unabashed triumph of Philip Morris.* New York: Knopf. Kluger presents a lengthy but fascinating account of the story of tobacco, the attempts to discourage its use, and the ultimate victory of the tobacco industry. This review of the leading theories of tobacco use includes a summary of relevant research.

Parascandola, M. (2001). Cigarettes and the U.S. Public Health Service in the 1950s. *American Journal of Public Health, 91*, 196–205. Public concern about the hazards of smoking began mostly with the 1964 Surgeon General's report. However, as shown in this article by Mark Parascandola, most scientists within the National Institutes of Health knew about the dangers of smoking by the mid 1950s, but they did not view their role as one of fighting against the tobacco industry. Thus, nearly a decade was lost before they began to battle against cigarette smoking.

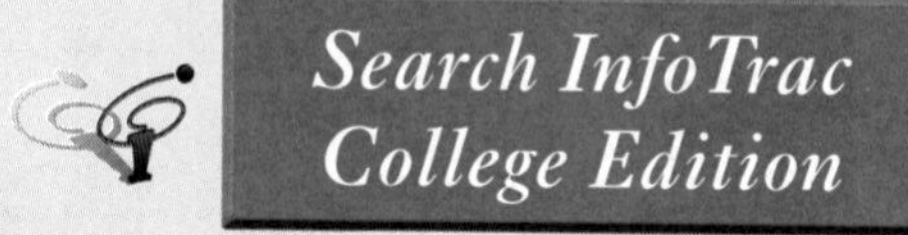

Search these terms to learn more about topics in this chapter:

- Tobacco and respiratory
- Smoking and demographic and United States
- Smoking and international
- Surgeon General and smoking
- Smoking and women and statistics
- Children and smoking and risks
- Adolescents and smoking and risk
- Nicotine addiction and smoking
- Smoking and genetic aspects
- Weight control and smoking
- Smoking and psychological effects
- Smoking and health risks
- Smoking and cancer risk
- Passive smoking and health
- Nicotine replacement
- Quitting smoking
- Smoking and relapse

14

Using Alcohol and Other Drugs

The Story of Chad

CHAPTER OUTLINE

QUESTIONS

This chapter focuses on six basic questions:

1. What are the major trends in alcohol consumption?
2. What are the health effects of drinking alcohol?
3. Why do people drink?
4. How can people change problem drinking?
5. What problems are associated with relapse?
6. What are the health effects of other drugs?

The Story of Chad

Chad, a European American college senior, classifies himself as a social drinker because he drinks only in social situations or when he is out with friends. He usually has just one drink per day and never more than four drinks. A year ago, however, his consumption was much higher. At that time, he was a member of a fraternity and frequently went out with his friends and drank heavily. About two or three times a year, he would get "stupid, falling down drunk," usually as a celebration for some occasion such as the completion of midterm exams.

Being part of a college fraternity shaped Chad's drinking habits. Unlike the majority of his peers in high school, he had no interest in experimenting with alcohol. In fact, he had a very negative attitude toward drinking, an attitude that started to change when he began to drink. His first experience with alcohol was just before his 18th birthday, when some friends took him out and got him drunk on beer. Although this episode resulted in a terrible hangover, Chad did not develop negative feelings about drinking.

As a freshman in college, Chad joined a fraternity, where drinking was a major part of the social life. Although he did not drink as much as many of his fraternity brothers, he began to drink at the fraternity house and at local clubs and bars. When one of the fraternity brothers had drunk too much, the other members would try to keep him from doing anything too embarrassing and to get him back to the fraternity house safely. Occasionally, Chad was the one in need of help, but more often, he provided assistance.

During college, Chad's level of alcohol consumption escalated to frequent moderate drinking combined with occasional binges. Presently, however, his drinking has decreased—partly because his fraternity has been dissolved but mostly because his last binge resulted in a "blackout" in which he did not remember the socially embarrassing behavior that got him thrown out of his favorite club. As a consequence of his embarrassment, he resolved never to get drunk again. However, he continues to be a light social drinker.

Chad believes that his reduction in drinking was the result of a natural process of "settling down." He has also noticed that his younger classmates and friends seem to be drinking less, mostly when the legal drinking age changed from 18 to 21.

Alcohol Consumption—Yesterday and Today

Is Chad's assessment of his drinking patterns accurate—is he a social drinker, or does he have problems associated with alcohol? Is his drinking typical for college students? What drinking patterns present problems? This chapter includes answers to these questions, but first, we examine the history of drinking.

A Brief History of Alcohol Consumption

The use of alcohol is not something that can easily be traced; it was discovered worldwide and repeatedly, dating back beyond recorded history. The yeast that is responsible for producing alcohol is airborne, and fermentation occurs naturally in fruits, fruit juices, and grain mixtures. Producing beverage alcohol requires no sophisticated technology, and there is evidence that most ancient cultures used beverage alcohol. Ancient Babylonians discovered both wine (fermented grape juice) and beer (fermented grain), as did the ancient Egyptians, Greeks, Romans, Chinese, and Indians. Pre-Columbian tribes in the Americas also used fermented products.

Ancient civilizations also discovered drunkenness, of course. In several of those countries, such as Greece, drunkenness was not only allowed but also practically required on certain occasions, but these occasions were limited to festivals. This pattern resembles present-day practices in the United States, where drunkenness is condoned at some parties and celebrations. Most societies

CHECK YOUR HEALTH RISKS

Check the items that apply to you.

- ☐ 1. I have had five or more alcoholic drinks in one day at least once during the past month.
- ☐ 2. I have had five or more alcoholic drinks on the same occasion on at least five different days during the past month.
- ☐ 3. When I drink too much, I sometimes don't remember a lot of the things that happened.
- ☐ 4. I sometimes ride with a driver who has been drinking.
- ☐ 5. On at least one occasion during the past year, I drove a motor vehicle after having more than two drinks.
- ☐ 6. I rarely have more than two drinks in one day.
- ☐ 7. I do not drive when I am intoxicated, but I have driven an automobile after having one or two drinks.
- ☐ 8. I sometimes play sports or go swimming after having a "couple" of drinks.
- ☐ 9. Some of my friends or family have told me that I drink too much.
- ☐ 10. I have tried to cut down on my drinking, but I never seem to succeed.
- ☐ 11. At least once in my life, I have tried to completely quit drinking, but I was not successful.
- ☐ 12. I believe that the best way to enjoy many activities (such as a dance or a football game) is to drink alcohol.
- ☐ 13. After waking up with a hangover, I sometimes have a drink to feel better.
- ☐ 14. There are some activities that I perform better after drinking.
- ☐ 15. I have drunk fewer than 10 alcoholic drinks in my lifetime.

Most of these items represent a health risk related to using alcohol by increasing risk for diseases and unintentional injuries. However, item #6 probably reflects a healthy pattern of consumption for most people, whereas #15 is not necessarily consistent with a healthy lifestyle. As you read this chapter, you will learn that some of these items are more risky than others.

condone drinking alcohol but not drunkenness, except on certain occasions.

Distillation was discovered in ancient China, and refined in 8th-century Arabia. Because the process is somewhat complex, the use of distilled spirits did not become widespread until they were commercially manufactured. In England, fermented beverages were by far the most common form of alcohol consumption until the 18th century, when England encouraged the proliferation of distilleries to stimulate commerce. Along with cheap gin came widespread consumption and widespread drunkenness. However, intoxication from distilled spirits was confined mostly to the lower and working classes; the rich drank wine, which was imported and, thus, expensive.

In colonial America, drinking was much more prevalent than it is today. Men, women, and children all drank, and it was considered acceptable for all to do so. This practice may not seem consistent with our present-day image of the Puritans, but nevertheless, the Puritans did not object to drinking. Rather, they considered alcohol one of God's gifts. Indeed, in those years, alcohol was often safer than unpurified water or milk, so the Puritans had a legitimate reason to condone the consumption of alcoholic beverages. What was not acceptable to them was drunkenness. They believed that alcohol should, like all things, be used in moderation. Therefore, the Puritans established severe prohibitions against drunkenness but not against drinking.

The 50 years following U.S. independence marked a transition in the way early Americans thought about alcohol (Edwards, 2000). An adamant and vocal minority came to consider

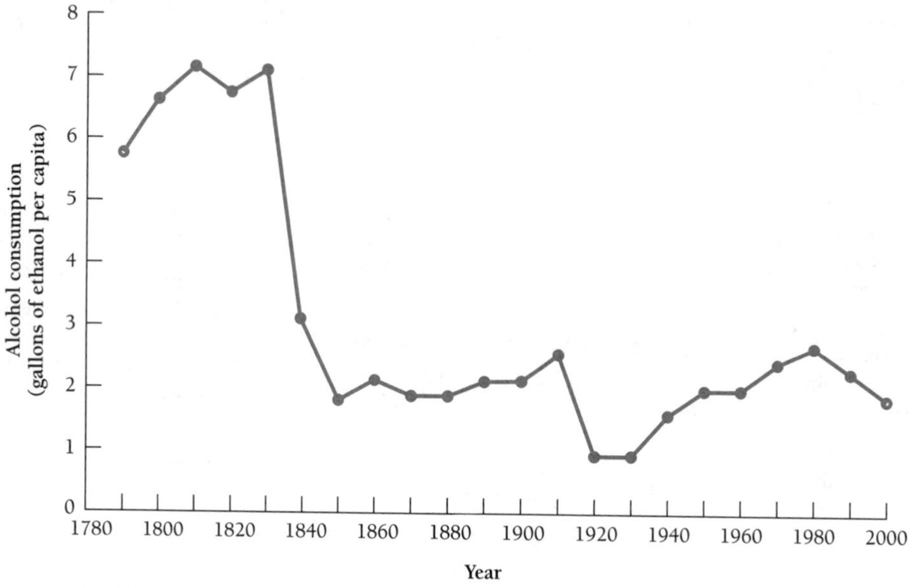

Figure 14.1 U.S. consumption of all alcoholic beverages, 1790–2000, ages 15 and older.

Source: From The Alcoholic Republic: An American Tradition *(p. 9) by W. J. Rorabaugh, 1979, New York: Oxford University Press. Copyright 1979 by Oxford University Press. Reprinted by permission. Also from* Apparent per capita ethanol consumption for the United States, 1850–1998. *Retrieved from the World Wide Web, July 2, 2002, www.niaaa.nih.gov/databases/consum01.txt.*

liquor a "demon" and to totally abstain from its use. Similar attitudes arose in Britain. This attitude was mostly limited to the upper and upper-middle classes. Later, abstention came to be an accepted doctrine of the middle class and people who aspired to join the middle class. Intemperance in drinking alcohol thus became associated with the lower classes, and "respectable" people, especially women, were expected not to be heavy drinkers.

Temperance societies proliferated throughout the United States during the mid-1800s. However, the term is a misnomer: the societies did not promote *temperance*—that is, the moderate use of alcohol. Rather, they advocated *prohibition,* the total abstinence from alcohol. Temperance societies held that liquor weakens inhibitions; loosens desires and passions; causes a large percentage of crime, poverty, and broken homes; and is powerfully addicting, so much so that even an occasional drink would put one in danger. Figure 14.1 shows a dramatic decrease in per capita alcohol consumption in the United States after 1830, a decrease due directly to the spread of the temperance (Prohibition) movement. Note also the more recent decline in consumption since about 1980.

In response to the growing temperance movement, both the demographics and the location of drinking changed. Rather than being consumed in a family setting or a respectable tavern, alcohol became increasingly confined to saloons, which were patronized largely by urban industrial workers (Popham, 1978). Portrayed by the temperance movement as the personification of evil and moral degeneracy, saloons served as a focus for growing Prohibitionist sentiment. Drinking became associated with the lower and working classes.

Prohibitionists were finally victorious in 1919 with the ratification of the 18th Amendment to the Constitution of the United States. This amendment outlawed the manufacture, sale, or transportation of alcoholic beverages and lowered per capita consumption drastically (as shown in Figure 14.1). This amendment was not popular and created a large illegal market for alcohol. The growing unpopularity of Prohibition resulted in the 21st Amendment, which repealed the 18th Amendment and ended Prohibition in 1934. Figure 14.1 shows that after the repeal of Prohibition, alcohol consumption rose sharply. Although the current per capita consumption of alcohol is considerably higher than during Prohibition, it is less than half the rate reached during the first 3 decades of the 19th century.

The Prevalence of Alcohol Consumption Today

About half of the adults in the United States are classified as current regular drinkers (defined as having at least 12 drinks during the past year), about 21% engage in binge drinking (five or more drinks on the same occasion at least once per month), and a little more than 5% are heavy drinkers (more than 14 drinks per week for men or 7 per week for women) (NCHS, 2001). These drinking rates—shown in Figure 14.2—reflect the leveling of a 20-year decline in alcohol consumption in the United States.

The frequency of drinking and the prevalence of heavy drinking are not equal for all demographic groups in the United States. As Figure 14.3 shows, drinking varies by ethnicity. European Americans tend to have higher rates of drinking than other ethnic groups, and Asian Americans have the lowest rates (Substance Abuse and Mental Health Services Administration [SAMHSA], 2001). Rates of binge and heavy drinking also vary with ethnicity, with Native Americans having higher rates of these drinking patterns.

Age is another factor in drinking. Adults 21 to 39 have the highest rates of drinking, but young adults 18 to 25 have the highest rates of binge drinking and heavy drinking. Nearly half of the drinkers 18 to 25 are binge drinkers and about one in five are heavy drinkers (NCHS, 2001). Many of Chad's friends were binge drinkers, and Chad, too, had several episodes of binge drinking during his earlier years at college. This increasing and then decreasing frequency of binge drinking during adolescence was one pattern that appeared in a study on adolescent binge drinkers (Tucker, Orlando, & Ellickson, 2003). However, many other patterns occur for binge drinking, including adolescents who accelerate their binge drinking beginning in their early teens and others who retain a stable pattern of binge drinking about once a month. Binge drinking can lead to a variety of hazards (especially for inexperienced drinkers), resulting in intoxication, poor judgment, and impaired coordination. Certain situations promote binge drinking, and college students are at particular risk. Chad chose to binge drink on "special occasions," such as homecoming or after midterm and final exams, and his fraternity brothers encouraged him to do so. Research confirms that Chad's experience is common: college students in fraternities and sororities drink more heavily than those not in these organizations, but their college drinking habits do not predict drinking problems after graduation (Jackson, Sher, Gotham, & Wood, 2001). During the college years, however, binge drinking is a persistent problem that creates many hazards (Wechsler et al., 2002).

Among adolescents 12 to 17, current use of alcohol dropped dramatically after the legal age

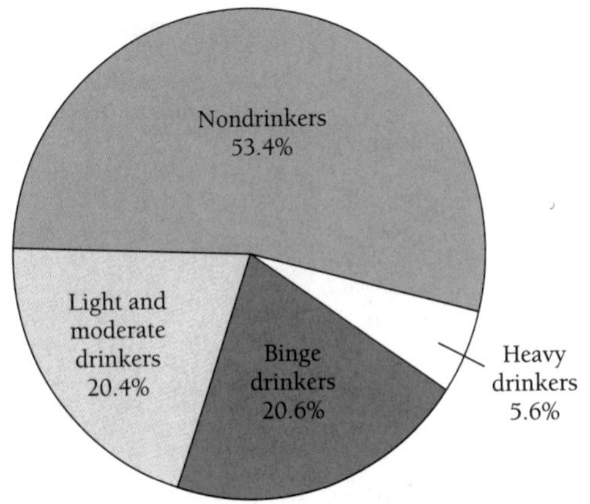

Figure 14.2 Alcohol consumption by type of drinker, adults, United States, 2000.

Source: SAMHSA, *www.samhsa.gov/oas/NHSDA/2kNHSDA.*

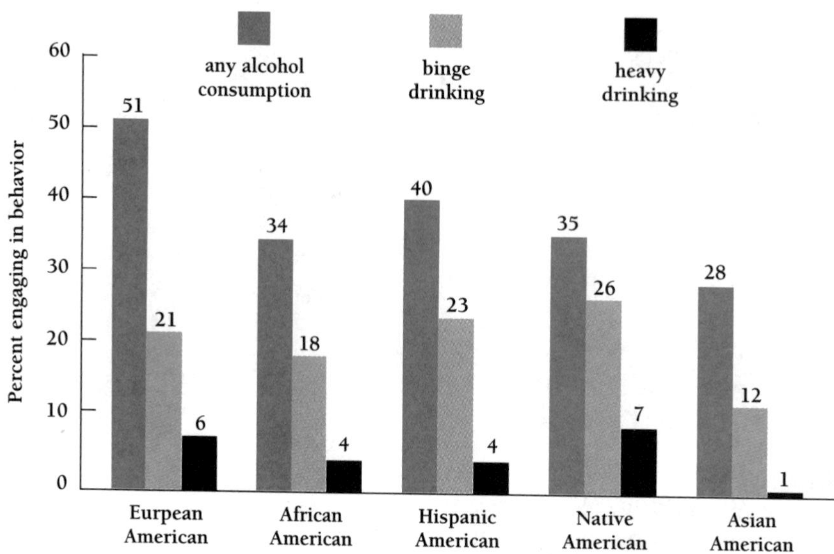

Figure 14.3 Percent of people age 12 and older who report monthly alcohol use, binge drinking, and heavy drinking, by ethnic group, United States, 2000.

Source: SAMHSA, 2001, Summary of findings from the 2000 National Household Survey on Drug Abuse. *(DHHS Publication No. 01–3549) Rockville, MD: U.S. Government Printing Office.*

for buying alcohol was raised to 21 in most states: in 1985, over 40% of the adolescents in this age group were current users, but by 1992, only 20% were current drinkers, a rate that has remained relatively stable since 1992 (USBC, 2001). Although binge drinking is still common among college and high school students, the percentage of students who engage in this drinking pattern has declined. Among male high school students, for example, binge drinking has declined from more than 50% during the early 1980s to about 33.5% in 1999 (Grunbaum et al., 2002). For female high school students, binge drinking also decreased to 28%.

Why are young people drinking less? One possibility is that they are replacing alcohol with illicit drugs. However, the evidence for this hypothesis is somewhat mixed. A report by Lloyd Johnston and his colleagues (Johnston, O'Malley, & Bachman, 2002) showed only a slight or no increase in high school students' use of most illicit drugs from 1991 to 2000. During the early 1990s, use of marijuana among high school students rose sharply but then leveled off. Thus, alcohol use has declined, but other drug use has not risen to compensate.

Alcohol consumption rates are lowest among older adults (NCHS, 2001). Some people decrease their alcohol consumption as they leave college and the social situations and pressures to drink (Jackson et al., 2001). In general, alcohol intake is inversely related to age—older ages are associated with lower levels of drinking (Eigenbrodt et al., 2001). This trend did not hold for African American women, whose drinking rate remained constant over the 6 years of the study. The general trend toward decreased alcohol consumption with increasing age may be a result of people quitting or drinkers lowering the amount they drink.

Gender and educational level are also related to alcohol consumption. Compared with women, men are more likely to be current drinkers (53% to 40%), binge drinkers (28% to 13.5%), and heavy drinkers (9% to 3%) (SAMHSA, 2001). These percentages suggest that men have more problems with binge and heavy drinking than do women. Educational level is another predictor of drinking behavior. In Chapter 13, we saw that the more education people have, the less likely they are to smoke cigarettes. With alcohol, however, the reverse is true: the more years of schooling, the greater the likelihood that people will drink alcohol. In 2000, about two thirds of college graduates were defined as current drinkers whereas only one third of people with less than a high school education were current drinkers. (SAMHSA, 2001). College graduates were less likely to be binge or heavy drinkers than any other educational group (SAMHSA, 2001), and high school dropouts were more likely to be heavy drinkers and to develop drinking problems when they reach their 30s (Muthen & Muthen, 2000).

In Summary

People have been consuming alcohol since before recorded history, and people have probably abused alcohol for almost as long. In most ancient societies—as well as modern societies—alcohol in moderation was condoned, but alcohol abuse and drunkenness were condemned.

Alcohol consumption per capita reached a peak in the United States during the first 3 decades of the 19th century. From about 1830 to 1850, consumption dropped dramatically due to the efforts of early Prohibitionists. Presently, alcohol consumption in the United States is going down among nearly all ethnic and age groups. Only about 47% of adults are current drinkers, of which, about 20% are light or moderate drinkers, 21% are binge drinkers, and 6% are heavy drinkers. European Americans have higher rates of alcohol consumption than Hispanic Americans and African Americans; adults 21 to 39 consume more than other age groups; and college graduates are much more likely to be drinkers than high school dropouts, who, nevertheless, are more likely to be heavy drinkers.

The Effects of Alcohol

Essentially the same thing happens to alcohol when you drink it as when you do not—it turns to vinegar (Goodwin, 1976). In the body, two enzymes turn alcohol into vinegar, or acetic acid. The first enzyme, **alcohol dehydrogenase,** is located in the liver and has no other known function except to metabolize alcohol. Alcohol dehydrogenase breaks down alcohol into aldehyde, a very toxic chemical. **Aldehyde dehydrogenase** converts aldehyde to acetic acid.

The process of metabolizing alcohol produces at least three health-related outcomes: (1) an increase in lactic acid, which correlates with anxiety attacks; (2) an increase in uric acid, which causes gout; and (3) an increase of fat in the liver and in the blood.

The specific alcohol used in beverages is called **ethanol.** Like other alcohols, ethanol is a poison. But cases of alcohol poisoning are rare and almost always involve inexperienced drinkers who have drunk very large amounts of distilled liquor in a very short time, often on a "dare." Chad reported that "funneling," putting a funnel in someone's mouth and pouring liquor into the funnel, was sometimes practiced at his fraternity. This method of drinking can provide so much liquor so rapidly that it can be lethal. Otherwise, ingesting beverage alcohol is self-limiting: intoxication usually yields to unconsciousness, preventing lethal poisoning.

Men and women are not equally affected by drinking alcohol. One factor is the difference in body weight; a 120-pound person will be more strongly affected by three ounces of alcohol than a 220-pound person. But body weight is not the only factor. Women are more strongly affected by alcohol because of differences in the absorption of alcohol in the stomach (Bode & Bode, 1997). These gender differences produce higher blood alcohol levels in women, even when they drink the same amount as men. Thus, women may be more vulnerable to the effects of alcohol than men are.

Among the problems associated with drinking are alcohol's ability to produce tolerance, dependence, withdrawal, and addiction. Although these concepts can be applied to many drugs, a consideration of the relevance to alcohol is necessary in evaluating alcohol's potential hazards.

Tolerance is a term applied to the effects of a drug when, with continued use, more and more of the drug is required to produce the same effect. Drugs with high tolerance potential are dangerous because people who build up tolerance need to take more of the drug to produce the effect they want and expect. If this amount is progressively larger, any dangerous effects or side effects of the drug will become more of a hazard. Alcohol is a drug with generally moderate tolerance potential, but it seems to affect people differentially. For some, heavy use of alcohol for an extended period is required before noticeable tolerance begins to develop. For others, tolerance can develop within a week of moderate daily consumption. With increased tolerance comes an increased risk of the physical damage that alcohol can cause.

Dependence is separate from tolerance, and it too is a term that can be applied to many drugs. Dependence occurs when a drug becomes so incorporated into the functioning of the body's cells that it becomes necessary for "normal" functioning. If the drug is discontinued, the body's dependence on that drug becomes apparent and **withdrawal** symptoms develop. These symptoms are the body's signs that it is adjusting to functioning without the drug. Dependence and withdrawal are physically determined and are manifested in physical symptoms. Generally, withdrawal symptoms are the opposite of the drug's effects. Because alcohol is a depressant, withdrawal from it produces symptoms of restlessness, irritability, and agitation.

The combination of dependence and withdrawal is often described as **addiction.** Addictive drugs are those that produce dependence and when discontinued, result in withdrawal. Many drugs produce notoriously unpleasant withdrawal, and alcohol is one of the worst. How difficult the process will be depends on many factors, including the length of use and the degree of dependence. In some cases, withdrawal from alcohol can be life threatening, and the dangers increase with repeated withdrawal episodes (Gonzalez, 1998). Usually the first symptom to appear is tremor—the "shakes." Sleep difficulties are also common. In those severely addicted, **delirium tremens** occurs, with hallucinations and disorientation. Convulsions may also occur during withdrawal, a process that usually lasts between 2 days and a week. The physical dangers are so severe that the process is often completed in a special facility devoted to alcohol treatment.

Tolerance and dependence are independent properties. A drug may produce tolerance but not dependence; also, a person can develop dependence on a drug that has little or no tolerance potential. In addition, some drugs have both a tolerance and a dependence potential. Some research (Zinberg, 1984) even indicates that tolerance and dependence are not inevitable consequences of taking drugs. Not everyone who drinks alcohol does so with sufficient frequency and in sufficient quantity to develop a tolerance, and most drinkers do not become dependent.

Some people speak of "psychological" dependence, but this term has little scientific meaning beyond the notion that some activities, including drinking alcohol, become part of one's habitual manner of responding. Giving up the activity is accomplished only through much difficulty because the person has become habituated to it. Psychological dependence could be extended to many behaviors that are difficult to change, such as gambling, overeating, jogging, or even watching television.

Hazards of Alcohol

Alcohol produces a variety of hazards, both direct and indirect. *Direct hazards* are all those harmful physical effects due to alcohol itself, exclusive of any psychological, social, or economic consequences. *Indirect hazards* include all those harmful consequences that result from psychological and physiological impairments produced by alcohol. These hazards produce an increased mortality rate for heavy drinkers (Rehm, Greenfield, & Rogers, 2001), and both direct and indirect hazards contribute to this increase

Direct Hazards Alcohol affects many organ system in the body, but the liver is mainly in charge of detoxifying alcohol. Thus, damage to the liver is the main health consideration for long-term, heavy drinkers. The oxidation that occurs during alcohol metabolism may be toxic, destroying cell membranes and causing liver damage in the form of scarring (Fernandez-Checa, Kaplowitz, Colell, & Garcia-Ruiz, 1997). With prolonged heavy drinking, scarring occurs, and this scarring is typically followed by **cirrhosis,** or the accumulation of nonfunctional scar tissue in the liver. Cirrhosis is an irreversible condition and a major cause of death among alcoholics, yet not all alcoholics develop it. Moreover, people with no history of alcohol abuse may also develop liver cirrhosis, but cirrhosis is significantly associated with heavy alcohol use (Friedman, 1997) and is one of the leading causes of death in the United States. For reasons not yet clearly understood, mortality from cirrhosis has declined, beginning in the early 1970s.

Chronic alcohol abuse is also a factor in developing several other disorders, including respiratory illness and severe neurological damage. Critically ill respiratory patients who are also chronic alcohol abusers have a much higher death rate than respiratory patients with no history of alcohol abuse (Moss, Bucher, Moore, Moore, & Parsons, 1996). Prolonged heavy drinking is also implicated in the development of a neurological dysfunction called **Korsakoff syndrome** (also known as Wernicke-Korsakoff syndrome). Korsakoff syndrome is characterized by chronic cognitive impairment, severe memory problems for recent events, disorientation, and an inability to learn new information. Alcohol is related to the development of this syndrome through its interference with the absorption of thiamin, one of the B vitamins (Langlais, 1995).

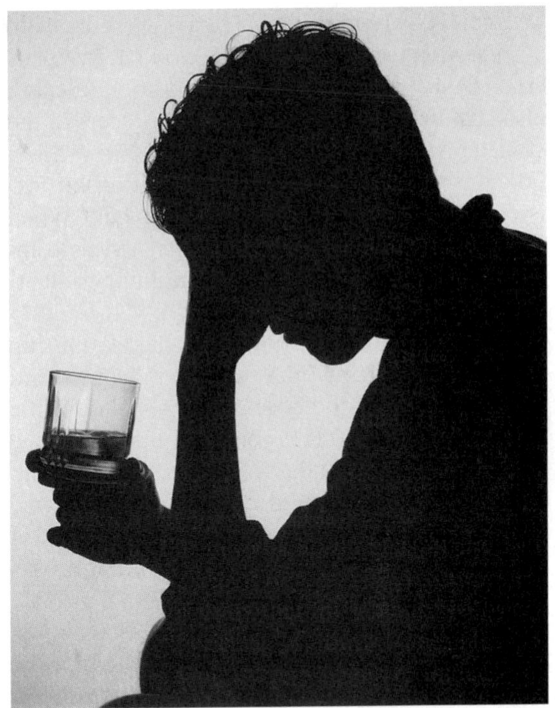
Corbis

The indirect effects of alcohol pose more dangers than the direct physiological effects.

Heavy drinkers can experience thiamin deficiency, which is worsened by their typically poor nutrition. Alcohol accelerates the progression of thiamin-related brain damage, and when this process has started, vitamin supplements do not reverse the progression. Moreover, most alcoholics do not receive treatment until the process is at an irreversible stage. Although heavy prolonged drinking is a risk factor for Korsakoff syndrome, light to moderate consumption does not seem to lead to cognitive impairment. Indeed, research suggests that people benefit from such levels of alcohol, and light to moderate drinking helps to prevent dementia of all types (Ruitenberg et al., 2002).

Does alcohol contribute to the development of cancer? A link between alcohol and cancer is not easy to establish because of many other factors that co-occur. However, a meta-analysis of over 200 studies (Bagnardi, Blangiardo, La Vecchia, &

Corrao, 2001) showed that drinking poses the strongest risk for cancer of the oral cavity, pharynx, esophagus, and larynx. In addition, alcohol also significantly raised the risk for cancers of the stomach, colon, rectum, liver, breast, and ovaries. For most sites, a dose-response relationship existed: heavier drinking meant higher risk. When drinkers also smoke cigarettes, their risk is compounded for cancers of the lung and upper digestive tract.

This meta-analysis confirmed the relationship between alcohol and breast cancer in women and also showed a strong dose-response relationship (Bagnardi et al., 2001). These results confirmed other large-scale studies (Singletary & Gapstur, 2001; Smith-Warner et al., 1998), which showed that any level of drinking presents some risk of breast cancer, and higher levels of drinking are related to higher risk.

Alcohol also affects the cardiovascular system, but the effects may not all be negative. (The next section looks at the possible positive effects of moderate alcohol consumption on cardiovascular functioning.) Heavy chronic drinking, however, does have a direct and harmful effect on the cardiovascular system. In large doses, alcohol reduces oxidation of fatty acids (the heart's primary fuel source) in the myocardium. The heart directly metabolizes ethanol, producing fatty acid ethyl esters that impair functioning of the energy-producing structures of the heart. Alcohol also can depress the myocardium's ability to contract, which can lead to abnormal cardiac functioning. In addition, alcohol consumption is related to increased systolic blood pressure, especially among African American women and men, although this association may be due to high levels of stress that contribute both to alcohol consumption and to increased blood pressure (Curtis, James, Strogatz, Raghunathan, & Harlow, 1997).

Alcohol has a direct and hazardous effect on pregnancy and the developing fetus in two basic ways. First, alcohol consumption reduces fertility, even at moderate levels of drinking (Jensen et al., 1998). Women who are chronic heavy users of alcohol experience amenorrhea, cessation of the menstrual cycle, which may be caused either by cirrhosis or by a direct effect of alcohol on the pituitary or the hypothalamus. Other possibilities include alcohol's effects on hormone production and regulation and interference with ovulation.

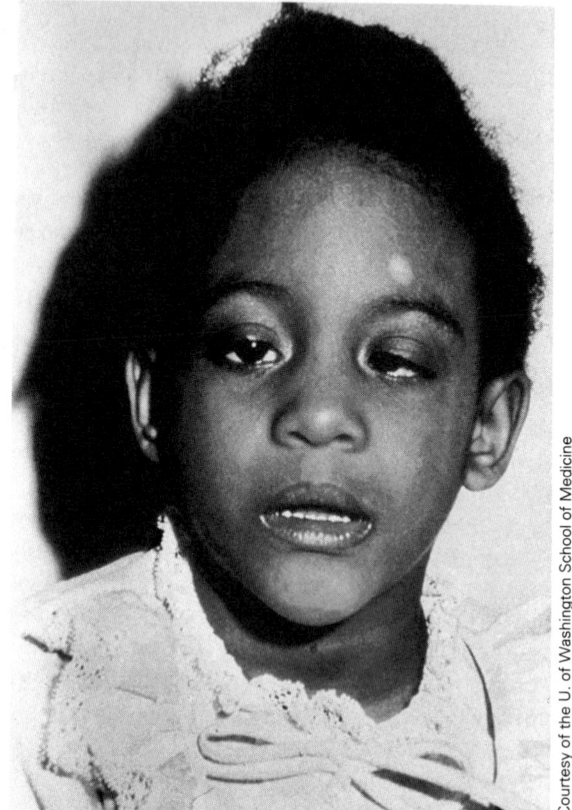

Courtesy of the U. of Washington School of Medicine

Facial abnormalities, growth deficiencies, central nervous system disorders, and mental retardation are symptoms of fetal alcohol syndrome.

The second direct, hazardous effect of excessive drinking during pregnancy is that it increases the risk of **fetal alcohol syndrome (FAS).** FAS affects many infants of mothers who drank excessively during pregnancy. Some tissues in the embryo are especially sensitive to alcohol, and exposure causes problems in developing embryos (Smith, 1997). These tissues give rise to specific facial abnormalities, growth deficiencies, central nervous system disorders, and mental retardation. The disorder has increased during recent years, climbing from an incidence of 0.1 per 1,000 births in 1979 to between 0.5 and 2.00 per 1,000 births during the 1990s (May & Gossage, 2001). Although heavy drinking is the main contributor to fetal alcohol syndrome, heavy smoking, stress, and poor nutrition are also involved, and combinations of these factors are not unusual in heavy drinkers.

What about moderate and even light drinking during pregnancy? Light to moderate drinking is not likely to cause fetal alcohol syndrome, but alcohol affects developing embryos. Even light drinking increased the risk for miscarriages and stillbirths (Kesmodel, Wisborg, Olsen, Henriksen, & Secher, 2002). Significant decreases in cognitive functioning have been observed in children of mothers who drank three or more drinks per day during pregnancy (Larroque et al., 1995). Slightly less alcohol consumption by pregnant mothers can lead to other health problems for the child. For example, children born to women who average two drinks a day have a lower average birth weight, and this condition, although not itself a danger, is related to many risks for newborns. Children of women who drank moderately during pregnancy showed somewhat slower reaction times and greater distractibility (Streissguth, Barr, Kogan, & Bookstein, 1996). Even small amounts of alcohol, especially during the early months of pregnancy, may have a direct and hazardous effect on the developing fetus.

Indirect Hazards In addition to these direct physiological damages, alcohol consumption is associated with several indirect hazards. Most of the indirect dangers arise from alcohol's effects on aggression, judgment, and attention. Alcohol also affects coordination and alters cognitive functioning in ways that contribute to increased chances of unintentional injury not only to the drinker but also to nondrinkers who live with a drinker (Rivara et al., 1997).

The most frequent and serious indirect hazard of alcohol consumption is the increased likelihood of unintentional injuries, the fifth leading cause of death in the United States and the leading cause of death for people under age 45. A dose-response relationship exists between alcohol consumption and unintentional fatal injuries; that is, the greater the number of drinks consumed per occasion, the greater the incidence of fatalities from unintentional injuries (Smith, 1999). As many as 42% of fatal unintentional injuries involve alcohol.

Motor vehicle crashes account for the largest number of alcohol-related fatalities. In the United States, more than 40,000 people die each year from injuries resulting from motor vehicle crashes, and about 40% of those deaths (about 16,000 per year) are related to alcohol-impaired driving (Smith, 1999). A self-report survey of adults in 49 states and the District of Columbia (Liu et al., 1997) found that alcohol-impaired driving was most frequent among young men 21 to 34 years old, but it was almost as common among men 18 to 20 who are not yet old enough to purchase alcohol legally. The survey also found that European Americans were most likely to report incidences of driving after drinking, followed by Hispanic Americans, then African Americans.

Alcohol consumption can also lead to more aggressive behavior for some drinkers. Both laboratory experiments and crime statistics have shown a relationship between alcohol and aggression. A review of laboratory studies (Taylor & Leonard, 1983) concluded that moderate and high doses of alcohol produce aggression in about 30% of drinkers, and more recent research (Parrott & Zeichner, 2002) has identified one important factor: trait anger. Not surprisingly, men with moderate or high trait anger behaved more aggressively than men with lower levels of anger. However, trait anger combined with alcohol to produce a variety of effects, including longer and higher levels of shock administered by men with moderate trait anger who had been drinking, compared to their sober counterparts. Thus, some people are more likely than others to become aggressive under the influence of alcohol.

Similarly, alcohol is related to crime. Two early studies (Mayfield, 1976; Wolfgang, 1957) indicated that either the victim or the offender or both had been drinking in two thirds of the homicides studied. Later research (Smith, 1999) has confirmed this relationship and extended the findings to assaults, including sexual assaults and incidents of domestic violence. Not only are people who commit homicides likely to be drinking, but consuming alcohol also relates to increased chances of being a crime victim. These relationships, however, do not demonstrate a causal relationship between alcohol and crime. In addition, the majority of crimes are committed by people who are not alcohol dependent, and the majority of alcohol abusers do not commit crimes.

Chad and his fraternity brothers were aware of the possible injuries that might follow from binge drinking. They tried not to drive while drunk and to take care of each other, but they did not designate a nondrinking driver. Instead, the designated driver role fell to the least intoxicated person. The fraternity members were not exempt from hazards; one member was killed in an automobile crash and one committed suicide while drinking and playing Russian roulette. Chad says that these tragedies did not slow the rate of drinking in the fraternity.

Finally, drinking alcohol can influence people's decision-making ability in sexual situations. College-aged men who were both intoxicated and sexually aroused reported more favorable attitudes and expressed greater intention of having unprotected sex than men who were sober (MacDonald, MacDonald, Zanna, & Fong, 2000). Other research (Dermen, Cooper, & Agocha, 1998) indicates that people who have been drinking carry through on those intentions: risky sex is associated with using alcohol and other drugs, especially among individuals who believe that alcohol will make them lose their inhibitions. (We discussed alcohol-related unsafe sex practices more fully in Chapter 11.)

Benefits of Alcohol

Is it possible that drinking might be good for you? This question was raised as a result of several early studies (Room & Day, 1974; Stason, Neff, Miettinen, & Jick, 1976) that reported a U-shaped or J-shaped relationship between alcohol consumption and mortality. In other words, light to moderate drinkers (one to five drinks per day) had the best prospects for good health, whereas nondrinkers and heavy drinkers had the greatest risk. Later evidence from several longitudinal studies supported the findings that light or moderate drinking was positively related to both reduced mortality and lower risk of disease. These early studies prompted further research, which has consistently found some health benefits for light to moderate levels of alcohol consumption.

Reduced Cardiovascular Mortality When researchers initially investigated the benefits of drinking, they discovered overall lower mortality for people who drink at light to moderate levels (Rehm, Bondy, Sempos, & Vuong, 1997). This advantage applied to men more strongly than to women, but women who are light drinkers also show lower mortality rates (Fuchs et al., 1995). This reduction in mortality was due mostly to lower heart disease deaths. Studies in the United States (Berkman, Breslow, & Wingard, 1983; Friedman & Kimball, 1986), Japan (Kitamura et al., 1998), and Australia (Cullen, Knuimon, & Ward, 1993) all showed advantages for light to moderate drinking compared to abstaining or heavy drinking. A meta-analysis of studies (Rimm, Williams, Fosher, Criqui, & Stampfer, 1999) concluded that two drinks per day could lower heart attack risk by 25%. A large-scale study on men (Mukamal et al., 2003) found that men who drank alcohol between three and seven times a week had a 30% lower risk of heart attack than men who drank less than once a week. In addition, this study demonstrated that type of alcoholic beverage made no difference—beer, wine, and distilled spirits were equally beneficial.

With heavy binge drinking (eight or more drinks at one sitting), both men and women lose their protection against heart disease. A recent study in Canada (Murray et al., 2002) compared the cardiovascular effects of both binge and nonbinge drinking and found that men with a pattern of binge drinking had more than double the risk for coronary heart disease, whereas women with a binge drinking pattern had only a slight increase in coronary heart disease. This study also found that binge drinking increased the risk for hypertension for men but not for women. Consistent with reports cited above, this study found that a nonbinge pattern of drinking offered both men and women significant protection against morbidity and mortality from cardiovascular disease.

The research evidence does not show as strong a protection against stroke as it does against heart disease (Ashley, Rehm, Bondy, Single, & Rankin, 2000). Indeed, some studies show an increased risk of stroke for people who drink. This discrepancy may be due to the different types of strokes. Similar to heart disease, people who drink at light to moderate levels derive some protection against ischemic strokes, those strokes caused by restriction of blood supply to the brain. On the other hand, drinking may pose a danger for hemorrhagic strokes, those strokes caused by rupture of a blood vessel that bleeds into the brain. Ischemic strokes are more common than hemorrhagic strokes; thus, the protection offered by drinking lowers the rate of death due to strokes. Another cardiovascular disorder, peripheral vascular disease, is also lower among drinkers.

The consistent findings that drinking alcohol reduces CVD risk led researchers to believe that alcohol produces changes in the course of atherosclerosis, the disease condition that underlies most CVD (Zakhari & Wassef, 1996). Alcohol alters cholesterol, raising specific subfractions of high-density lipoprotein known as HDL_2 and HDL_3, which seem to offer some protection against coronary heart disease and stroke, and also reducing the probability of blood clot formation (Rimm et al., 1999). Both of these actions protect against death from CVD.

Other Benefits of Alcohol Cardiovascular disease is not the only condition that is lower among those who drink. Chances of developing Type 2 diabetes are lower among men who drink one or two drinks per day than those who abstain (Ajani, Hennekens, Spelsberg, & Manson, 2000), and this protective effect may extend to women as well (Ashley et al., 2000). Alcohol affects glucose tolerance and insulin resistance, which makes this effect comprehensible. The role of alcohol in cholesterol metabolism and its effect on bile acids suggests that drinkers may be at lowered risk for gallstones (Ashley et al., 2000). Epidemiological research bears out this conjecture: moderate drinkers experienced gallstones at about half the rate as those who did not drink.

Alcohol also has some effect on *H. pylori,* a bacterium that infects the gastrointestinal system and is involved in gastritis, ulcer development, and possibly gastric cancers. People who drink have lower concentrations of this bacterium in their digestive tracts (Ashley et al., 2000). (See Chapter 6 for a discussion of H. pylori and ulcer formation.) Reductions in the levels of this infection may decrease risk, but more research is necessary to determine if drinking is beneficial in this way.

Some surpassing evidence (Ruitenberg et al., 2002) suggests that drinking may protect against cognitive deficits. This effect is unexpected because heavy drinking is associated with Korsakoff syndrome, which produces memory problems and other cognitive deficits. However, drinking is related to decreased risk for Alzheimer's disease, the most common form of dementia associated with advancing age. As Chapter 11 explained, Alzheimer's disease is a devastating degenerative brain disorder, and few protective measures have been identified. Should other research confirm the protective effect of alcohol, that information would offer hope of a way to combat this disease in an aging population.

For all of the diseases for which alcohol has shown some protective effect, the amount of alcohol is an important factor. At high levels of drinking, alcohol becomes a risk for these disorders. At light to moderate levels, it offers some protection. Individual differences are important in calculating who may benefit from drinking how much. Women gain the protective effects of alcohol at lower levels of drinking than men and

WOULD YOU BELIEVE

What Your Doctor Never Told You about Alcohol

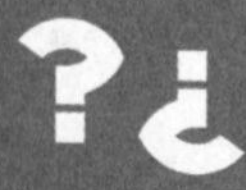

Would you believe that drinking may be good for you, but health care professionals are reluctant to admit it? Addiction authority Stanton Peele (1993) contended that medical investigators, public health officials, and health educators are uneasy about research findings concerning alcohol's beneficial health effects. He suggested that the United States has been so influenced by what he called the "temperance mentality" that medical authorities have trouble accepting their own findings about alcohol. "A cultural preoccupation with alcoholism and the negative effects of drinking works against frank scientific discussions in the United States of the advantages for the cardiovascular system of alcohol consumption" (Peele, 1993, p. 805).

Peele contended that the negative effects of alcohol dominate discussions at professional conferences and meetings. No official medical organization in the United States has made a recommendation concerning the positive effects of drinking alcohol, and the American Medical Association continues to issue official announcements about the dangers of drinking (AMA, 2002). Peele pointed out that the benefits of light to moderate drinking are similar to those obtained by following a low-fat diet in decreasing the risk for coronary heart disease, and many medical groups have made official statements concerning the wisdom of adopting a low-fat diet, but the only statements about alcohol concern the dangers of drinking.

Scientific evidence accumulated during the 1980s suggesting that moderate drinking might improve cardiovascular disease risk, but recommendation against drinking continued in the 1990 revision of the *Dietary Guidelines for Americans* due to the personal beliefs of the Surgeon General and the pressure brought on him by organizations opposed to drinking (Nestle, 1997). After a good deal of controversy and heated debate, the first official statement about the benefits of light drinking came in 1996 from a joint committee of the Agriculture Department and the Department of Health and Human Services that issues *Dietary Guidelines for Americans* (Nestle, 1997). The changes in the *Guidelines* came about as a result of mounting scientific evidence and political pressure, this time from the liquor industry. The current version of the dietary *Guidelines* allows for the possibility that drinking can be a positive health habit, but the move from Prohibition to moderation has not occurred throughout the medical establishment.

feel the hazards at lower levels (Ashley et al., 2000). For both women and men, the pattern of abstainers being at higher risk than drinkers applies as well as the dangers of heavy drinking.

If moderate drinking has a beneficial effect on the development of many diseases, it could also be related to better health. Investigators in the Alameda County study (Camacho & Wiley, 1983) found that moderate alcohol consumption (17 to 45 drinks per month) was most closely associated with good health scores. Abstinence was negatively related to subsequent health, and heavy drinkers, especially women, reported somewhat lower health scores than the average. However, heavy drinkers were not as unhealthy as the nondrinkers, suggesting that drinking is related to overall physical health.

The conclusion that drinking offers more health benefits than hazards is controversial, and many doctors are reluctant to recommend moderate drinking to their patients (see Would You Believe . . . ? box). About half of the people in the United States consume alcohol, and most of them do so in a manner more conducive to health rather than disease.

In Summary

Alcohol consumption has both harmful and beneficial effects on health. In addition, it has some negative indirect effects on society that reach beyond an individual's physical health. The direct hazards of prolonged and heavy drinking include cirrhosis of the liver and a brain dysfunction called Korsakoff syndrome. In addition, some evidence suggests that alcohol may contribute to the development of some cancers. Also, heavy drinking during pregnancy increases the risk of fetal alcohol syndrome, a serious disorder that often includes growth deficiencies and severe mental retardation. In addition, alcohol is a risk factor for many types of violence, both intentional and accidental. The level of alcohol consumption necessary to increase the risk is not as high as the level necessary to produce legal intoxication, but the more heavily people drink, the more likely they will be involved in accidents and violent crimes. Finally, alcohol consumption may also lead to poor decisions regarding sexual behavior.

The principal positive aspect of alcohol consumption is its buffering effect against mortality and morbidity from cardiovascular disease, including heart disease, stroke, and peripheral vascular disease. Other health benefits of light to moderate drinking may include lowered risks for diabetes, gallstones, H. pylori infection, and Alzheimer's disease. In addition, many light to moderate drinkers enjoy drinking and the sociability they associate with alcohol.

Why Do People Drink?

Investigators trying to understand drinking and alcohol abuse have proposed several models to explain behavior related to alcohol consumption. These models go beyond the pharmacological effects of alcohol and even beyond the research findings to integrate and explain drinking. To be useful, a model for drinking behavior must address at least three questions. First, why do people start drinking? Second, why do most people maintain moderate rather than excessive drinking levels? Third, why do some people drink so much as to develop serious problems?

Until the 19th century, drinking was well accepted in the United States and Europe, but drunkenness was unacceptable under most circumstances. This attitude makes drinking the norm, thus requiring no explanation for it, but leaves drunkenness unexplained. Two models have been proposed to explain drunkenness: the moral model and the medical model (McMurran, 1994).

The moral model appeared first, holding that people have free will and choose their behaviors, including excessive drinking. Thus, those who do so are either sinful or morally lacking in the self-discipline necessary to moderate their drinking. The moral model of alcoholism began to fade in the late 19th century, when the medical model started to gain prominence. Unacceptable behaviors that were formerly seen as moral problems became medical problems and, thus, subject to scientific explanation and medical treatment. The medical model of alcoholism conceptualized problem drinking as symptomatic of underlying physical problems, and the notion that alcoholism is hereditary grew from this view. The first form of this hypothesis took the view that a "constitutional weakness" ran in families and that this weakness produced alcoholics.

Problem drinking does run in families, but the relative contributions of heredity and environment remain the subject of heated debates. Most authorities agree that both genetic and environmental influences play a role in shaping alcohol abuse. Children of problem drinkers are more likely than children of nonproblem drinkers to abuse alcohol as well as other drugs (McGue, 1999). These children grow up in an environment marked by marital discord, tolerance for early initiation of alcohol use, and lack of parental warmth and communication. Such an environment, combined with an inherited vulnerability for alcohol abuse, greatly increases a child's likelihood of becoming a problem drinker. However, most children reared in this type of environment are resilient to those environmental effects and do not become problem drinkers (Ohannessian, Stabenau, & Hesselbrock, 1995). How can investigators learn about the relative effects of environment and heredity on the development of problem drinking?

To determine the contribution of genetic factors, researchers have taken several approaches, including the degree of agreement in drinking behavior in twins or adopted children and parents (McGue, 1999). Twin studies ordinarily involve measuring the degree of agreement between pairs of identical twins, with comparisons in the amount of agreement between pairs of fraternal twins. If identical twins are more similar to each other than fraternal twins are, the difference is assumed to be due to genetics. Indeed, research generally shows a closer concordance of problem drinking for identical twins than for fraternal twins. This greater concordance between identical twins supports the idea of at least some genetic component in alcohol abuse. A second test of a hereditary factor in alcohol abuse is the study of adopted children. Adoption studies investigate the frequency of alcohol abuse in adoptees whose biological parent was alcoholic. Results from several large-scale studies using this approach also indicate a genetic component for problem drinking (McGue, 1999). Both types of studies indicate a stronger component for genetics in the problem drinking of men than in women.

Genes do not determine drinking. Indeed, genes do not produce any behavior. Instead, genes govern protein synthesis, and there are a number of steps between genes and behavior. Research has begun to explore the molecular basis of how genes affect drinking. Many possibilities exist, including effects on alcohol metabolism and the function of neurotransmitters in the brain when alcohol in present (Fromme & D'Amico, 1999). One effect of genes on alcohol metabolism is fairly well understood, but this type of inheritance protects against problem drinking (McGue, 1999). When individuals inherit a gene that results in deficient activity of one of the enzymes that break down alcohol, they experience an unpleasant "flushing" reaction when they drink. This gene is more common among people of Asian ancestry than other ethnic groups, and people with this gene rarely develop problem drinking.

The genetic component of problem drinking is likely to be more complex than the gene that produces the flushing reaction in combination with alcohol. That is, problem drinking is unlikely to be traceable to one gene pair (Schuckit, 2000). Indeed, current research has located a number of possible gene sites that may contribute to problem drinking. Considering the complexity of alcohol effects on brain neurochemistry, researchers now expect their search to yield multiple gene locations that underlie a vulnerability to problem drinking and not a simple genetic determination of alcoholism. This situation makes problem drinking a good example of the diathesis-stress view of disease development, with certain genetic configurations furnishing the diathesis and experiential and environmental factors creating the precipitating events.

The Disease Model

The disease concept of alcoholism is a variation of the medical model, holding that people with problem drinking have the disease of alcoholism. Throughout history, isolated attempts have been made to describe alcohol intoxication as a disease brought about by the physical properties of alcohol, but not until the late 1930s and early 1940s did this view begin to become popular. In psychiatric and other medically oriented treatment programs in the United States, the disease model still predominates, but it is less influential in psychologically based treatment programs and in treatment programs in Europe and in Australia.

The disease model of alcoholism was elevated to scientific respectability by the pioneering work of E. M. Jellinek (1960), who identified several different types of alcoholism and described various characteristics of these types. The two most common types are **gamma alcoholism,** or loss of control once drinking begins, and **delta alcoholism,** or the inability to abstain. Any model that conceptualizes alcoholism as an incurable unitary disorder is too simplistic, even if it allows for different varieties of alcoholism (Miller, 1993).

The Alcohol Dependency Syndrome Dissatisfaction with Jellinek's disease model led Griffith Edwards and his colleagues (Edwards, 1977; Edwards & Gross, 1976; Edwards, Gross, Keller, Moser, & Room, 1977) to advocate the alcohol dependency syndrome, which rejects the term *alcoholism* and the notion that problem drinking is a disease. The word *syndrome* adds flexibility to the disease model by suggesting a group of concurrent behaviors that accompany alcohol dependence. The behaviors need not always be observed in an individual, nor do they need to be observable to the same degree in everyone who is alcohol dependent. Edwards and his colleagues modified several of Jellinek's concepts, including the notion that alcoholics experience loss of control. Rather, the alcohol dependency syndrome holds that those who are alcohol dependent have *impaired control,* suggesting that people drink heavily because, at certain times and for a variety of reasons, they do not exercise control over their drinking.

Edwards and Milton Gross (1976) described seven essential elements of the alcohol dependency syndrome. First is a *narrowing of drinking repertoire,* suggesting that a person tends to drink the same beverage the same time of day and the same day of the week. Second is a *salience of drink-seeking behavior,* meaning that drinking begins to take priority over all other aspects of life. A third element of the alcohol dependency syndrome is *increased tolerance.* As noted earlier, alcohol does not produce as much tolerance as do some other drugs, but some drinkers gradually become accustomed to going about their daily routine "at blood alcohol levels that would incapacitate the non-tolerant drinker" (Edwards & Gross, 1976, p. 1059).

A fourth element of the alcohol dependency syndrome is *withdrawal symptoms.* As previously mentioned, the severity of withdrawal depends on length and amount of use. Those who are alcohol dependent *avoid withdrawal symptoms by further drinking,* the fifth characteristic of the alcohol dependency syndrome. A mildly dependent person might relieve the morning "blues" by having a drink with lunch, but some drinkers use the strategy of avoiding withdrawal symptoms by maintaining a steady alcohol level.

The sixth element is the *subjective awareness of the compulsion to drink.* The final element of the alcohol dependency syndrome is *reinstatement of dependence after abstinence.* Edwards and Gross believe that time of reinstatement is inversely related to the degree of dependence. Moderately dependent people may not reinstate drinking for months, whereas severely dependent patients may resume full dependence in as little as 3 days.

Evaluation of the Disease Model Despite the continuing popularity of the disease model of alcoholism, the concept has only limited research support. This model fails to address our first question: "Why do people begin to drink?" Its answer to the second question about why some people continue to drink at moderate levels is hardly adequate: people who are not alcoholic can drink with impunity (Miller, 1993).

One key concept in the disease model is loss of control or impaired control—the inability to stop or moderate alcohol intake once drinking begins. Research has not supported this key concept. G. Alan Marlatt and his colleagues (Marlatt, Demming, & Reid, 1973; Marlatt & Rohsenow, 1980) have conducted experiments suggesting that many effects of alcohol, including impaired control, are due more to expectancy than to any pharmacological effect of alcohol. Their experimental design, called the *balanced placebo design,* included four groups, two of which expect to be given alcohol and two of which do not. Two groups actually received alcohol, and two did not. Figure 14.4 shows all four combinations.

Using the balanced placebo design, several studies (Marlatt et al., 1973; Marlatt & Rohsenow, 1980) showed that people who think they have received alcohol behave as though they have (whether they have or not). Even for those who had been in treatment for problem drinking, expectancy appeared to be the controlling factor

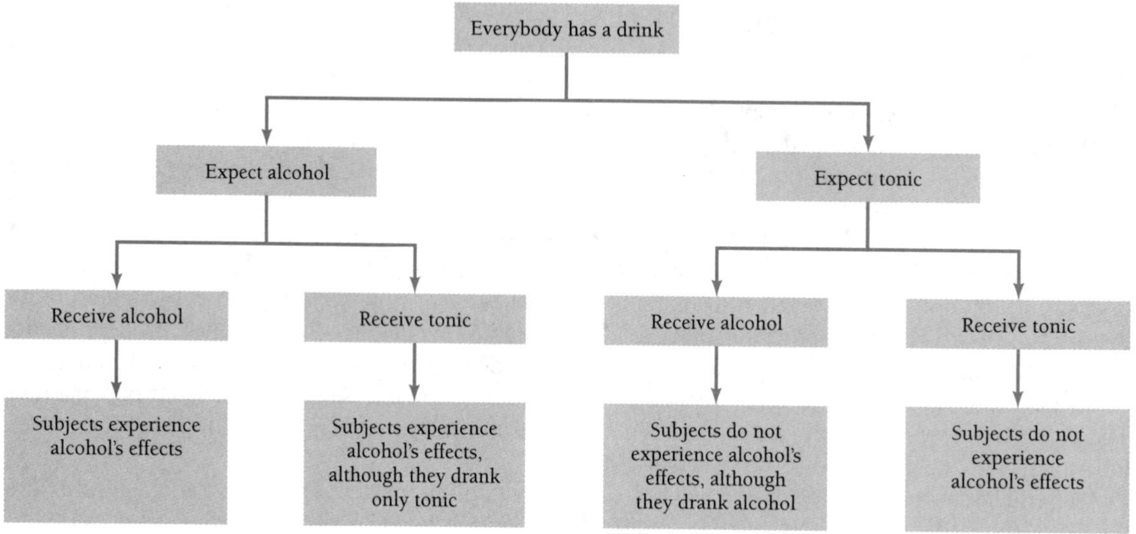

Figure 14.4 Balanced placebo design.

in the craving for alcohol and in the amount consumed. These findings suggest that loss of control and craving for alcohol result from expectancy rather than from some physical property of alcohol. The difference between severely dependent drinkers and moderately dependent drinkers is interesting because it suggests some possible differences between those whose dependence is severe and those with less serious drinking problems. Although this study did not provide strong support for the disease model of alcoholism, it is one of the few well-controlled studies to have found any support for the model.

Some investigators (Marlatt, 1987; Miller, 1993) have criticized the disease model of alcohol, arguing that it does not adequately consider environmental, cognitive, and affective determinants of abusive drinking; that is, in its emphasis on the physical properties of alcohol, the disease model neglects the cognitive and social learning aspects of drinking.

Cognitive-Physiological Theories

Alternatives to the disease model exist, several of which emphasize the combination of physiological and cognitive changes that occur with alcohol use. Rather than hypothesizing that alcohol use and misuse are based only on the chemical properties of alcohol, these models contend that alcohol use also depends on the cognitive changes experienced by drinkers.

The Tension Reduction Hypothesis As the name suggests, the tension reduction hypothesis (Conger, 1956) holds that people drink alcohol because of its tension-reducing effects. This hypothesis has much intuitive appeal because alcohol is a sedative drug that leads to relaxation and slowed reactions.

Despite its consistency with popular belief, experimental evidence from human studies shows little support for the tension reduction hypothesis (Greeley & Oei, 1999). Studies that have manipulated tension or anxiety to observe their effects on participants' readiness to consume alcohol have yielded contradictory results; some participants experience tension reduction, whereas others do not. One factor that complicates assessments of the tension reduction hypothesis is expectancy. When people expect to experience tension reduction, they tend to get what they expect. Thus, tension reduction is one of many effects that may occur as a result of drinking, and expectancy may be more important than alcohol in these effects.

The realization that alcohol's effects on physiological processes are not simple led to a reformulation of the tension reduction hypothesis. A group of researchers at Indiana University (Levenson, Sher, Grossman, Newman, & Newlin, 1980; Sher, 1987; Sher & Levenson, 1982) discovered that high levels of alcohol consumption decrease the strength of responses to stress. They labeled this decrease the **stress-response-dampening (SRD) effect.** People who had been drinking did not respond as strongly as nondrinking participants to either physiological or psychological stressors. People whose personality profile suggested a high risk of developing problem drinking showed the strongest SRD effect, and those whose profile indicated a low risk showed a weaker effect (Sher & Levenson, 1982). Later research has confirmed this pattern (Greeley & Oei, 1999). The largest SRD effects seem to occur in people with the highest risk, which may account for at least part of the variability that people exhibit to alcohol. Perhaps the tension-reducing effects occur for individuals who are susceptible to alcohol's effects, mediating the SRD effect and the dangers that alcohol poses for these individuals (Greeley & Oei, 1999). However, neither the original tension reduction hypothesis nor stress response dampening provides general explanations for initiating or nonproblem drinking.

The Self-Awareness Model A second approach, proposed by Jay Hull, is based on social psychological theories of self-awareness (Hull, 1981, 1987; Hull & Bond, 1986). Hull built a model of drinking behavior on the observation that alcohol consumption indirectly affects behavior through changes in cognitive processes. He then hypothesized that alcohol can interfere with cognition to make thought more superficial and to decrease negative self-feedback. Negative self-feedback consists of statements such as "I can't do anything very well" or "I shouldn't be such a coward." By making cognitions more superficial, alcohol enables people either to reduce or to avoid these kinds of tension-producing self-statements and thus to think better of themselves than when they are not drinking.

Hull's explanation of drinking is therefore based on changes in self-awareness. By inhibiting the use of normal, complex information-processing strategies, such as memory and information acquisition, drinking makes people less self-aware. Decreased self-awareness leads to decreased monitoring of behavior, resulting in the disinhibition that commonly occurs among drinkers.

The self-awareness model also proposes that drinkers become less self-critical as they become less self-aware because they fail to process information that reflects badly on them. Hull (1987) hypothesized that this effect may be the reason that some people consume alcohol—to avoid self-awareness. Reduced self-awareness might also be rewarding through decreased self-censure for inappropriate (but personally attractive) social behavior. Therefore, loss of self-awareness can offer some rewards, which explains why people drink and why some people drink unwisely. What this model fails to elaborate is who will fall into each category. The self-awareness model has gathered some research support but also some failures (Sayette, 1999). The difficulties in assessing self-awareness limit this model's potential for research support.

Alcohol Myopia Claude Steele and his colleagues (Steele & Josephs, 1990) have developed a model of alcohol use and abuse based on alcohol's psychological and physical properties. This model hypothesizes that alcohol use creates effects on social behaviors that produce *alcohol myopia,* "a state of shortsightedness in which superficially understood, immediate aspects of experience have a disproportionate influence on behavior and emotion, a state in which we can see the tree, albeit more dimly, but miss the forest altogether" (Steele & Josephs, 1990, p. 923). According to this view, alcohol blocks out insightful cognitive processing and alters thoughts related to the self, stress, and social anxiety.

Part of alcohol myopia is *drunken excess,* the tendency for those who drink to behave more excessively. This tendency appears as increased aggression, friendliness, sexiness, and many other exaggerated behaviors. Tendencies to behave in such extreme ways are usually inhibited, but when people drink, they experience less inhibition, and their behavior becomes more extreme.

Another aspect of alcohol myopia is *self-inflation,* a tendency to inflate self-evaluations. When asked to rate the importance of 35 trait dimensions for their real and ideal selves, drunken participants rated themselves higher on traits that were important to them and on which they had rated themselves low when sober (Banaji & Steele, 1989). Thus, drinking allowed participants to see themselves as better than they did when they were not drinking, confirming the ability of alcohol to inflate a person's self-evaluation.

A third aspect of alcohol myopia is *drunken relief* (Steele & Josephs, 1990, p. 928): that is, people who drink tend to worry less and pay less attention to their worries. When consumed in large quantities, alcohol alone may produce drunken relief, but in smaller quantities and combined with distracting activity, it can also produce a powerful stress reduction effect (Steele, Southwick, & Pagano, 1986). Drunken relief is not entirely an effect of alcohol but of alcohol in combination with other factors in the social environment that provide distraction.

Several pieces of research have supported the alcohol myopia model. One study (MacDonald, Zanna, & Fong, 1995) showed that intoxicated people analyze information at a more superficial level than sober people; drinkers were more likely than nondrinkers to go along with a suggestion that it is acceptable to drive a short distance after drinking. Intoxicated college men who were sexually aroused reported more positive feelings about having unprotected sex than men who were sexually aroused but had not been drinking (MacDonald et al., 2000). Their sexual arousal constituted a very salient cue that led them to focus myopically on sex rather than think through the wisdom of condom use. However, when intoxicated people received strong cues concerning risky sex, their intentions to use condoms were higher than their sober counterparts (MacDonald, Fong, Zanna, & Martineau, 2000). That is, drinkers' tendency to process information in a limited way is influenced by what cues are present rather than by a general tendency for disinhibition. Thus, alcohol myopia has growing research support.

The Social Learning Model

The social learning model provides an explanation for why people begin to drink, why they continue to drink in moderation, and why some people drink in a harmful manner. Social learning theory conceives of drinking as learned behavior, acquired in the same manner as other behaviors.

According to social learning theory, people begin to drink for at least three reasons. First, the taste of alcohol and its immediate effects may bring pleasure (positive reinforcement); second, a person may decide earlier that drinking alcohol is consistent with personal standards (cognitive mediation); and third, the person may learn to drink through observing others (modeling). Research on the reason for drinking (MacLean & Lecci, 2000) indicates that three reasons for college students' drinking were to increase social rewards and to enhance their mood (positive reinforcement) as well as to conform to social pressure (modeling). Social learning was a prominent feature of drinking for Chad. He began to drink with his friends and continued to drink in the company of fraternity brothers who also drank. Now that he is not around his fraternity friends so much, he drinks less.

The social learning model also offers three explanations for why people drink too much. First, excessive drinking may serve as a coping response; that is, the initial effect of small doses may be interpreted by drinkers as enhancement of their ability to cope. This response can give drinkers a sense of power and also a feeling of avoiding responsibility or minimizing stress. Peo-

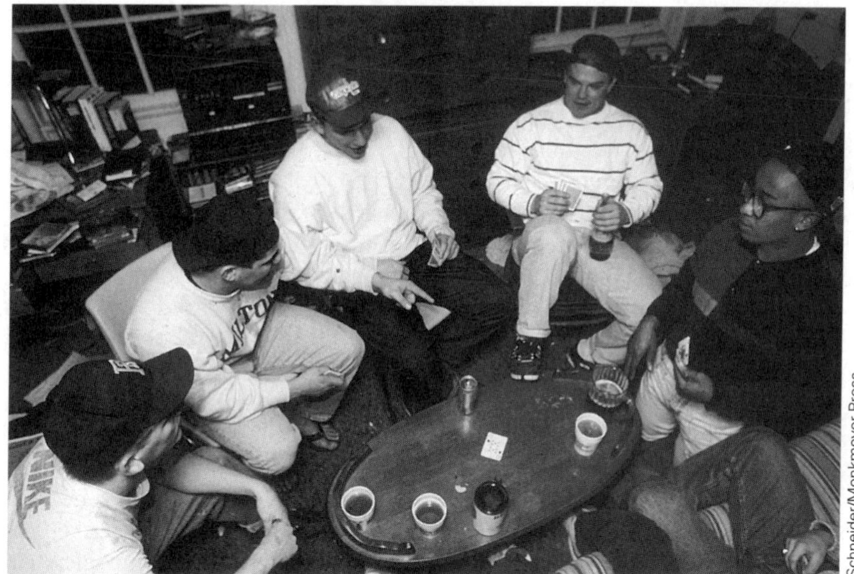
Schneider/Monkmeyer Press

College social gatherings may encourage binge drinking.

ple will then continue to drink as long as they perceive that alcohol has desirable effects.

Second, drinkers tend to adjust their level of alcohol according to the amounts they see others consuming. Research with children of alcoholics (Brown, Tate, Vik, Haas, & Aarons, 1999) showed that both modeling and family history predicted the effects these young people expected from drinking. Individuals who saw their parents abuse alcohol formed their expectancies on the basis of this modeling. Thus, modeling can explain the initiation of drinking and relates to the tendency of some people to drink to excess.

A third explanation for excessive drinking offered by the social learning model is based on the principles of negative reinforcement. Most heavy drinkers have learned that they can avoid or reduce the painful effects of withdrawal symptoms by maintaining blood alcohol concentrations at a particular level. As this level begins to drop, the alcohol addict feels the discomfort of withdrawal. These symptoms can be avoided by ingesting more alcohol; thus, negative reinforcement increases the probability that heavy drinking will continue.

Social learning theory provides an explanation for why people start drinking, why some continue to drink in moderation, and why others become problem drinkers. In addition, social learning theory also suggests a variety of treatment techniques to help people overcome excessive drinking habits. Because drinking behavior is learned, it can be unlearned or relearned, with either abstinence or moderation as a goal of therapy.

In Summary

The question of why people drink has three components: (1) Why do people begin drinking? (2) Why do some people drink in moderation? (3) Why do others drink to excess? Theories of drinking behavior should be able to offer explanations for each of these questions. This section discussed three theories or models, each of which has some potential explanatory ability. The disease model assumes that people drink excessively because they have the disease of alcoholism. One variation of the disease model—the alcohol dependency syndrome—assumes that alcohol dependent people have impaired control and drink heavily for a variety of reasons. Cognitive-physiological models, including the tension reduction hypothesis, the self-awareness model, and alcohol myopia, propose that people drink because alcohol produces alterations in cognitive function that allow people to escape tension and negative self-evaluations. Social learning theory assumes that people acquire drinking behavior in the same manner that they learn other behaviors—that is, through positive or negative reinforcement, modeling, and cognitive mediation. All three models offer some explanation of why some people continue to drink, but none of them has a satisfactory explanation for why some people start or why some can drink in moderation.

Changing Problem Drinking

Despite a recent and steady decline in the percentage of drinkers in the United States, an increasing number of people seek help for problem drinking, with over half a million people receiving treatment each year (USBC, 2001). People between ages 25 and 44 years are the most likely to seek treatment, and men outnumber women by a ratio of over 2 to 1 (USBC, 2001). However, the prevalence of women who seek treatment may be partially shielded by their greater tendency to seek help in non-alcohol-specific settings, such as mental health treatment services (Weisner & Schmidt, 1992). Five out of six people who receive treatment do so on an outpatient rather than inpatient basis (USBC, 2001). Although private for-profit facilities emphasize inpatient treatment, these programs may have benefits that are limited to people with the most serious problems, but the costs are much higher (Pettinati et al., 1999). In addition to the various treatment settings, the majority of alcoholics are able to quit drinking without formal treatment (Brink, 2001; Sobell, Cunningham, & Sobell, 1996).

Change without Therapy

Some problems (and even some diseases) disappear without formal treatment, and problem drinking is no exception. When a disease disappears without treatment, the term spontaneous remission is used to describe the cure. Many authorities in the field of problem drinking do not accept the term **spontaneous remission;** they prefer the term *unassisted change* to describe a switch from problem to nonproblem drinking (McMurran, 1994). Even the term *unassisted change* may be misleading because people who change their drinking patterns may have the help and support of many people, including family members, employers, and friends. Many people are able to change from problem to nonproblem drinking without formal treatment (Sobell et al., 1996; Walters, 2000).

Although many problem drinkers are able to quit on their own or to moderate their drinking, others seek professional help or the assistance of traditional groups such as Alcoholics Anonymous. Presently, nearly all treatment programs in the United States are oriented toward abstinence; a few in other countries allow for the possibility that some problem drinkers can moderate their alcohol intake.

Treatments Oriented toward Abstinence

All formal treatments—even those that permit the possibility of resuming drinking—seek immediate abstinence as their goal. This section examines several treatment programs aimed at total and permanent abstinence.

Alcoholics Anonymous Alcoholics Anonymous (AA) is one of the most widely used alcohol treatment programs, and it is often a component in other treatment programs. Founded in 1935 by two former alcoholics, AA has become the best known of all approaches to problem drinking. The organization follows a very strict version of the disease model and combines it with quasi-religious meetings that are designed to bring the problem drinker into the group. To adhere to the AA doctrine, a person must maintain total abstinence from alcohol. Part of the AA philosophy is that those who are in need of joining AA can never drink again and that problem drinkers are addicted to alcohol and have no power to resist it. According to AA, alcoholics never recover but are always in the process of recovering. They will be alcoholics for a lifetime, even if they never take another drink.

AA and other 12-step programs have become increasingly popular, attracting large numbers of people. A survey of U.S. adults (Room & Greenfield, 1993) revealed that nearly 5% of adults had sought help at some time during their lives for drinking problems, and for those who had sought help, 60% of the men and 80% of the women had attended AA meetings (Weisner, Greenfield, & Room, 1995).

The anonymity offered to those who attend AA meetings presents serious barriers to researchers wishing to conduct studies on the effectiveness of this program. Some evidence (Cunningham & Breslin, 2001) indicates that people who attend AA achieve the goal of abstaining from drinking, but few maintain lifelong abstention, and many drop out of AA. Alternative self-help organizations, such as Secular Organization for Sobriety, Women for Sobriety, SMARTRecovery, Rational Recovery, and Moderation Management, offer the value of support and group discussions without the inflexible philosophy and religious orientation of AA.

Psychotherapy Nearly as many psychotherapeutic techniques have been used to treat alcohol abuse as there are psychotherapies. This variety should not be surprising because a variety of psychiatric and behavioral problems often accompany alcohol abuse. Whether these disorders are the cause or the effect of heavy drinking, the immediate goal of all treatment approaches is sobriety, because no psychotherapy is successful with intoxicated patients. For this reason, psychotherapeutic approaches are often combined with detoxification, AA, or some form of chemical treatment aimed at stopping drinking.

In terms of setting, treatment may be centered in Veterans Administration hospitals, care units in other hospitals, private treatment clinics, offices of psychiatrists and psychologists, halfway houses, or one of a variety of other treatment facilities. In terms of form, psychotherapeutic treatment can be divided into group procedures and individual therapy, with patients frequently participating in both within a single treatment regimen.

Group therapy for alcoholics has both advantages and disadvantages. Observing others who have successfully stopped drinking can raise expectancies for achieving the same goal, and patients within a group setting are more likely to receive praise and recognition from other group members for staying away from problem drinking. Another advantage for group treatment is the opportunity that groups provide to allow the patient a chance to give help. The experience of being helpful is, itself, often therapeutic, and AA members who reach the final step of their program often sponsor a new member, which may be helpful in their own recovery as well as the new member's.

However, group therapy is sometimes rather superficial in dealing with individual problems, so individual psychotherapy may be preferable. How effective are the various individual therapy programs for alcohol abuse? Unfortunately, reports of success are frequently exaggerated, with some private treatment centers claiming a greater than 90% recovery rate (Miller, Walters, & Bennett, 2001). Well-controlled studies, however, usually yield somewhat lower success rates, depending on the sample composition (healthy, middle-social class, married, employed alcoholics have the highest improvement rates), the definition of success (abstinence versus improvement), and the interval before follow-up (longer periods before follow-up report lower success rates).

In an analysis that combined seven studies, each conducted with a large group of participants in a variety of treatment types and locations (Miller et al., 2001), an average of 25% attained and maintained abstinence for at least 1 year after treatment. Those drinkers who failed to quit often cut their drinking; about 10% drank at levels that no longer qualified as problem drinking. For the variety of treatment programs, drinking declined by 87% and problems caused by drinking decreased by 60%. Therefore, a variety of treatments can be effective in decreasing problem drinking, but no treatment approaches 100% effectiveness.

Chemical Treatments Many treatment programs for problem drinking include administering drugs that interact with alcohol to produce a range of unpleasant effects. The most commonly used of these drugs is **disulfiram** (Antabuse). The unpleasant effects include flushing of the face, chest pains, a pounding heart, nausea and vomiting, sweating, headache, dizziness, weakness, difficulty in breathing, and a rapid decrease in blood pressure. These effects do not occur unless disulfiram and alcohol are both ingested. Disulfiram does have side effects of its own, including skin eruptions, fatigue, drowsiness, headache, and impotence. As with all side effects to drugs, these vary from person to person, and some individuals have few or none. The possibility of liver damage and compliance to the required daily dosage present problems that make this approach unattractive (*Harvard Mental Health Letter,* 2000). People are not eager to take a drug that will make them sick if they drink. Noncompliance, of course, lowers the effectiveness of this treatment because low levels of the drug may not cause the unpleasant effects after a person drinks alcohol.

An alternative drug treatment is naltrexone, a drug that attaches to opiate receptors in the brain and prevents their activation. Several studies showed that patients who received naltrexone as part of their treatment were better able to maintain abstinence and experienced reduced craving for alcohol than patients who received a placebo, but other studies failed to replicate these positive findings (Krystal, Cramer, Krol, Kirk, & Rosenheck, 2001). This negative finding from a large, well-controlled study casts doubt on the benefits of this chemical treatment.

Aversion Therapy Drugs like disulfiram, which produce nausea when combined with alcohol, are intended to produce an aversion to drinking or to act as a punishment for drinking. Thus, they would technically be considered aversion therapies. However, the term **aversion therapy** is more commonly applied to the classical conditioning technique of using an electric shock, an emetic drug, or some other aversive stimulus to countercondition the patient's response to alcohol. In the classical conditioning paradigm, the unconditioned stimulus (shock or the emetic drug) is paired one or more times with the conditioned stimulus (sight, smell, taste, or image of alcohol) so that it will elicit the unconditioned response (aversion or withdrawal from alcohol). Through this process, drinking should come to be associated with an aversive condition and thus be avoided.

Rather than relying on electric shock, many aversive conditioning treatment programs use a pharmacological agent such as **emetine,** a drug that induces vomiting, as the aversive stimulus. This aversive therapy procedure pairs the pharmacological agent with the sight, smell, taste, and thought of alcohol. One evaluation of the effectiveness of emetine treatment (Wiens & Menustik, 1983) found that 63% of patients were not drinking at the end of 1 year, but only 31% were abstinent after 3 years. A later report (Howard, 2001) indicated that the conditioning procedure built an aversion to alcohol and increased alcoholics' evaluations of their ability to resist drinking. The conditioning was not as successful for drinkers with prior nausea connected with drinking or for drinkers who experienced more serious behavior problems connected with their drinking. Thus, aversion therapy may be least useful for drinkers who need the most help.

In addition, the high dropout rate for this approach limits its use.

Controlled Drinking

Until the late 1960s, all treatments for problem drinking were aimed at total abstinence. Then something quite unexpected happened. In 1962 in London, D. L. Davies found that 7 of the 93 recovered alcoholics whom he studied were able to drink "normally" (defined as consumption of up to three pints of beer or its equivalent per day) for at least a 7-year period following treatment. These moderate drinkers represented less than 8% of those Davies studied, but this finding was still remarkable because it opened up the possibility that diagnosed alcoholics could successfully return to nonproblem drinking. All seven of the controlled drinkers had been completely abstinent for at least a few months following treatment, yet all had been able to resume "normal" drinking without relapsing into a heavy, harmful pattern of drinking.

Prompted by Davies's results, several studies conducted in the United States (Armor, Polich, & Stambul, 1976; Polich, Armor, & Braiker, 1980) showed that controlled drinking occurred in a small percentage of patients who received treatment oriented toward abstinence. Publicity about this study produced a waive of criticism from those holding the position that alcoholics can never drink again, and this controversy became more heated when researchers began to design treatment programs with controlled drinking as the goal.

Abstinence-oriented programs usually teach that the urge to drink will always be present and that if it is indulged even for a single drink, total relapse is inevitable. In contrast, controlled drinking programs do not have such a self-fulfilling prophecy built into them. Instead, they emphasize moderating patients' behavior and finding environmental supports that will reinforce moderation. They teach patients to monitor their intake, set weekly goals for total consumption, intersperse nonalcoholic drinks with alcoholic ones, and dilute drinks. In addition, behaviorally oriented controlled drinking programs train patients in a variety of human relations skills so they can modify all their self-destructive behaviors (Alden, 1988).

Problem drinkers can become moderate drinkers. Several studies have found that controlled drinking occurs as a result of abstinence-oriented treatment programs (Sobell et al., 1996; Miller et al., 2001) and in drinkers who quit on their own (Pukish & Tucker, 1994). Despite the evidence, most treatment centers in the United States have resisted the possibility that former problem drinkers can learn to moderate their use of alcohol. Many of the people who provide treatment services are people who have experienced problems themselves, providing indoctrination to the disease model and making them committed to the programs that helped them (Shavelson, 2001). This attitude does not extend to other countries; in Britain, nearly all treatment centers accept the principle of controlled drinking treatment (McMurran, 1994).

What type of drinker might be a good candidate for controlled drinking? One factor that predicts success is belief: drinkers who believe in the possibility of controlled drinking are better candidates than those who believe that control over drinking is not possible (Rosenberg, 1993). In addition, people with a spouse and a job, shorter histories of problem drinking, and low levels of physical damage from alcohol are better candidates. People who quit on their own have a better chance of becoming controlled drinkers than those who seek treatment for their drinking problems, possibly because most treatment programs teach that alcoholics cannot ever drink moderately.

Even advocates of controlled drinking accept that controlled drinking is not a treatment goal for *all* alcohol abusers. We cannot state too strongly that *controlled drinking is not for everyone.* Some former alcohol addicts must abstain completely, and even those drinkers who are candidates for controlled drinking must apparently undergo at least 1 month of complete abstinence to allow the toxic effects of excessive drinking to diminish. In addition, former alcohol abusers who initially learn control may gradually or even abruptly escalate their consumption until they reach complete relapse.

The Problem of Relapse

Problem drinkers who successfully complete either an abstinence-oriented or a moderation-oriented treatment program do not necessarily maintain their goals. As we saw with smoking, people who complete a treatment program usually improve quite a bit, but the problem of relapse is often substantial. Interestingly, the time course and rate of relapse is similar for those who complete treatment programs for smoking, alcohol abuse, or opiate abuse (Hunt et al., 1971). Most relapses occur within 90 days after the end of the program. At 12 months after the end of treatment, only about 35% of those completing the programs are still abstinent.

Improved treatment programs lead to lower relapse rates. One factor in this improvement is the knowledge that relapse is so frequent; programs now prepare clients for relapse and include provisions for follow-up and additional treatment (McCrady, 1994). Another factor is the definition of relapse. Holding to the standard that any drinking constitutes a relapse, then the success rate for treatment programs is only 25% to 35% (Miller et al., 2001). However, if the standard is improvement and a lower level of problems caused by drinking, then relapse is not as common; as many as 60% of people who complete a treatment program achieve this level of success.

Most behavior-based treatment regimens include training for relapse prevention, taking the view that a relapse is an opportunity for learning and not a complete failure (*Harvard Mental Health Letter,* 2000). As discussed in Chapter 13, relapse prevention training is aimed at changing cognitions so that the addict comes to believe that one slip does not equal total relapse. Programs that focus on long-term goals and incorporate relapse prevention into their regimen tend to have the highest rates of success (McLellan, Lewis, O'Brien, & Kleber, 2000).

In Summary

Despite a decline in the percentage of drinkers in the United States, the number of people seeking help for their drinking problems has continued to grow. In addition to formal treatment programs, many problem drinkers are able to quit without therapy. Traditional alcohol treatment programs have been oriented toward abstinence, but most have had only moderate success. The effectiveness of the AA programs is difficult to assess because members are anonymous. Psychotherapeutic approaches to changing problem drinking usually deal with a wide range of personal problems and are not limited to the problem of drinking. People most likely to be helped by psychotherapy are healthy, middle class, married, and employed. Chemical treatments such as the drug disulfiram have been used for some time to curb alcohol consumption, but its drastic effects hinder its usefulness. Aversion therapy with electric shock and emetine have been used with limited success.

Controlled drinking might be a reasonable goal for a substantial minority of all problem drinkers. However, many abstinence-oriented therapists do not consider controlled drinking a viable alternative to abstinence, which may keep them from accepting the success of therapy programs that result in the decrease but not elimination of drinking. Treatment produces only about 25% abstinence 1 year after treatment, but drinking levels drop substantially, and so do alcohol-related problems.

With all alcohol treatment approaches, relapse has been a persistent problem. Most relapses occur within 3 months after the end of treatment, and after 12 months, only 25% of those who complete the program are still abstinent. Relapse training, especially programs teaching that one slip does not equal complete relapse, can help

TABLE 14.1 *Lifetime, Past Year, and Past Month Use of Various Drugs, Including Nonmedical Use of Legal Drugs, Persons Aged 12 Years and Older, United States, 2000*

Drug	Lifetime Use	Use during Past Year	Use during Past Month
Alcohol	81.3%	61.9%	46.6%
Cigarettes	66.5	29.1	24.9
Smokeless Tobacco	18.5	4.5	3.4
Sedatives	3.2	0.3	0.1
Tranquilizers	5.8	1.2	0.4
Heroin	1.2	0.1	0.1
Pain Relievers	8.6	2.9	1.2
Stimulants	6.6	0.9	0.4
Cocaine	11.2	1.5	0.5
Crack cocaine	2.4	0.3	0.1
Marijuana	34.2	8.3	4.8
LSD	8.8	0.8	0.2

Source: *Summary Findings from the 2000 National Household Survey on Drug Abuse* by Substance Abuse and Mental Health Services Administration, 2001, (DHHS Publication No. SMA 01-3549) Rockville, MD: U.S. Government Printing Office.

people to stop abusing alcohol, but complete abstinence probably occurs in a very small percent of problem drinkers.

Other Drugs

Illicit drugs have created many serious problems in the United States, but these problems are mainly social and not related to physical health. Compared with the effects of smoking cigarettes, drinking alcohol, eating unwisely, and failing to exercise, relatively few people die from the effects of illegal drugs. For example, cocaine, the deadliest of the illicit drugs kills only one person for every 1,000 killed by tobacco products (Rouse, 1998). Even one death from illicit drugs, of course, is too many, and this section addresses some of the negative health consequences of both legal and illegal drugs. Table 14.1 shows the rates of use of various drugs, including alcohol and nicotine.

Researchers are beginning to understand how drugs function in the brain to alter mood and behavior. Alcohol and other drugs produce effects on neurotransmitters, the chemical basis of neural transmission. Several neurotransmitters are involved in drug actions, but the neurotransmitter **dopamine** is especially important (Fromme & D'Amico, 1999). Dopamine is the most important neurotransmitter in a brain subsystem that relays messages from the ventral tegmental area in the midbrain to the nucleus accumbens in the forebrain (*NIDA Research Report,* 1999). Researchers have known for years that this area is involved in the brain's experience of reward and pleasure. However, the same system seems to underlie the actions of many drugs (Spanagel & Weiss, 1999).

Psychoactive drugs do not all act in the same way in this subsystem, but all increase the availability of dopamine and affect the function of other neurotransmitters such as glutamate and GABA. Alterations of these neurotransmitters produce temporary changes in brain chemistry but rarely damage neurons. Changing the brain's chemistry, however, is not without risks, but brain damage is not a health effect associated with most drugs.

Health Effects

Even though they do not damage neurons, both legal and illegal drugs pose potential health hazards. However, illegal drugs present certain risks not found with legal drugs, regardless of pharmacological effects. Illegal drugs may be sold as one drug when they are actually another; buyers have no insurance as to dosage; and illegally manufactured drugs may have impurities that can be dangerous chemicals themselves. In addition, the sources of illegal drugs can be dangerous people. Legal drugs are free from these risks, but they are not always safe or harmless.

All drugs have potential hazards, but drugs termed *safe* are tested by the federal Food and Drug Administration (FDA) and defined as safe. The FDA considers a drug safe if its potential benefits outweigh its potential hazards. Many drugs, such as antibiotics, have been approved although they produce severe side effects in some people. The more potentially beneficial a drug, the more likely it is to be labeled safe despite unpleasant side effects.

The FDA classifies drugs into five categories, based on their potential for abuse and their potential medical benefits. Schedule I includes drugs judged to be high in abuse potential and with no accepted medical use. Included in this category are heroin, LSD, and marijuana. Schedule II includes drugs that have high abuse potential, capable of causing severe psychological or physical dependence but having some medical use. In this category are most opiates, some barbiturates, amphetamines, and cocaine. Schedule III consists of drugs judged to produce moderate or low physical dependence or high psychological dependence but with accepted medical uses, such as some opiates and some tranquilizers. Schedule IV drugs, such as Phenobarbital and most tranquilizers, are judged to have low abuse potential, limited dependence properties, and accepted medical uses. Schedule V contains drugs with less abuse potential than those in Schedule IV.

Drugs in Schedule V do not require a prescription and are available over the counter in drug stores, drugs in Schedule I are not legally available, and those in Schedules II, III, and IV are available only by prescription. This classification has evolved somewhat haphazardly over the past 100 years and represents legislative and social convention rather than scientific findings.

Sedatives **Sedatives** are drugs that induce relaxation and sometimes intoxication by lowering the activity of the brain, the neurons, the muscles, and the heart, and even by slowing the metabolic rate. In low doses, these drugs tend to make people feel relaxed and even euphoric. In high doses, they cause loss of consciousness and can result in coma and death due to their inhibitory effect on the brain center that controls respiration. Sedatives include barbiturates, tranquilizers, opiates, and methadone, but the most commonly used drug in this category is alcohol.

Depressant effects are a major problem with sedative drugs, and these effects are additive when sedatives are taken in combination. The effect of mixing two or more of these drugs can be depression of the respiratory system to a dangerously low level. Some people mix alcohol with tranquilizers or other depressants, providing a potentially lethal combination. Furthermore, sedatives and stimulants have opposite effects, but these effects do not cancel each other; instead, both sets of effects occur. For example, caffeine (the stimulant drug in coffee) will not sober a person intoxicated on alcohol (a sedative). Rather, caffeine merely makes a drunken person more alert and less sleepy—not less drunk.

Barbiturates are synthetic drugs used medically to induce sleep. Taken recreationally, barbiturates produce effects similar to alcohol: relaxation and intoxication in small doses, drunkenness and unconsciousness in larger doses. Because they are ingested in pill form, barbiturate overdoses are more common than alcohol overdoses. Barbiturates produce both tolerance and dependence, although the tolerance properties are difficult to assess. Many people can take barbiturates in the form of sleeping pills over an extended time without increasing the dose, whereas others rapidly escalate their dosage to dangerous levels. People who use barbiturates as sleeping pills on a regular basis are not able to sleep without them, and they manifest withdrawal symptoms when they stop taking them—two definite indications of dependence. Withdrawal is similar to that from alcohol, lasting up to a week and including tremor, nausea, vomiting, sweating, sleep disturbances, and sometimes hallucinations and deliriums.

Tranquilizers are relatively recent, dating only to the 1960s. The most prominent variety of these chemical compositions is the *benzodiazepine* group. Like barbiturates, tranquilizers induce depression, but they are less likely to produce sleep and more likely to suppress anxiety. Recognition of the dangers of this class of drug has led to decreased prescriptions and fewer health problems.

Benzodiazepines produce both tolerance and dependence, but only over an extended period. Neither tolerance nor dependence is particularly severe if the drug is taken in small or even moderate amounts. In large amounts, however, these drugs not only produce tolerance and dependence but also cause disorientation, confusion, and even rage, a paradoxical effect for a tranquilizer.

Another category of depressants is the **opiates,** drugs derived from the opium poppy. Opium can also be refined into *morphine,* which can be further chemically treated to produce *heroin.* Synthetic and semisynthetic compounds, including *meperidine, methadone,* oxycodone (OxyContin), and hydrocodone (Vicodin), are chemically similar to the opiates and produce similar effects.

Opium has been used for centuries for both medical and recreational purposes. It can be ingested by swallowing, sniffing, smoking, or injecting under the skin, into a muscle, or intravenously, making it one of the most versatile drugs for transmission into the body. In the 19th century in the United States, physicians prescribed opiates frequently and for a variety of conditions. Today, the principal medical use of opiates is to relieve pain. Because they act on the central nervous system and the digestive system, opiate drugs are also prescribed for cough and for diarrhea. Opiates cross the blood–brain barrier and attach to receptors in the brain, altering the interpretation of pain messages. The physical condition responsible for the pain is not halted, of course, but the person's subjective experience of pain diminishes. Opiate drugs, therefore, have important medical uses.

Opiates produce both tolerance and dependence after only a brief time, sometimes as little as 24 hours, thus making opiates such as heroin easily abused. However, heroin use is not common in the United States (see Table 14.1). Johnston et al. (2001, 2002) reported significant increases in the annual use of heroin and other opiates among high school seniors from 1979 to 1996, with most of the increase occurring in the mid-1990s. The growing popularity of oxycodone and hydrocodone were part of that trend. In addition, young people began using heroin by means other than injection. The trend toward increased use of opiates is more prominent among teenagers than young or older adults (Johnston et al., 2001), and use remains very low (1% or less) for adults.

Stimulants Stimulant drugs tend to make some people feel more alert and energetic, more able to concentrate, and more able to work long hours. They make other users feel jittery, anxious, and unable to sit still. More specifically, stimulants tend to produce alertness, reduce feelings of fatigue, elevate mood, and decrease appetite. They are synthetic but are similar in chemical structure to norepinephrine, the neurotransmitter identified as the brain's main excitatory chemical. After a decline in the nonmedical use of stimulants from 1975 to the early 1990s, there was a slight increase in the use of illegal stimulants in the United States by high school seniors (Johnston et al., 2002) but little change in use among college students and young adults from 1991 to 2000 (Johnston et al., 2001).

Amphetamines are stimulant drug that are often abused due to their mood-altering effects. In addition, amphetamines produce such physical symptoms as increased blood pressure, slower heart rate, increased respiration, relaxation of bronchial muscles, dilation of pupils, increased

BECOMING HEALTHIER

1. Avoid binge drinking, that is, drinking five or more drinks on any one occasion. This level of drinking confers more risks than benefits.
2. Avoiding alcohol may not be the healthiest choice, and light to moderate drinkers have health advantages over those who abstain as well as over those who drink unwisely.
3. One or two drinks per day can confer health benefits, but impaired judgment and coordination can present dangers for even low levels of alcohol consumption.
4. Occasional light drinking presents some risks but does not convey as many benefits as more regular drinking.
5. Do not drive, operate machinery, or swim after drinking.
6. Do not escalate your drinking but keep to one or two drinks per day.
7. The safest level of alcohol for pregnant women is none.
8. If one or both of your parents experienced drinking problems, you may be at elevated risk. Manage this risk by moderating your drinking.
9. If you have an extremely pleasant experience with any drug (including alcohol) the first time you try it, be aware that this drug may present problems for you with future use.
10. Drugs that produce dependence are more dangerous than those that do not. Be aware and cautious about using such drugs, including alcohol and nicotine as well as opiates, barbiturates, and amphetamines.
11. Illegal drugs, even those without tolerance or dependence potential, can be dangerous because they are illegal.

EEG activity, and increased blood supply to the muscles. These effects can be dangerous to the cardiovascular system, especially for people who have heart problems or other cardiovascular diseases. Amphetamines can also produce psychological effects, including hallucinations and paranoid delusions. High energy levels combined with paranoid delusions can make amphetamine users dangerous to society. In addition to these physical, psychological, and social effects, amphetamines produce both tolerance and dependence. Thus, they are undesirable as diet pills, despite their appetite suppressant effects.

Another stimulant drug, **cocaine,** is extracted from the coca plant, which grows in the Andes Mountains in South America. In the 1880s, several European physicians, including Sigmund Freud, discovered that cocaine was capable of blocking neural transmission at the site of application and therefore was useful for **anesthesia.** For a time, cocaine was used as an anesthetic for surgery, especially eye surgery. In the 1890s, it became a popular drug in America and was widely available in tonics, wines, and soft drinks. Soon, however, people began to recognize the dangers of cocaine, and the passage of U.S. federal drug laws restricted its use. Today, the medical uses of cocaine are quite limited because more effective anesthetics have been developed.

Cocaine acts as a stimulant to the nervous system, and the strength and duration of its action depend not only on dose but also on mode of administration. Although South American Indians take cocaine orally by chewing the coca leaves, this method is seldom used elsewhere. Instead, cocaine is snorted through the nasal passages, smoked (in the "freebase" or crack form), or injected intravenously. The stimulant effects of cocaine are short, lasting only 15 to 30 minutes. During this time, the user often feels a powerful euphoria, a strong sense of well-being, and heightened attention. But when the effects wear off, the user frequently feels fatigued, sluggish, and anxious and is left with a strong craving to repeat the experience. Frequently the user will increase the dose in a futile effort to make the euphoria last

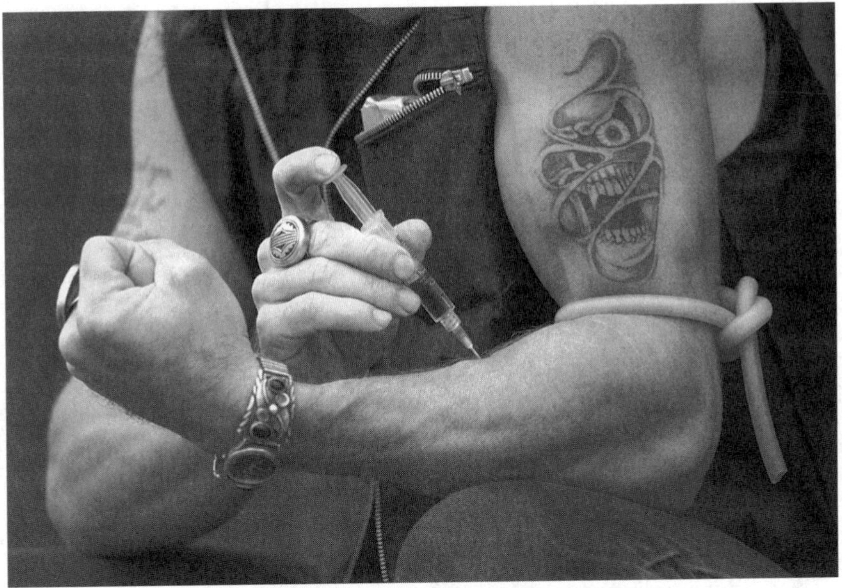
Corbis

Injection drug use can pose health hazards from the drug and from unsterile needles.

longer the next time. The stimulant effects of increased doses of cocaine can endanger the cardiovascular system. The health effects of prolonged heavy use of cocaine are still not clearly understood, but a study of lifetime cocaine use among young adults (Braun, Murray, & Sidney, 1997) found no relationship between prolonged heavy use of cocaine and various cardiovascular risk factors. Longitudinal studies are required to determine if continued use of cocaine might be related to cardiovascular risk factors later in life.

During the early 1990s, a group of neuropharmacology researchers (Hearn et al., 1991) discovered that cocaine and alcohol interact in the body to form a third chemical, *cocaethylene,* which produces or enhances the euphoria that cocaine users experience. However, the mixture of cocaine and alcohol is potentially lethal and accounts for a higher death rate and a greater rate of emergency room admissions than either drug alone.

Crack cocaine became a serious social problem in the United States in the 1980s, when this form of cocaine became cheap and widely available. Crack, a form of freebase cocaine, is ingested by smoking. The use of crack among high school seniors declined during the mid-1980s (from 4.1%) to a low of 1.5% in 1991, but its use has increased slightly to 2.1% in 2001 (Johnston et al., 2002). For young adults, the rates of annual use have fallen steadily from the mid-1980s through 2000, to 1.2% (Johnston et al., 2001). The annual use of both cocaine and crack cocaine is quite low in the general population (see Table 14.1).

Use of methylenedioxymethamphetamine (MDMA)—"Ecstasy"—has risen more rapidly than any other illicit drug in the United States, both among high school students (Johnston et al., 2002) and young adults (Johnston et al., 2001). This drug is a derivative of methamphetamine, but its effects are not mainly those of stimulation or excitation. Instead, MDMA produces feelings of peace, joy, and empathy with others. These feelings come from the massive release of the neurotransmitter *serotonin.* This action depletes the brain of serotonin, resulting in a deficient amount for normal functioning and possibly long-lasting problems with serotonin regulation in the brain (Reneman et al., 2001).

These problems are more likely to occur in women than in men. More immediate dangers involve problems in regulating body temperature, which can be fatal. Despite its dangers, this drug showed increasing popularity worldwide, beginning in the late 1990s. About 12% of high school seniors and young adults have tried Ecstasy, and about 3% of high school seniors and 2% of young adults use this drug at least monthly (Johnston et al., 2001, 2002).

Marijuana The most commonly used illegal drug in the United States is *marijuana* (see Table 14.1). Its potential for serious health consequences is still debated, but few authorities regard it as a major health risk. In fact, Stephen Sidney and his associates (Sidney, Beck, Tekawa, Quesenberry, & Friedman, 1997) found no increased death rates for marijuana users, except for men who died of AIDS. Although this study does not determine cause and effect, it seems safe to assume that marijuana did not cause death from AIDS, but rather that men receiving a diagnosis of AIDS may have subsequently increased their use of marijuana.

Marijuana is composed of the leaves, flowers, and small branches of *Cannabis sativa,* a plant that flourishes in almost every climate in the world. The intoxicating ingredient in marijuana, delta-9-tetrahydrocannabinol (THC), comes from the resin of the male plants and especially the female plants. The most reliable physiological effect of THC is increased heart rate, which occurs with the consumption of heavy doses. Although a rapid heartbeat may present health hazards to users with coronary problems, no evidence exists that marijuana in small or moderate doses causes any organic damage. Nevertheless, any drug used chronically and in heavy doses poses a danger to health. Thus, marijuana, like nicotine, alcohol, or aspirin, has some potential to impair health, and, if smoked as frequently as cigarettes, it would be at least as harmful to the respiratory system as tobacco.

Marijuana has been used medically to treat glaucoma and to prevent the vomiting and nausea associated with chemotherapy. THC and the cannaboids that are the active ingredients in marijuana are capable of reducing nausea and vomiting in cancer patients treated with chemotherapy (Tramer et al., 2001). Marijuana also has analgesic properties that are similar to the pain-relieving properties of codeine (Campbell et al., 2001). In the 1970s, researchers noticed that healthy young marijuana smokers experienced a lessening of pressure within their eyes, decreasing glaucoma (Hepler & Frank, 1971). In 1992, however, the Drug Enforcement Administration rejected all pleas for reclassifying marijuana to Schedule II. Nevertheless, marijuana continues to be used illegally for nausea, glaucoma, muscle relaxation, and as an appetite stimulant for AIDS patients (Grinspoon & Bakalar, 1995).

The desired psychological effects of marijuana are euphoria, a sense of well-being, feelings of relaxation, and heightened sexual responsiveness, and these are usually attained by experienced smokers who expect to attain them. On the negative side, marijuana also has an effect on short-term memory, judgment, and time perception. These effects can be persistent in long-term, heavy users (Solowij et al., 2002). Even the slight effects of light and occasional marijuana use may be hazardous when a person is operating an automobile or engaging in any other potentially dangerous activity (Sadovsky, 2000).

People involved in providing treatment to long-term, heavy marijuana users have contended that marijuana is capable of producing dependence and withdrawal. Research has confirmed that withdrawal symptoms occur in such users (Budney, Hughes, Moore, & Novy, 2001). However, very few users experience these symptoms, and most of the people who have tried or used marijuana do not continue to use this drug (Johnston et al., 2001). The psychological effects of marijuana, like those of alcohol and other drugs, seem to depend partially on setting and expectation.

Recreational use of marijuana in the United States is a relatively recent phenomenon. Only 2% of people born between 1930 and 1940 used marijuana before age 21, but more than half the people born during the 1970s used this drug before their 21st birthday (Johnson & Gerstein, 1998). Unlike the use of most other illicit drugs, marijuana use among young people has recently increased in the United States. Johnston et al. (2002) reported a rise in marijuana among 8th graders, 10th graders, and 12th graders from 1991 to 1997, after more than a decade of slow decline. For example, from 1991 to 2001, both annual and monthly use of marijuana among 10th grade students almost doubled, increasing from 22% to 40% for annual use and from 12% to 22% for monthly use (Johnston et al., 2002). Lifetime use among college students and young adults is more than 50%, but that number has not changed much since 1991. During the early 1990s, monthly use among college students and young adults remained relatively constant—at around 14% to 15%, but in the mid-1990s, that rate increased, a possible result of increased marijuana smoking among high school students during the early 1990s (Johnston et al., 2001).

Anabolic Steroids In recent years, many athletes have used **anabolic steroids (AS)** to increase their muscle bulk and to decrease body fat. Is this practice a potential health hazard? Before addressing this question, we briefly describe anabolic steroids and discuss their positive effects.

Steroids can be either endogenous (manufactured by the body) or synthetic. Endogenous steroids are produced by the adrenal glands, which secrete cortisone, and by the ovaries and testes, which secrete estrogen and testosterone. The effects of anabolic steroids include thickening of vocal cords, enlargement of the larynx, increase of muscle bulk, and decrease of body fat. These last two properties make AS attractive to athletes, bodybuilders, and people who wish to alter their appearance. Anabolic steroids have some medical uses, including reduction of inflammation and control of some allergic reactions.

On the other hand, anabolic steroids are potentially dangerous. They can upset the chemical balance in the body, produce toxicity, and shut off the body's production of its own steroids, leaving the person more susceptible to stress and infection and altering reproductive functioning. Other hazards include increased coronary risk factors, heart attack, abnormal liver function, stunted height, and breast development in men. Some authorities (*NIDA Research Reports,* 2000) contend that the use of steroids leads to dependence in some circumstances and produces behavioral problems in many more. These behavioral problems include aggression, euphoria, mood swings, distractibility, and confusion.

Monthly use of steroids is around 1% for high school students, but only 0.1% for young adults (Johnston et al., 2001, 2002). These overall percentages do not reflect the extent of use among selected groups. Young men are three to five times more likely than young women to use anabolic steroids (Johnston et al., 2001); use among athletes is much higher.

Drug Misuse and Abuse

Most people believe that some drugs are acceptable and even desirable because of the medical benefits they confer. But all *psychoactive* drugs—drugs that cross the blood–brain barrier and alter mental functioning—are potentially harmful to health. Most have the capacity for tolerance or dependence (see Table 14.2). Even drugs that are not psychoactive have the potential for unpleasant side effects. For example, penicillin can cause nausea, vomiting, diarrhea, swelling, and skin eruptions. In addition, people who have allergies to penicillin can die from ingesting it. Also, caffeine, a commonly found drug in coffee and cola drinks, can produce effects that meet the DSM-IV criteria of substance dependence. For example, one study (Strain, Mumford, Silverman, & Griffiths, 1994) found that a high percentage of people who believed that they were dependent on caffeine had been unsuccessful in quitting or cutting down, showed withdrawal symptoms when denied caffeine, and continue to use the drug despite knowledge that its use may cause persistent or recurrent physiological and psychological

TABLE 14.2 *Summary of the Characteristics of Psychoactive Drugs*

Name	Source	Medical use	Mode of ingestion	Effects	Duration of effects	Tolerance	Dependence
Stimulants							
Caffeine	Natural (tea, coffee, etc.)	Anti-depressant	Swallowed	Increases alertness, reduced fatigue	1–2 hrs.	Yes	No
Cocaine	Natural (coca plant)	Local anesthetic	Swallowed, injected, sniffed	Produces euphoria, suppresses appetite	15–30 mins.	?	?
Amphetamines	Synthetic	Appetite suppressant	Swallowed, injected	Produces alertness, reduces fatigues	4 hrs.	Yes	Yes
Nicotine	Natural (tobacco plant)	None	Smoked, sniffed, chewed	Elevates blood pressure	30 mins.	Yes	Yes
Depressants							
Barbiturates	Synthetic	Sedative	Swallowed	Relaxes, intoxicates	Varies depending on type	Yes	Yes
Tranquilizers	Synthetic	Anxiety reducer	Swallowed	Relaxes, intoxicates	3–4 hrs.	Yes	Yes
Opiates	Natural (opium poppy) semi-synthetic	Analgesic	Swallowed, sniffed, smoked, injected	Produces euphoria, sedates	4–6 hrs.	Yes	Yes
Methadone	Syntheic	Treatment for heroin addiction	Swallowed	Prevents heroin withdrawal	12–24 hrs.	Yes	Yes
Alcohol	Natural (fruits, grains)	External antiseptic	Swallowed	Relaxes, intoxicates	1–2 hrs.	Yes	Yes
Marijuana	Natural (cannabis)	Treatment for glaucoma, antiemetic	Smoked	Relaxes, intoxicates	2–3 hrs.	?	No
Steroids	Natural, synthetic	Agent for reducing inflammation and rashes	Swallowed, injected, applied to skin	Builds muscles, increases blood pressure, reduces immune system functioning	7–14 days	Yes	No

problems. Therefore, even a drug that is safe for most people will not be without substantial risks for some.

Almost all drugs that have potential medical or health benefits also have the potential for misuse and abuse. The moderate use of alcohol, for instance, is related to decreased cardiovascular mortality. The *misuse* of alcohol—defined as inappropriate but not health-threatening levels of consumption—can result in social embarrassment, violent acts, and injury. And *abuse* of alcohol—defined as frequent heavy consumption to the point of addiction—can lead to cirrhosis, brain damage, heart attack, and fetal alcohol syndrome.

Treatment for Drug Abuse

Treatment for the use and abuse of illegal drugs is similar to the treatment of alcohol abuse, both in the philosophy and the administration of treatment. The goal of treatment for all types of illegal drug use is total abstinence. In many cases, the programs that treat drug abusers often coexist physically with treatment programs for alcohol abuse, and patients who are receiving treatment for their drug problems participate in the same therapy as those who are receiving therapy for their alcohol problems. The philosophy that guides Alcoholics Anonymous led to the development of Narcotics Anonymous, an organization devoted to helping drug users abstain from using drugs.

The reasons for entering drug abuse treatment programs are often similar to those for entering treatment for alcohol abuse. These reasons are primarily social. The abuse of illegal drugs leads to legal, financial, and interpersonal problems, as does alcohol abuse. Like alcohol, most illegal drugs produce impairments of judgment that lead to accidents, making accidental injury the leading health risk for drug abuse. Unlike alcohol abuse, the abuse of illegal drugs does not often directly damage health. However, when health problems occur, they are likely to be major and life threatening. Such crises may precipitate a person's decision to seek treatment or lead family members to enforce treatment.

Inpatient treatment programs for drug abuse are strikingly similar to those designed to treat alcohol abuse, but they do differ from programs for alcohol abuse in several minor ways. The detoxification phase of inpatient hospitalization is typically shorter and less severe for most types of drug use than it is for alcohol, for which withdrawal can be life threatening. Alcohol is a depressant drug, as are barbiturates, tranquilizers, and opiates. Therefore, all these drugs have similar symptoms during withdrawal, including agitation, tremor, gastric distress, and possibly perceptual distortions. Stimulants such as amphetamines and cocaine produce different withdrawal symptoms, namely lethargy and depression. These differences necessitate different medical care during detoxification.

One similarity between drug and alcohol abuse treatment is the high rate of relapse. As noted earlier, alcohol, smoking, and opiate treatment all share a high rate of relapse (Hunt et al., 1971), and the first 6 months after treatment are critical. To ameliorate this problem, drug treatment programs, like alcohol treatment interventions, typically include some aftercare or "booster" sessions. Frequently, this continued care comes from joining a support group such as Narcotics Anonymous. However, evidence exists that more comprehensive psychosocial services boost the effectiveness of drug treatment (McLellan, Arndt, Metzger, Woody, & O'Brien, 1993).

Preventing and Controlling Drug Use

Chapter 13 presented information on attempts to decrease smoking in children and adolescents by various interventions aimed at discouraging their experimentation with cigarettes and smokeless tobacco. Similar efforts have been applied to the use of other drugs (Goldberg et al., 1996), but programs aimed at children and adolescents are not the only approach to controlling drug use.

A more common control technique is the limitation of availability. This strategy is common in all Western countries through the existence of laws that limit the legal access to drugs. However, legal restriction of drugs has a number of side effects, some of which create other social problems (Robins, 1995). For example, when the United States legally prohibited the manufacture and sale of alcohol, illegal manufacture and distribution flourished, creating a large criminal enterprise, huge profits, loss of tax revenue, and corruption among law enforcement agencies. Therefore, the limitation of availability has negative as well as positive consequences, and the extent to which this approach should be enacted remains controversial (Spillane, 1999).

The prevention attempts aimed at keeping children and adolescents from experimenting with drugs are intended to delay or inhibit the initiation of drug use (Ammerman, Ott, Tarter, & Blackson, 1999). As with the efforts at preventing smoking (see Chapter 13), those aimed at preventing drug use do not have an impressive success rate (Botvin, 1999). Some programs have been counterproductive, increasing drug use or increasing adolescents' beliefs that drug use is more prevalent than it is (Donaldson, Graham, Piccinin, & Hansen, 1995). As with smoking prevention programs, drug prevention programs that rely on scare tactics, moral training, factual information about drug risks, and boosting self-esteem generally are ineffective (Donaldson et al., 1995). Indeed, a meta-analysis of the effectiveness of Project DARE (Drug Abuse Resistance Education), a widely used school-based drug education program, showed that this popular intervention is not very effective, even in the short term (Ennett, Tobler, Ringwalt, & Flewelling, 1994).

Some types of prevention programs are more effective than others. Peer programs that involve peers or older adolescents are more effective than those using adults as counselors (Botvin, 1999). These programs typically involve developing social skills necessary to resist social pressure to use drugs. In addition, research (Chilcoat, Deshion, & Anthony, 1995) has demonstrated that parental monitoring of children's activities and whereabouts decreased the risk for drug involvement among children of elementary school age.

Another strategy is the control of the harm of drug use. This strategy involves the assumption that people will use psychoactive drugs, sometimes unwisely, but that reduction of the health consequences of drug use should be the first priority (McMurran, 1994; Peele & Brodsky, 1996). Rather than taking a moralistic stand on drug use, this strategy takes a practical approach to minimizing the dangers of drug use. An example of the harm reduction strategy is to help injection drug users exchange used needles for sterile ones and, thus, slow the spread of HIV infection or to encourage moderate drinking that is compatible with health promotion. The controversy surrounding such programs is representative of the debate over the harm reduction strategy.

In Summary

Abuse of alcohol is a serious health problem in most developed nations, but other drugs—including depressants, stimulants, cocaine, marijuana, ecstasy, and anabolic steroids—also are potentially harmful to health. At one time, many of these drugs have been available over the counter or through a physician's prescription. Although the abuse of these drugs often leads to a number of social problems, their health risks are much less than those associated with nicotine or alcohol. Treatments for drug abuse are similar to those for alcohol abuse, and programs aimed at prevention are similar to those aimed at preventing smoking. A new strategy called harm reduction aims at decreasing the social and health risks of taking drugs by changing drug policies.

Answers

This chapter addressed six basic questions.

1. **What are the major trends in alcohol consumption?**
People have consumed alcohol worldwide and before recorded history. Alcohol consumption in the United States reached a peak during the first 3 decades of the 19th century, dropped sharply during the mid-1800s as a result of the "temperance" movement, and continued at a steady rate until it declined even more during Prohibition. Currently, rates of alcohol consumption in the United States are holding steady after a period of slow decline. About half of adults are classified as current drinkers, including 21% as binge drinkers and 6% as heavy drinkers. Adult European Americans have higher rates of drinking than members of other ethnic groups.

2. **What are the health effects of drinking alcohol?**
Drinking has both positive and negative health effects. Prolonged heavy drinking of alcohol often leads to cirrhosis of the liver and other serious health problems, such as heart disease and brain dysfunction. Moderate drinking may have certain long-range health benefits in reduced heart disease and lowered probability of developing gallstones, Type 2 diabetes, and Alzheimer's disease.

3. **Why do people drink?**
Models for drinking behavior should be able to explain why people begin drinking, why some can drink in moderation, and why others drink to excess. The disease model assumes that people drink excessively because they have the disease of alcoholism. Cognitive-physiological models, including the tension reduction hypothesis, the self-awareness model, and alcohol myopia, propose that people drink because alcohol allows them to escape tension and negative self-evaluations. Social learning theory assumes that people acquire drinking behavior through positive or negative reinforcement, modeling, and cognitive mediation.

4. **How can people change problem drinking?**
Many problem drinkers seem to be able to quit without therapy, but treatment programs are moderately effective in helping people who do not succeed in quitting on their own. About 25% of treated alcoholics are abstinent at the end of 1 year, but many others have decreased their drinking to a level that is no longer a problem. In the United States, most treatment programs are oriented toward abstinence, and those drinkers who do not quit are often considered treatment failures. Alcoholics Anonymous is the most popular treatment program, but despite its prominence, its effectiveness is difficult to establish. Chemical treatments to curb drinking have been of limited usefulness. Controlled drinking remains controversial as a treatment goal, although some problem drinkers are capable of attaining this type of drinking.

5. **What problems are associated with relapse?**
Relapse is common among heavy drinkers who have quit, although many are able to maintain abstinence or to drink in a controlled manner. Most relapses occur during the first 3 months. After a year, about 65% of all successful quitters have resumed drinking, some in a harmful manner. Relapse rates are reduced in programs that include "booster" sessions or follow-up treatment.

6. **What are the health effects of other drugs?**
Other drugs—including depressants, stimulants, ecstasy, cocaine, marijuana, and anabolic steroids—have had some medical use, but they also are potentially harmful to health. The principal problems from most of these drugs are social, not physical. Treatments for drug abuse are similar to those for alcohol abuse, and programs aimed at prevention are similar to those aimed at preventing smoking.

Suggested Readings

Edwards, G. (2000). *Alcohol: The world's favorite drug.* New York: Thomas Dunne Books. Griffin Edwards, prominent researcher and authority on alcohol, examines the history, use, misuse, and treatment of drinking in this nontechnical book.

McMurran, M. (1994). *The psychology of addiction.* London: Taylor & Francis. Mary McMurran is a British psychologist whose background is in treatment of drug and alcohol problems. Her book is an interesting review of the history, legislation, theory, treatment, and prevention of drug use. Writing in Great Britain, she offers a different view of substance abuse from that of most U.S. therapists and theorists.

Nestle, M. (1997). Alcohol guidelines for chronic disease prevention: From prohibition to moderation. *Nutrition Today, 32*(2), 86–92. Marion Nestle tells about the experience of being a member of the panel that recommended moderate alcohol consumption in the most recent *Dietary Guidelines for Americans.* That advice for moderation is a departure from the Prohibitionist sentiment that has ruled official pronouncements concerning drinking.

Shavelson, L. (2001). *Hooked: Five addicts challenge our misguided drug rehab system.* New York: New Press. Emergency room physician and journalist Lonny Shavelson examined San Francisco's drug treatment system. His critical book follows the story of five individuals with drug problems and their interactions with the organizations that provide treatment.

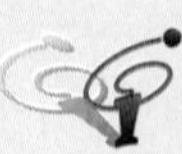

Search InfoTrac College Edition

Search these terms to learn more about topics in this chapter:

Alcohol consumption and demographic

Alcohol consumption and statistics

Binge drinking and statistics

Korsakoff syndrome and alcohol

Fetal alcohol syndrome

Alcohol and injury

Alcohol and violence

Alcohol and crime

Alcohol and health benefits

Alcoholism and genetic aspects

Disease model of alcoholism

Alcoholics Anonymous and philosophy

Alcoholics Anonymous and effectiveness

Tension reduction and alcohol

Alcoholism and psychological treatment

Controlled drinking

Relapse and alcoholism

Drug use and risk and health

Drug use and statistics

Drug use and demographics

Stimulant and health

Marijuana and health aspects

MDMA and health

Drug abuse and treatment programs

Drug abuse and prevention programs

15

Eating to Control Weight

The Stories of Jessica and Elise

CHAPTER OUTLINE

The Digestive System

Factors in Weight Maintenance

Overeating and Obesity

Dieting

Eating Disorders

QUESTIONS

This chapter focuses on six basic questions:

1. How does the digestive system function?
2. What factors are involved in weight maintenance?
3. What is obesity and how does it affect health?
4. Is dieting a good way to lose weight?
5. What is anorexia nervosa and how can it be treated?
6. What is bulimia and how can it be treated?

The Stories of Jessica and Elise

Jessica, a 20-year-old college junior majoring in psychology, was a model student. She worked hard, earned excellent grades, and had high ambitions for a future career. Like many young college women, Jessica wanted to lose a few pounds—8 or 10. However, unlike most other college women, she was already dangerously thin—five feet four inches tall and weighing 81 pounds. Jessica had **anorexia nervosa,** an eating disorder that includes intentional starvation and a distorted body image.

At age 15, Jessica weighed 130 pounds, ate well, and was a normal teenager. In 4 years all this had changed. When she was 16, Jessica took a job as a dance instructor. Her employer suggested that she lose a few pounds, so Jessica began a conscientious program to lose weight. When her weight dropped to 110 pounds, her parents, boyfriend, and girlfriends all complemented her on how good she looked. However, Jessica continued to diet, and her eating habits became extreme as her concern with weight intensified. She would skip breakfast but drink five or six cups of coffee every morning. Her only food of the day was lunch, which consisted of a slice of low-calorie cheese on a half piece of diet bread. She would pick at her lunch for 20 to 30 minutes and eventually consume about half of it. After eating, she would go to the dance studio, where she exercised strenuously for 6 or 7 hours. After work, if daylight permitted, she would ride her bike for several miles or play a couple sets of tennis. In addition to her morning coffee, she would drink one or two cups of hot tea and three or four diet drinks a day.

As her weight continued to drop, Jessica began to hide her weight loss beneath large, loose-fitting clothing. She weighed herself several times a day and spent a good deal of time looking at herself in a mirror. Where others saw an emaciated body, Jessica always saw a figure that seemed too fat. She also worried that her parents or doctor would put her in a hospital and force her to gain weight.

When her weight dropped below 90 pounds, Jessica began noticing soft black hair growing on parts of her body. At the same time, she began to feel cold all the time, even on hot summer days. Despite constantly feeling sick, Jessica was neither concerned nor displeased about her loss of weight. Except for believing that she was a little too fat, she liked her body as it was and had no desire to reverse the downward spiral of weight loss. On the contrary, she became even more determined to lose additional weight and began to fast completely for 4 or 5 days at a time.

Elise was a senior in high school who had always been an excellent student. She made good grades and was involved in many school-related activities, but like many other young women, she was unhappy with her weight. Elise wanted to weigh less than 100 pounds, a weight she felt was reasonable for her 5′2″ frame, but she weighed over 120 pounds. She began eating less—not eating at all during the day, missing dinner due to school-related activities, and fooling her family into thinking that she was eating. Like Jessica, she tended to wear baggy clothing, so at first her family and friends did not notice her weight loss. Unlike Jessica, Elise found fasting difficult and did not feel like exercising to lose weight, so she began to vomit as a way to compensate for eating. Soon she added laxatives as an additional technique. She kept both practices secret from her family, whom she believed would have tried to stop her.

It was not her disordered eating that resulted in Elise receiving treatment, but rather, it was signs of depression—she cried easily, was always tired, and didn't seem to enjoy anything. Elise's family insisted that she go to a psychiatrist, who recognized her eating problems and tried to get Elise to recognize them, too. Elise listened to her psychiatrist and trusted her, forming a positive relationship, but she resisted the notion that she had an eating problem.

Denying any eating problems, Elise continued to vomit and abuse laxatives as ways to lose weight. By the time she graduated from high school, she had lost more than 15 pounds (but still weighed 104 pounds, 5 pounds away from her goal). Her weight began to be an issue with her family and friends, who told her that she was too thin and that she looked terrible. Despite the amount of weight she had lost, she did not meet the criteria to be diagnosed as anorexic according to the *Diagnostic and Statistical Manual of Mental Disorders* (APA, 2000). Those criteria include weight loss to the point that the person is 15% below ideal weight, which Elise was not. However, she exhibited the distorted body image, fear of gaining weight, and

amenorrhea (cessation of menstrual periods), all of which are symptoms of anorexia.

Elise's diagnosis was **bulimia,** an eating disorder consisting of binge eating followed by some method to compensate for the binge, such as fasting, excessive exercising, or purging through either vomiting or using laxatives. Elise exhibited these symptoms, forcing herself to vomit and abusing laxatives, even when the amount of food she had eaten was not excessive.

Elise's eating problems got worse when she began college. She purged by both vomiting and using laxatives. But the more laxatives she consumed, the less effective they became. So she increased the dosage to the point that she once took 45 tablets in less than 2 days. This precipitated a medical crisis, resulting in her being hospitalized and receiving psychotherapy. Her therapist tried to convince Elise to accept a reasonable body image, to eat reasonably, and to stop purging.

Elise tried hard to get better over the next 5 years, but her distorted body image continued. She is still unhappy with her weight, but she continues to work on her recovery. She purged for years but says that the urge to do so has decreased.

Like millions of Americans, Jessica and Elise suffer from some form of **eating disorder.** An eating disorder is any serious and habitual disturbance in eating behavior that produces unhealthy consequences. This definition excludes starvation resulting from the inability to find suitable food supplies and also unhealthy eating resulting from inadequate information about nutrition. Also excluded are disturbances in eating behavior such as pica, or the eating of nonnutritive substances such as plastic and wood, and the rumination disorder of infancy—that is, regurgitation of food without nausea or gastrointestinal illness. Neither of these latter disorders presents serious health problems to adults, and they are of relatively minor importance in health psychology. This chapter examines in detail the three major problems of eating—overeating and dieting, anorexia nervosa, and bulimia—each related to certain difficulties in weight maintenance. To put these in context, we first consider the organs and functions of the digestive system.

The Digestive System

The human body can digest a wide variety of plant and animal tissues, converting these foods into usable proteins, fats, carbohydrates, vitamins, and minerals. The digestive system takes in food, processes it into particles that can be absorbed, and excretes the undigested wastes. The particles that are absorbed through the digestive system are transported through the bloodstream so as to be available to all body cells. These molecules nourish the body by providing the energy for activity as well as the materials for body growth, maintenance, and repair.

The digestive tract is a modified tube, consisting of a number of specialized structures. Also included in the digestive system are several accessory structures connected to the digestive tract by ducts. These ducted glands produce substances that are essential for digestion, and the ducts provide a way for these substances to enter the digestive system. Figure 15.1 shows the digestive system.

In humans and other mammals, some digestion begins in the mouth. The teeth tear and grind food, mixing it with saliva. Several **salivary glands** furnish the moisture that allows the food to be tasted. Without such moisture, the taste buds on the tongue do not function. Saliva also contains an enzyme that digests starch, and so some digestion actively begins before food particles leave the mouth.

Swallowing is a voluntary action, but once food is swallowed, its progress through the **pharynx** and **esophagus** is largely involuntary. **Peristalsis** propels food through the digestive system, beginning with the esophagus. Peristaltic movement is the rhythmic contraction and relaxation of the circular muscles of structures in the digestive system. In the stomach, rhythmic contractions mix the food with **gastric juices** secreted by the stomach and the glands that empty into the stomach. The major digestive activity of the stomach is protein digestion,

CHECK YOUR HEALTH RISKS

Check the items that apply to you.

- ☐ 1. I feel comfortable with my present weight.
- ☐ 2. Although I don't eat much, I stay heavier than I would like to be.
- ☐ 3. I have lost 15 pounds or more over the past 2 years.
- ☐ 4. I have gained 15 pounds or more over the past 2 years.
- ☐ 5. I am more than 30 pounds overweight.
- ☐ 6. My weight has fluctuated about 5 or 10 pounds during the past 2 years, but I'm not concerned about it.
- ☐ 7. If I were thinner, I would be happier.
- ☐ 8. My waist is as big or bigger than my hips.
- ☐ 9. I have been on at least 10 different diet programs in my life.
- ☐ 10. I have fasted, used laxatives, or used diet drugs to lose weight.
- ☐ 11. My family has been concerned that I am too thin, but I disagree.
- ☐ 12. A coach, instructor, or trainer has suggested that weighing less could improve my athletic performance.
- ☐ 13. I sometimes lose control over eating and eat far more than I planned.
- ☐ 14. I would like to have liposuction surgery to remove fat from my body.
- ☐ 15. I have vomited after eating as a way to control my weight.
- ☐ 16. Food is a danger that can be managed by careful thought and mental preparation in order not to eat too much.

Items 1 and 6 reflect a healthy attitude toward weight, but each of the other items represents a health risk from improper eating or unhealthy attitudes concerning eating. Unhealthy eating not only relates to the development of several diseases, but preoccupation with weight and frequent dieting can also be unhealthy.

initiated by the action of the enzyme **pepsin.** Little absorption of nutrients occurs in the stomach; only alcohol, aspirin, and some fat-soluble drugs are absorbed through the stomach lining. The major function of the stomach is to mix food particles with gastric juices, preparing the mixture for absorption in the small intestine.

The mixture of food particles and gastric juices moves into the small intestine a little at a time. The high acidity of the gastric juices results in a very acidic mixture, and the small intestine cannot function in high acidity. To reduce the level of acidity, the pancreas secretes several acid-reducing enzymes into the small intestine. These **pancreatic juices** are also essential for digesting carbohydrates and fats.

The digestion of starch that begins in the mouth is completed in the small intestine. The upper third of the small intestine absorbs starch and other carbohydrates. Protein digestion, initiated in the stomach, is also completed when proteins are absorbed in the upper portion of the small intestine. Fats, however, enter the small intestine almost entirely undigested. **Bile salts** produced in the **liver** and stored in the **gall bladder** break down fat molecules into a form that is acted on by a pancreatic enzyme. Absorption of fats occurs in the middle one third of the small intestine. The bile salts that aid the process are reabsorbed later in the lower third of the small intestine.

Large quantities of water pass through the small intestine. In addition to the water that people drink, digestive juices increase the fluid volume. Of all the water that passes into the small intestine, 90% is absorbed. This absorption process also causes vitamins and electrolytes to pass into the body at this point in digestion.

From the small intestine, digestion proceeds to the large intestine. As with other portions of

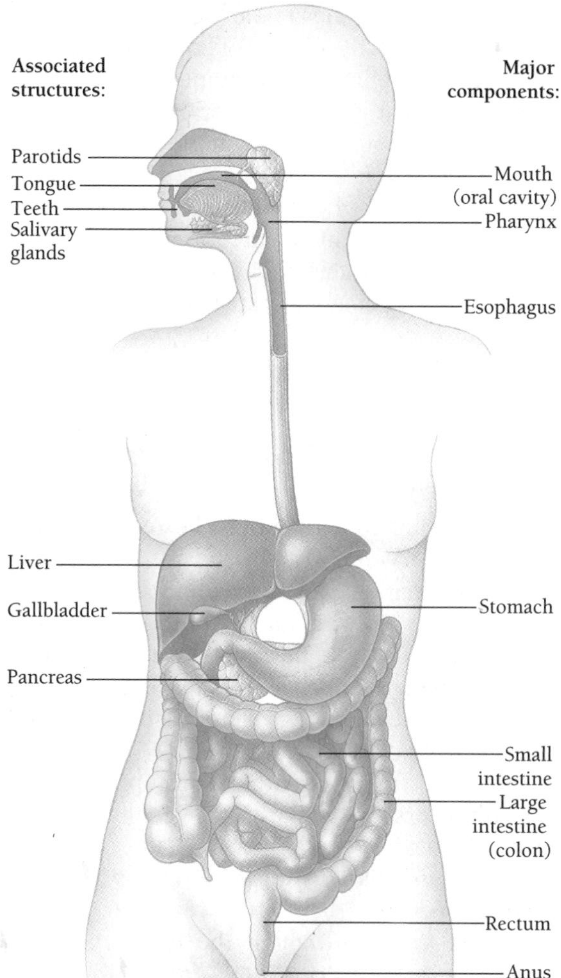

Figure 15.1 The digestive system.

Source: Introduction to Microbiology *(p. 556) by J. L. Ingraham & C. A. Ingraham, 1995, Belmont, CA: Wadsworth. Copyright 1995 by Wadsworth Publishing Company. Reprinted by permission.*

the digestive system, movement through the large intestine occurs through peristalsis. However, the peristaltic movement in the large intestine is more sluggish and irregular than in the small intestine. Bacteria inhabit the large intestine and manufacture several vitamins. Although the large intestine has absorptive capabilities, it typically absorbs only water, a few minerals, and the vitamins manufactured by its bacteria.

Feces consist of the materials left after digestion has taken place. Feces are composed of undigested fiber, inorganic material, undigested nutrients, water, and bacteria. Peristalsis carries the feces through the large intestine, through the **rectum,** and finally through the **anus,** where they are eliminated.

In summary, the digestive system turns food into nutrients by a process that begins in the mouth with the breakdown of food into smaller particles. Digestive juices continue to act on food particles in the stomach, but digestion of most types of nutrients occurs in the small intestines. Digestion is completed with the elimination of the undigested residue. The digestive system is plagued by more diseases and disorders than any other body system. Many digestive disorders are not of active concern to health psychology, but several, such as obesity, anorexia nervosa, and bulimia, have important behavioral components. In addition, maintaining a stable weight depends on behaviors—eating and activity.

Factors in Weight Maintenance

A stable weight is maintained when the calories absorbed from food equal those expended for body metabolism plus physical activity. This balance is not a simple calculation bur rather the result of a complex set of actions. Caloric content varies with foods, with fat having more calories per volume than carbohydrates or proteins. The degree of absorption depends on how rapidly food passes through the digestive system and even the nutrient composition of the foods. Furthermore, differences exist in metabolic rates from person to person and from time to time. Activity level is another source of variability, with greater activity requiring greater caloric expenditures.

To obtain calories, people (and other animals) eat, and eating and weight balance have components in the nervous system. Several hormones and neurotransmitters are important for regulating eating and weight. **Leptin,** a protein hormone discovered in 1994 (Bowles & Kopelman, 2001), is produced by adipose tissue (fat) and acts on receptors in the central nervous system. Genetically obese mice (Pelleymounter

hormones:
leptin -> protein hormone
-> produced by adipose tissue
-> not cause of obesity
-> obese people have ↑ levels
insulin -> ↑ insulin leads to intake of more glucose than cells can use & converted to fat
ghrelin -> peptide hormone
-> rises before & after meals
-> produced in stomach
-> acts on hypothalamus to activate neuropeptide
cholecystokinin -> produced by intestines
-> feelings of satiation

Insulin is a second hormone involved in weight maintenance. This hormone allows body cells to take in glucose for their use. (Deficiency in insulin production or use results in diabetes, which is covered in Chapter 11.) High insulin production leads to the intake of more glucose than cells can use, and the excess is converted into fat. Like leptin, insulin levels are correlated with body fat. The brain contains receptors for both hormones through several pathways (Woods, Schwartz, Baskin, & Seeley, 2000).

A third hormone called *ghrelin* is a peptide hormone discovered in 1999, which also seems to be involved in eating (Cummings, Purnell, et al., 2001). The level of this hormone rises before and falls after meals; its levels change along with changes in leptin levels. Produced in the stomach, ghrelin acts in the **hypothalamus** to activate neuropeptide Y, a neurotransmitter that is involved in eating. Researchers believe that ghrelin prompts eating. In addition, the hormone **cholecystokinin (CCK),** a peptide hormone produced by the intestines, is also a neurotransmitter in the brain. Its production is related to feelings of satiation. Therefore, the picture of hormone and neurotransmitter action is very complex in relation to hunger and eating, with several hormones involved and various pathways in the brain that underlie their action.

To understand the complexities of weight metabolism and weight maintenance, consider an extreme example, an experiment in which participants were systematically starved.

Experimental Starvation

Nearly 60 years ago, Ancel Keys and his colleagues (Keys, Brozek, Henschel, Mickelsen, & Taylor, 1950) published a study on the physical effects of human starvation. The research took place during World War II, and the participants were conscientious objectors who volunteered to be part of a study as an alternative to military service. In most ways these volunteers were quite normal young men; their weights were normal, their IQs were in the normal to bright range, and they were emotionally stable.

For the first 3 months of the project, the 36 volunteers ate regularly and established their normal caloric requirements. Next, the men were put on half their previous rations, with the goal of reducing their body weight to 75% of previous levels. Although the researchers cut the participants' caloric intake in half, they were careful to give them adequate nutrients so that the men were never in any danger of actually starving.

At first these men lost weight rapidly. They were constantly hungry, but the initial pace of weight loss did not last. To continue losing weight, the men had to consume even fewer calories, which led to considerable suffering. Nevertheless, most stayed with the project through the whole 6 months, and most met their goal of losing 25% of their body weight.

The behaviors that accompanied the semistarvation were quite surprising to Keys and his colleagues. At the beginning, the men were optimistic and cheerful, but these feelings soon van-

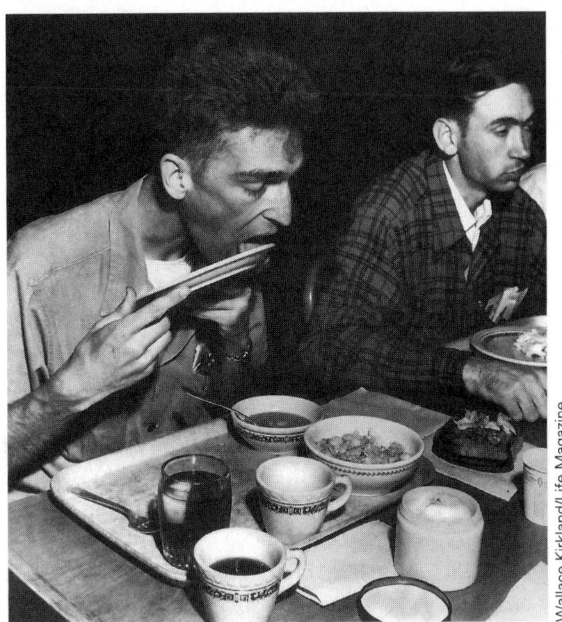

Wallace Kirkland/Life Magazine

Experimental starvation produced an obsession with food and a variety of negative changes in the behavior of these volunteers.

ished. The men became irritable, aggressive, and began to fight among themselves, behavior that was completely out of character. Although the men continued this bellicose behavior throughout the 6 months of starvation, they also became apathetic and avoided as much physical activity as they could. They became neglectful of their dormitory, their own physical appearance, and their girlfriends.

The men were, of course, hungry, and they became increasingly obsessed with thoughts of food. Mealtimes became the center of their lives, and they tended to eat very slowly and to be very sensitive to the taste of their food. At the beginning of the period of caloric reduction, the researchers saw no need to place physical restrictions to prevent the men from cheating on their diets. But about 3 months into the starvation, the men felt that they would be tempted to cheat if they left the dormitory alone. As a result, they were allowed to go out only in pairs or in larger groups. These dedicated, polite, normal, stable young men had become abnormal and unpleasant under conditions of semistarvation.

Obsession with food and continued negative outlook also characterized the refeeding phase of the project. During refeeding, the plan was for the men to regain the weight they had lost. This phase was to have lasted 3 months, with food introduced at gradually increasing levels, but the men objected so strongly that the pace of refeeding was accelerated. As a result, the men ate as much and as often as they could, some as many as five large meals a day. By the end of the refeeding period, most men had regained their preexperimental weight. In fact, many were even slightly heavier. About one half were still preoccupied with food, and for many, their prestarvation optimism and cheerfulness had not completely returned.

Experimental Overeating

A study in experimental starvation does not seem attractive to volunteers, but an experiment on overeating might sound like fun to many people. Ethan Allen Sims and his associates (Sims, 1974, 1976; Sims et al., 1973; Sims & Horton, 1968) found a group of people who should have been especially interested and appreciative—prisoners. Inmates at the Vermont State Prison volunteered to gain 20 to 30 pounds as part of an experiment on overeating. Sims's interest was analogous to Keys's—an understanding of the physical and psychological components of overeating. Special living arrangements were made for these prisoners, including plentiful and delicious food. In addition, the experiment included a restriction of physical activity to make weight gain easier.

Did these men gain weight? With an increase in calories and a decrease in physical activity, weight gain was nearly assured. At first they gained fairly easily. But soon the rate of weight gain slowed, and the participants had to eat more and more to continue gaining. As with the men in the starvation study, these men needed about 3,500 calories to maintain their weight at normal levels, but many had to double that amount to continue gaining. Not all the men were able to attain their weight goals, regardless of how much they ate. One man did not reach his goal even though he ate over 10,000 calories per day.

Were the overeating prisoners as miserable as the starving conscientious objectors? No, but they did find overeating unpleasant. Food became repulsive to them, despite the excellent quality and preparation. They had to force themselves to eat, and many considered dropping out of the study.

When the weight-gain phase of the study was over, the prisoners cut down their food intake dramatically and lost weight. Not all lost as quickly as others, and two had some trouble returning to their original weight. An examination of these two men's medical backgrounds revealed some family histories of obesity, although the men themselves had never been overweight. These results indicate that normal-weight people have trouble increasing their weight substantially and that, even if they do, the increased weight is difficult to maintain.

In Summary

Weight maintenance depends largely on two factors: the number of calories absorbed through food intake and the number expended through body metabolism and physical activity. Underlying this balance is a complex set of hormones and neurotransmitters that have selective effects on various brain sites, including the hypothalamus. Weight gain occurs when more nutrients are present than are required for maintenance of body metabolism and physical activity. Weight loss occurs when insufficient nutrients are present to furnish the necessary energy for body metabolism and activity. An experiment in starvation showed that loss of too much weight leads to irritability, aggression, apathy, lack of interest in sex, and preoccupation with food. Another experiment in overeating showed that gaining weight can be almost as difficult as losing it for some people.

Overeating and Obesity

Overeating is not the sole cause of obesity, but it is part of the weight maintenance equation. Obese people usually eat more than normal weight people (Wing & Polley, 2001), although many overweight people say that they eat less than others. These self-reports, however, are not very accurate, and objective measurements usually indicate that obese people eat more. They are especially likely to eat food rich in fat, which has a higher caloric density than carbohydrates or protein. Thus, they may eat less food but more calories. Overweight individuals also have a tendency to be less physically active than leaner people, which contributes to overweight.

As the studies on experimental starvation and overeating show, metabolic level changes with food intake as well as with energy output to alter the efficiency of nutrient use by the body. Therefore, individual variations in body metabolism allow some people to burn calories faster than others. Two people who eat the same amount may have different weights, but most overweight people eat more calories and perform less physical activity than normal weight people. These behaviors contribute to obesity and its related health consequences, but the definition and underlying reasons for obesity remain the source of controversy.

What Is Obesity?

What is obesity? Answers to this question vary by personal and social standards. Should obesity be defined in terms of health? Appearance? Body mass? Percentage of body fat? Weight charts? Total weight? No good definition of obesity would consider only body weight, because some individuals have a small skeletal frame, whereas others are larger, and some people's weight is in muscle, whereas others carry weight in fat. Muscle tissue and bone weigh more than fat, so some people can be heavier yet leaner, as athletes often are.

TABLE 15.1 *Metropolitan Life Insurance Company's Desirable Weights*

	Small frame		*Medium frame*		*Large frame*	
Height	1959	1983	1959	1983	1959	1983
Women						
4 ft. 10 in.	92-98 lb.	102-111 lb	96-107 lb.	109-121 lb.	104-119 lb.	118-131 lb.
4 11	94-101	103-113	98-110	111-123	106-122	120-134
5 0	96-104	104-115	101-113	113-126	109-125	122-137
5 1	99-107	106-118	104-116	115-129	112-128	125-140
5 2	102-110	108-121	107-119	118-132	115-131	128-143
5 3	105-113	111-124	110-122	121-135	118-134	131-147
5 4	108-116	114-127	113-126	124-138	121-138	134-151
5 5	111-119	117-130	116-130	127-141	125-142	137-155
5 6	114-123	120-133	120-135	130-144	129-146	140-159
5 7	118-127	123-136	124-139	133-147	133-150	143-163
5 8	122-131	126-1[illegible]	128-143	136-150	137-154	146-167
5 9	126-135	129-[illegible]	[illegible]	[illegible]	141-158	149-170
5 10	130-140	132-[illegible]	[illegible]	[illegible]	145-163	152-173
5 11	134-144	135-[illegible]	[illegible]	[illegible]	[illegible]	155-176
6 0	138-148	138-[illegible]	[illegible]	[illegible]	[illegible]	158-179
Men						
5 ft. 2 in.	112-120 lb.	128-[illegible]	[illegible]	[illegible]	[illegible] lb.	138-150 lb.
5 3	115-123	130-[illegible]	[illegible]	[illegible]	[illegible]	140-153
5 4	118-126	132-[illegible]	[illegible]	[illegible]	[illegible]	142-156
5 5	121-129	134-[illegible]	[illegible]	[illegible]	[illegible]	144-160
5 6	124-133	136-[illegible]	[illegible]	[illegible]	[illegible]	146-164
5 7	128-137	138-[illegible]	[illegible]	[illegible]	[illegible]	149-168
5 8	132-141	140-[illegible]	[illegible]	[illegible]	[illegible]	152-172
5 9	136-145	142-[illegible]	[illegible]	[illegible]	[illegible]	155-176
5 10	140-150	144-[illegible]	[illegible]	[illegible]	[illegible]	158-180
5 11	144-154	146-[illegible]	[illegible]	[illegible]	[illegible]	161-184
6 0	148-158	149-[illegible]	[illegible]	[illegible]	[illegible]	164-188
6 1	152-162	152-[illegible]	[illegible]	[illegible]	[illegible]	168-192
6 2	156-167	155-[illegible]	[illegible]	[illegible]	[illegible]	172-197
6 3	160-171	158-[illegible]	[illegible]	[illegible]	[illegible]	176-202
6 4	164-175	162-176	172-190	171-187	182-204	181-207.

Source: From "New Weight Standards for Men and Women," by Metropolitan Life Insurance Company, 1959, *Statistical Bulletin, 40,* p. 1. Copyright © 1959, 1983 by The Metropolitan Life Insurance Company. Adapted by permission.

Traditionally, charts that provide normal weight ranges for various heights and body frame sizes were the standard for determining normal weight and overweight. The charts, published by the Metropolitan Life Insurance Company, are based on statistics from the Society of Actuaries and thus reflect weight ranges with the lowest mortality. Table 15.1 shows both the 1959 and the 1983 charts, and a comparison shows that being overweight has been redefined in an upward direction.

Despite the convenience of weight charts, an accurate measure of percentage of body fat is a better index of obesity than total weight. Determining percentage and distribution of body fat is not as easy as consulting a chart, and several different methods exist to assess body fat. Many new technologies for imaging the body—computer

TABLE 15.2 *Body Mass Index Scores and Their Corresponding Heights and Weights*

	Body Mass Index, kg / m²							
	17.5*	21	23	25	27	30	35	40**
Height in Inches				**Weight in Pounds**				
60″	90	107	118	128	138	153	179	204
61	93	111	122	132	143	158	185	211
62	96	115	126	136	147	164	191	218
63	99	118	130	141	142	169	197	225
64	102	122	134	145	157	174	202	232
65	105	126	138	150	162	180	210	240
66	109	130	142	155	167	186	216	247
67	112	134	146	159	172	191	223	255
68	115	138	155	164	177	197	230	262
69	118	142	155	169	182	203	236	270
70	122	146	160	174	188	207	243	278
71	125	150	165	179	193	215	250	286
72	129	154	169	184	199	221	258	294
73	132	159	174	189	204	227	265	302
74	136	163	179	194	210	233	272	311
75	140	168	184	200	216	240	279	319
76	144	172	189	205	221	246	287	328

*BMI of 17.5 after intentional starvation meets one DSM-IV definition of anorexia nervosa.

**BMI of 40 is considered morbid obesity by Bender, Trautner, Spraul, & Berger, 1998.

tomography, ultrasound, and magnetic resonance imaging—can be applied to assessing fat content, but these methods have the drawbacks of being very expensive and relatively inaccessible. Simpler methods are less accurate but more accessible. The skinfold technique involves measuring the thickness of a pinch of skin. Although this method is relatively easy and inexpensive, it is not very accurate (Bray, 1992). The water immersion technique is awkward, requiring a person to be lowered into water to determine the amount of displacement.

Another method is the **body mass index (BMI),** defined as body weight in kilograms (kg) divided by height in meters squared (m^2), that is, BMI = kg / m^2. Although BMI does not consider a person's age, gender, or body build, this measurement began to gain popularity in the early 1990s (Bray, 1992). The National Task Force on the Prevention and Treatment of Obesity (2000) acknowledged that neither the weight charts nor BMI measures body fat but contended that this index can provide a standard for measuring overweight and obesity. This group defined overweight as a BMI of 25 through 29.9 and obesity as a BMI of 30 or more. (A 5′10″ man with a BMI of 30 would weigh 207 pounds, and a 5′4″ woman with a BMI of 30 would weigh 174.) These numbers are approximately 20% above the weights in the 1983 Metropolitan Life Insurance Company's height-weight charts for people with a medium frame. Table 15.2 shows a sample of BMI levels and their corresponding heights and weights.

Another measure that can be useful in assessing overweight is fat distribution, measured as the ratio of waist to hip size. People who have waists that approach the size of their hips tend to have fat distributed around their middles, whereas people who have large hips compared to their waists have lower hip-to-waist ratios.

Regardless of the definitions that researchers have used to study obesity, overweight is often defined in terms of social standards. These definitions usually have little to do with health and are subject to variations over culture and time. Examples are numerous during human history (Rozin, 1999). During times when food supply was uncertain (the most frequent situation throughout history), carrying some supply of fat on the body was a type of insurance and thus often considered attractive (Polivy & Herman, 2002). Fat could also be considered a mark of prosperity; fat advertised to the world that a person could afford an ample supply of food. Only in very recent history has this standard changed. Before 1920, thinness was considered unattractive, possibly due to the association between thinness and diseases or poverty.

Thinness is no longer considered unattractive. In fact, today it is as highly desirable as [illegible] accepted that even normal weight women [illegible] consider themselves too heavy. A national survey (Biener & Heaton, 1995) revealed that many women of normal weight were concerned that they weighed too much. Clearly, obesity, like beauty, is in the eye of the beholder, and the ideal body has become thinner over the past 50 years.

Despite the emphasis on thinness, obesity in the United States continues to grow. From the early 1980s to the late 1990s, adult obesity increased by 50% (Brown, 2001). Researchers have proposed several reasons for the steady increase in obesity over the past 2 decades, including an increase in fast-food consumption, growing portion sizes, and a decrease in physical activity. Robert Jeffery and Simone French (1998) cited evidence that Americans are eating more of their meals in fast-food restaurants and are viewing more television and videos. Both behaviors are related to a larger body mass index and to weight gain—at least in some people. Another factor that has contributed to increased weight is large portion size (Young & Nestle, 2002). Restaurant portion sizes grew, and people were supersized.

If obesity is defined as having a BMI of 30 or higher, then 25% of U.S. women and 20% of men are obese. An additional 25% of women and 39% of men in the United States are overweight, defined as a BMI of 25.0 to 29.9 (Wadden, Brownell, & Foster, 2002). Obese and overweight people are found in both genders, all ethnic groups, all geographic regions, and all educational levels (Mokdad et al., 1999). As. Figure 15.2 shows, however, the rates of obesity and overweight differ by gender and ethnic background. The United States is not alone; in many industrialized countries a majority of adults are overweight, including the United Kingdom, Russia, and Germany.

Why Are Some People Obese?

Many eating patterns may result in obesity, but binge eating is a definite risk. Binge eating consists of episodes of consuming large quantities of food coupled with a feeling of being out of control while doing so. Many people experience times when they eat too much, such as holidays, but binge eating that occurs on a weekly basis (or more frequently) poses problems. Binge eating combined with purging is a characteristic of bulimia nervosa (described in a later section), but binge eating without purging is not currently classified as a disorder (APA, 2000). However,

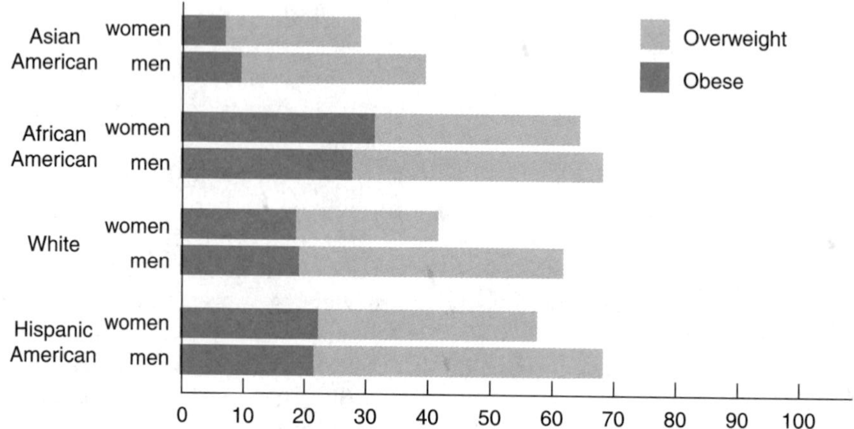

Figure 15.2 Percent of U.S. women and men who are overweight and obese, by ethnic group.

Source: Data based on Statistical Abstract of the United States, 2001 *by U.S. Bureau of the Census, 2001, Washington, DC: U.S. Government Printing Office, Table 197, p. 126.*

this pattern of eating is related to obesity (Stice, Presnell, & Spangler, 2002).

Although binge eating contributes to obesity, it is not an explanation for it; an explanation must include an underlying mechanism that specifies why people engage in this behavior. Several models attempt to explain why some people are obese and others maintain a normal weight. These models, which should be able to explain both the development and the maintenance of obesity, include the setpoint model and the positive incentive model.

The Setpoint Model The setpoint model holds that weight is regulated around a **setpoint,** a type of internal thermostat. When fat levels rise above or fall below a certain level, physiological and psychological mechanisms are activated that encourage a return to setpoint. The findings from the study on experimental starvation and the studies on experimental overeating are consistent with the concept of a setpoint, which predicts that deviations from normal weight in either direction are achieved only with difficulty. When fat levels fall below setpoint, the body takes action to preserve fat levels. Part of that action includes slowing the metabolic process to require fewer calories, thus making the body more conservative in its energy expenditures. People on diets have difficulty in continuing to lose weight because their bodies fight against depletion of fat stores. With conditions of prolonged and serious starvation, this slowed metabolism is expressed behaviorally as listlessness and apathy—both of which were exhibited by Keys's starving volunteers.

Increased hunger is the body's other corrective action when fat supplies fall below setpoint. Again, this mechanism seems to be consistent with the results of the Keys et al. study on starvation. The men who dieted to 75% of their normal body weight became miserable and hungry, and they stayed that way until they were back to their original weight. During the entire time they were below their normal weight (which would be below setpoint), they were obsessed with food. When they were allowed to eat, they preferred the high-calorie foods that tended to increase their fat stores most rapidly, a situation that is consistent with setpoint theory.

The experiment on overeating also fits with setpoint theory. The prisoners who tried to gain more than their normal weight were fighting their natural setpoint. According to the setpoint concept, the bodies of the overfed prisoners should have sent messages that they had enough fat stored already and did not need more. This message should have translated into something like "Stop eating," which seems to have happened because the prisoners found eating unpleasant.

The setpoint hypothesis is also consistent with a study of how people adjusted to weight loss and weight gain (Leibel, Rosenbaum, & Hirsch, 1995). This study involved underfeeding obese men and women until they lost 10% to 20% of their baseline body weight and overfeeding normal weight men and women until they gained 10% of their baseline body weight. Participants who lost weight also lost energy, expending 15% less than before they were underfed; participants who gained weight increased their total expenditure of energy. Like Keys's conscientious objectors, the people who lost weight became increasingly hungry, and this hunger along with decreased energy made it very difficult for them to maintain weight loss. On the other hand, the increased energy and decreased hunger of the overfed participants hampered their ability to maintain weight gain.

Questions remain concerning the usefulness of the setpoint model, including why setpoint should vary so much from person to person and why some people have a setpoint that is set at obese. One answer may be that the setpoint is at least partly established through a hereditary component. Evidence from studies of adopted children (Stunkard et al., 1986) and of identical twins reared together or apart (Stunkard, Harris, Pedersen, & McClean, 1990) have suggested a role for heredity in weight. Adopted children's weights were more similar to their biological parents than to their adoptive parents, and the weights of twins were highly correlated, even when the twins had not been raised together.

Concluding that weight has a genetic component is not the same as saying that weight is genetically determined; genes influence fat only indirectly through effects on eating and metabolism. For individuals with faulty genes for controlling leptin, obesity may be controlled in a simple way, but this situation applies to very few obese people. Researchers have come to realize that the genetics of obesity are very complex, controlled by 30 or more genes that influence hormones, neurotransmitters, and metabolism (Watanabe, 2002). In addition, genes have not changed over the past 25 years, yet the levels of obesity have.

Although the setpoint concept is consistent with many of the findings about weight maintenance, some pieces of information do not fit with this model (Pinel, Assanand, & Lehman, 2000). Why would the setpoint be set at the level of obesity for some people but not others? A setpoint that dictates obesity for some and thinness for others makes very little sense. For example, variations in setpoint should not occur disproportionately in the United States. That is, setpoints should not differ from decade to decade or country to country, but obesity has grown in industrialized (and even some developing) countries. Indeed, when animals have a plentiful food supply, they tend to overeat (Pinel et al., 2000). This situation is not consistent with the setpoint model but instead supports an alternative: the positive incentive model.

The Positive Incentive Model The failure of setpoint theory to explain some factors related to eating and weight maintenance has led to the formulation of the positive incentive model. This model holds that the positive reinforcers of eating have important consequences for weight maintenance. This view suggests that people have several types of motivation to eat, including personal pleasure, social context, and biological factors (Hetherington & Rolls, 1996; Pinel et al., 2000). The personal pleasure factors concentrate on the pleasures of eating, including the taste of food and how pleasurable eating will be at any given time. The social context of eating includes cultural background of the person eating as well as the people present and whether or not they are eating. Biological factors involved in eating include such factors as the length of time since eating and blood glucose levels. In addition, some proponents of the positive incentive theory (Pinel et al., 2000) take an evolutionary view, contending that humans have an evolved tendency to eat in the presence of food. Food scarcity has built animals that survived when they laid on fat, making eating and the selection of food an important evolved ability. Therefore, this model includes biological factors in eating but holds that people learn to regulate their eating rather than having a setpoint that controls food intake (Ramsay, Seeley, Bolles, & Woods, 1996).

The setpoint model ignores the factors of taste, learning, and social context in eating, and these factors are unquestionably important (Rozin, 1996, 1999). For each person in each instance, the act of choosing something to eat has a long history of personal experience and cultural learning. A preferred food will not be equally appealing under all circumstances. For example, some foods do not seem to go together, even if each food is individually tasty. Various cultures have restrictions (and requirements) on what to eat and when. People tend to get hungry on a schedule that corresponds to mealtimes, but people in the United States are much more likely to eat cereal for breakfast than for dinner. In contrast, people in Spain do not eat cold cereal, and the lack of cultural tradition for this type of food made marketing it difficult in that country (Visser, 1999). These cultural and learned factors also affect the caloric value of chosen foods and how much a person eats; these choices influence body weight. For example, a woman who is dieting might desire a brownie but choose a diet soda instead.

The positive incentive view predicts a variety of body weights, depending on food availability, individual experience with food, cultural encouragement to eat various foods, and the cultural ideal for body weight. The availability of an abundant food supply is necessary but not sufficient to produce obesity. People must overeat to become obese, and the quantity of food a person eats is related to how palatable the food is. Some tastes, such as sweet, are innately determined through the action of taste buds, but preference for flavor combinations seems to be the result of learning (Capaldi, 1996). In industrialized countries, a huge food industry promotes food products as desirable through massive advertising campaigns, and many of these foods are high in fat and sugar. This situation influences individual food choices that promote population-wide obesity.

Another factor that promotes overeating in industrialized countries is the availability of a variety of foods. Eating a very desirable food leads to a decreased evaluation of how pleasant that food is (Hetherington & Rolls, 1996). That is, people become satiated for any particular food. When food supplies are limited in variety (but not in quantity), this factor can lead to lower levels of food consumption, but a new taste can tempt someone who is full to eat more. Indeed, if eating a sufficient amount terminated a meal, dessert would not be so popular (Pinel, 2003).

Variety is important in boosting eating, even in rats. A large body of research (Raynor & Epstein, 2001) indicates that variety is important in the amount eaten. With a variety of foods available, humans (and other animals) eat more. An early study (Sclafani & Springer, 1976) showed that a "supermarket" diet produced weight gains of 269% in laboratory rats. The diet consisted of a changing variety of foods chosen from the supermarket, including chocolate chip cookies, salami, cheese, bananas, marshmallows, chocolate, peanut butter, and sweetened condensed milk. The combination of high fat and high sugar plus the changing variety led to enormous weight gain. Are humans very different? The availability of a wide variety of tasty food should produce widespread obesity, which is exactly the situation that exists in the United States and other industrialized countries today. This wide variety of foods allows people to always have some foods that furnish a new taste, and people in such situations never become satiated for all available foods.

Some evidence not consistent with the setpoint model fits better with the positive incentive theory of eating and weight maintenance, including individual food preferences, cultural influences in eating, cultural influences on body composition, and the relationship between food availability and obesity. Both the setpoint and

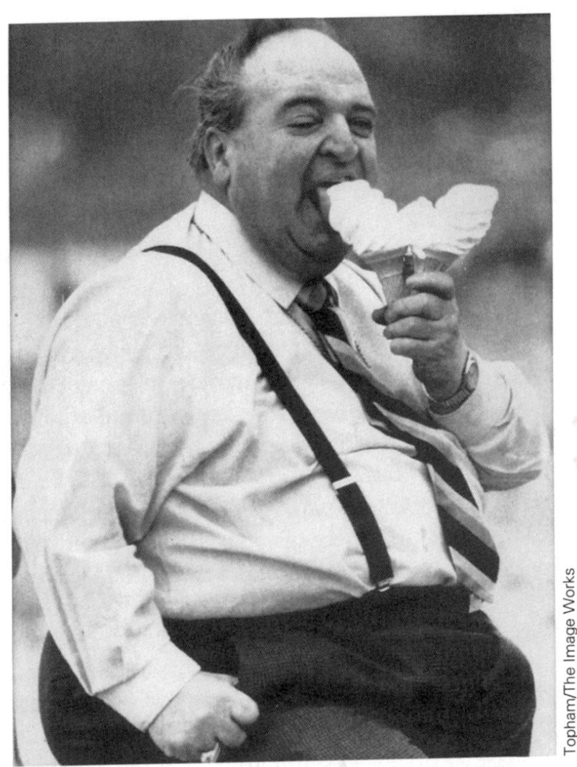
Topham/The Image Works

The weight maintenance equation is complex, but overeating is a cause of obesity.

positive incentive models suggest that some people will be obese, and this situation is disturbing to those who want to adhere to fashion and those who believe that obesity constitutes a serious health problem.

Is Obesity Unhealthy?

Obesity is undesirable from a social point of view, but the question of its effect on health is less clear. The answer depends partly on one's degree of obesity and distribution of fat. Some early research indicated that cycles of weight loss and gain presented risks for blood pressure and cardiovascular disease (Brownell & Rodin, 1994), but later research (Field et al., 1999) led to the conclusion that weight cycling is not an independent risk factor for hypertension or cardiovascular disease. Weight gain, however, was strongly related to the risk of developing hypertension. Therefore, gaining weight is a risk, but how much weight must one gain to be at increased risk for disease and death? Research is not clear in its implication of being slightly overweight as a health risk. However, being severely obese places a person at an elevated risk for several types of health problems and premature death.

A U-shaped relationship has appeared between weight and poor health; that is, the very thinnest and the very heaviest people seem to be at greatest risk for all-cause mortality. However, many studies have failed to control for smoking and preexisting disease conditions, which are related to low body weight and to high mortality (Visscher et al., 2000). Thus, low body weight may not be a risk. Indeed, some researchers (Pinel et al., 2000) have argued that low body weight can be healthier than normal weight. However, overweight is a health risk.

The degree of overweight that is necessary to raise risks is not entirely clear. Without any question, extreme obesity is a risk, but those who are overweight yet not obese may not experience much more risk than those in the normal weight range. For example, a large-scale study from Germany (Bender, Trautner, Spraul, & Berger, 1998) showed no relationship between obesity and all-cause mortality for men with BMI scores up to 32 and only a very weak relationship for women in this range (see Table 15.2 for weights and BMIs). When BMI scores rose above 40, both men and women more than doubled their risk for all-cause mortality. A summary of these levels of risk appears in Table 15.3. Other studies show similar results: obesity is associated with increased mortality (Allison, Fontaine, Manson, Stevens, & Van-Itallie, 1999) and increased morbidity, especially the development of Type 2 diabetes, gallbladder disease, and high blood pressure (Must et al., 1999), but also sleep apnea, respiratory problems, liver disease, osteoarthritis, reproductive problems in women, and colon cancer (National Task Force on the Prevention and Treatment of Obesity, 2000). Mortality risk is lowest for women with BMIs between 22 and 23.4 and for men with BMIs

TABLE 15.3 *Categories of Obesity and Risks for All-Cause Mortality Based on Body Mass Index (BMI)*

Degree of Obesity	BMI Range	Risk for Men	RR	Risk for Women	RR
Moderate	25 to 32	None	1.0	Very low	1.1
Obese	32 to 36	Low	1.3	Low	1.2
Gross	36 to 40	High	1.9	Low	1.3
Morbid	40+	Very high	3.1	Very high	2.3

Information based on Bender et al. (1998).

between 23.5 and 24.9 (Calle, Thun, Petrelli, Rodriguez, & Heath, 1999).

Both age and ethnicity complicate the interpretation of risk from obesity. For young and middle-aged adults, being overweight is a risk for all-cause mortality and especially for death due to cardiovascular disease (Stevens et al., 1998). After age 65, the relationship no longer exists (Baik et al., 2000), and losing weight after age 50 increases risk (Diehr et al., 1998). For African American men and women, the healthiest BMI levels were around 27, which is in the range considered overweight.

Another weight-related factor associated to morbidity and mortality is a person's distribution of weight. During the past 20 years, evidence has suggested that people who accumulate excess weight around their abdomen are at greater risk than people who carry their excess weight on their hips and thighs. Recent research (Price, Li, & Kilker, 2002) has suggested that the pattern of carrying fat around the midsection may have a genetic component. A variety of studies have shown that patterns of body weight and the waist-to-hip ratio are good predictors of a variety of health problems (see the "Would You Believe . . . ?" box).

In conclusion, obese people have heightened risks of developing certain health problems, especially diabetes, gallstones, and cardiovascular disease. Table 15.4 summarizes studies showing

TABLE 15.4 *The Relationship between Weight and Disease or Death*

Study	Sample	Results
		Effects of Obesity
Field et al., 1999	female nurses	Weight gain is a risk for developing hypertension.
Visscher et al., 2000	middle-aged and older men	BMI of 25–30 not related to increased mortality; >30 is.
Allison et al., 1999	overweight and obese adults	BMI of >30 accounts for over 80% of obesity-related deaths.
Must et al., 1999	overweight and obese adults	Obesity is related to diabetes, gallbladder disease, and hypertension.
Bender et al., 1998	obese men	No increase in all-cause mortality up to BMI of 32. Morbid obesity carries a threefold risk for men and more than a double risk for women.
		Effects of Abdominal Fat
Hartz et al., 1984	middle-aged and older men	Large waist is a risk for diabetes, hypertension, and gallbladder disease.
Sjöström, 1992	men and women	High waist/hip ratio increases the risk for heart disease.
Folsom et al., 2000	middle-aged and older women	Waist/hip ratio is a better predictor than BMI of all-cause mortality.
Rexrode et al., 1998	female nurses	High waist/hip ratio increases risk for coronary heart disease threefold.
Freedman et al., 1995	African American women	Central fat does not predict heart disease.
Freedman et al., 1995	All other groups	Central fat predicts heart disease.

WOULD YOU BELIEVE

A Big Butt Is Healthier Than a Fat Gut

Would you believe that a big butt is better than a fat gut, at least in terms of health risks? All fat is not equal: abdominal fat creates more of a health risk than fat in the thighs and hips. Women generally have lower waist-to-hip ratios than men, and they also have lower rates of heart disease. A woman with a waist of 28 inches and a hip measurement of 36 would have a ratio of 0.78, whereas a man with 36-inch waist and a 41-inch hip measurement would have a ratio of 0.88. Each of these ratios is considered to be in the healthy range for women and men respectively. However, a ratio of 1.0 or higher, indicating a waistline larger than the hip measurement, could be dangerous, especially for women.

Early studies showed that both women (Hartz, Rupley, & Rimm, 1984) and men (Sjöström, 1992a; 1992b) were at elevated risk of diabetes, hypertension, and gallbladder disease when their waist-to-hip ratio was large. The amount of fat was not as important as its distribution. Although "beer bellies" are associated with middle age, the accumulation of fat around the middle is related to risk factors for heart disease, even during adolescence and early adulthood (van Lenthe, van Mechelen, Kemper, & Twisk, 1998).

Weight around one's middle may be a better predictor of all-cause mortality than body mass index. A study on women's risk of cardiovascular disease (Noble, 2001) showed that waist-to-hip ratio was much more strongly related to CVD than BMI was. Similarly, the Nurses' Health Study (Rexrode et al., 1998), after adjusting for body mass index, found that women with a waist-to-hip ratio of 0.88 or higher had more than a threefold risk for coronary heart disease compared with women with a ratio less than 0.72. Fat around the midsection is also related to all-cause mortality; that is, people with this pattern of fat distribution are more likely to die than people with other body types (Folsom et al., 2000). Therefore, waist-to-hip ratio is an independent risk factor for mortality, with an especially strong relationship to cardiovascular disease.

However, the health risk of a big gut may not be equal for all people. Examining the distribution of body fat and its relation to heart disease in African American and European American men and women revealed differences (Freedman, Williamson, Croft, Ballew, and Byers, 1995). The relationship between fat around one's middle and ischemic heart disease appeared, but this risk did not extend to African American women. The relative risk for African American men and European American men was essentially identical, and the risk for European American women was highest of all. However, African American women with weight distributed around the middle had no extra risk of heart disease. Some evidence (Biener & Heaton, 1995) indicates that African American women are less concerned about losing weight than European American women, and this reduced concern may be justified. For other subgroups, however, a fat gut is more dangerous to health than a big butt.

that gross obesity and fat distributed around the waist all relate to increased mortality rates, especially from heart disease.

In Summary

Obesity can be defined in terms of health or social standards, and the two are not always the same. The ideal weight for health can be seen in the Metropolitan Insurance Company weight charts or reflected in the body mass index (BMI). Social standards, however, have dictated a standard of thinness with a lower body weight than is ideal for health.

Obesity has been explained by the setpoint model and by the positive incentive model. Setpoint theory explains obesity in terms of a high setpoint for body weight, whereas positive incentive theory holds that people gain weight when they have an abundant supply of tasty food.

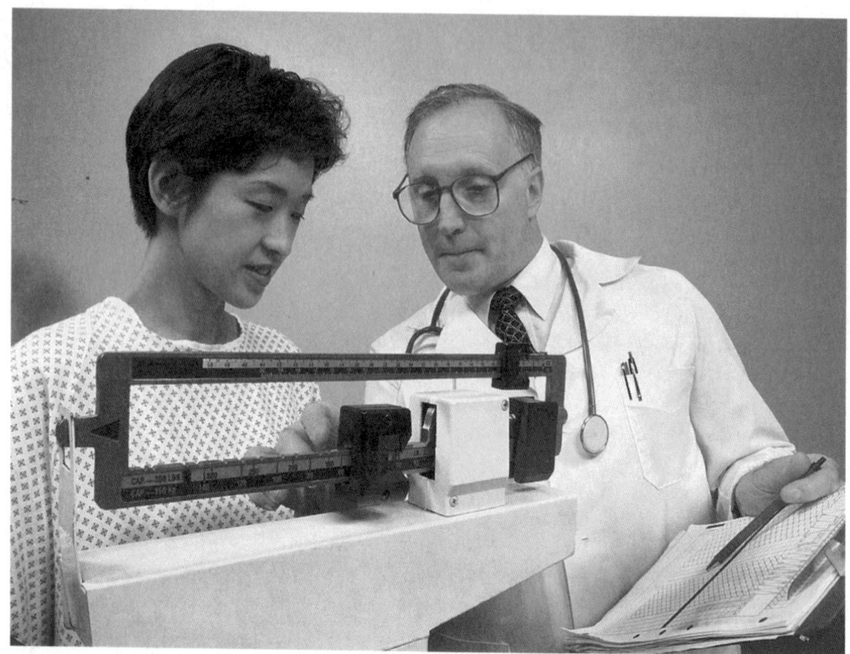

Dieting is increasingly common among those who do not need to lose weight for health reasons.

Obesity is associated with increased mortality, heart disease, Type 2 diabetes, and gallstones. Although very thin people are also at increased risk for disease, they are often ill or smokers and thus not healthy. Most people who are moderately overweight and who have no coronary risk factors are not at an increased risk for heart disease or all-cause mortality. Nevertheless, severe obesity is a risk for morbidity and mortality. In addition, the pattern of fat distribution is an important factor in the risk, with those carrying excess weight around the waist rather than hips at increased risk.

Dieting

Many people in the United States have some knowledge of the risks of obesity and an unfavorable waist-to-hip ratio, but even more are influenced by the media portrayals of idealized thin bodies (King, Touyz, & Charles, 2000). Nevertheless, obesity in the United States has risen sharply during the past 10 years (Mokdad et al., 1999). Accepting the ideal body as thin, combined with the growing prevalence of overweight, produces a situation in which dieting and weight loss are the subject of a great many people's concern. What are people doing to try to lose weight and how well do these strategies work?

Many people have concentrated on cutting the amount of fat in their diet, but they have failed to attend to their sugar consumption. People in the United States have reduced dietary fat from about 40% of energy intake to 33%, but they have increased their intake of sugar from 120 pounds per person to about 150 pounds (Connor & Connor, 1997). The exchange of fat for sugar is not a good dieting choice. A low-fat, high-carbohydrate diet may contribute to reduced total cholesterol, but it tends to do so largely by lowering HDL cholesterol (Katan,

Grundy, & Willett, 1997), and the calories may be equivalent or higher. Many people believe that they are making a healthy choice by reducing fat, but they are mistaken. Thus, people may not have the necessary information to make wise choices in their dieting.

Unwise decisions abound in dieting, both in terms of the number of people dieting and the methods they use. The trend toward dieting has become more severe in the past few decades. During the mid-1960s, only 10% of the overweight adults were dieting (Wyden, 1965), but during subsequent years those percentages steadily increased; in 2001, 70% of high school girls and more than 30% of high school boys were trying to lose weight (Grunbaum et al., 2002). Adults too are increasingly likely to diet. A survey of adolescents and adults (Serdula et al., 1999) showed that almost 80% of the women and almost two thirds of the men were trying either to lose or not gain weight, making weight concerns a common experience to a majority of people in the United States. However, many of these dieters do not have sufficient excess weight to put them at risk for disease or death, and most failed to follow the best approaches to losing weight (Serdula et al., 1999).

Approaches to Losing Weight

To lose weight or keep from gaining weight, people have several choices. They can (1) reduce portion size, (2) restrict the types of food they eat, (3) increase their level of exercise, (4) rely on drastic medical procedures, or (5) use a combination of these approaches. Regardless of the approach, keep in mind that *all diets that prompt weight loss do so through restriction of calories.*

Restricting Types of Food Maintaining a diet consisting of a variety of foods with smaller portions is a reasonable and healthy strategy, but many people find it difficult simply to eat less. A variety of foods is necessary for adequate nutrition, but the approach of restricting types of foods has been a popular dieting strategy. Although severely restricting or eliminating a food category may be nutritionally unwise, this approach is the basis of several prominent diets.

Restricting carbohydrates has been a popular approach, mostly because low-carbohydrate diets usually allow dieters to eat high-fat foods, which most people find tasty. Examples of this diet come from Dr. Atkins and Sugarbusters. Low-carbohydrate diets are open to severe criticism for being both ineffective and potentially dangerous. Such diets tend to produce fatigue and depression as frequent side effects, which some people develop after a few days on such diets (Schenker, 2001). The primary danger of a high-fat diet is the increases in serum cholesterol. People who lose weight on such diets do so for the same reason that people on any diet lose weight: they consume fewer calories.

High-carbohydrate, low-fat diets have also had their advocates (Ornish, 1993). These diets strive to increase the amount of foods with "complex" carbohydrates while lowering fat intake. Fruits, vegetables, and whole-grain cereals contain complex carbohydrates, but sugar does not. Fats come from animal and vegetable fats such as oils and butter, but many types of meat contain a high proportion of fats. Therefore, low-fat, high-carbohydrate diets are often vegetarian or modified vegetarian diets. Some dieters find these programs easy to follow, because they allow a greater volume of food (carbohydrates are lower in calories per volume, so a person can eat more and still consume fewer calories). However, for some dieters, the food choices are not their favorites, and the feeling of constantly being deprived of preferred foods often leads to "cheating" and failure. Nutritionally, high-carbohydrate diets are safe and can be effective programs for controlling weight, especially if the carbohydrates are consumed in the form of complex carbohydrates such as fruits and vegetables rather than simple carbohydrates such as refined flour and sugar.

Some diets are more extreme, restricting the dieter to a limited group of foods or even a single food. All-fruit diets, egg diets, cabbage soup diet, and even the ice cream diet fall into this category. Of course, such diets are nutritional disasters. They produce weight loss by restricting calories; dieters get tired of the monotony of one food and eat less than they would if they were eating a variety. "All the hard-boiled eggs you want" turns out to be not many!

Taking monotony a step further are the liquid diets, which exist in a variety of forms and under various brand names. Liquid diets have the advantage of being nutritionally more balanced than most restricted food diets. Still, liquid diets and their equivalent meals in the form of puddings or bars have the disadvantage of being monotonous and repetitive, and they tend to be low in fiber. Like all other diets, these work by restricting calorie intake. Although current researchers may disagree on the advantages of low-fat or low-carbohydrate diets, they are likely to agree that diets high in fiber from fruits and vegetables are good choices (Schenker, 2001).

In conclusion, all food restriction strategies can be successful in producing weight loss, but most are a bad approach to weight loss. None of these diets teach new eating habits that people can maintain over the long term. Thus, people who lose weight on one of these diets will be likely to regain that weight, and they will have the experience of a period of unhealthy eating, which may have health consequences.

Behavior Modification Programs Although dieting should be seen as a permanent modification in one's eating habits, such a change is a difficult task. The behavior modification approach toward treating obesity was originated by Richard Stuart (1967), who reported a much higher success rate than with previous approaches. Most behavior modification programs focus on eating and exercise goals, helping overweight people to monitor and change their behavior. Clients in these programs often keep eating diaries to focus their awareness on the types of foods they eat and under what circumstances as well as to provide data the therapist can use to devise a personal plan for changing unhealthy eating habits that often include calorie and fat consumption goals. In addition, exercise goals are a typical component of a behavior modification program. The most common format for these programs is a group setting with weekly meetings that include instruction in nutrition and in self-monitoring to attain the individual goals (Wing & Polley, 2001).

Because weight loss is not a behavior, these programs tend to reinforce good eating habits rather than the numbers of pounds lost. In other words, the behaviors, not the consequences, are rewarded. People who are overweight to moderately obese may be fairly successful in these types of programs. The goal is typically gradual weight loss and maintenance of that loss. The average amount of weight lost is about 20 pounds over 6 months, but dieters maintain only about 60% of that loss over a year (Wing & Polley, 2001). Therefore, even moderate, gradual weight loss may be difficult to maintain.

Exercise The importance of exercise in weight loss has become increasingly apparent. Because metabolic rate slows down when food intake decreases, some form of physical activity is necessary to speed up metabolism. Exercise is known to counteract metabolic slowdown and thus may be an indispensable part of weight reduction programs. In a large-scale survey of dieters (*Consumer Reports,* 2002), exercising at least three times a week was a strategy shared by 73% of successful dieters. Exercise can also decrease body mass index (Kahn et al., 1997), making it a valuable contribution to weight control programs. (The role of exercise is more fully discussed in Chapter 16.)

Drastic Methods of Losing Weight People sometimes take drastic measures to lose weight, and physicians sometimes recommend drastic measures for severely obese patients. Even with medical supervision, some weight reduction programs present risks, sometimes to the point of being life threatening.

One approach that turned out to be more dangerous than initially believed was taking drugs to reduce appetite. In the 1950s and 1960s, diet pills were widely prescribed. These drugs were amphetamines, stimulant drugs that increase the activity of the nervous system, speed up metabolism, and suppress appetite. Unfortunately, these drugs lose their appetite-suppressing effect within a few weeks, so the dosage must be increased to maintain the desired effect. These drugs can be effective for a short time, but for people who need to lose a considerable amount of weight and who therefore must continue taking amphetamines, dependence may become a more serious problem than obesity.

Increasing evidence of the dangers of amphetamines led to the development of other diet drugs. Most were chemically similar to amphetamines and shared their disadvantages, including the possibility of abuse. Two of these alternatives, fenfluramine and phenylpropylalamine were once believed to be safe and effective. However, in the fall of 1997, the Food and Drug Administration warned people to stop taking these two drugs—known collectively as fen-phen—because their combination may contribute to damaging heart valves. A variety of over-the-counter and herbal preparations are available, but the evidence of their effectiveness is limited (Egger, Cameron-Smith, & Stanton, 1999). Other diet pills continue to be developed and will be available as long as people desire an easy solution to weight loss.

Fasting is another weight loss measure that can be dangerous. Under conditions of severe food deprivation, people tend to lose stores of carbohydrate stored as glycogen, along with the water stored with it; after this weight loss (which seems easy), people begin to metabolize stored fat and muscle tissue about equally. If people continue to cut food intake drastically or to fast, the muscle tissue loss may present a health threat to internal organs. However, the *protein-sparing modified fast* averts this problem. In this type of program, patients eat high-protein food in very limited amounts. Under careful supervision, this program may be a successful approach for very obese individuals. For others, this strategy is a dangerous choice.

Other drastic measures to control obesity include several types of surgery. One procedure consists of wiring the jaws so that the person is unable to chew. Caloric intake can thus be severely restricted, but such body functions as coughing can be very painful, and vomiting could be deadly. For good reason, this approach is rare.

Surgery has also been a strategy to deal with extreme obesity. One type of surgery removes part of the intestines, preventing food from being absorbed and cutting down on the calories metabolized, but surgical techniques that reduce the size of the stomach are a more common approach (Dixon, Dixon, & O'Brien, 2001). People are candidates for this surgery only if their BMI is 35 or higher and they have health problems that make weight loss imperative. This surgery may implant a mesh cover or band that wraps around the stomach, or the surgery may involve stapling part of the stomach to restrict the amount the stomach can hold. These procedures may be successful in promoting weight loss and in improving quality of life for people who were extremely obese (Dixon et al., 2001).

Another surgical approach to weight loss is to remove adipose tissue through a fat-suctioning technique called liposuction. The technique allows for a recontouring of the body rather than an overall weight loss. This procedure is not useful in controlling obesity; rather, it is a cosmetic procedure to change body shape. Despite the discomfort and expense of the surgery, liposuction has become a very common type of plastic surgery. However, it presents risks; the mortality risk for liposuction is higher than for motor vehicle accidents (*Medical Update,* 2000).

Therefore, drastic means of losing weight are poor solutions to obesity but are not uncommon. High school and college women reported using drastic strategies for weight loss, such as fasting (39.4%) and appetite suppressant drugs (8.1%), and a majority (60%) admitted chronic dieting or purging (Tylka & Subich, 2002). Severe food restriction presents nutritional problems. All these drastic means of losing weight can be dangerous. In addition, all are difficult to maintain long enough to produce significant weight loss. Even when dieters succeed with these strategies, they usually regain the weight they have lost because these approaches do not allow dieters to learn how to make good diet choices for permanent weight loss. Indeed, keeping weight off is a major problem. Regardless of weight loss method, maintaining weight loss is a challenge.

Maintaining Weight Loss In Chapters 13 and 14, we saw that about two thirds of the people who initially quit smoking or stop drinking will eventually relapse. For people who successfully lose weight, maintaining that loss is equally difficult. A large number of studies have confirmed the difficulty of maintaining weight loss (National Heart, Lung, and Blood Institute, 1998). However, most of these studies looked at highly selected dieters, including those who were extremely obese and those who sought professional help in losing weight. For those people, weight control should probably be treated as a chronic illness, with continued professional assistance in maintaining weight loss (Kubetin, 2001).

Effective formal weight reduction interventions typically include posttreatment programs to help dieters maintain lost weight. These programs are usually more successful than those that lack a posttreatment phase. For example, after completing a behavioral program of weight loss, the women who also completed a follow-up program of problem-solving therapy were more successful in maintaining their weight loss than those who received no additional treatment (Perri et al., 2001). A novel approach to providing follow-up care involves the Internet (Harvey-Berino, Pintauro, & Gold, 2002); dieters who used an Internet support group after weight loss made as many contacts with group members and maintained their weight loss as well as dieters who met in a group in person.

A survey by *Consumer Reports* (2002) supplied information about a wide selection of dieters, both successful and unsuccessful. This survey included over 32,000 dieters, 25% of whom had lost at least 10% of their starting weight and kept it off for at least a year. This number confirmed that people have problems both with losing and with maintaining weight loss, but it also showed that some people are successful.

Most of the dieters in the *Consumer Report* survey lost weight on their own rather than through a formal weight loss program. Indeed, more of the unsuccessful dieters (26%) tried a program such as Weight Watchers or Jenny Craig than those who were successful (14%). About 10% of the successful dieters sought advice from a psychologist or nutritionist, and those who did rated this advice as very effective. Those who were successful tended to use a variety of approaches, including exercise and increased physical activity, eating fewer fatty and sweet foods, increasing consumption of fruits and vegetables, and cutting down on portion size. Not surprisingly, those dieters who were successful in maintaining their weight loss rarely used any of the drastic means of losing weight reviewed in the prior section. That is, people who lose weight and keep it off tend to alter their eating and physical activity, forming new habits that they are able to maintain.

In contrast to the difficulty that adults have in keeping off lost weight, obese children who lose weight are more likely to maintain that loss. A program of family-based behavioral treatment resulted in good weight loss and maintenance (Epstein, 1996). For example, a 10-year follow-up of formerly obese children who had participated in such a program (Epstein, Valoski, Wing, & McCurley, 1994) demonstrated that more than one third of the children decreased the degree of obesity, and another 30% were no longer obese at the follow-up. Children who adopted a more active lifestyle were the most successful in maintaining weight loss.

Is Dieting a Good Choice?

Although dieting can produce weight loss, it may not be a good choice for all dieters. Dieting has psychological costs, may not be effective in improving health, and may be a signal of body dissatisfaction that is a risk for eating disorders.

Dieters often behave like starving people: they are irritable, obsessed with food, finicky about taste, easily distractible, and hungry. These behavioral abnormalities make dieting foolish for those who are close to the best weight for their health (Polivy & Herman, 1995). Dieting may be a good choice for those who are sufficiently overweight to endanger their health, but most dieters are not. Developing reasonable and healthy eating patterns is a far better choice for those who are not obese.

Ironically, weight loss may be a health risk for some people. Several studies (Dyer, Stamler, & Greenland, 2000; Williamson & Pamuk, 1993) have explored the mortality risks of weight loss and found an increased risk for those who lost weight. For thin women who lost weight, risk for cardiovascular disease increased (Harris, Ballard-Barbasch, Madans, Makuc, & Feldman, 1993). Involuntary weight loss is often associated with disease, so the association between unintentional weight loss and mortality is no surprise. However, even voluntary weight loss was associated with increased mortality in a group of older men (Wannamethee, Shaper, Whincup, & Walker, 2000). For middle-aged and elderly men who lose weight, mortality risk increased slightly (Yaari & Goldbourt, 1998). Indeed, Reubin Andres (1995) criticized all weight charts that do not consider age as a factor. Acknowledging the existence of a U-shaped relationship between weight and mortality, he insists that the nadir of the U-shaped curve increases with age. After looking at the research, he stated that many people would be healthier if they gained some weight as they age—up to seven pounds a decade.

Of course, some people who lose weight voluntarily benefit from their weight loss. Research on obese people who lost weight (Oster, Thompson, Edelsberg, Bird, & Colditz, 1999) indicates that a 10% loss is sufficient to produce significant decreases in lifetime health risks and personal health-related expenditures. Therefore, even modest weight loss can be important for those who are obese.

In Summary

The near obsession with thinness in our culture has led to a plethora of diets, many of which are neither safe nor permanently effective. Most diets will produce some initial weight loss in response to the restriction of caloric intake, but maintaining the reduced weight levels is a matter of permanent changes in basic eating habits and activity levels. Despite a recent decline in fat consumption, people in the United States are now heavier than ever because they have increased the number of calories consumed.

Losing weight is easier than maintaining weight loss, but programs that include posttreatment and frequent follow-up can be successful in helping people maintain a healthy weight. Whether part of a formal program or a personal attempt, diets that include a variety of healthy foods and increases in physical activity are more likely to result in long-term weight loss than more drastic programs. In addition, behavior modification programs with obese children have greater success in promoting permanent weight loss than similar programs with adults.

Dieting is a good choice for some people but not for others. Morbidly obese people and those with a high waist to hip ratio should try to lose weight and keep it off. However, most people who diet for cosmetic reasons would be healthier if they did not lose weight.

Eating Disorders

The eating disorders that have received the most attention, both in the popular media and in the scientific literature, are anorexia nervosa and bulimia. The term *anorexia nervosa* literally means lack of appetite due to a nervous or physiological condition; *bulimia* means continuous, morbid hunger. Neither meaning, however, is quite accurate. People with anorexia nervosa have not lost their appetite. Ordinarily, they are perpetually hungry, but they insist that they do not wish to eat. Like Jessica, our first case study, these people become preoccupied with losing weight, and their self-induced starvation may result in a life-threatening condition. Similarly, bulimia has come to mean more than continuous morbid hunger. The chief identifying mark of this eating disorder is repeated bingeing and purging, the purge usually coming after eating huge quantities of food, typically high in calories and loaded with carbohydrates, fat, or both. Like Elise, our second case study, people with bulimia ordinarily purge by vomiting, but fasting and using laxatives and diuretics are also purging methods.

These two eating disorders obviously have much in common. Indeed, some authorities regard them as two dimensions of the same illness. Others see them as two separate but related illnesses (Polivy & Herman, 2002). The core components of these two disorders are the same: body dissatisfaction combined with preoccupation with food, weight, and body shape. The basis for body dissatisfaction is easy to understand: overweight and obesity have become more common, yet the ideal body is thin. This combination has created a discontent that touches everyone in the culture. Children as young as 7 years old express body dissatisfaction (Kostanski & Gullone, 1999; McCabe & Ricciadelli, 2003), and discontent with body shape is so common among women that it is the norm (Rodin, Silberstein, & Striegel-Moore, 1985). However, only a small percentage of people with body dissatisfaction develop eating disorders, indicating that other factors operate to produce anorexia and bulimia.

Janet Polivy and Peter Herman (2002) suggested that body dissatisfaction constitutes an essential precursor to the development of eating disorders, but those who develop eating problems must also come to see being thin as a solution to other problems in their lives. People who channel their distress into body concerns and focus on their bodies as a way to change their dissatisfaction have the cognitions that lead to eating disorders. Other risks for eating disorders include family and personality correlates such as a great deal of negative family interaction, a history of sexual abuse during childhood, low self-esteem, and high levels of negative mood. In addition, some genetic or neuroendocrine predisposition may contribute to the development of eating disorders. A test of factors related to unhealthy weight control strategies (Neumark-Sztainer, Wall, Story, & Perry, 2003) revealed that concern about body weight was the most important factor in this risky behavior.

Anorexia Nervosa

This chapter opened with a description of Jessica, a college junior who showed classic symptoms of anorexia. When first interviewed, her weight had dropped from 130 to 81 pounds, but Jessica's story was far from over. In this section, we continue with the case of Jessica, pointing out how it matches or deviates from a composite model of hundreds of cases of anorexia nervosa.

Despite recent publicity on anorexia, neither the disorder nor the term is new. The first two documented cases of intentional self-starvation were reported by Richard Morton in 1689 (Sours, 1980). Morton wrote about an 18-year-old English girl who had died of the effects of anorexia some 25 years earlier and about an 18-year-old boy who had survived. Both had shown a remarkable indifference to starvation, and both had been described as sad and anxious. Over the next 2 centuries, several other cases were reported, but often these were not clearly distinguished from tuberculosis or consumption.

In London, Sir William Gull (1874) studied several cases of intentional self-starvation during the 1860s. He regarded the condition as a psychological disorder and coined the term *anorexia nervosa* to indicate loss of appetite due to "nervous" causes—that is, psychological factors. From that time until about 1910, Gull's psychopathological conception pervaded the psychological and psychiatric literature. From about 1910 until the late 1930s, some medical authorities tried to link anorexia nervosa with atrophy of the anterior lobe of the pituitary gland, but this medical view soon lost favor.

During the 1940s and 1950s, speculation proliferated concerning the causes and cures of anorexia nervosa. Some psychiatrists hypothesized that the ailment was a denial of femininity and a fear of motherhood. Other theorists suggested that it represented an attempt on the part of the young woman to reestablish unity with her mother. Unfortunately, none of these hypotheses proved fruitful in expanding the scientific understanding of anorexia nervosa. The last 3 decades have seen a shift away from this sort of speculation and a turn toward the view that anorexia is a complex of sociocultural, family, and biological factors (Polivy & Herman, 2002). Recent emphasis has been on describing the disorder in terms of the behaviors and physiological effects, the demographic correlates, and the effective treatment procedures.

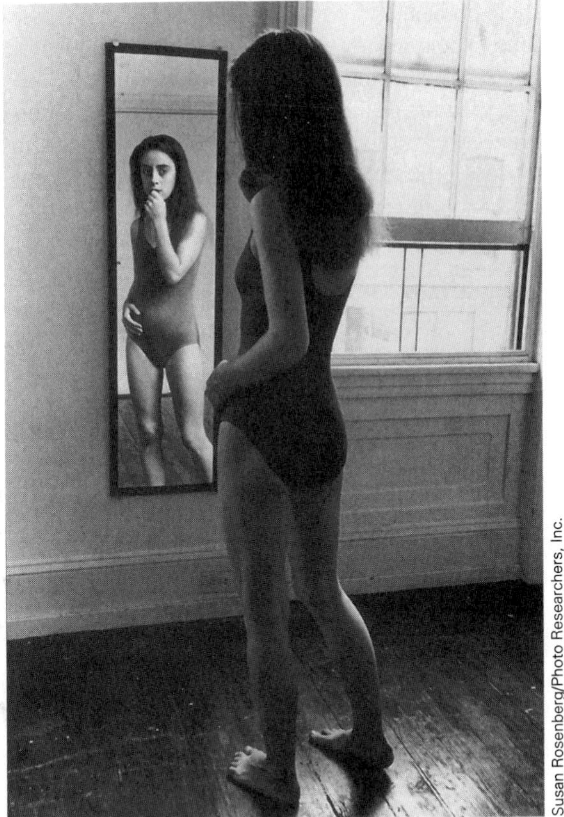

Susan Rosenberg/Photo Researchers, Inc.

No matter how thin they get, anorexics continue to see themselves as too fat.

What Is Anorexia? Anorexia nervosa is an eating disorder characterized by intentional self-starvation or semistarvation, sometimes to the point of death. People with anorexia are extremely afraid of gaining weight and have a distorted body image, seeing themselves as being too heavy even though they are exceedingly thin. The *Diagnostic and Statistical Manual of Mental Disorders* (4th edition, text revision [DSM-IV-TR]) of the American Psychiatric Association (APA, 2000) defined anorexia nervosa as intentional weight loss to a point that a person weighs less than 85% of weight considered normal by the Metropolitan Life Insurance tables or has a body mass index of 17.5 or less, a fear of being fat, a distorted body image, and for women, the cessation of menstrual periods for at least three cycles.

Two subtypes of anorexia exist: the restricting type and the binge-eating/purging type (APA, 2000). Anorexics with the restricting type eat almost nothing, losing weight by dieting, fasting, exercising, or a combination of these strategies. Those with the binge-eating/purging type may eat large quantities of food and use vomiting or laxatives to purge the food they have eaten. Alternatively, these anorexics may eat small amounts of food and purge. Purging is typical of bulimia, but bulimics use purging to maintain a normal body weight, and anorexics purge to lose weight.

Jessica is typical of the restricting type of anorexia; she ate almost nothing and did not purge. She also shares other characteristics typical of many anorexics, who are often young, White women who are outwardly compliant and high achievers in school. They are preoccupied with food, usually like to cook for others (Jessica didn't), insist that others eat their food, but eat almost nothing themselves. They lose from 15% to 50% of their body weight yet continue to see themselves as overweight. Like Jessica, they tend to be ambitious, perfectionistic, unhappy with their bodies, and come from high-achieving families. Their preoccupation with body fat usually leads to a strenuous program of exercise—dancing, jogging, doing calisthenics, or playing tennis. Excessively active and energetic behavior continues until their weight loss reaches a level that produces fatigue and weakness, making further activity impossible.

After substantial weight loss has occurred, individual differences tend to disappear, and accounts of the disorder itself are remarkably similar. Interestingly, most of the descriptions are also consistent with the sketch of starving conscientious objectors drawn by Keys et al. (1950). Thus, these conditions are probably an effect of starvation and not its cause. As weight loss becomes more than 25% of one's previous normal weight, the person constantly feels chilled, grows a soft, downy covering of body hair, loses scalp hair, loses interest in sex, and develops an unusual preoccupation with food. As starvation nears a perilous level, the anorexic becomes more hostile toward family and friends who try to reverse the weight loss.

Many authorities, including Hilde Bruch (1973, 1978, 1982), have regarded anorexia nervosa as a means of gaining control. Bruch, who spent more than 40 years studying eating disorders and the effects of starvation, reported that prior to dieting, anorexics typically are troubled girls who feel incapable of changing their lives. These young women often see their parents as overdemanding and in absolute control of their life, yet they remain too compliant to rebel openly. They try to seize control of their life in the most personal manner possible: by changing the shape of their body. Short of force-feeding, no one can stop these young women from controlling their own body size and shape. They take great pleasure and pride in doing something that is difficult and often compare their superior willpower with that of others who are overweight or who shun exercise. Bruch (1978) stated that anorexics enjoy being hungry and eventually regard any food in the stomach as dirty or damaging.

Who Is Anorexic? Anorexia nervosa cuts across ethnic groups (Arriaza & Mann, 2001). This diagnosis is more common among upper-middle-class and upper-class White women in North America and Europe, but this description matches individuals who have better access to health care and thus are more likely to receive a diagnosis. In terms of incidence, most clinicians and researchers believe that anorexia has become more common in the United States than it was 50 years ago, but anorexia nervosa is still a very rare disorder in the general population. The DSM-IV-TR (APA, 2000) estimated the lifetime prevalence of anorexia at 0.5% for women and one- tenth that for men. However, among some populations the incidence rates are much higher. Young women between the ages of 15 and 19 are at elevated risk (Steinhausen, Winkler, & Meier, 1997), and young women who attend ballet classes or modeling academies are at especially high risk. The competitive, weight-conscious atmosphere of professional schools for dance and modeling prompt the development of anorexia, and 6.5% of dance students and 7% of modeling students met the diagnostic criteria for anorexia nervosa (Garner & Garfinkel, 1980). Athletes are also at increased risk, especially female athletes. The risk increases with higher levels of competition and appears in programs for all sports, especially those that emphasize appearance, thin body type, or low body fat (Picard, 1999).

Individuals with anorexia often report family difficulties, but it is difficult to determine if the difficulties precede the onset of eating problems or are a result of them (Polivy & Herman, 2002). Families with children who have eating disorders tend to include a lot of negative emotion and little emotional support. Physical or sexual abuse is a more common experience in the history of those who are anorexic than for individuals who eat normally. In addition, mothers of anorexic girls are often critical of their daughters' appearance and praise their weight loss, even when the weight loss is extreme (Hill & Franklin, 1998).

Over the years, a large majority of those diagnosed as anorexic have been women, and research and treatment have focused on women. Men make up about 10% of all anorexics (APA, 2000). This estimate—that 90% or more of all anorexics are women—has remained constant over a period of years, but it is based mostly on clinical impressions rather than complete population data. A survey of eating attitudes and behaviors among college students (Nelson, Hughes, Katz, & Searight, 1999) found that 20% of the women and 10% of the men showed symptoms of anorexia, leading to the conclusion that this eating disorder may be more common among men than the clinical impressions suggest.

Male anorexics are quite similar to female anorexics in terms of social class and family configuration, symptoms, treatment, and prognosis, but they differ in terms of the factors that pushed them toward disordered eating (Crosscope-Happel, Hutchins, Getz, & Hayes, 2000). The ideal body for boys is muscular, and escaping this indoctrination is as difficult as avoiding the thin body ideal is for girls. However, both ideals share the abhorrence of fat. Boys and young men may take drastic measures to achieve their ideal body, just as girls and young women do. Some theorists (McCaughey, 1999) have argued that the same type of concern with the body is expressed in men as bodybuilding and compulsive exercising and in women as self-starvation. Therefore, both women and men have concerns about body shape and size that may appear as disordered eating.

In addition, sexual orientation is a factor that differs for male and female anorexics (Carlat, Camargo, & Herzog, 1997). Gay men are slightly overrepresented among the anorexics, but more than half of male anorexics identified themselves as asexual, a finding consistent with loss of sexual interest among female anorexics.

Treatment Treatment for anorexia suffers from an unfortunate dilemma: this disorder has the highest mortality rate of any psychiatric diagnosis, but treatment does not show a high success rate (Brown, Mehler, & Harris, 2000). Between 5% and 10% of all anorexics die from their disorder. Most die of cardiac arrhythmia, but suicide is also a frequent cause of death. Despite the very real possibility of death, anorexia nervosa remains one of the most difficult behavior disorders to treat. About 50% of anorexics recover, 30% improve but struggle with eating-related or body image problems, and 20% experience continued pathology.

An initial complication for treatment is that most anorexics see nothing wrong with their eating behavior, resent suggestions that they are too thin, and resist any attempt to change their eating. Therefore, parents and friends have great difficulty motivating anorexics to seek treatment. Short of force, family and friends have few options. The one aspect of the environment that anorexics can control is their own body. As long as they refuse to eat, their control remains sovereign.

As starvation continues, anorexics eventually reach the point of fatigue, exhaustion, and possible physical collapse. At that point, some sort of treatment is usually forced on them. After 2 years of self-imposed starvation and weighing only 52 pounds, Jessica was forced by her parents to seek treatment. She was then hospitalized and fed intravenously. Forced treatment seems unlikely to be effective, but research (Watson, Bowers, & Andersen, 2000) indicates that anorexics who underwent involuntary treatment regained weight at similar rates to anorexics who volunteered for treatment.

The immediate aim of almost any treatment program for anorexia is medical stabilization of any danger due to physical symptoms of starvation (Goldner & Birmingham, 1994). Then, anorexics need to work toward restoration of normal weight, healthy eating, and good body image. Recommendations concerning the methods of achieving these goals are not universally accepted. Some authorities believe that hospitalization is required, especially for medical stabilization and restoration of weight, whereas others believe that psychological treatments can be effective.

Since the mid-1970s, cognitive behavior therapy has become increasingly popular as a treatment for anorexia nervosa, and it has shown some success in changing both cognitive distortions that accompany body image problems and eating behavior. Cognitive behavior therapists attack these irrational beliefs while maintaining a warm and accepting attitude toward patients. Anorexics are taught to discard the absolutist, all-or-nothing thinking pattern expressed in such self-statements as "If I gain one pound, I'll go on to gain a hundred." Patients are also encouraged to stop centering all attention on themselves and to realize that others do not have the same high standards for their behavior that they do. Finally, therapists need to point out the errors in superstitious food beliefs such as "Any sweet is instantly converted into fat" or "Laxatives prevent the absorption of calories" (Thompson & Sherman, 1993). When patients understand the superstitious nature of these beliefs, they can become more realistic about the effects of food on body composition.

Many hospital-based programs consist of individual and group cognitive behavioral therapy plus supervised meals, meal planning, and nutrition education (Williamson, Thaw, & Varnado-Sullivan, 2001). However, cognitive behavioral therapy is underutilized as a therapy for eating disorders (Mussel et al., 2000). Despite a great deal of evidence for its effectiveness, this approach is not among the most frequent that therapists use, which may partially explain why anorexia treatment success rates are as low as they are.

For adolescents, parents may or may not be actively involved in cognitive behavioral treatment program, but another approach emphasizes the role of parents in treatment. Developed at the Maudsley Hospital in London, this approach is family based (Locke, Le Grange, Agras, & Dare, 2001). Rather than treating parents as part of the problem, this approach accepts them as an essential part of the solution. Acknowledging that it is relatively easy to get anorexics to gain weight in the hospital, this approach focuses on helping them eat at home by equipping parents with strategies to get their children to eat. This family-centered approach has shown promise of being more effective than some other programs, but its applicability is limited to adolescents.

Relapse always remains a possibility. Even with intensive therapy that targets irrational eating patterns and distorted body image, some anorexics retain elements of these maladaptive thought processes. Some slip back to self-starvation, others attempt suicide, some become depressed, and some develop bulimia (Goldner & Birmingham, 1994). Follow-up care is often included in comprehensive programs, and this element can be helpful. In addition, the drug fluoxetine (Prozac) has shown some benefit. This drug is not very effective in helping anorexics gain weight or change distorted cognitions or body image (Peterson & Mitchell, 1999), but some research (Kaye et al., 2001) has indicated that it can be useful in preventing relapse for anorexics who have returned to the normal range of body weight.

Jessica's treatment was not adequate to address her body image problems or to train her to adopt healthy eating patterns. However, after being hospitalized and her weight restored, Jessica became convinced that continuing self-starvation threatened her life. With almost no psychological or psychiatric intervention, she gradually began a weight restoration program, and within 6 months her weight was up to 110 pounds. Her appearance was normal, but she had suffered severe and permanent damage to her heart and intestinal tract due to her laxative abuse. In addition, she continued to see herself as overweight, a view quite similar to that of an anorexic.

Bulimia

Bulimia is often regarded as a companion disorder to anorexia nervosa. Unlike anorexics, who rely mostly on strict fasts to lose more and more weight, bulimics engage in binge eating; that is, they consume huge quantities of food in an uncontrolled manner. The seemingly bizarre practice of binge eating followed by purging is not new. The ancient Romans sometimes indulged in very similar eating rituals. After they had feasted

BECOMING HEALTHIER

1. Get good information about nutrition and use that information in deciding on a healthy diet.
2. Be more concerned with eating a healthy diet than with what you weigh.
3. Consult a chart that contains height-weight recommendations or body mass index rather than a fashion magazine to determine what is the correct weight for you.
4. Give up dieting. Instead, consider any dietary change as a permanent change in the way you eat.
5. Concentrate less on food restriction and more on exercise as a way to change your body shape.
6. Understand that losing weight will not solve all your problems.
7. If you lose weight, know when to stop. Listen to people who tell you that you have lost enough.
8. Do not hide how little you weigh from friends or family by wearing baggy clothing.
9. When you make dietary changes, find ways to keep eating a pleasurable activity. Feelings of deprivation and going without favorite foods can make you too miserable to care about eating correctly.
9. Do not use diet drugs, fast, or go on a very low-calorie diet to lose weight, even if you are very obese.
10. Do not vomit as a way to keep from gaining weight.
11. Learn how to see someone who is normal weight or slightly overweight as attractive. Look for such people in the news and in the media.

on great quantities of rich food, these Romans would retire to the vomitorium, empty their stomachs, and then return to eat some more (Friedländer, 1968). The ancient Romans were neither the first nor the last to binge and purge, but theirs was perhaps the only society to have elevated this practice to such a refined state. Today, bulimia is defined as an eating disorder and affects millions of people.

What Is Bulimia? As defined by the *Diagnostic and Statistical Manual of Mental Disorders (DSM-IV-TR)* of the American Psychiatric Association (APA, 2000), bulimia nervosa involves recurrent episodes of binge eating, a sense of lack of control over eating, and inappropriate, drastic measures to compensate for the binge. Some bulimics fast or exercise excessively, but most use self-induced vomiting and maintain a relatively normal weight. Binge eating may occur without any attempts to purge, but this pattern is not yet part of DSM diagnoses.

In many ways, Elise, our second case study, was not typical of people with bulimia, but in other ways she was. As a woman, Elise was typical of bulimics; about 90% of bulimics are women. Like most other bulimics, she began purging as part of a weight control strategy. The common pattern for bulimia involves binge eating compensated by fasting, with this pattern developing into one of vomiting or laxative abuse or both as methods of purging. Unlike most bulimics, Elise's binges were never a central part of her eating problem, but her purging behavior was. Like most bulimics, Elise felt guilty about her bingeing and purging and after several years and therapeutic intervention, managed to end this cycle.

One factor that distinguishes bulimia from anorexia is impulse control (Polivy & Herman, 2002). Bulimics often experience other problems that relate to impulsivity, such as a history of alcohol or drug abuse, sexual promiscuity, suicide attempts, and stealing or shoplifting. This factor may be critical; a person may become bulimic rather than anorexic if she or he cannot resist the impulse to eat and yet feels the body dissatisfaction that is common to both of these disorders. Elise's behavior did not reflect any of these problems. Like many college students, Elise's alcohol use was not always wise, but her drinking never got her into serious trouble, and, except for laxatives, she did not misuse drugs.

Childhood experiences with sexual abuse, physical abuse, and posttraumatic stress are additional correlates of bulimia (Welch, Doll, & Fairburn, 1997). Stephen Wonderlich's team of researchers (Wonderlich, Wilsnack, Wilsnack, & Harris, 1996) surveyed a nationally representative sample of bulimic women and reported that nearly one fourth of all female victims of childhood sexual abuse displayed bulimic behaviors later on. A later review of more than 50 studies (Wonderlich, Brewerton, Jocic, Dansky, & Abbott, 1997) showed that childhood sexual abuse is more closely associated with bulimia than it is with anorexia. Although not all victims of childhood sexual abuse become bulimic and not all bulimics are victims of childhood abuse, there is a relationship between the two.

A relationship also exists between bulimia and depression, but childhood sexual abuse is also related to depression, as are suicide attempts. Depression and negative mood are more common among bulimics than others. Some research (Stice & Bearman, 2001) showed that body image and eating disorders precede the development of depression in adolescent girls. This research suggests a developmental sequence and may allow the establishment of a chain of causality for the development of bulimia. Bulimics also tend to react strongly to negative events and to experience sustained negative reactions that interfere with effective coping. Using food for comfort is a maladaptive coping strategy that requires countermeasures for those who have extreme body concerns, which bulimics solve by purging. Establishing the binge-purge pattern makes eating distressing rather than comforting, producing more negative feelings.

Elise felt a lot of stress in her life when she started purging, and her life centered around controlling her eating. When she ate more than she thought she should (and her criteria were very strict), she would vomit or take laxatives. Indeed, she often took laxatives in anticipation of eating and feared her stomach being full for long. Unlike most bulimics, Elise did not plan eating sprees in advance or collect special types of food for her binges. Also unlike most bulimics, she was not completely secretive about vomiting or laxative abuse. On the other hand, Elise was like many other bulimics in her continued belief that she was too heavy. She thought that if she could weigh less than 100 pounds, she would be happier. This continued dissatisfaction of one's body reflects the distorted thinking that is even more typical of both bulimics than of anorexics (Cash & Deagle, 1997).

Who Is Bulimic? In at least one way, the population of bulimics is quite similar to that of anorexics. Both eating disorders occur far more often in women than in men, with about 90% to 95% of those diagnosed in both groups being women (APA, 2000). Whereas anorexia appears primarily among upper-middle- and upper-class Whites, bulimia is always more democratic, occurring with equal prevalence in various social classes and ethnic groups.

How prevalent is bulimia? Is its incidence increasing or decreasing? Early surveys generally found high prevalence rates, much higher than the rates for anorexia. Studies conducted during the 1980s (Pope, Hudson, & Yurgelun-Todd, 1984; Pyle et al., 1983) found that between 8% and 13% of women and 1.4% of men met the DSM diagnostic criteria for bulimia at that time. Those diagnostic criteria became more stringent, which lowered prevalence estimates for bulimia. Approximately 1% to 3% of women and 0.2% of men meet the current diagnostic criteria for bulimia (APA, 2000).

Is prevalence of bulimia on the increase? One early review (Fairburn, Hay, & Welch, 1993) noted not only higher rates of bulimia in younger women but also a higher lifetime occurrence. That is, women born after 1960 were at higher risk to have ever been bulimic than women born before 1950, indicating that the prevalence of bulimia is increasing. A survey of high school students (Grunbaum et al., 2002) indicated that 7.8% of girls and 2.9% of boys said that they had vomited or used laxatives to lose or to prevent gaining weight. These percentages reflect a high rate of these behaviors, which suggests a growing prevalence of bulimia.

Is Bulimia Harmful? To many people, bingeing and purging may seem to be an acceptable means of controlling weight. To others, guilt is a nearly inevitable part of bulimia, and some mental health problems accompany this disorder. However, the question remains: Is bulimia harmful to physical health? Unlike anorexia nervosa, which has a mortality rate of 5% to 10% (Brown et al., 2000), bulimia is very seldom fatal. Nevertheless, there are serious detrimental consequences to both bingeing and purging.

Binge eating is harmful in several ways. First, the intake of large quantities of sweets can result in **hypoglycemia,** or a deficiency of sugar in the blood. This may seem paradoxical because the typical binge eater consumes huge amounts of sugar. However, high sugar intake activates the pancreas to release excessive amounts of insulin, and insulin drives down blood sugar levels. Low blood sugar results in dizziness, fatigue, and depression. The low blood sugar level frequently produces cravings for more sugar, which in turn prompt the person to eat more cake, candy, ice cream, and other sweets. Second, binge eaters seldom eat a balanced diet. They usually lack sufficient fatty acids, a major energy source, and consequently they may experience lethargy and depression. Third, binge eating is expensive. Bulimics can spend more than $100 a day on food, and this expense can lead to other problems, such as financial difficulties or stealing. Also, binge eaters are almost invariably preoccupied with food. They nearly constantly think of the next binge and have little time or energy for other activities. This obsession may leave bulimics with limited time to attend to other activities (Polivy & Herman, 2002).

Purging also leads to several physical problems (McGilley & Pryor, 1998). One of the most common consequences of frequent vomiting is damaged teeth; hydrochloric acid from the stomach erodes the enamel that protects the teeth. Many longtime bulimics need extensive dental work, and thus dentists are sometimes the first health care professionals to see evidence of bulimia. Hydrochloric acid is also implicated in damage to other parts of the digestive system, particularly the mouth and esophagus. Unlike the stomach, they are not naturally protected against hydrochloric acid. Bleeding and tearing of the esophagus are not common among bulimics but are very dangerous. Some longtime sufferers report reverse peristalsis, a spontaneous regurgitation of food, often after eating quite moderately.

Besides damage to teeth, mouth, and esophagus, other potential dangers of frequent purging include anemia, electrolyte imbalance, and alkalosis. **Anemia,** a reduction in the number of red blood cells, leads to generalized weakness and a lack of vitality. **Electrolyte imbalance** is caused by the loss of such body minerals such as sodium, potassium, magnesium, and calcium and leads to muscle cramps and weakness. **Alkalosis,** an abnormally high level of alkaline in the body tissues due to the loss of hydrochloric acid, results in generalized fatigue and frequent headaches. In addition, purging through excessive use of laxatives and diuretics may lead to kidney damage, dehydration, and a spastic colon or the loss of voluntary control over excretory functions. In summary, bulimia is not a benign eating practice but a serious disorder with a multitude of harmful consequences.

Treatment In one important respect, the treatment of bulimia has a critical advantage over therapy programs for anorexia nervosa. Anorexics cling to their dangerous eating behaviors, but bulimics usually do not approve of their own eating habits, and many of them would like to change. Unfortunately, this motivation does not guarantee that bulimics will seek therapy.

Cognitive behavior therapy is an effective treatment for bulimia (Wilson, Fairburn, Agras,

Walsh, & Kraemer, 2002). Cognitive behavior therapists work toward changing both distorted cognitions, such as obsessive body concerns, and in altering behavior, such as bingeing, vomiting, and laxative use. Specific techniques may include keeping a diary on the factors related to bingeing and on their feelings after purging; monitoring their caloric intake and purging; eating slowly; eating regular meals; and clarifying their distorted views of eating and weight control. A review of the effectiveness of cognitive behavioral treatment for bulimia (Compas et al., 1998) found that the average reduction in the frequency of binge eating was 80%, an unusually high percentage of success for any type of therapy.

Interpersonal psychotherapy has also been used successfully in treating bulimics (Wilson et al., 2002). Interpersonal psychotherapy is a nonintrospective, short-term therapy that was originally applied to depression. It focuses on present interpersonal problems and not on eating, taking the approach that eating problems tend to appear in late adolescence when interpersonal issues present major developmental challenges. In this view, eating problems represent maladaptive attempts to cope. The success rate of interpersonal therapy is comparable to cognitive behavioral therapy (Wilson et al., 2002), but it does not work as quickly.

Drugs, especially antidepressants, have been used for some time in the treatment of bulimia. Controlled studies using these drugs tend to show decreases in frequency of binges, but drugs are not a substitute for psychotherapy for most patients (Peterson & Mitchell, 1999). Indeed, cognitive behavioral therapy is more effective than antidepressant drugs in managing bulimia, and drugs alone are not as good a choice as this type of psychotherapy (Compas et al., 1998)

A combination of educational and cognitive psychology programs can be effective in treating women at risk for bulimia who have not yet developed the disorder (Kaminski & McNamara, 1996). The risks include low self-esteem, poor body image, a strong need for perfectionism, a history of repeated dieting, and other dysfunctional eating behaviors or attitudes. College women with such attitudes and behaviors were randomly assigned to receive no treatment or a 7-week treatment consisting of educational information about realistic weights and healthy eating habits as well as cognitive strategies for enhancing self-esteem, challenging negative thinking styles, improving body image, and combating social pressures for thinness. The treatment group showed significantly greater improvement in self-esteem and body satisfaction than those in the control group and manifested fewer destructive dieting practices and less need for perfectionism. Results of this study are encouraging, suggesting that intervention can change the attitudes and risky behaviors that are symptomatic of bulimia before the appearance of the disorder.

In Summary

Some people begin a weight loss program that seemingly gets out of control and turns into an almost total fasting regimen. This eating disorder, called anorexia nervosa, is uncommon but most prevalent among young, high-achieving women who have high body dissatisfaction and believe that being thin will lead to a solution to their problems. Anorexia is very difficult to treat successfully because people with this disorder continue to see themselves as too fat and thus they lack any motivation to change their eating habits. A type of family therapy and cognitive behavioral therapy is more effective than other approaches, and fluoxetine (Prozac) may be useful in preventing relapse, which is a substantial problem for anorexics.

Bulimia is an eating disorder characterized by uncontrolled binge eating, usually accompanied by guilt and followed by vomiting or other purgative methods. Although people with bulimia differ from one another in some ways, many of them share certain personal characteristics. In general terms, bulimics, compared with other people, are more likely to be depressed and impulsive, which may lead to alcohol and other drug abuse and stealing. In addition, they are more likely to have been victims of childhood sexual abuse, to be dissatisfied with their bodies, and to use food as a coping strategy.

Treatment for bulimia has generally been more successful than treatment for anorexia partly because of bulimics' greater motivation to change. The more successful programs for eating disorders are those that include cognitive behavioral techniques, which seek to change not only eating patterns but also the pathological concerns about weight and eating, and interpersonal therapy, which focuses on relationship issues. Antidepressant drugs have been used with limited success to treat bulimia.

Answers

This chapter addressed six basic questions.

1. **How does the digestive system function?**
   The digestive system turns food into nutrients by breaking down food into particles that can be absorbed. The process of breaking down food begins in the mouth and continues in the stomach, but absorption of most nutrients occurs in the small intestines. Hormones such as leptin, insulin, ghrelin, and cholecystokinin (CCK) affect eating, and the hypothalamus and other brain structures are involved in eating in complex ways.

2. **What factors are involved in weight maintenance?**
   Weight maintenance depends largely on two factors: the number of calories absorbed through food intake and the number expended through body metabolism and physical activity. Experimental starvation has demonstrated that losing weight leads to irritability, aggression, apathy, lack of interest in sex, and preoccupation with food. Initial weight gain may be easy, but the slowing of metabolic rate makes drastic weight loss difficult. Experimental overeating has demonstrated that gaining weight can be almost as difficult and unpleasant as losing it.

3. **What is obesity and how does it affect health?**
   Obesity can be defined in terms of percent body fat, Body Mass Index, or social standards, which yields different estimates for the prevalence of obesity. Over the past 20 years, obesity has become more common in the United States and the ideal body has become thinner, leading to questions about the causes for obesity. The difficulty of either losing or gaining weight has led several investigators to adopt the notion of a natural setpoint for weight maintenance, but an alternative view holds that positive aspects of eating lead people to overeat when a variety of tasty foods is available. This latter model is more compatible with the growing rate of obesity in the United States and other industrialized countries.

   Obesity is associated with increased mortality, heart disease, Type 2 diabetes, and digestive tract diseases, and the very thinnest and the very heaviest people are at the greatest risk for death. Severe obesity and carrying excess weight around the waist rather than hips are both risks of death from several causes, especially heart disease.

4. **Is dieting a good way to lose weight?**
   A cultural obsession with thinness has led to a plethora of diets, many of which are neither safe nor permanently effective. Changing to healthier eating patterns and incorporating exercise are wise choices for weight change, whereas surgery, diet drugs, fasting, and very low-calorie diets are not.

5. **What is anorexia nervosa and how can it be treated?**
   Anorexia nervosa is an eating disorder characterized by self-starvation. This disorder is most

prevalent among young, high-achieving women with body image problems but is uncommon, affecting only about 1% of the population. Anorexics are very difficult to treat successfully because they continue to see themselves as too fat and thus they lack any motivation to change their eating habits, but a specific type of family therapy and cognitive behavioral therapy are more effective than other approaches.

6. **What is bulimia and how can it be treated?** Bulimia is an eating disorder characterized by uncontrolled binge eating, usually accompanied by guilt and followed by vomiting or other purgative methods. Bulimia is more common than anorexia, affecting between 1% and 3% of the population. Their motivation to change eating patterns has made bulimics better therapy candidates than anorexics. Treatment for bulimia, especially cognitive behavioral therapy and interpersonal therapy, has generally been successful.

Suggested Readings

Bruch, H. (1978). *The golden cage: The enigma of anorexia nervosa.* Cambridge, MA: Harvard University Press. Written by one of the leading authorities on anorexia nervosa, this nontechnical book describes anorexia and suggests methods of treating this eating disorder.

Consumer Reports. (2002, June). The truth about dieting. *Consumer Reports, 67*(6), 26–31. This article in a popular magazine reports on the results of a survey of over 30,000 dieters—both successful and unsuccessful. The article evaluates some of the latest research about dieting and presents it in a readable way, along with suggestions about how to change eating patterns for permanent weight loss.

Rozin, P. (1999). Food is fundamental, fun, frightening, and far-reaching. *Social Research, 66,* 9–30. In this clever article, Paul Rozin examines the psychological, biological, social, and cultural importance of food and eating.

Wadden, T. A., Brownell, K. D., & Foster, G. D. (2002). Obesity: Responding to the global epidemic. *Journal of Consulting and Clinical Psychology, 70,* 510–525. Thomas Wadden, Kelly Brownell, and Gary Foster view obesity as a major epidemic, one that threatens the health of millions of people in the United States. These authors call for research aimed at changing society's attitude toward food consumption.

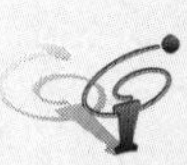

Search InfoTrac College Edition

Search these terms to learn more about topics in this chapter:

Body weight and regulation
Weight and leptin
Ghrelin
Obesity and causes of
Obesity and demographic aspects
Obesity and statistics
Obesity and measurement of
Obesity and genetic aspects
Obesity and mortality risk
Weight loss and health benefits
Weight loss and demographic aspects
Weight loss and evaluation
Weight loss and maintenance
Weight loss and physical activity
Weight loss and risks
Eating disorders and statistics
Eating disorders and demographic aspects
Eating disorders and causes of
Eating disorders and genetic aspects
Eating disorders and diagnosis
Eating disorders and treatment

16

Exercising

The Story of Jim Fixx

CHAPTER OUTLINE

Types of Physical Activity

Reasons for Exercising

Physical Activity and Cardiovascular Health

Other Health Benefits of Physical Activity

Hazards of Physical Activity

How Much Is Enough but Not Too Much?

Maintaining a Physical Activity Program

QUESTIONS

This chapter focuses on six basic questions:

1. What are the different types of physical activity?
2. Does physical activity benefit the cardiovascular system?
3. What are some other health benefits of physical activity?
4. Can physical activity be hazardous?
5. How much is enough but not too much?
6. What are some problems in maintaining an exercise program?

The Story of Jim Fixx

At age 35, Jim Fixx was 50 pounds overweight, smoked two packs of cigarettes a day, and except for an occasional game of tennis or touch football, generally lived a sedentary existence as a magazine editor. But at that point, his life changed dramatically. By his account, the impetus for this transformation was a pulled leg muscle he incurred while playing tennis. To rehabilitate his leg and avoid another muscle pull, Fixx began a modest running program. Painfully he jogged half a mile or so three or four times a week. Gradually he increased both his distance and his speed, and running began to play an increasingly important role in his life.

His exercise routine slowly altered both his physical appearance and his attitude toward his health. He lost weight, stopped smoking, felt physically rejuvenated, and came to believe strongly in the preventive and curative powers of running. Perhaps too much so. On a warm July day in 1984, Jim Fixx died while returning from his afternoon run. The cause of death was listed as sudden **cardiac arrhythmia** due to coronary artery disease.

Because Jim Fixx, like some other runners, died during or immediately after exercising, some controversy arose over the potential hazards of strenuous physical activity. However, Fixx had a family history of heart problems; his father suffered a heart attack at age 35 and died of another one at 43. Fixx, then, outlived his father by 9 years—so perhaps his 17 years of long-distance running produced more benefits than risks. Some people conclude that exercise is hazardous to health. Others, however, argue that Fixx would have died earlier if he had not become a runner.

Although Jim Fixx died 20 years ago, his popular books on the joy of running motivated others to begin a running program (Fixx, 1977, 1980). In the intervening years since Fixx's death, most people in the United States became aware of the health benefits of regular exercise. However, most of the people do not engage in the strenuous running that Fixx advocated; nevertheless, a substantial portion of the population now believe that regular physical activity—along with not smoking, moderate drinking, and wise eating—play an important role in people's health.

During the past 20 years, scientists and lay people alike have asked several questions about the benefits and dangers of vigorous physical activity. Does exercise reduce heart disease? Does it contribute to longevity? Can physical activity protect against cancer? Does it enhance personal well-being and psychological health? How much is necessary to maintain good health? How much is too much? Can physical activity be a health hazard? This chapter examines the available evidence on these issues and attempts to reach some conclusions about the health effects of both moderate and strenuous physical activity.

Types of Physical Activity

Although exercise can include hundreds of different kinds of physical activity, physiologically there are only five different types of exercise: isometric, isotonic, isokinetic, anaerobic, and aerobic. Each has different goals, different activities, and different advocates. Each can contribute to some aspect of fitness or health, but only aerobic exercise benefits cardiorespiratory health.

Isometric exercise is performed by contracting muscles against an immovable object. Although the body does not move in isometric exercise, muscles push hard against each other or against an immovable object and thus gain strength. Pushing hard against a solid wall is an example of isometric exercise. Because joints do not move, it may not be apparent that exercise is occurring, but the contraction of muscles produces gains in strength—and little else. This type of physical activity can improve muscle strength, which can be especially important for older people in preserving independent living (Tanji, 1997).

Isotonic exercise requires the contraction of muscles and the movement of joints. Weight lifting and many forms of calisthenics fit into this category. Programs based on isotonic exercise can improve muscle strength and muscle endurance if the program is sufficiently lengthy. Again, older

CHECK YOUR HEALTH RISKS

Check the items that apply to you.

- ☐ 1. Whenever the urge to exercise comes over me, I sit down until the urge goes away.
- ☐ 2. My family history of heart disease means that I am going to have a heart attack whether I exercise or not.
- ☐ 3. When it comes to exercise, I subscribe to the motto "No pain, no gain."
- ☐ 4. I have changed jobs in order to have more time to train for competitive athletic events.
- ☐ 5. I use exercise along with diet as a means of controlling my weight.
- ☐ 6. People have advised me to start an exercise program, but I just never seem to have the time or energy.
- ☐ 7. One of the reasons I exercise is that I believe that a person can't be too thin and that exercise will help me continue to lose weight.
- ☐ 8. I may begin an exercise program when I'm older, but now I'm young and in good shape.
- ☐ 9. I'm too old and out of shape to begin exercising.
- ☐ 10. I'd probably have a heart attack if I started to jog or run.
- ☐ 11. I'd like to exercise, but I can't run and walking doesn't help.
- ☐ 12. I try not to let injuries interfere with my regular exercise.

Except for item #5, each of these items represents a health risk from either too little or too much exercise. Count your check marks to evaluate your risks. As you read this chapter, you will learn that some of these items are riskier than others.

people can profit from this isotonic exercise, but most people in a weight-lifting program are bodybuilders interested in improving the appearance of their body rather than improving health.

In **isokinetic exercise,** exertion is required for lifting, and additional effort is required to return to the starting position. This type of exercise requires specialized equipment that adjusts the amount of resistance according to the amount of force applied. Isokinetic exercise is frequently used to restore muscle strength and muscle endurance in people who have suffered muscle injuries. It is an important adjunct in physical rehabilitation, helping injured people to regain strength and flexibility with more safety than other types of exercise.

Anaerobic exercises include short-distance running, some calisthenics, softball, and other exercises that require short, intensive bursts of energy but do not require an increased amount of oxygen use. Such short, strenuous exercises improve speed and endurance, but they may be dangerous for people with coronary heart disease.

Aerobic exercise is any exercise that requires dramatically increased oxygen consumption over an extended period of time. Aerobic exercise includes jogging, walking at a brisk pace, cross-country skiing, dancing, rope skipping, swimming, cycling, and other activities that increase oxygen consumption.

The important characteristics of aerobic exercise are intensity and duration. Exercise must be intense enough to elevate the heart rate into a certain range, which is computed from a formula based on age and the maximum possible heart rate. In general, the heart rate should stay at this elevated level for 12 to 20 minutes for the aerobic benefits to accrue. This type of program requires elevated oxygen use and provides a workout for both the respiratory system, which furnishes the oxygen, and the coronary system, which pumps the blood. Of the various approaches to fitness, aerobic activity is superior to other types of exercise in developing cardiorespiratory fitness, provided a person engages in some aerobic exercise at least three times a week.

Kenneth Cooper (1968, 1982, 1985), one of the early advocates of aerobic exercise, was also one of the first to recommend caution in adopting an aerobic exercise program. First, he recommended a medical examination before beginning a program of aerobic exercise, because potentially dangerous coronary abnormalities can exist without any apparent symptoms. Second, he strongly suggested the use of an exercise electrocardiogram, known as a *stress test,* to detect any abnormal cardiac activity during exercise. Third, Cooper suggested less strenuous activity than some of his contemporaries. For example, Jim Fixx advocated running long distances 6 or 7 days a week. whereas Cooper maintained that jogging or speed walking three miles a day for 5 days a week confers an optimum level of cardiovascular fitness. For Cooper, more frequent exercise or greater distance does not confer much additional benefit and may increase the chances for injuries. In a later section of this chapter, we examine the question of how much exercise is enough and how much is too much.

Reasons for Exercising

People exercise for a variety of reasons, some that are consistent with good health and some that are not. Reasons for adhering to a physical activity program include physical fitness, weight loss, cardiovascular health, increased longevity, protection against cancer, prevention of osteoporosis, control of diabetes, aid to sleep, enhanced self-esteem, and a buffer against depression, anxiety, and stress. This chapter looks at evidence relating to each of these reasons as well as to the potential hazards of physical activity.

Physical Fitness

Does physical activity help people become physically fit? The effects of exercise on fitness depend both on the duration and intensity of the exercise and on the definition of fitness. To most exercise physiologists, fitness is a complex condition consisting of muscle strength, muscle endurance, flexibility, and cardiorespiratory (aerobic) fitness. Each of the five types of exercise can contribute to these four different aspects of fitness, but no one type fulfills all the requirements.

In addition, fitness can be considered in terms of both organic and dynamic fitness. *Organic fitness* is the capacity for action and movement that is determined by inherent characteristics of the body. These organic factors include genetic endowment, age, and health limitations. *Dynamic fitness,* which is determined by experience, is probably what most people think of in connection with the term *fitness.* Dynamic fitness is affected by exercise, whereas organic fitness is not. A person can have a good level of organic fitness and yet be "out of shape" and perform poorly. Another person may train and improve dynamic fitness but still be unable to win races because of relatively poor organic fitness. Athletes who want to be champions need to have been very selective about choosing their biological parents in order to have inherited a high level of organic fitness. Aspiring champions also need to train to gain the dynamic fitness necessary for optimal athletic performance. The following discussion is concerned almost exclusively with dynamic fitness and its components, because this type of fitness can be modified through exercise.

Muscle Strength and Endurance Two components of physical fitness are muscle strength and muscle endurance. Muscle strength is a measure of how strongly a muscle can contract. This type of fitness can be achieved through isometric, isotonic, isokinetic, and to a lesser extent, anaerobic exercise. All these types of exercise have the capability to increase muscle strength, because they contract muscles.

Muscle endurance differs from muscle strength in that it requires continued performance. Some strength is necessary for muscle endurance, but the opposite is not true: a muscle may be strong but not have the endurance to continue its performance. Exercises that improve strength require greater exertion for limited repetitions; exercises that improve endurance require less exertion but are performed many times. Both muscle strength and muscle endurance are improved by similar types of exercises, including isometric, isotonic, and isokinetic.

Flexibility Flexibility is the range-of-motion capacity of a joint. The types of exercises that develop muscle strength and muscle endurance generally do not improve flexibility. Moreover, flexibility is specific to each joint, so that exercises designed to develop flexibility tend to be quite varied. In addition to being a component of fitness, flexibility also decreases the likelihood of injury in other types of physical activity, especially aerobic and anaerobic exercise.

Flexibility is best attained through slow, sustained stretching exercises. Fast, jerky, bouncing movements are not recommended, because they can cause soreness and injury. Also, flexibility training should not be as intense as strength and endurance training.

Aerobic Fitness Of all the types of physical activity, aerobic exercise contributes most to cardiorespiratory fitness. Aerobic exercise greatly increases the body's requirement for oxygen, thereby causing the respiratory system to work harder and the heart to pump blood at a higher rate. Research suggests that exercise increases aerobic fitness and helps protect both men and women from heart disease (Lakka et al., 1994; Lee, Rexrode, Cook, Manson, & Buring, 2001).

When people acquire aerobic fitness, they improve cardiorespiratory health in several ways. First, they increase the amount of oxygen that can be used during strenuous exercise, and second, they increase the amount of blood pumped with each heartbeat. These changes result in a lowering of both resting heart rate and resting blood pressure and increase the efficiency of the cardiovascular system (Pollock, Wilmore, & Fox, 1978).

Weight Control

Does physical activity contribute to weight control? Many people exercise to lose weight or to sculpt a more ideal body by improving their body composition—that is, the percentage of fat tissue on the body or the ratio of fat to muscle. Exercise increases muscle tissue and can therefore change this ratio.

In recent years, young people in the United States have adopted a sedentary lifestyle, spending much of their time watching television, viewing videos, playing computer games, and talking on the telephone. At the same time, pediatric obesity has become a serious health problem. Would children and preteen adolescents lose weight by taking up a more physically active lifestyle? A study of 8- to 12-year-old children (Epstein, Paluch, Gordy, & Dorn, 2000) showed that a physically active lifestyle yielded significant reductions in the percent of overweight children. However, children who were simply encouraged to change to a less sedentary lifestyle did just as well. This finding indicates that childhood obesity may be decreased merely by reducing the number of minutes children engage in sedentary activities.

Exercise is not recommended for people who are looking for a method of spot reduction. Despite some exercise promoters' claims, a particular callisthenic exercise will not reduce fat in a specific part of the body. Muscle and fat have little to do with one another, and it is possible to have both in the same part of the body. When weight is lost, both fat and muscle tissue are depleted. If people exercise during weight reduction, they build muscle tissue while losing fat. Spot reduction appears to be the result, because fat tends to be lost from the places where it was most abundant. Because fat distribution is under strong genetic control, people with large hips or

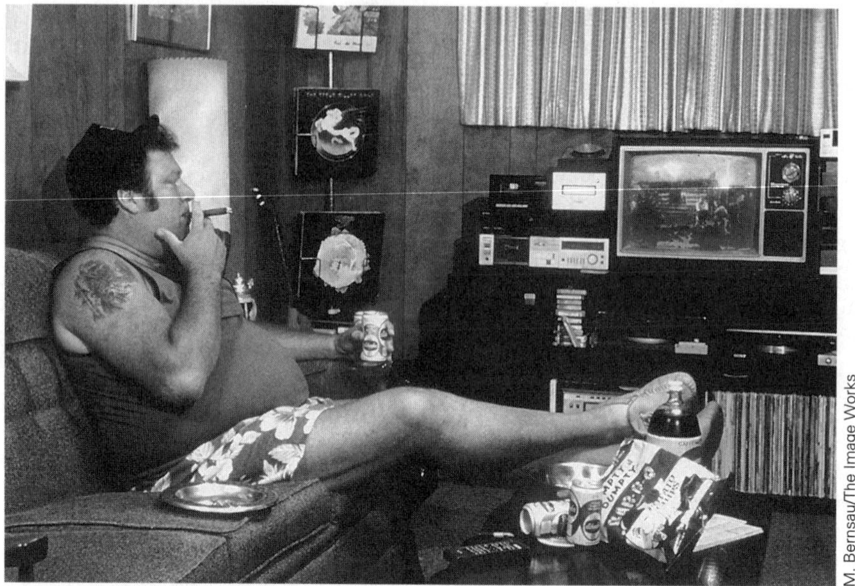
M. Bernsau/The Image Works

Sedentary lifestyle is a risk for several chronic illnesses.

thighs before they gained weight will, in relation to other body parts, have large hips or thighs after they lose weight.

Increased physical activity is recommended for people who wish to stop smoking but who are concerned about gaining too much weight—and research confirms this recommendation. One study (Marcus et al., 1999) divided healthy, sedentary female smokers into an exercise group and a control group, with both groups receiving a cognitive-behavioral smoking cessation program. In addition, women in the exercise group attended three exercise programs per week, whereas those in the control group received three health lecture programs per week. Compared with women in the control group, those in the exercise group achieved higher smoking cessation rates at 12-months follow-up—12% versus 5% for the control group. Also, women in the exercise group gained an average of about 6 pounds, whereas those in the control group gained about 11 pounds. This study confirmed an earlier study (Kawachi et al., 1996) that found that women who increased their level of physical activity after quitting smoking gained less weight than those who quit but did not become more physically active. These studies suggest that women who use weight concerns as an excuse to continue smoking will be much healthier if they stop smoking and initiate a moderate exercise program.

Whether one quits smoking or not, physical activity is recommended for weight control. Indeed, exercise is at least equal to dieting in controlling weight and much better than dieting in changing the ratio of fat to muscle tissue. In an early study (Wood et al., 1988), sedentary obese men were randomly assigned to one of three groups: dieters, runners, or controls. The dieters did not exercise, the runners did not diet, and the controls did neither. After a year, the exercise group and the dieting group had both lost weight, whereas people in the control group had not. However, some important differences emerged in comparing the dieters and the runners. Although both groups had lost an equal amount of weight, the dieters lost both fat and lean tissue, whereas the runners lost only fat tissue and retained more lean muscle tissue.

Exercise does not produce much weight loss through burning calories; for example, more than 30 minutes of tennis is required to work off the calories in two doughnuts. However, sitting and eating doughnuts is a risk for obesity in two ways—the sitting and the eating. For physically active people, weight loss may come not only from spending time on activities that burn calories but also in avoiding sedentary activities that may lead to consuming calories, such as watching television while eating snacks (Andersen, Crespo, Bartlett, Cheskin, & Pratt, 1998; Ching et al., 1996).

Most of the weight loss associated with exercise does not come from consuming fewer calories, but from the elevation of metabolic rate, the rate at which the body metabolizes calories. Regular exercise may prompt changes in basal metabolism, allowing an adjustment of how many calories are burned. Thus, exercise may be capable of increasing metabolic rate, which would produce changes in weight that exceed the number of calories spent in any activity.

How much exercise is enough to bring about weight loss? Research evidence (Kahn et al., 1997) indicates that moderate physical activity is sufficient to help control weight. Women who walk as little as 4 hours a week decrease their body mass index as well as improve their waist to hip ratio. Men who jog or run 1 to 3 hours a week are able to control their weight and improve body composition. Thus, although strenuous exercise will also bring about loss of weight, even moderate physical activity can be a helpful ingredient in weight loss programs.

Is exercise helpful for people who are already thin, or will it make them too thin? One review (Forbes, 1992) concluded that if people have a low body mass index at the beginning of an exercise program, they may have a tendency to lose some lean body weight. However, thin exercisers can maintain lean body mass through proper diet. The review also found that moderate exercisers who do not decrease total weight often increase lean body weight, suggesting that even when exercisers fail to lose weight, they increase lean body mass and decrease body fat.

In Summary

All physical activity can be subsumed under one or more of five basic categories: isometric, isotonic, isokinetic, anaerobic, and aerobic. Each of these five exercise types has advantages and disadvantages for improving physical fitness, but only aerobic exercise benefits cardiorespiratory health.

People have a variety of reasons for maintaining an exercise regimen, including physical fitness, aerobic health, and weight control. The various types of exercise can increase dynamic fitness, strengthen muscles, improve endurance, and add flexibility. Aerobic fitness reduces death not only from cardiovascular disease but also from all causes.

One popular reason for remaining physically active is to control weight and achieve a sculpted body. Physical activity can help people lose weight, but its ability for spot reduction is very limited. Adopting a regular exercise program can help ex-smokers avoid unwanted weight. Overweight people can lose weight through moderate physical activity, highly active thin people can maintain lean body mass through proper diet, and people of moderate weight can increase lean body weight without an overall weight gain.

Physical Activity and Cardiovascular Health

During the earlier years of the 20th century, physicians often advised patients with heart disease to avoid strenuous physical activity, based on the belief that too much physical activity could damage the heart and threaten a person's life. Some cardiologists, however, began to rethink this advice and to recommend aerobic exercise both as an adjunct to standard treatment and as a protection against heart disease. At about the same time, many people began running, not only for cardiovascular health, but also for a variety of other reasons. Later in this section, we examine the evidence for the cardiovascular benefits of exercise, but first we look briefly at the history of exercising for cardiovascular health.

Early Studies

The history of the positive cardiovascular effects of physical activity began in England during the early 1950s and involved London's famous double-decker buses. Jeremy Morris and his colleagues (Morris, Heady, Raffle, Roberts, & Parks, 1953) discovered that physically active male conductors differed from less active bus drivers in the incidence of heart disease. This study, of course, did not prove that physical activity decreases the chances of coronary heart disease (CHD), because these two groups of workers may have been selected for jobs on the basis of body type, personality, or some other factor associated with a high or low risk of CHD.

Ten years later, Harold Kahn (1963) investigated the relationship between physical activity and heart disease among postal workers in Washington, D.C. When Kahn compared the death rates among sedentary postal workers versus the more active mail carriers, he found lower CHD death rates among the active men. A more important finding was that the potential benefits from past activity disappeared after a few years. When mail carriers switched to more sedentary clerical jobs, their rates of CHD changed. After more than 5 years of working as a clerk, former carriers had an incidence of death from CHD equal to that of men who had always been clerks. This finding suggested that exercise should be incorporated into one's lifestyle on a continuing basis.

These studies seemed to indicate that workers who are physically active have a reduced risk of coronary heart disease. However, the studies did not address the problem of self-selection that clouds any conclusion about exercise benefits. Furthermore, none of the early studies measured the workers' activity levels off the job. Most of these issues have been addressed in more recent studies, including a series of investigations by Ralph Paffenbarger, a professor of epidemiology at the Stanford University School of Medicine. Paffenbarger investigated the relationship between physical activity and health in two large populations of participants: San Francisco longshoremen and Harvard alumni.

In the early 1970s, Paffenbarger and his associates (Paffenbarger, Gima, Laughlin, & Black, 1971; Paffenbarger, Laughlin, Gima, & Black, 1970) published several reports of a study involving a large number of San Francisco longshoremen whom they had followed since 1951. In general, they found that CHD death rates were much higher for workers with low versus high activity. In these studies, the problem of initial self-selection was not a major factor, because all workers in both the high- and low-activity groups had begun their employment with at least 5 years of strenuous cargo handling. From these and other studies, Paffenbarger concluded that high-intensity exercise produces a training effect that protects against coronary heart disease.

In the late 1970s, Paffenbarger and his associates (Paffenbarger, Wing, & Hyde, 1978) published a landmark epidemiological investigation that avoided most of the flaws found in earlier studies. These investigators found extensive medical records of former Harvard University students dating back to 1916 and sent detailed questionnaires to the men who were still living.

To measure the weekly total energy expenditure of these men, the investigators used a composite physical activity index that took into account all activity, both on and off the job. By asking these men such questions as how many flights of stairs they climbed, how far they walked, and what sports they played and for how long, the investigators were able to arrive at an estimate of energy expenditure per week, measured in kilocalories (kcal). For example, walking up one flight of 10 stairs per day was equated to 28 kcal, light sports such as golf or softball were rated at 5 kcal per minute, and strenuous sports such as running, skiing, or swimming were rated at 10 kcal per minute.

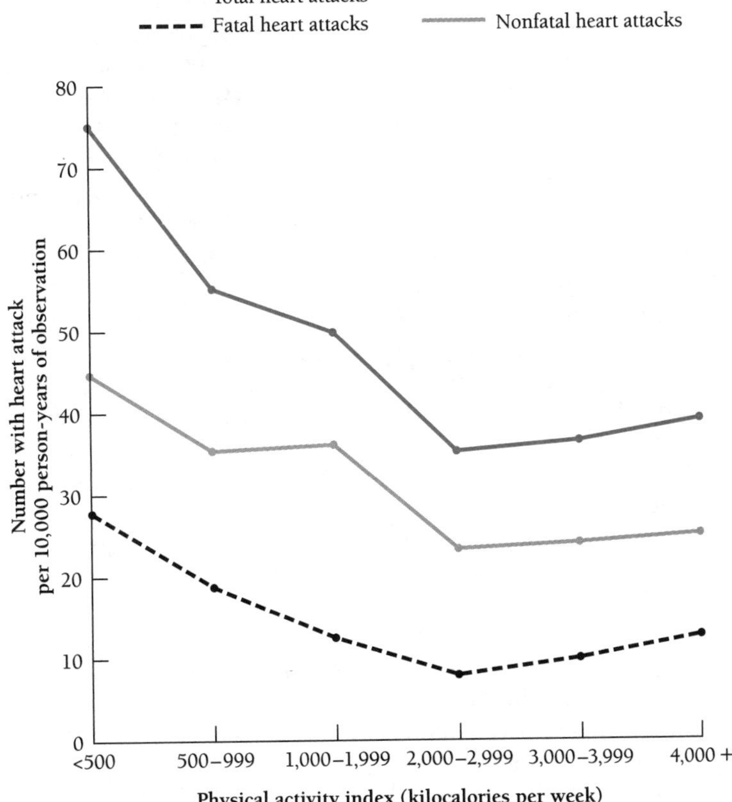

Figure 16.1 Age-adjusted first heart attack rates by physical activity index in a 6- to 10-year follow-up of male Harvard alumni.

Source: Adapted from "Physical activity as an index of heart attack risk in college alumni," by R. S. Paffenbarger, Jr., A. L Wing, and R. T. Hyde, 1978, American Journal of Epidemiology, 108, *p. 166. Copyright © 1978 by The Johns Hopkins University School of Hygiene and Public Health. Adapted by permission of the publisher and Dr. Paffenbarger.*

Paffenbarger et al. then divided the Harvard alumni into high- and low-activity groups. Of those men whose energy levels could be determined, about 60% expended fewer than 2,000 kcal per week and were thus placed in the low-activity group; the 40% who expended more than 2,000 kcal made up the high-activity group. (Note that 2,000 kcal of energy is approximately that expended in 20 miles of jogging or its equivalent.)

Paffenbarger et al. (1978) reported that the least active Harvard alumni had an increased risk of heart attack over their more physically active classmates, with 2,000 kcal per week as the breaking point. In addition, exercise benefited men who smoked and/or had a history of hypertension. Beyond the 2,000 kcal. per week expenditure, increased exercise paid no dividends in terms of reduced risk of fatal or nonfatal heart attacks. Figure 16.1 shows this relationship.

Later Studies

In October of 2000, an international panel of scientists met in Toronto to hold a symposium on evidence for a dose-response relationship between physical activity and several measures of health, including cardiovascular disease and all-cause mortality (Bouchard, 2001; Kesaniemi et al., 2001). Recall that a dose-response relationship is a direct, consistent association between an independent variable, such as physical activity, and a dependent variable, such as heart disease or all-cause mortality. Panelists at this conference evaluated existing research, giving most weight to randomized, controlled trials. In general, a review of the research found a consistent inverse association between levels of physical activity and cardiovascular disease for both women and men (Kohl, 2001). This review found that even minimal levels of exercise provided some protection against cardiovascular disease. Another review from this symposium (Lee & Skerrett, 2001) concluded that a strong dose-response relationship existed between physical activity and premature death and that higher levels were proportionately related to lower death rates.

Steven Blair and his team from the Cooper Institute in Dallas (Blair, Cheng, & Holder, 2001) presented yet another review from the Toronto symposium, one that included both physical fitness and physical activity. Their review of 67 well-designed studies showed an inverse, dose-response relationship between both fitness and activity with coronary heart disease and stroke. However, Blair et al. were not able to learn whether physical fitness or physical activity provided the better protection against cardiovascular disease. These reports yield compelling evidence that physical activity, even small amounts, has therapeutic value.

Evidence is also beginning to show cardiovascular benefits among people in a variety of nations and different ethnic groups. For example, a group of researchers in Nigeria (Forrest et al., 2001) found that a lack of occupational and leisure-time physical activity was related to an unfavorable body mass index, high blood pressure, and high cholesterol, all known risk factors for heart disease. Many Mexican Americans are at risk for obesity, high cholesterol, and other cardiovascular risk factors, which suggests that they can probably profit from a routine exercise program. A study of Mexican Americans in the San Antonio Heart Study (Rainwater et al., 2000) found that changes in physical activity over a 5-year period tended to mirror changes in CVD risk factors. The evidence was somewhat stronger for men than for women and for participants who were lean at the beginning of the study than for heavy ones.

Finally, Jonathan Myers (2000) reviewed 4 decades of studies and provided several important pieces of information on the association between physical activity and cardiovascular disease. First, people who are already active received some gains by increasing their level of activity, but the largest cardiovascular gains occurred when people went from a sedentary lifestyle to an active one. Second, walking, especially for older people, has been found to confer protection against CVD. Third, an inactive lifestyle was shown to be equal to diabetes, cholesterol level, smoking, and high blood pressure as a CVD risk factor. Fourth, physically fit men and women in all age groups reduced their CVD risk through leisure-time activities. Fifth, exercise accumulated several years ago does not provide much current protection against all-cause mortality. Similarly, people who survived a heart attack and who included physical activity as part of their cardiac rehabilitation program decreased their all-cause mortality as well as their risk for a subsequent heart attack. However, those benefits disappeared after 5 years, if participants stopped exercising. Thus, because previous physical activity loses its benefit after a few years, heart attack survivors should maintain an exercise program.

These and other recent reports suggest that a lifestyle that includes at least some physical activity can help protect people against premature cardiovascular disease. Even small amounts of activity can help, but more is better, at least to a point. (In a later section, we discuss how much is enough without being too much.)

Do Women and Men Benefit Equally?

All the earlier studies on the cardiovascular effects of exercise had one important limitation: they focused exclusively on men. To complete the picture of the health benefits of exercise, later researchers extended their investigations to women. Gender differences in degree of physical activity, leisure-time activity, and job-related activity might suggest differences between men and women in their level of protection against cardiovascular disease and all-cause mortality.

A number of recent studies have looked exclusively at women to see if benefits of physical activity extend equally to them. For example, a study of postmenopausal women in Iowa (Kushi, et al., 1997) found that older women who exercised moderately at least four times a week had much lower rates of all-cause mortality than women who were sedentary. Even moderate physical activity once a week significantly reduced the chances of death from CVD. In this study, vigorous activity also reduced death rates but was not superior to moderate physical activity. A report from the Nurses' Health Study (Rockhill et al., 2001) showed that active middle-aged and older women can reduce their risk for death by 20% to 30% and that the benefits of exercise is stronger for cardiovascular disease than it is for cancer.

Palph Paffenbarger and his associates (Oguma, Sesso, Paffenbarger, & Lee, 2002) looked at 37 prospective cohort studies and one retrospective study that dealt with the association between all-cause mortality and both physical activity and physical fitness in women. This review attempted to answer five questions pertaining to women and physical activity and fitness. First, do highly active women postpone death by their activity? Second, do gender differences exist regarding physical activity and all-cause mortality? Third, is there a dose-response relationship between levels of activity in women and mortality? Fourth, how much physical activity is required for women to benefit? Fifth, does age play a role in the relationship between physical activity and all-cause morality in women?

How does current research answer these five questions? The review by Oguma et al., generally found that women can gain about as much as men from physical activity. First, active women were 34% less likely than the least active (or least fit) women to have died during the study period. Second, studies with men yielded almost exactly the same results as that of women. Third, evidence is not robust for a dose-response relationship between levels of physical activity and all-cause mortality in women. Fourth, the reviewers estimated that an energy expenditure of about 1,000 kcal per week is probably adequate to avoid premature death. (See Figure 16.1 for a relationship between level of kcal and first heart attack in men.) Fifth, women below age 55 probably benefit more from exercise than do older women.

In summary, both women and men can improve their cardiovascular health and live longer by light to moderate exercise. Physically activity people can expect an average increase in longevity of about 2 years (Blair et al., 2001; USDHHS, 1996). A cynic might criticize this finding by pointing out that a person would need to jog a total of about 2 years between the ages of 20 and 80 to increase longevity by 2 years. Why live another 2 years if one spends that time exercising? However, physical activity does not merely extend the life span 2 years at the end, but it adds quality years throughout a person's life. Remaining physically active not only protects against disability, disease, and death but also contributes to enhanced health in all age groups. People who are overweight, who smoke, and who have high cholesterol levels can lower their risks of heart disease by light to moderate exercise, for example by walking at least 1 hour a week (Vita, Terry, Hubert, & Fries, 1998).

Physical Activity and Cholesterol Levels

How does exercise protect against cardiovascular disease? Some evidence, from both animal and human studies, suggests that exercise may increase high-density lipoprotein (HDL), the so-called "good" cholesterol. In addition, a program of regular physical activity may actually lower LDL, the "bad" cholesterol. If both processes occurred, total cholesterol might remain the same, but the ratio of total cholesterol to HDL would become more favorable, and the risk for heart disease would decrease. Some investigators have conducted experiments on animals to determine the effects of exercise on cholesterol and atherosclerosis. For example, one study (Kramsch et al., 1981) demonstrated that exercise can have a beneficial effect on the cardiovascular system of monkeys fed a diet high in cholesterol. Compared with sedentary monkeys, physically active monkeys had significantly higher HDL levels, lower LDL levels, less narrowing of arteries, and fewer sudden deaths.

Studies with humans have generally found that moderate levels of exercise, with or without dietary changes, bring about a favorable ratio of total cholesterol to HDL. Reviews of studies from the Toronto symposium (Leon & Sanchez, 2001; Williams, 2001) generally found moderate exercise, such as walking and gardening, increases HDL and less frequently decreases both LDL and triglycerides. Thus, moderate activity may lead to a favorable ratio of total cholesterol to HDL, but prolonged strenuous physical activity does not seem to confer additional protection against heart disease; that is, there is inconsistent evidence for a dose-response relationship between varying levels of physical activity and death from heart disease (Leon & Sanchez, 2001).

If adults can improve their lipid numbers through moderate exercise, could children and adolescents also benefit from regular physical activity? A study of male and female 12-, 15-, and 18-year-olds (Raitakari et al., 1994) found differences in lipid profiles of the physically active and the physically inactive. Physically active male participants had lower triglycerides, higher HDL, and a lower total cholesterol to HDL ratio. Similarly, physically active female participants had lower triglycerides and lower body fat than their inactive peers. These studies suggest that regular aerobic exercise may protect against heart disease by increasing HDL and by improving the ratio of total cholesterol to HDL and that prolonged vigorous activity is unnecessary.

Physical Activity and Stroke

Physical activity does not seem to be as strong a protector against stroke as it is against heart disease, or at least the evidence is less clear. For example, evidence from one study (Gillum, Mussolino, & Ingram, 1996) indicated that being sedenary doubled the risk for European American women for both fatal and nonfatal stroke. However, the risk was only slight for African American women, African American men, and European American men. On the other hand, the Framingham study (Kiely, Wolf, Cupples, Beiser, & Kannel, 1994) found almost the opposite results: physical activity did not seem to lower women's risk but significantly reduced men's risk of stroke. Yet another study (Abbott, Rodriguez, Burchfiel, & Curb, 1994) found that older sedentary men, compared with active men of the same age, were three to four times more likely to have a stroke, but this relationship did not hold true for middle-aged men. Recent studies have not clarified the relationship between physical activity and stroke. Researchers from the Nurses' Health Study (Hu, Stampfer, Colditz, et al., 2000) found that the most active women, compared with sedentary women, reduced their risk of death from ischemic stroke but not other types of stroke.

In summary, physical activity seems to offer some protection against stroke for middle-aged and older men and women, but the evidence remains inconsistent. Because stroke is far less common than coronary heart disease among middle-aged people, exercise does not save as many lives lost to stroke as it does to heart disease. However, as people become older and more prone to stroke, the benefits of physical activity become more dramatic.

In Summary

For 50 years, evidence has accumulated suggesting a positive relationship between physical activity and reduced incidence of coronary heart disease. The early studies had many flaws and tended to include only men. However, later research has confirmed a strong association between a regimen of moderate physical activity and coronary health. Regular activity also protects both women and men against stroke, but this protection is not as strong as it is for heart disease. In addition, physical activity can raise HDL, thereby improving the ratio of total cholesterol to high-density lipoprotein. In addition, regular activity may add as much as 2 years to one's life while decreasing disability, especially in later years.

Other Health Benefits of Physical Activity

Besides contributing to physical fitness, weight control, and cardiovascular health, regular exercise confers several other health benefits, including protection against some kinds of cancer, prevention of bone density loss, control of diabetes, and improved sleep. In addition, regular physical activity appears to offer several psychological benefits, including a defense against depression, a reduction of anxiety, a buffer against stress, and a contributor to high self-esteem.

Protection against Cancer

Although most people who exercise do so for physical fitness, weight control, or cardiovascular health, recent studies have associated physical activity with reduced chances of some cancers. Two recent, comprehensive reviews (Batty & Thune, 2000; Thune & Furberg, 2001) have summarized much of the literature on the connection between physical activity and various cancers. Several key findings emerged from these reviews.

First, of more than 200 studies during the past decade, most have examined cancers of colon and rectum, breast, endometrium, prostate, testes, and lung. Second, measures of both occupational activity and leisure-time activity yielded an inverse relationship with cancer of all sites, and findings showed a dose-response relationship for both genders. Third, both meta-analyses and systematic reviews indicate an inverse dose-response relationship between physical activity and colon cancer, with physically active women and men having only about half the risk as their sedentary counterparts. Fourth, evidence for a relationship between physical activity and breast cancer is less clear and depends on age at diagnosis, body mass index, and whether or not the women are pre- or postmenopausal. Young, premenopausal, thin women probably gain most from physical activity. Fifth, although most studies show an inverse relationship between physical activity and both prostate and testicular cancers, the evidence remains inconsistent. Sixth, the few case-control, prospective studies that looked at lung cancer generally revealed an inverse dose-response relationship for physical activity and lung cancer in men, but additional studies need to be conducted on both men and women before this relationship becomes more firmly established.

More recent research in different cultures has added to growing evidence for an inverse relationship between physical activity and cancer. For example, a study in the Netherlands (Van der Kooy, Rookus, Verloop, Van Leeuwen, & Peterse, 2001) of lifetime physical activity (recreational, occupational, and housekeeping) found women's risk of breast cancer reduced by 25%, and a study from Alberta, Canada (Friedenreich, Bryant, & Courneya, 2001) also found benefit for lifetime physical activity as a protection against postmenopausal breast cancer. Finally, vigorous physical activity reduces breast cancer in both Hispanic and non-Hispanic white women, especially postmenopausal women (Gilliland et al., 2001).

To review, recent research suggests that physical activity may protect against many cancers, including cancer of all sites. The inverse relationship between physical activity and colon cancer is at least as strong as the association between physical activity and cardiovascular mortality. Exercise also protects women against breast cancer, whereas evidence for protection against prostate, testicular, and lung cancer remains somewhat inconsistent.

Prevention of Bone Density Loss

Exercise has also been recommended as a protection against **osteoporosis,** a disorder characterized by a reduction in bone density due to calcium loss and resulting in brittle bones. Is this recommendation valid? An early review of research (Harris, Caspersen, DeFriese, & Estes, 1989) concluded that physical activity offers strong protection against osteoporosis in postmenopausal women but is less effective in preventing this disorder in premenopausal women.

Since this review, evidence has accrued suggesting that physical activity can protect both men and women against loss of bone mineral density, especially if they have a history of lifetime activity. For example, a retrospective study (Greendale, Barrett-Connor, Edelstein, Ingles, & Halle, 1995) asked a group of older men and women to recall their level of physical activity as teenagers, at age 30, and at age 50. They found that both men and women with a history of physical activity had more bone mineral density than the more sedentary people but about the same number of bone fractures. Other retrospective studies (Jagal, Kreiger, & Darlington, 1993; Zhang, Feldblum, & Fortney, 1992) found a relationship between lifetime physical activity and current levels of bone mineral density, suggesting that people who exercised regularly continued to be protected against loss of bone mineral density.

A study in Denmark (Høldrup et al., 2001) found that moderate exercise reduced hip fractures in both men and women by about 25%, but that more vigorous physical activity did not add to the protective effect. Also, people who were formerly active, but who reduced their level of activity to the point of being sedentary, lost their protection. Also, the NHANES III study (Mussolino, Looker, & Orwoll, 2001) reported that men who jogged nine or more times a month had significantly higher levels of bone mineral density than men who jogged one to eight time per month.

Starting an exercise program may help older women retain bone mineral density. An experimental study of previously sedentary women ages 50 to 70 (Nelson, Fiatarone, et al., 1994) divided participants into a control group that remained sedentary and an exercise group that began moderate physical activity. Women in the exercise group preserved their bone mineral content, whereas those in the sedentary control group experienced a decrease in bone mineral density. Moreover, the exercise group increased muscle mass and muscle strength.

This body of research suggests that children and adolescents should begin a regular exercise program and continue moderate physical activity into old age as a protection against a variety of disorders, including loss of bone mineral density and osteoporosis.

Control of Diabetes

Because obesity is a factor in Type 2 diabetes and because exercise is an established means of controlling weight, it follows that physical activity may be a useful weapon in the control of diabetes.

Frank Hu and his associates (Hu, Leitzmann, et al., 2001) recorded the amount of TV viewing in middle-aged and older men and discovered two important findings. First, physical activity has an inverse dose-response relationship with Type 2 diabetes, and second, the risk for developing Type 2 diabetes is positively related to number of hours watching television. Men who watched 40 or more hours of TV per week were nearly three times as likely to develop diabetes, compared with men who watched less than an hour per week. Again, a clear dose-response relationship emerged; the more TV these men watched, the more likely they were to become diagnosed with Type 2 diabetes. Even after adjusting for body mass index, a strong relationship remained. Researchers in England (Wannamethee, Shaper, & Alberti, 2000) found that physical activity had an inverse dose-response relationship with the development of diabetes but only an inverse relationship with coronary heart disease. In other words, more physical activity is better for preventing Type 2 diabetes but more is not better with regard to heart disease.

Does physical activity protect Type 1 diabetics against early death? One study (Moy et al., 1993) followed insulin-dependent mostly European American male and female children and adolescents and found that sedentary male diabetics were three times more likely to die than more active male diabetics. However, the trend for female diabetics was not as pronounced.

Although these studies reported a modest protective benefit for physical activity, they do not suggest that exercise is a panacea for the control of diabetes. Nevertheless, they do indicate that physical activity can be a useful adjunct in the treatment of insulin-dependent diabetes and can offer some protection against the development of noninsulin-dependent diabetes.

Aid to Sleep

Can physical activity help people sleep better? Emerging evidence suggests that the answer is yes. One study (King, Oman, Brassington, Bliwise, & Haskell, 1997) found that moderate exercise can help at least some people improve their sleep. Participants in this investigation were sedentary men and women, 50 to 76 years of age with moderate sleep complaints; that is, they took at least 25 minutes to fall asleep and then slept for only about 6 hours.

The researchers divided participants into an experimental (exercise) group and a wait-list (control) group. Participants in the experimental group engaged in 30 to 40 minutes of brisk walking four times a week, whereas those in the control group remained sedentary. After 16 weeks, people in the exercise group showed significant improvements in sleep; they decreased sleep onset by 15 minutes and increased sleep duration by 45 minutes. The authors concluded that 8 weeks of moderate, regular exercise may be needed to obtain these benefits.

Physical activity also helps people with more severe sleep disorders to sleep better. Researchers from the Tucson Epidemiological Study of Obstructive Airways Disease (Sherrill, Kotchou, & Quan, 1998) defined sleep disorders as difficulty in maintaining sleep, excessive daily sleepiness, nightmares, and any other sleep problems. Relying on self-reports of both sleep problems and level of physical activity, the authors found that both men and women could significantly reduce their sleep disorders by walking at a normal pace six blocks a day. Although these studies show promise, more research is needed before physical activity can be prescribed as treatment for sleep disorders.

Psychological Benefits of Physical Activity

The physiological benefits of physical activity are well established, but what about the psychological benefits? Can exercise lessen depression, reduce anxiety, lower stress levels, and enhance self-esteem? People who exercise list psychological reasons nearly as often as physiological ones when asked about the benefits they receive from exercise. Does the evidence support these claims?

William P. Morgan, one of the leading authorities in this area, believes that physical activity has great potential for treating and preventing some psychological disorders. Nevertheless, Morgan (1997) insists that most of the current research on this topic has serious methodological problems and that some enthusiastic conclusions are based more on wishful thinking than on scientific evidence. In general, the link between physical activity and psychological functioning is less clearly established than the one between physical activity and physiological health. In addition, any evaluation of the therapeutic effects of exercise on psychological disorders must consider the problems raised by the placebo effect. Few studies on the psychological benefits of physical activity have sufficiently controlled for the 35% to 38% improvement that might be expected from a

WOULD YOU BELIEVE

It's Never Too Late—Or Too Early

Physical activity is a healthy habit at any point in the lifespan, but would you believe that it's never too late to start exercising? Or too early?

Older adults benefit from being physically active in many ways. Cardiovascular benefits include lower blood pressure, improved symptoms of congestive heat failure, and decreased risk for cardiovascular disease (Karani, McLaughlin, & Cassel, 2001). In addition, physically active older adults have lower risk for diabetes, osteoporosis, osteoarthritis, and depression. All of these benefits result in lowered sickness and death among physically active older adults.

Despite these many benefits, 75% of older adults in the United States are sedentary. People tend to become less active as they age, and they also reduce their exercising when they experience pain (Nied & Franklin, 2002). For example, arthritis causes knee and hip joint pain that makes older people less willing to exercise. Also, people who have had a stroke may experience balance or weakness problems that make them feel uneasy about even normal levels of activity. Older people are more likely than younger ones to fall, and resulting broken bones may make a permanent change in their mobility and independence. Although all of these concerns have some foundation, the risks are manageable. Physical activity offers more benefits than risks for older people, even for those over age 85 and for those who are frail. They may need supervision for their exercise and profit from consulting a professional to obtain a personally tailored program, but almost all older people decrease health risks and gain mobility from exercising.

Very young children may not seem to be at any risk from inactivity, but they are. To maintain their goals of safety and convenience, parents and caregivers often confine infants in strollers, infant seats, or playpens that limit their movement (National Association for Sport and Physical Education, 2002). These experiences not only limit mobility during infancy but may also delay developmental goals such as crawling and walking and lay the foundation for a sedentary life. As toddlers and preschoolers, inactive children may also lag in developing motor skills and join the growing number of overweight and obese children in the United States (Strauss & Pollack, 2001).

The National Association for Sport and Physical Education (NASPE, 2002) proposed guidelines for physical activity, beginning during infancy. For all children, NASPE emphasized supervision and safety. The recommendations for infants include allowing them to experience settings in which they can move while maintaining safety and playing a variety of games such as peekaboo. For toddlers, NASPE recommends at least 30 minutes a day of structured physical activity and 60 minutes for preschool children. Scott Roberts (2002) went a step farther, recommending workouts for children. He argued that the prohibitions against weightlifting and other types of strength training for children have no research basis. On the contrary, Roberts maintained that children experience the same benefits from this type of exercise as adults, including protection against cardiovascular disease, hypertension, and obesity as well as improved strength, flexibility, and posture.

Would you believe that age—any age—is not an excuse to be inactive. It's never too late to benefit from exercise, and it's also never too early to begin an active lifestyle. Physical activity furnishes lifetime benefits, so anytime during the lifespan is a good time to start.

placebo effect alone. Although a causal relationship between physical activity and improved psychological health has not yet been firmly established, some correlational evidence suggests that a regular exercise regimen can decrease depression, reduce anxiety, buffer stress, and raise self-esteem.

Decreased Depression The *Diagnostic and Statistical Manual of Mental Disorders (DSM-IV-Text Revision)* of the American Psychiatric Association (2000) defines a major depressive episode as "a period of at least 2 weeks during which there is either depressed mood or the loss of interest or pleasure in nearly all activities"

(p. 349). During a lifetime, as many as 25% of women and 12% of men may suffer from major depression (APA, 2000). If physical activity can relieve major depression, then millions of people can benefit from a therapy that is easily available to nearly everyone.

People who exercise regularly are generally less depressed than sedentary people. When groups of exercisers are compared to groups of sedentary people on different measures of depression, highly active people are usually less depressed, but such data do not reveal the direction of causation. Depressed people may simply be less motivated to exercise.

However, a randomized, controlled trial with older depressed participants (Singh, Clements, & Singh, 2001) presented strong evidence that noninstitutionalized depressed individuals can lower their depression scores by a program of weight lifting. Participants in the experimental group received 10 weeks of supervised weight lifting followed to 10 weeks of unsupervised exercise; participants in the control group received 10 weeks of lecture followed by no contact with the experimenters. Depression for both groups was measured by standardized depression inventories both before and after the exercise intervention. After 20 weeks, participants in the unsupervised weight-lifting group, compared with those in the lecture group, had significantly lower depression scores. This suggests the relationship between physical activity and depression is not simply due to higher levels of motivation by nondepressed people. Additional evidence for direction of the inverse relationship between physical activity and depression comes from a study of rats (Moraska & Fleshner, 2001). In this study, rats that were allowed to exercise showed fewer stress-related behaviors than those that did not exercise, indicating that exercise may buffer the negative aspects of depression.

Can physical activity, either alone or as an adjunct to drug therapy and psychotherapy, reduce clinical depression? One pioneer in running therapy is John Greist, who along with his associates (Greist, 1984; Greist, Eischens, Klein, & Linn, 1981; Greist & Greist, 1979; Greist et al., 1978, 1979), has found tentative evidence supporting the use of running as a treatment for depression. In a pilot study, Greist et al. (1978) assigned moderately depressed men and women either to a running group or to one of two kinds of individual psychotherapy—time limited or time unlimited. Patients in the running group received no conventional psychotherapy and were not permitted to talk about their depression during running therapy. As a whole, patients who received the running treatment were somewhat less depressed after treatment than those in either the time-limited or the time-unlimited therapy group.

Since this early study, several other investigators have examined the usefulness of running as a psychotherapeutic tool. For example, Greist (1984) randomly assigned depressed patients to one of three treatment groups: aerobic exercise, Benson's (1975) relaxation training, or group psychotherapy. At the end of a 3-month follow-up, only the exercise and relaxation groups showed improvement. A later study (Bosscher, 1993) randomly assigned depressed inpatients to either a short-term running program or to a treatment-as-usual program, which included both physical and relaxation exercises. Patients in the running program increased their self-esteem and lowered their depressive symptoms, whereas patients in the treatment-as-usual group showed no significant improvements.

A review of research on the effectiveness of physical activity as treatment for clinical depression (Martinsen & Morgan, 1997) led to the conclusions that: (1) aerobic exercise is more effective than no treatment; (2) physical activity is at least as effective as psychotherapy; (3), aerobic and nonaerobic exercise seem to be equally effective in treating depression, (4) no dose-response relationship exists between aerobic exercise and decreased amounts of depression; that is, depressed patients do not continue to benefit from increasing levels of physical activity; (5) to date, no evidence exists showing the therapeutic value of exercise for severe forms of major depression, and (6) evidence does not yet exist that exercise can prevent relapse into a major depression. In addition, there are no well-controlled studies comparing the effectiveness of physical activity and drug therapy for depressed patients.

Martinsen and Morgan (1997, p. 105) concluded that "physical exercise may be an alternate or adjunct to traditional forms of treatment in mild to moderate forms of unipolar depression." Despite this therapeutic potential, few health psychologists possess the training in exercise physiology and cardiovascular medicine to supervise exercise programs without the aid of physicians, athletic trainers, or others trained in this area.

Reduced Anxiety Many people report that they exercise to feel more relaxed and less anxious. Does exercise play a role in anxiety reduction? The answer may depend on the type of anxiety. **Trait anxiety** is a general personality characteristic or trait that manifests itself as a more or less constant feeling of dread or uneasiness. **State anxiety** is a temporary, affective condition that stems from a specific situation. Feelings of worry or concern over a final examination or a job interview are examples of state anxiety. This type of anxiety is usually accompanied by physiological changes, such as increased perspiration and rapid heart rate.

Research on the effects of physical activity on trait and state anxiety suffers from many of the same methodological limitations as research on physical activity and depression: that is, only a few of the studies have had an adequate number of participants and have used random assignment to experimental, placebo, or control groups (Dunn, Trivedi, & O'Neal, 2001).

Nevertheless, sufficient evidence suggests that a moderate program of physical activity can reduce both trait and state anxiety, at least in some people (Raglin, 1997). Moreover, exercise need not be aerobic or vigorous to be effective. As one would expect, highly anxious people experience a greater decrease in anxiety than do people with lower levels, but both groups can profit from moderate physical activity. A report from the Toronto symposium (Dunn et al., 2001) looked at more than 100 studies on physical activity and anxiety and found significant benefit for aerobic exercise. However, the review found little evidence for a dose-response effect, largely due to a lack of randomized controlled trials.

How does physical activity help reduce anxiety? One hypothesis is that exercise simply provides a change of pace—a chance to relax and forget one's troubles. In support of this change of pace hypothesis, exercise demonstrated no stronger therapeutic effect than meditation (Bahrke & Morgan, 1978). Studies that have shown that other techniques to reduce anxiety, including biofeedback, transcendental meditation, "time out" therapy, and even beer drinking in a pub atmosphere, can also be effective (Morgan, 1981). Each of these interventions provides a change of pace and all have been demonstrated to be associated with reduced levels of state anxiety.

Although any one of a variety of interventions that break into a stressful daily routine may help relieve anxiety, physical activity seems particularly suitable. From a practical standpoint, walking and jogging have several advantages over most other forms of treatment: they can be done by almost anyone, nearly anywhere, and with very little expense.

Buffer against Stress Can exercise reduce stress? More importantly, can it protect people against the harmful effects of stress? Research on the first question has generally produced an affirmative answer. For example, many people view exercise as the most effective strategy for reducing tension and eliminating a bad mood (Thayer, Newman, & McClain, 1994).

Answers to the second question are more difficult, because a direct causal link between stress and subsequent illness has not yet been firmly established. Thus, no conclusive evidence exists for exercise's buffering effects. However, several studies suggest that physical activity helps people deal with stress. One study (Sonnentag, 2001) showed that leisure activities, including sports participation, were one factor that helped protect people against workplace stress. Another study (Carmack, Boudreaux, Amaral, Brantley, & de Moor, 1999) investigated the role of exercise as a moderator in the stress-illness relationship. The results suggested a buffering effect for participation in leisure physical activities. Thus, these naturalistic studies suggest that exercise plays a buffering role against stress.

More controlled studies have also indicated that exercise can ameliorate stress. Exercise can moderate the effects of laboratory stressors—such as video games or mental arithmetic tasks—on cardiovascular reactivity in mildly hypertensive people (Perkins, Dubbert, Martin, Faulstich, & Harris, 1986). Another study (Castro, Wilcox, O'Sullivan, Bauman, & King, 2002) tested the effects of exercise on women who provided primary caregiving for people with dementia by assigning half to an exercise program. After a year, those in the exercise group reported that exercise improved their perceived stress.

Therefore, both naturalistic and controlled studies demonstrate that exercise can help people with stress. Even more promising, the duration of exercise required to produce positive effects is not extreme: as little as 10 minutes of moderately strenuous exercise is capable to elevating mood (Hansen, Stevens, & Coast, 2001). The results of the studies on stress buffering do not indicate a strong effect for exercise, but physical activity is a strategy that many people use to help them manage stress. Figure 16.2 shows some of the positive effects of exercise.

Increased Self-Esteem Do people who exercise regularly increase their self-esteem? Do they have more self-confidence and improved feelings of self-worth? In the previous sections, we saw that exercise is associated with decreases in both depression and anxiety and that it may have some ability to buffer stress. This section considers the possibility that exercise might be related to increases in self-esteem.

Reviews of the literature dealing with the relationship between exercise and self-esteem (Sonstroem, 1984, 1997) revealed that the majority of studies showed a significant positive relationship between self-esteem and exercise. Although these studies suggested that exercise raises self-esteem, their methodological limitations prevent this conclusion. Few of the studies employed an experimental design, with random assignment to experimental, placebo, or control groups. Also, no single definition of self-esteem was used. Many studies adopted a global definition, defining self-esteem as having a positive feeling about oneself. Such broad definitions confound any relationship between exercise and self-esteem. That is, adherence to a regular exercise program may improve physical health, enhance body image, raise physical fitness, boost feelings of self-mastery, increase social support, bolster feelings of self-control, or improve physical self-efficacy. Any one or combination of these factors can lead to better feelings about oneself. Despite attempts to identify a more precise pathway through which physical activity relates to self-esteem (Sonstroem, 1997), it may not be necessary to know the exact variables responsible for improved self-esteem as long as increased feelings of self-worth and self-confidence are associated with an exercise program.

We have seen that people who regularly exercise decrease their risk of cardiovascular disease, cancer, and diabetes; improve their cholesterol ratio; sleep better and longer; have lower levels of depression; decrease anxiety; and have fewer stress-related illnesses. Exercise may not be the direct cause of enhanced feelings of self-esteem (Sonstroem, 1984), but it may contribute indirectly through each of these factors, in addition to achieving weight loss, improved appearance, increased levels of physical energy, and greater self-discipline. Participation in an exercise program is strongly associated with feeling good about oneself.

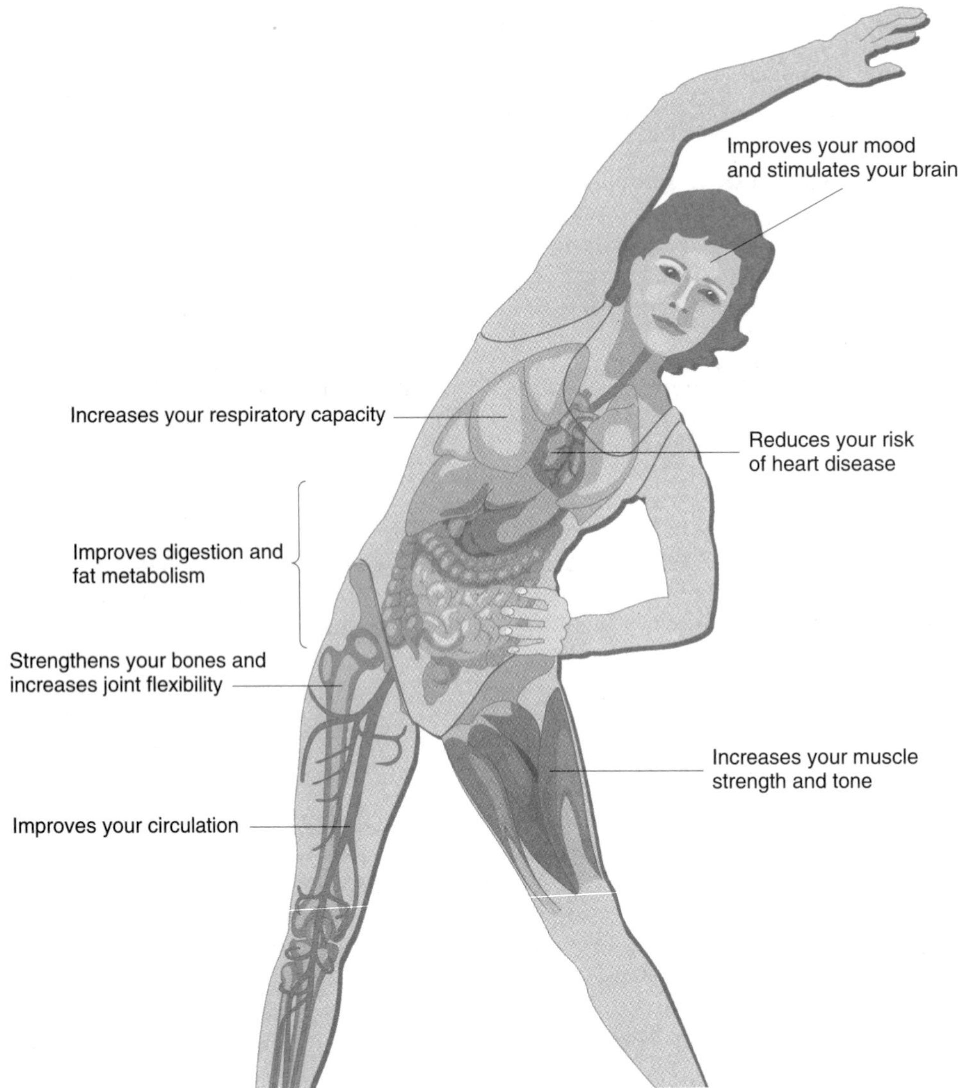

Figure 16.2 Some of the physical and psychological benefits of exercise.

Source: An Invitation to Health *(7th ed. p. 493) by D. Hales, 1997, Pacific Grove, CA: Brooks/Cole. Copyright © 1997 by Brooks/Cole Publishing Company. Reprinted by permission.*

In Summary

During the past 40 years, research has accumulated to support the hypothesis that physical activity is associated with both cardiovascular health and improved psychological functioning. The first Surgeon General's report on physical activity and health (USDHHS, 1996) examined much of that research and found that regular moderate physical activity can reduce the incidence of cardiovascular disease, diabetes, colon cancer, and high blood pressure. Moreover, physical activity can reduce symptoms of depression and anxiety, increase feelings of well-being, and enhance ability to perform daily tasks. The Inter-

TABLE 16.1 *Reasons for Exercising and Research Supporting These Reasons*

Reasons for Exercising	Findings	Principal Source(s)
Physical fitness	Exercise improves several kinds of physical fitness, including cardiovascular fitness.	Lakka et al., 1994; Lee et al., 2001; Blair et al., 2001
Weight control	Exercise is a slow way to burn calories, but it may change setpoint.	Epstein et al., 2000; Marcus et al., 1999; Andersen et al., 1998; Kahn et al., 1997
Increased longevity	Exercise may increase longevity by 2 years or more.	Lee et al., 1995; Oguma et al., 2002; Vita et al., 1998
Protection against cancer	Physical activity has a dose-response effect with colon cancer and an inverse relationship with breast and prostate cancer.	Batty & Thune, 2000; Thune & Furberg, 2001; Blair et al., 2001
Protection against loss of bone mineral density	Lifetime activity protects both men and women against osteoporosis.	Harris et al., 1989; Høldrup et al., 2001; Mussolino et al., 2001
Control of diabetes	Physically active men have an inverse dose-response relationship with Type 2 diabetes.	Hu, Leitzmann et al., 2001; Wannamethee et al., 2000
Aid to sleep	Exercise can reduce sleep disorders, including nightmares.	King et al., 1997; Sherrill et al., 1998
Decreased depression	Exercise can reduce mild and moderate levels of depression.	Singh et al., 2001; Greist et al., 1978; Bosscher, 1993
Reduced anxiety	Moderate amounts of exercise can reduce both state and trait anxiety.	Raglin, 1997; Dunn et al., 2001; Bahrke & Morgan, 1978
Buffer against stress	Exercise may reduce stress, but it probably does not reduce CHD through this mechanism.	Castro et al., 2002; Perkins et al., 1986; Carmack et al., 1999
Enhanced self-esteem	Some studies show a positive relationship between exercise and self-esteem.	Sonstroem, 1997

national Society of Sport Psychology (1992) issued a position statement delineating the benefits of physical activity on both short-term and long-term personal well-being and self-esteem. The society also suggested that physical activity can reduce anxiety and stress and can have a positive effect on hypertension, osteoporosis, and adult-onset diabetes. Moreover, regular exercise is as effective as any form of psychotherapy in lessening depression.

An earlier section of this chapter examined several reasons why people exercise. Table 16.1 lists some of these reasons, summarizes research evidence, and cites at least one study pertaining to each reason.

No strong causal relationship has been established between physical activity and health, because people who exercise regularly generally engage in other health-related activities, such as eating more fruits and vegetables, wearing seat belts, and not smoking (Pate, Heath, Dowda, & Trost, 1996). Nevertheless, sufficient correlational evidence exists to suggest that regular physical activity can be an effective adjunct in the treatment or prevention of cardiovascular disease, some types of cancer, diabetes, osteoporosis, insomnia, depression, anxiety, and stress. In addition, moderate exercise is related to enhanced feelings of well-being, self-esteem, and improved body image.

Hazards of Physical Activity

Although physical activity can enhance physical functioning, reduce anxiety, stress, and depression, and increase feelings of self-esteem, it also poses hazards to one's physical and psychological health. Some athletes overtrain to the point of **staleness** and, as a consequence, suffer from negative mood, fatigue, and depression (O'Connor, 1997). In addition, some highly active people suffer from exercise-related injuries and others allow exercise to assume an almost addictive importance. In this section, we look at some of these potential hazards related to physical activity.

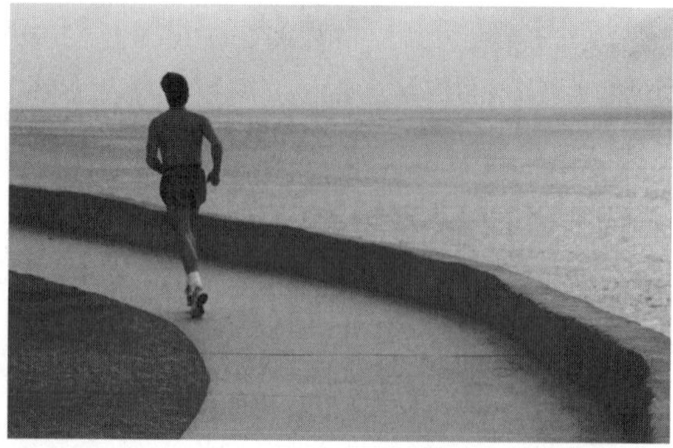

Corbis

Exercise poses hazards as well as benefits for those who exercise vigorously.

Exercise Addiction

Some people become so involved with exercise that they ignore injuries to continue exercising or allow their exercise regimen to interfere with other parts of their lives such as work or family responsibilities. These people are often labeled as having an *exercise addiction,* but their behavior may not match the description of an addiction. In Chapter 14, we saw that addictions produce tolerance, dependence, and withdrawal symptoms.

William Morgan (1979) compared the process of excessive exercising to the development of other addictions. Initially, the tolerance for running is low, and it has many unpleasant side effects. But persistence eases the unpleasant aspects, and the pleasure of meeting goals becomes a powerful reinforcer. Like most social drinkers who have a casual, nonobsessive relationship with alcohol, most exercisers are able to incorporate physical activity into their lives without drastic changes in lifestyle (Rodgers, Hall, Blanchard, & Munroe, 2001). Other exercisers, however, can not. Those who continue to increase their exercise must make changes in their lives to accommodate the time required, with consequences for other responsibilities and activities.

Some people's exercise habits fit the description for dependence: they show a strong emotional attachment to exercise (Ackard, Brehm, & Steffen, 2002) and exhibit withdrawal symptoms such as depression and anxiety when prevented from exercising (Hausenblas & Symons Downs, 2002a). The physiological basis for any addiction to exercise remains unconfirmed, leading some authorities to prefer the term *obligatory exercise* or *exercise dependence* rather than exercise addiction.

Obligatory exercisers share several characteristics that make them similar to anorexics. For example, they continue their chosen activity even when they are injured, continuing behavior that is harmful and even self-destructive. They also show a progressive self-absorption, with a great deal of concentration on internal experiences. In addition, many obligatory exercisers exhibit the type of concentration on thinness and body image that anorexics do. Researchers who noticed these similarities (Yates, Leehey, & Shisslak, 1983) considered the possibility that female anorexics and addicted male runners were analogous; both show the need for mastery of the body, unusually high expectations of self, tolerance or denial of physical discomfort and pain, a single-minded commitment to endurance, and preoccupation with exercise and body image.

Later research revealed a complex relationship between obligatory exercise and eating disorders: not all people with eating disorders exercise excessively, and not all obligatory exercisers have characteristics of eating disorders. Research has confirmed the characteristic of absorption in imagery for obligatory exercisers

(Rodgers et al., 2001). This imagery is not necessarily oriented toward body image, and men are more subject to its influence than are women (Hausenblas & Symons Downs, 2002b). However, some obligatory exercisers have eating disorders. One study (Davis, Kennedy, Ravelski, & Dionne, 1994) looked at women hospitalized for eating disorders and found that more than three fourths of the patients had engaged in excessive exercise, with 60% involved in competitive athletics. Other research (Ackard et al., 2002) found that obligatory exercising has two dimensions. The first describes people who exhibit body obsession, eating disorders, and other psychological problems. For these individuals, the connection between exercising and eating disorders was a strong emotional attachment to exercise. The second dimension includes exercisers who engage in high levels of activity, but who do not show the same problems.

Therefore, a subgroup of obligatory exercisers exhibit eating disorders, but not all do. Even normal eating does not remove the danger from obligatory exercising; these individuals experience injuries yet continue to exercise, neglect their personal relationships, and shortchange their jobs to devote time to exercise. Perhaps this fanaticism can be best expressed in the words of one obligatory runner:

> One day last spring I was having an exceptionally good run. I was running about 10 miles a day at that time and on this particular day I had decided to extend my workout. I was around the 14-mile point and I was preparing to cross a one-lane bridge when all of a sudden a large cement mixer turned the corner and began to cross the bridge. I never thought for a second about stopping and letting the truck pass. I simply continued and said to myself, "Come on you son-of-a-bitch and I'll split you right down the middle—there will be concrete all over the road!" The driver slammed on the brakes and swerved to the side as I sailed by. That was really scary afterward, but at the time I really felt good. I have felt equally strong and indestructible many times since, but never have taken on a cement truck again. (Morgan, 1979, pp. 63, 67)

Injuries from Physical Activity

Excluding head-to-head challenges with cement trucks, what are the chances of experiencing injuries from exercise? Many people with a regular exercise program accept minor injuries and soreness as an almost inevitable component of their program. However, irregular exercise produces even more injuries and more discomfort, with "weekend athletes" accounting for a disproportional number of injuries.

Musculoskeletal injuries are common, and the greater the frequency and intensity of exercise, the more likely people will injure themselves (Cooper, 2001). The Surgeon General's report (USDHHS, 1996) found that about half of runners had experienced an injury during the past year. This review also found, as expected, that the injury rate was lower for walkers than for joggers and that previous injury is a risk factor for subsequent injury. Physical activity is the source of 83% of all musculoskeletal injuries, and at least one fourth of exercisers must interrupt their regimen due to such injuries (Hootman et al., 2002). The decision to decrease exercise in response to injury is a wise one; "working through the pain" is an exercise myth that is associated with further injury (Cooper, 2001).

Besides muscular and skeletal injuries, avid exercisers encounter a number of other health hazards. Heat, cold, dogs, and drivers can all be sources of danger. During exercise, body temperature rises. It can be maintained at 104° F with no danger (Pollock et al., 1978). Fluid intake before, after, and even during exercise can protect against overheating by allowing cooling through sweating. However, conditions of extremely high air temperature, high humidity, and sunlight can combine to raise body temperature and prevent sweat from evaporating from the skin surface. If the body is prevented from cooling itself, dangerous overheating may occur.

Cold temperatures can also be dangerous for outdoor exercising, but proper clothing can provide protection. Layered clothing for the body and gloves, hat, and even a face mask can protect against temperatures of 20° F and below (Pollock et al., 1978). Temperatures below zero, especially when combined with wind, can be dangerous even to people who are not exercising.

Death during Exercise

Many patients who have had a heart attack are put into cardiac rehabilitation programs that include an exercise program, which generally includes close supervision. Although these coronary patients are at an elevated risk during exercise, the cardiovascular benefit they receive from exercising ordinarily outweighs the risk (USDHHS, 1996). Nevertheless, individuals who have been diagnosed as having coronary heart disease should undertake exercise only with a physician's permission and under the supervision of specialists in cardiac rehabilitation.

What about people who have no known disease? Heart-related deaths are more likely during exercise, but those people experience a predictable risk. Is it possible for a person who looks and feels well to die unexpectedly during exercise? Yes—but it is also possible to die unexpectedly while watching TV or sleeping. However, exercise increases the risk of such sudden death. A 12-year follow-up analysis of male physicians (Albert et al., 2000) showed that sudden death was over 16 times more likely during or immediately after vigorous physical exertion than during other times. However, the risk was very low for any specific episode of exercise—1 death per 1.5 million episodes of exercise. This study also showed that the benefits for exercise outweighed the risks: men who exercised regularly were less likely to die during exercise than those who were unaccustomed to exertion. In addition, not all types of exertion are equally risky. Downhill skiing (Burtscher, Pachinger, Mittleman, & Ulmer, 2000) is more likely than sexual activity (Moller et al., 2001) to provoke a fatal heart attack.

Although the men in this follow-up study (Albert et al., 2000) did not identify themselves as having cardiovascular disease when the study began, either they were affected without their knowledge or developed this disease during the 12 years of the study. Most sudden deaths during exercise are the result of some type of heart disease, but people may be unaware of their risks.

Even young people may be vulnerable to sudden cardiac death during exercise (Virmani, Burke, & Farb, 2001). For children, adolescents, and young adults, the cause of sudden cardiac death is most often congenital heart abnormalities or arrhythmias (abnormal heart beat patterns). For adults, about 60% of sudden cardiac deaths are caused by blood clots that precipitate heart attacks, the typical case of the most frequent cause of death in the United States. Thus, most sudden deaths during exercise are individuals who have underlying cardiovascular problems, whether they know it or not.

Reducing Exercise Injuries

Adequate caution can decrease the probability of injury. For people who have or are at risk for cardiovascular disease, supervised training is a wise precaution, especially when initiating an exercise program. Others may also benefit from supervision or training, such as people who have been sedentary for a long time. With the guidance of a trainer, people will be less likely to attempt exercise that is inappropriate for their fitness level or to continue to exercise for too long as they start a program. In addition, an exercise professional will teach proper warm-up and stretching routines that are important in preventing injuries (Cooper, 2001).

Regardless of the level of fitness, the use of appropriate equipment decreases injuries. For example, proper running shoes are a necessity for running, jogging, or even exercise walking (Cooper, 2001). The correct type and amount of clothing are also important either to allow for cooling or to retain heat.

In addition to dressing properly for heat or cold, exercisers need to recognize the symptoms of heat stress (Barber, 2001). Exercise raises body temperature, so hot, humid weather is not a requirement for exercisers to experience trouble. However, exercising during the hottest time of the day is unwise. These risks are greater for children, older individuals, and people whose fitness levels are low, but all exercisers should recognize that dizziness, weakness, nausea, muscle cramps, and headache are symptoms that should signal them to stop exercising. Recognizing when one should stop or decrease the intensity of a workout is a strategy that can prevent many injuries (Cooper, 2001). Exercisers are often so fixed on meeting their daily goals that they lose sight of the moderation that is wise in attaining and retaining overall fitness.

In Summary

Exercise has hazards as well as benefits. Potential hazards include exercise addiction, that is, a compulsive need to devote long periods of time to strenuous physical activity. Also, exercise may lead to injuries, the majority of which are musculoskeletal and relatively minor. Exercisers should also avoid working out in extremes temperatures, and they should know how to avoid dogs, drivers, and darkness. Death during exercise is a possibility. The people who are most vulnerable are older individuals with cardiovascular disease, but young people with heart abnormalities are also at risk. Nevertheless, people who exercise regularly are much less likely than sporadic exercisers to die of a heart attack during intense physical exertion. Exercise-related injuries can be reduced by appropriate preparation such as choosing the appropriate level of exercise, using appropriate equipment, and recognizing signs of trouble and reacting appropriately.

How Much Is Enough but Not Too Much?

During the 1980s, many people, perhaps led by devoted runner/writers such as Jim Fixx, believed that they had to achieve aerobic fitness through vigorous exercise if they were to enhance their health. At the same time, Ralph Paffenbarger and his colleagues were reporting that high levels of physical activity were more beneficial than moderate levels. Based on research at that time, health professionals were advising people to structure their exercise program around at least 20 minutes of sustained activity at an intensity level of 50% to 85% of their maximum heart rate for 4 or 5 days a week. At the apex of the running epoch, Kenneth Cooper (1985) said that anyone who ran more than 15 miles a week was running for reasons other than health. That statement, which seemed quite moderate at the time, remains valid. If anything, the amount of exercise needed to enhance health is probably less than the equivalent of running 15 miles per week.

How much physical activity is enough but not too much? In recent years, experts have emphasized the value of moderate physical activity, including walking, gardening, bicycling, climbing stairs, and swimming (Pratt, 1999). Evidence now suggests that the amount of physical activity necessary for health depends on one's reason for exercising. For cardiovascular health, almost any level of physical activity is better than none. Brisk walking three hours a week or six miles a week can reduce women's risk of heart attack by 30% to 40% (Manson et al., 1999; Sesso, Paffenbarger, Ha, & Lee, 1999). No strong evidence exists that more than 3 or 4 hours of brisk walking further enhances cardiovascular health.

In 1995, a 20-member panel of experts reviewed this and other evidence on frequency and intensity of physical activity (Pate et al., 1995) and recommended that every adult should accumulate 30 minutes of moderate physical activity a day, or at least on most days. These experts also suggested that sedentary people should begin a program of moderate, regular physical activity.

> If Americans who lead sedentary lives would adopt a more active lifestyle, there would be enormous benefit to the public's health and to individual well-being. An active lifestyle does not require a regimented, vigorous exercise program. Instead, small changes that increase daily physical activity

> will enable individuals to reduce their risk of chronic disease and may contribute to enhanced quality of life. (Pate et al., 1995, p. 406)

Patricia Dubbert (2002) has referred this change in emphasis from vigorous physical activity to moderate lifetime activities as nothing less than a paradigm shift, a momentous and enduring new way of viewing physical activity.

Recent research has supported the notion that people can benefit from a moderate exercise program. For example, one report from the Honolulu Heart Program (Hakim et al., 1998) found that older men who included a daily walk of two or more miles cut their risks for sudden cardiac death in half. Another study from the Cooper Clinic in Dallas (Stofan, DiPietro, Davis, Kohl, & Blair, 1998) included both women and men and found much the same results. Small changes in lifetime activity are probably as effective as a vigorous, structured program of exercise in helping overweight men and women increase their physical activity and their cardiorespiratory fitness (Dunn et al., 1999). Also, obese women have lost as much weight through diet plus moderate physical activity compared with diet plus a structured aerobic exercise program (Andersen, et al., 1999). These studies suggest that moderate levels of physical activity can confer cardiovascular health as effectively as vigorous exercise.

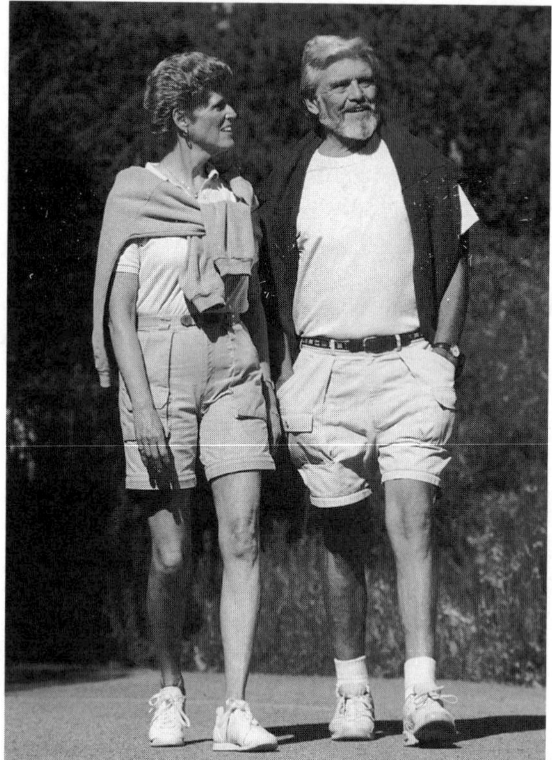

Corbis

Walking is one form of physical activity that offers more advantages than hazards for most people.

Maintaining a Physical Activity Program

Adherence to nearly all medical and health regimens is a serious problem (see Chapter 4), and exercise is no exception. Only 25% of adults in the United States meet physical activity requirements for health (USBC, 2001). This low rate of physical activity reflects a developmental trend toward lower activity levels with age. About 70% of children younger than 12 years old are physically active, but the rate drops sharply during adolescence (Sullum, Clark, & King, 2000). This decline is more dramatic among women than men; only 30% of 21-year-old women are active, yet 42% of 21-year-old men are. The age trend toward a sedentary lifestyle extends to older people, almost half of whom are physically inactive (USBC, 2001). For individuals who participate in prescribed exercise regimens, the dropout rates closely parallel the relapse rates reported in smoking and alcohol cessation programs.

Predicting Drop-Outs

When people consider an exercise program, they weigh the advantages and disadvantages of exercise. For those who move from contemplation to action, the advantages outweigh the disadvan-

BECOMING HEALTHIER

1. If you don't exercise, make plans to start a program of regular physical activity.
2. If you are overweight or over 40, consult a physician before beginning.
3. Don't start too fast. Once you have determined that you are ready to begin an exercise program, start slowly. The first day you may feel as though you can run a mile. Don't give in to that temptation.
4. Exercising too vigorously on the fist day will result in injuries or at least sore muscles. If you are stiff and sore the next day, you overdid it, and you won't feel like exercising on the second day.
5. If you are exercising for weight control, don't weigh yourself every day, and try not to become preoccupied with your weight or body shape.
6. If you are in the process of quitting smoking, use exercise as a way to prevent weight gain.
7. Choose and use correct equipment when you exercise.
8. If you exercise in a location unfamiliar to you, check out your surroundings before you begin. Several types of potential dangers may be in your path.
9. Remember that in order to receive maximum health benefits from your exercise program, you must stick to it. Don't expect quick or dramatic results.
10. To acquire muscle tone as well as aerobic fitness, include a combination of types of exercise such as working out with weights or other isotonic exercise as well as aerobics.

tages (Sullum et al., 2000). To maintain their exercise regimen, the advantages must continue to dominate; otherwise, people will relapse into a sedentary lifestyle. Unrealistic expectations about exercise may contribute to the judgment that the disadvantages predominate; that is, exercise is not worth the effort (Polivy & Herman, 2000). When people's expectations (including unrealistic expectations) about the benefits of exercise are unmet, then they begin to reassess their reasons for exercising and begin to see more disadvantages than advantages to their exercise program. This reassessment can lead to dropping out.

The factors that contribute to discontinuing exercise may be divided into personal, social-environmental, and exercise program variables. The assessment that exercise is not worth the effort is a personal factor. In a review of research, Rod Dishman and Janet Buckworth (1997) identified several additional personal attributes that predict adherence to physical activity. The demographic variables that characterize those most likely to stick to an exercise plan include being male, being younger, having a past history of physical activity, and attaining a higher levels of education and income. Smokers, blue-collar workers, and people with low self-efficacy for maintaining an exercising program are most likely to drop out. Women cited self-consciousness about their physical appearance as a barrier to exercise (King et al., 2000). People who see themselves as having poor health are reluctant to enter a physical activity program and have a high rate of quitting if they do. Also, people who experience a higher number of stressful life events are more likely than those with a lower number to discontinue exercising (Oman & King, 2000). Therefore, a number of personal factors form obstacles to continuing with an exercise program.

Environmental conditions may also present barriers to continuing an exercise program. People cited lack of time and energy as reasons for not exercising (Dishman & Buckworth, 1997);

women added the reason that their caregiving duties made it difficult for them to exercise (King et al., 2000). Finding the time to exercise is a challenge for many people, and therefore convenience makes adherence easier. This effect appeared in a study in which some participants received exercise equipment they could use at home, which boosted their adherence to the program (Jakicic, Winters, Lang, & Wing, 1999). A study that included Hispanic American, African American, Native American, and European American women (King et al., 2000) confirmed the importance of convenience as a factor in exercise maintenance.

Among the exercise program variables, the most common reason for stopping is injury. Of the people who engage in high-intensity physical activity, as many as 50% per year develop injuries serious enough to force them to stop (Dishman & Buckworth, 1997; USDHHS, 1996). As noted earlier, the more frequent and more intense the activity, the greater the chance that an injury will lead to temporary or permanent drop-out. Thus, intense, frequent physical activity is one of the best predictors of noncompliance.

Increasing Maintenance

The second step in increasing adherence to physical activity is establishing an intervention strategy for all participants, with special attention for those at greatest risk of dropping out. Behavior modification and cognitive behavioral methods have had some success in reducing the drop-out rate of exercisers. These programs ordinarily rely on reinforcement for healthy behaviors, contracting, self-monitoring, instruction, modeling, goal setting, increased self-efficacy, relapse prevention, and a variety of other strategies. Most of these have been discussed in earlier chapters and need no additional elaboration here. In general, psychological interventions have improved adherence to physical activity programs by about 15% to 20% (Dishman & Buckworth, 1997). In other words, if a program without an intervention has a 40% compliance rate, adding a psychological intervention may increase compliance to about 55% to 60%.

An important part of relapse prevention is protection against slips leading to full relapse. G. Alan Marlatt and Judith Gordon (1980) called this phenomenon the *abstinence violation effect* (see Chapter 13). With physical activity, people do not violate their abstinence, but rather they go a few days without any exercise behavior. Injury, illness, travel, or other breaks in daily routine can lead to an abstinence violation effect if people use four or five days of inactivity as an excuse to give up their physical activity regimen. Research with drop-outs from an exercise program (Sears & Stanton, 2001) indicated that failures to achieve the expected effects and expectancy violations characterized these individuals. Relapse prevention programs attempt to warn participants that they may be tempted to permanently quit exercising after a period of inactivity, but resuming exercise is a better choice than continuing inactivity. Although behavioral and cognitive behavioral strategies have demonstrated some success, especially when used in combination, maintenance remains a serious problem in most health-related exercise programs.

In Summary

In the United States, a sedentary lifestyle is more common than a physically active one; about 75% of adults fail to comply with recommendations for regular, vigorous exercise. Maintaining an exercise program may be difficult if the person's expectations for exercise are not fulfilled by the program. In addition, personal and environmental barriers exist, such as time constraints and alternative obligations. People are more likely to maintain an exercise program that is convenient; avoiding injuries is also important in continuing to exercise. Programs designed to improve adherence to physical activity programs are able to boost maintenance by about 15% to 20%.

Answers

This chapter addressed six basic questions.

1. **What are the different types of physical activity?**
All physical activity can be subsumed under one or more of five basic categories: isometric, isotonic, isokinetic, anaerobic, and aerobic. Each of these five exercise types has advantages and disadvantages for improving physical fitness. Most people who exercise do so for one or another of these five types of physical activity, but no one type of exercise promotes all types of fitness.

2. **Does physical activity benefit the cardiovascular system?**
Most results on the health benefits of exercise have confirmed a positive relationship between regular physical activity and enhanced cardiovascular health, including weight control and a favorable cholesterol ratio. This research suggests that a regimen of moderate, brisk physical activity should be prescribed as one of several components in a program of coronary health.

3. **What are some other health benefits of physical activity?**
In addition to improving cardiovascular health, regular physical activity may protect against some kinds of cancer, especially colon cancer; help prevent bone density loss, thus lowering one's risk of osteoporosis; control adult-onset diabetes, especially in those men most at risk; and help people sleep better and live longer.
Besides improving physical fitness and health, regular exercise can confer certain psychological benefits. Specifically, research has demonstrated that aerobic and nonaerobic exercises can decrease depression, reduce anxiety, buffer against the harmful effects of stress, and enhance feelings of self-esteem.

4. **Can physical activity be hazardous?**
Several hazards accompany both regular and sporadic exercise. Some runners appear to be addicted to exercise, becoming obsessed with body image and fearful of being prevented from following their exercise regimen. Injuries are frequent among veteran runners, but the most serious hazard is sudden death while exercising. However, people who exercise regularly are much less likely than sporadic exercisers to die of heart attack during heavy physical exertion.

5. **How much is enough but not too much?**
During the past 25 years, "experts" have gradually decreased their estimation of the amount of physical activity necessary to benefit cardiovascular health. The latest recommendation was provided by a 20-member panel of experts who recommended that every adult should accumulate 30 minutes of moderate physical activity a day, or at least on most days. For cardiovascular health, however, almost any amount of exercise is better than no exercise.

6. **What are some of the problems in maintaining an exercise program?**
About 50% of adolescents and 75% of adults in the United States are too sedentary for good health. Many of those who begin an exercise program will drop out, and personal factors such as unfulfilled expectations for exercise benefits, environmental factors such as time constraints and alternative obligations, and program factors such as injuries, all contribute to relapse to a sedentary lifestyle. Behavioral interventions have had some limited success in improving compliance with health-related exercise programs.

Suggested Readings

Blair, S. N., Cheng, Y, & Holder, J. S. (2001). Is physical activity or physical fitness more important in defining health benefits? *Medicine and Science in Sports & Exercise, 33,* S379–S399. In this article, Steven Blair and his associates from the Cooper Institute review the literature on the effects of physical activity and physical fitness on heart disease and cancer and conclude that a sedentary lifestyle and poor physical fitness are important risk factors for both heart disease and cancer.

McAuley, E. (1994). Physical activity and psychosocial outcomes. In C. Bouchard, R. J. Shephard, & T. Stephens (Eds.), *Physical activity, fitness, and health: International proceedings and consensus statement* (pp. 551–568). Champaign, IL: Human Kinetics. An authority on the psychosocial outcomes of exercise, Edward McAuley reviews the literature and concludes that the area suffers from methodologically weak designs, imprecise outcome measures, lack of sufficient follow-up, and confusion between physical fitness and physical activity.

Plymire, D. C., & Bennett, S. J. (2002). Running, heart disease, and the ironic death of Jim Fixx. (History and philosophy). *Research Quarterly for Exercise and Sport, 73,* 38–46. Darcy Plymire and Simon Bennett provide an interesting look at factors underlying the death of Jim Fixx and discuss the potentially deadly way of life of some obligatory runners.

U.S. Department of Health and Human Services (USDHHS). (1996). *Physical activity and health: A report of the Surgeon General.* Atlanta, GA: Centers for Disease Control and Prevention. With this first Surgeon General's report on physical activity, the U.S. Government officially recognized the health-related benefits of exercise. This volume discusses the effects of physical activity on cardiovascular disease, cancer, diabetes, arthritis, osteoporosis, and psychological health.

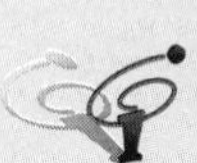

Search InfoTrac College Edition

Search these terms to learn more about topics in this chapter:

- Isometric exercise and fitness
- Aerobic exercise and fitness
- Physical activity and weight control
- Physical activity and heart disease
- Physical activity and diabetes
- Physical activity and cancer
- Physical activity and osteoporosis
- Physical activity and health benefits
- Physical activity and psychological
- Physical activity and hazards
- Exercise and sudden death
- Exercise addiction
- Physical activity and barriers
- Physical activity and maintenance

17

Future Challenges

CHAPTER OUTLINE

Healthier People

The Profession of Health Psychology

Outlook for Health Psychology

QUESTIONS

This chapter focuses on three basic questions:

1. What role does health psychology play in contributing to the goals of *Healthy People 2010*?
2. What type of training do health psychologists receive and what kinds of work do they do?
3. What is the outlook for the future of health psychology?

As Americans have become increasingly health conscious, they have come to realize that their physical well-being is not solely in the hands of medical professionals and that they have an important share of the responsibility in maintaining their own health. They are aware of the dangers of smoking, abusing alcohol, eating improperly, and not exercising regularly. They know that they should learn to cope better with stress, make and keep regular medical and dental appointments, and follow the advice of their health care professionals. This knowledge does not always translate into action, and people have difficulty in making changes in their behavior and lifestyle. But over the past 30 years, U.S. residents have managed to make some healthy changes in their behavior. The percentage of smokers has fallen, the amount of alcohol consumed has decreased, and the use of seatbelts and other safety measures has increased. People have started to become more conscious of what they eat and to consume more fruit and vegetables and less red meat and other saturated fats.

These positive changes are reflected in declining mortality for heart disease, stroke, cancer, homicide, and unintentional injuries (USBC, 2001), but unhealthy and risky behaviors continue to contribute to an increasing rate of obesity, diabetes, and lower respiratory disease. This chapter looks at the nation's health goals and at the role and status of health psychology in confronting the principal challenges facing the field.

Healthier People

An example of the influence of health consciousness on a national policy level was *Healthy People 2000* (USDHHS, 1991), a report that detailed three broad goals, 22 priority areas, and 300 main objectives for improving the health of people in the United States. The broad goals included increasing the span of healthy life, reducing health disparities among Americans, and achieving access to preventive services for all people in the United States. This report was followed by *Healthy People 2010: Understanding and Improving Health* (2nd ed., USDHHS, 2000), which built on the successes and shortcomings of the previous goals to establish health objectives for the first decade of the 21st century. These objectives include 28 focus areas and 467 specific goals, but two overarching goals summarize the focus of this report. They are to increase quality and years of healthy life and to eliminate health disparities. Those goals are ambitious and hold many challenges.

Increasing the Span of Healthy Life

The first goal—to increase the span of healthy life—is a different from increasing life expectancy. Rather than striving for longer lives, many people are now trying to increase their number of well-years. A **well-year** is "the equivalent of a year of completely well life, or a year of life free of dysfunction, symptoms, and health-related problems" (Kaplan & Bush, 1982, p. 64). This concept has grown in acceptability since 1946, when the World Health Organization charter defined health in terms of positive states of mental and physical well-being.

In addition to striving to increase well-years, health psychologists advocate the concept of **health expectancy,** defined as that period of life a person spends free from disability (Robine & Ritchie, 1991). For example, the life expectancy at age 65 is about 16 additional years for men and 19 years for women, but health expectancy is only 8 more years for men and 10 years for women, leaving both men and women with a discrepancy that represents years of disability (Robine & Ritchie, 1991; USBC, 2001). That is, health expectancy has not grown as rapidly as life expectancy. Furthermore, U.S. residents are not benefiting from increases in healthy life expectancy as much as residents of many other countries (Mathers, Sadana, Salomon, Murray, & Lopez, 2001). Although people in the United

States may expect 70.0 years of healthy life, this figure ranks 24th in the world in terms of disability-free life expectancy. The United States trails most other countries because of high rates of smoking-related disease, violence, and AIDS-related health problems. Table 17.1 shows the healthy life expectancy for countries with both high and low values.

The differences between life expectancy and health expectancy are even larger when comparing the richest and poorest segments of the population. Wealthy people not only live longer but also have more years of healthy life. In addition, the disorders that shorten life are not necessarily the same as those that compromise health. For example, circulatory disorders head both lists, but disorders producing restricted movement and respiratory disorders are responsible for producing lost health expectancy, whereas cancer and accidents are major sources of lost life expectancy. Therefore, interventions aimed at increasing life expectancy will not necessarily improve health expectancy and quality of life.

The need to increase the health of the elderly is important not only to improve their quality of life but also to help manage health care costs. Due to their tendency to have chronic illnesses, older people use health care services more heavily than younger people, with a rate of physician contacts twice as high for those over 75 compared with those between ages 15 and 44 (NCHS, 2001). In an editorial in the *New England Journal of Medicine,* Andrew Kramer (1995) advocated a change in emphasis for health care for the elderly. Rather than concentrating on acute care delivered in hospitals, Kramer argued for the promotion of primary care and long-term care, strategies that might help improve quality of life for the elderly. Following this suggestion, several types of programs have demonstrated effectiveness in improving quality of life for chronically ill older people (Boult, Kane, & Brown, 2000). These programs include strategies such as providing care from an interdisciplinary team of health care providers rather than exclusively through physicians, teaching self-management skills so that older people are better able to care for themselves, making group rather than individual physician appointments, and providing in-home services rather than hospital-based services. Unfortunately, implementation of these innovative programs has been slow, and resistance among hospitals and physicians has been high. Without innovative changes, the goal of increasing healthy years of life will not be attained.

TABLE 17.1 *Healthy Life Expectancy for Selected Nations*

Ranking	Country	Healthy Life Expectancy
1	Japan	74.5
2	Australia	73.2
3	France	73.1
4	Sweden	73.0
12	Canada	72.0
14	United Kingdom	71.7
22	Germany	70.4
23	Israel	70.4
24	USA	70.0
36	Jamaica	67.3
46	Yugoslavia	66.1
55	Mexico	65.0
81	China	62.3
91	Russian Federation	61.3
94	Belize	60.9
111	Brazil	59.1
116	Viet Nam	58.2
124	Pakistan	55.9
134	India	53.2
153	Haiti	43.8
160	South Africa	39.82
180	Mozambique	34.4
188	Zambia	30.3
191	Sierra Leone	25.9

Source: "Healthy life expectancy in 191 countries, 1999," by C. D. Mathers et al., 2001, *Lancet, 357,* pp. 1685–1690.

Reducing Health Disparities

The United States made progress toward achieving the objectives of *Healthy People 2000,* and set higher goals for *Healthy People 2010.* However,

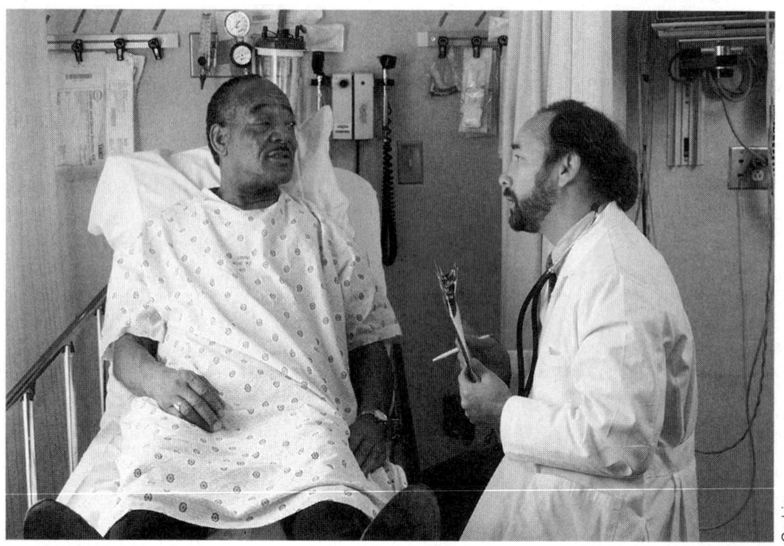
Corbis

Reducing health disparities is one of the goals included in *Healthy People 2010.*

most of those improvements have been among higher socioeconomic groups. Hugh discrepancies in health status continue to exist among various socioeconomic and ethnic groups (USDHHS, 2000). When *Healthy People 2000* was published in 1991, the plan for reducing ethnic and socioeconomic disparities was to target minority groups separate from the general population. However, with *Healthy People 2010* (USDHHS, 2000), the emphases had shifted away from targeting special groups and toward high standards of improved health for everyone. With such a plan, the Department of Health and Human Services hopes to eliminate disparities in infant mortality, cancer screening, cardiovascular disease, diabetes, HIV/AIDS, sedentary lifestyle, obesity, and other health areas that now show large discrepancies between the general population and at least one ethnic group.

In the United States, ethnicity is not separable from social, economic, and educational factors that contribute to disease as well as to seeking and receiving health care (USDHHS, 2000). Being poor with a low educational level elevates risks for many diseases and provides a poorer prognosis for those who are ill. African Americans, Hispanic Americans, and Native Americans have lower average educational levels and incomes than European Americans and Asian Americans (USDHHS, 2000). Thus, the factor of ethnicity is difficult to separate from income and education, complicating the interpretation of the underlying reasons for health disparities among people of different ethnic backgrounds.

For example, African Americans, compared with European Americans, have shorter life expectancy as well as a higher infant mortality rate, more homicide deaths, increased cardiovascular disease rate, higher cancer mortality, and more tuberculosis and diabetes (USBC, 2001). Inadequate medical treatment and lack of health education may be responsible for much of this disparity, but even when equating for income (De Lew & Weinick, 2000) and access to health care (Schneider, Zaslavsky, & Epstein, 2002), African Americans have poorer outcomes than European Americans.

The poorer health outcomes for African Americans present the possibility that discrimination is an additional reason for African Americans receiving less adequate treatment than European Americans (Smiles, 2002). For example, African Americans receive less aggressive treatment for symptoms of coronary heart disease and are less likely to be referred to a cardiologist than European Americans, are less likely to receive kidney dialysis, and are less likely to receive the most effective treatments for HIV infection (Institute of Medicine, 2002).

Low economic status and the lack of access to medical care affect Native Americans at least as strongly as African Americans. Native Americans have shorter life expectancy, higher mortality rate, higher infant mortality, and higher rates of infectious illness than European Americans (Hayes-Bautista et al., 2002). Many Native Americans receive health care from the Indian Health Service, but that organization has a history of poor funding as well as mistreatment of Native American patients that has led to mistrust (Lawrence, 2000). Both circumstances may contribute to decreased access to health care, which is related to poor health.

Socioeconomic status and limited access to health care, however, are not the only contributors to the health discrepancy between Native Americans and European Americans. One study (Cheadle et al., 1994) showed that even with socioeconomic status adjusted, Native Americans had a higher prevalence of risk-taking behaviors and poorer health status than people who were not Native Americans. Native Americans, then, are one of the groups poorly served by the current system of health care and health education in the United States.

Many Hispanic Americans also experience low income and educational status. However, not all groups of Hispanic Americans are affected equally, and their health and longevity tend to vary accordingly. Cuban Americans generally have higher education and economic levels than Mexican Americans or Puerto Ricans; and Cuban Americans are more likely to have access to regular health care and physician visits (LaVeist, Bowie, & Cooley-Quille, 2000).

For Hispanic Americans without insurance coverage, their ethnic background and geographic location may affect the health care they receive. Compared with Mexican Americans living near the U.S.–Mexican border, Puerto Ricans are more likely to live in places that offer better accessibility to Medicaid and thus more opportunity for frequent visits to physicians (Apodaca, Woodruff, Candelaria, Elder, & Zlot, 1997). Both Puerto Ricans and Mexican Americans have lower life expectancy than other Hispanics in the United States.

Hispanic Americans are much more likely to develop diabetes, obesity, and hypertension than non-Hispanic Whites (USDHHS, 2000). Hispanic American young men are at sharply increased risk of violent death (Hayes-Bautista et al., 2002), which may be the reason for the overall lower life expectancy for Hispanic Americans. In other age groups, Hispanics fare about the same as or better than European Americans on some health and mortality measures. Hispanic Americans have a lower death rate than European Americans (LaVeist et al., 2000), including death from heart disease, stroke, and lung cancer. These low death rates are puzzling, given the high rates of smoking, obesity, and hypertension among Hispanic Americans. The poor health habits of Hispanic Americans, combined with their low disease prevalence, may reflect a transition in which immigrants are adopting European American lifestyles but have not yet developed the chronic diseases typical of the United States.

This same trend applies to all immigrant groups—those who adopt the lifestyle of the United States soon have the patterns of disease and death characteristic of the United States. For example, adolescent obesity increased significantly in the second and third generations of children of Asian American and Hispanic American immigrants compared to their parents and grand parents (Popkin & Udry, 1998). Similarly, Hispanic and Asian American adolescents who speak English at home were more likely to smoke than those who did not speak English at home (Unger et al., 2000). Speaking English represents one measure of acculturation, which was related to increases in access to cigarettes and peer influences to smoke. Thus, Asian Americans who have adopted Western habits increase their risks, but Asian Americans still have more favorable health status and life expectancy than other ethnic groups (USDHHS, 2000).

Asian Americans have lower infant mortality, longer life expectancy, lower lung and breast cancer deaths, and lower cardiovascular death rates than other ethnic groups. Some factors in Asian cultures promote good health, such as strong social and family ties, whereas other factors present barriers to seeking health care. For example, the value of caring for family members at home may slow or prevent a person from seeking professional sources for health care (McLaughlin & Braun, 1998). Overall, Asian Americans have the longest life expectancy and best health of any ethnic group in the United States.

Low income has an obvious connection to lower standards of health care, and people without health insurance and access to a physician are at increased risk. However, universal access to health care does not remove the disparities among socioeconomic groups (Martikainen, Valkonen, & Martelin, 2001). Even in countries that have universal access to health care, health disparities between poor and wealthy people continue to exist, suggesting that factors other than receiving health care are involved in maintaining health.

Education and socioeconomic level are two factors that may influence health status—independent of access to health care. Across ethnic groups, people who have higher education and income also have better health and longevity than those with lower education and income (Crimmins & Saito, 2001). As the Chapter 1 Would You Believe . . . ? box detailed, people who attend college have many health advantages. Compared to those who have a high school education or less, those who attend college live longer and healthier, including lower rates of infectious and chronic diseases and unintentional injuries (NCHS, 2001). These advantages should not be surprising, considering the low rate of smoking among those who attend or graduate from college; smoking is a leading contributor to ill health and death. People with fewer than 12 years of education are much more likely to smoke than those with college degrees.

In addition, people with low education and low socioeconomic status are more likely to have risky health habits, such as eating a high-fat diet and leading a sedentary life, than people with higher incomes and more education (USDHHS, 2000). Improved access to health care and decreased discrimination in health care delivery will probably eliminate some of the health disparities among ethnic groups, but changes in health-related behaviors and improved living conditions will also be necessary to achieve the goal of eliminating health disparities in the United States.

In Summary

People in the United States and other industrialized countries are becoming more health conscious, and both government policy and individual behavior reflect this concern. *Healthy People 2010* built upon the success of *Healthy People 2000* and stated two overarching goals for the U.S. population: (1) to increase the quality and years of healthy life and (2) to eliminate health disparities. The first goal includes increasing the number of well-years or healthy life expectancy, that is, years free of dysfunction, disease symptoms, and health-related problems. The goal also includes the concept of health expectancy, that is, the period of life a person spends free from disability. The second goal—eliminating disparities in health care—is far from being met, in part because people in the upper socioeconomic level continue to make greater gains in health status than do those in the lower levels and ethnicity remains a factor in health and health care.

WOULD YOU BELIEVE

Terence Was Right

Would you believe that Terence, the Roman playwright who lived during the second century (BCE) was mostly right when he advised moderation in all things? Except for cigarette smoking, most of your health behaviors should follow Terence's counsel.

In Chapter 14, we discussed evidence that moderation in alcohol consumption was healthier for people's hearts than either heavy drinking or complete abstinence. For example, a recent meta-analysis (Rimm et al., 1999) found that neither abstinence nor heavy binge drinking have any cardiovascular benefits. However, both men and women can substantially reduce their deaths from heart disease by light to moderate drinking, defined as about two drinks a day.

In Chapter 15, we reviewed research by Reina Wing and Betse Polley (2001) showing a relationship between overeating and obesity. Next, we examined the association between obesity and health and found evidence for a U-shaped relationship between weight and poor health. That is, the heaviest people and the thinnest people had a greater risk for poor health than people who have avoided extremes of weight. Confirmation of these findings (Calle et al., 1999) showed that women who have a body mass index (BMI) around 23 and men who have a BMI of about 24 have the lowest risk for mortality. As body mass index moves substantially in either direction away from these moderate levels, mortality rate goes up.

In Chapter 16, we saw that the devoted runners of 20 years ago were not improving their health through excessive physical activity but were running for reasons other than health. Although marathon running may not be harmful to cardiovascular health, it can lead to other types of health problems, including serious injuries (Dishman & Buckworth, 1997). But if long-distance running can be harmful, a sedentary lifestyle is even more dangerous. In 1995, a panel of experts (Pate et al., 1995) recommended that every adult accumulate 30 minutes of moderate physical activity a day through such activities as brisk walking, gardening, bicycling, climbing stairs, or swimming. In other words, sedentary people can improve their cardiovascular health by beginning moderate exercise.

Could moderation also apply to eating candy? Consuming candy may seem like a guilty pleasure, but if you are not diabetic and you eat moderately, you may live longer than people who do not eat candy. This statement is consistent with the results of a study conducted by I-Min Lee and Ralph Paffenbarger (1998), who began their article saying, that "our attitude towards candy—'if it tastes that good, it can't be healthy'—betrays society's puritanical stance towards pleasure" (p. 1683). As with most things in life, however, moderation is the key.

Lee and Paffenbarger asked male participants in the Harvard Health study (thus limiting any generalization of these findings) to fill out a survey on consuming candy. Seven years later, these researchers obtained death certificates for the men who had died during that interim. People who ate candy one to three times a months had a longer life span than people who consumed much larger quantities of candy, as well as those who ate no candy. Interestingly, men at all levels of candy consumption lived longer than those who ate no candy. How much longer? After adjusting for age and cigarette smoking, Lee and Paffenbarger found that men who indulged in candy consumption lived nearly one year longer than those who ate no candy.

Once again, Terence was right. Moderation is the key to good health. People who use alcohol, eat, and exercise in moderation are generally healthier than those who are less moderate. Indeed, people who eat moderate amounts of candy live longer than those who eat lots of candy and even longer than those who abstain from this pleasure.

The Profession of Health Psychology

During the 125 years of its history in the United States, psychology has developed a science-based body of knowledge and several unique skills that allow it to make major contributions to the field of health. Among these contributions are sophistication in statistics and measurement, techniques for behavior change, and a large array of models and theories that permit psychologists to explain and predict human behavior. Psychology's development and use of a variety of research designs and statistical procedures has led to a large body of health-related information. In addition, its historical involvement in changing human behavior places it in a position to help people eliminate unhealthy practices as well as to incorporate healthy behaviors into an ongoing lifestyle.

The prevalence of such chronic disorders as asthma, arthritis, Alzheimer's disease, AIDS, cancer, cardiovascular disease, diabetes, headaches, and stress has created challenges for psychology—and specifically, health psychology. How successfully has health psychology progressed toward meeting this challenge?

Progress in Health Psychology

Since the founding of health psychology, the field has grown rapidly, and this growth has been apparent both in the amount of research published by psychologists on health-related topics and in the growing number of psychologists who work in health care settings.

In 1969, William Schofield published an article in the *American Psychologist* that provided a major impetus to health psychology. Analyzing the research publications in psychology that dealt with health, he found that only 19% of the research articles dealt with topics other than the traditional mental health concerns of psychology. This finding brought about a call for a wider scope of psychological services and research. The American Psychological Association (APA) appointed a task force to perform a further analysis, and this task force concluded that health was not a common area of research for psychologists (APA Task Force on Health Research, 1976). However, during the past 25 years, psychology research on health issues has accelerated to the point where health psychology has changed the field of psychology, making health-related issues common topics in psychology journals.

In addition to the increasing amount of research publications, the growth of health psychology is seen by the number of employment opportunities available to health psychologists. Our examination of the September, 2002 *APA Monitor* found more than 60 advertisements for psychologists to work in health-related fields. Several of these descriptions specifically included the term *health psychologist,* and the others listed either the field of *behavioral medicine* or the area of *behavior health.* Some of these advertisements mentioned specific topics of health psychology, including pain management, fitness and health, interventions to reduce risky behaviors, substance abuse, eating disorders, and physical rehabilitation. These advertisements represented a wide variety of positions, including university faculty appointments, medical schools, hospitals, and clinics. Thus, psychologists trained to work in health-related areas have a wide assortment of possible employment opportunities.

The Training of Health Psychologists

This training for health psychologists includes grounding in psychological principles and substantial preparation in neurology, endocrinology, immunology, public health, epidemiology, and other medical subspecialties. Standards for the preparation of health psychologists follow the Boulder model of 1949 that views psychologists as both scientists and practitioners. These standards also are consistent with those established by the National Working Conference on Education and

Training in Health Psychology of 1983 that defined the core program in psychology to which health psychologists should be exposed. Although this training program was established 20 years ago, health psychologists continue to receive a solid core of graduate training in such areas as (1) the biological bases of behavior, health, and disease; (2) the cognitive and affective bases of behavior, health, and disease; (3) the social bases of health and disease, including knowledge of health organizations and health policy; (4) the psychological bases of health and disease, with emphasis on individual differences; (5) advanced research, methodology, and statistics; (6) psychological and health measurement; (7) interdisciplinary collaboration; and (8) ethics and professional issues (Belar, 1997). In addition to this core, many health psychologists have recommended postdoctoral training, with at least 2 years of specialized training in health psychology to follow a Ph.D. or Psy.D. in psychology (Belar, 1997; Matarazzo, 1987a). This training might include some combination of internships and residencies in which health psychologists would learn to provide treatment in hospitals and other traditional health care settings.

Linda Travis (2001) has continued to emphasize interdisciplinary training for psychologists who wish to become health care professionals. No single discipline in the health care field has the capacity to solve all the problems of health promotion and disease prevention. Nevertheless, the training and education of a new generation of health psychologists must develop teamwork skills that enhance cooperation with other health-related disciplines. This situation suggests an interdisciplinary training that accepts and welcomes the contributions of other disciplines. Travis has suggested techniques for enhancing teamwork among different disciplines. For example, students of different disciplines can discuss different formulations of the same case, followed by group discussion of the case. A second technique emphasizes diversity issues. Teams can be constituted to maximize diversity and to enhance creativity in solving problems in health care. Such procedures can benefit not only students from the health psychology field but those from other disciplines as well.

The Work of Health Psychologists

Health psychologists work in a variety of settings and perform many different functions, including universities, hospitals, clinics, health maintenance organizations (HMOs), and private practice. In addition, federal agencies such as the Centers for Disease Control and Prevention and the National Institutes of Health employ health psychologists. They teach, conduct research, and provide a medley of services to individual patients as well as private and public agencies. As with the training of health psychologists, much of their work is collaborative in nature; that is, health psychologists frequently work with a team of health professionals, including physicians, nurses, physical therapists, and counselors.

The services provided by health psychologists working in clinics and hospitals fit into several categories. One type of service provides alternatives to pharmacological treatment; for example, biofeedback might be an alternative to analgesic drugs for headache patients. Another type of service is the primary treatment of physical disorders that respond favorably to behavioral interventions, such as chronic pain and some gastrointestinal problems. Several other types of services that psychologists might provide are related to traditional clinical psychology and include ancillary psychological treatment for patients who are hospitalized, such as cardiac or cancer patients. Health psychologists employed in hospitals and clinics also help improve the rate of patient compliance with their medical regimens and provide some assessments using psychological and neuropsychological tests. Those who concentrate on prevention and behavior changes are more likely to be employed in health maintenance organizations, school-based prevention programs, or worksite wellness programs. All these organizations use services that trained health psychologists can perform.

Most health psychologists engage in several activities. The combination of teaching and research is common among those in educational settings. Health psychologists who work in medical centers may teach medical students, conduct research, perform clinical services, or carry out some mixture of these activities. Those who work in service delivery settings are much less likely to teach and do research and are more likely to spend the majority of their time providing diagnosis and therapy.

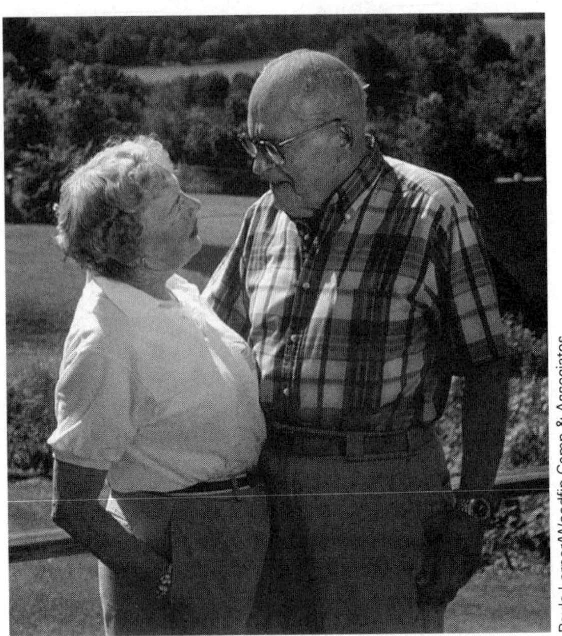

Paula Lerner/Woodfin Camp & Associates

Increasing the span of healthy life is a goal for health psychologists.

In Summary

To maximize their contributions to health care, health psychologist must be both broadly trained in the science of psychology and specifically trained in the knowledge and skills of such areas as neurology, endocrinology, immunology, epidemiology, and other medical subspecialties. Health psychologists with a solid background in generic psychology and specialized knowledge in medical fields are currently employed in a variety of settings, including universities, hospitals, clinics, private practice, and health maintenance organizations. They typically collaborate with other health care professionals in providing services for physical disorders rather than for traditional areas of mental health care. Research in health psychology is also likely to be a collaborative effort that may include the professions of medicine, epidemiology, nursing, pharmacology, nutrition, and exercise physiology.

Outlook for Health Psychology

Despite the growth of health psychology and its ability to contribute to health care, the field faces several challenges. One major challenge is acceptance by other health care practitioners, an acceptance that continues to grow. Health psychologists will be challenged by the most serious problem within health care, namely, escalating costs. In an environment of limited resources, psychologists will be forced to justify the costs that their services add to health care. Although the diagnostic and therapeutic techniques used by health psychologists have demonstrated effectiveness, these procedures also have financial costs. Health psychology must meet the challenges of justifying its costs by offering services that meet the needs of individuals and society while fitting within a troubled health care system.

Future Challenges for Health Care

Health care in the United States faces many challenges. The two goals of *Healthy People 2010*—to add years of healthy life and to eliminate disparities in providing health care—pose substantial challenges for the United States. Adding years of healthy life to an aging population is a

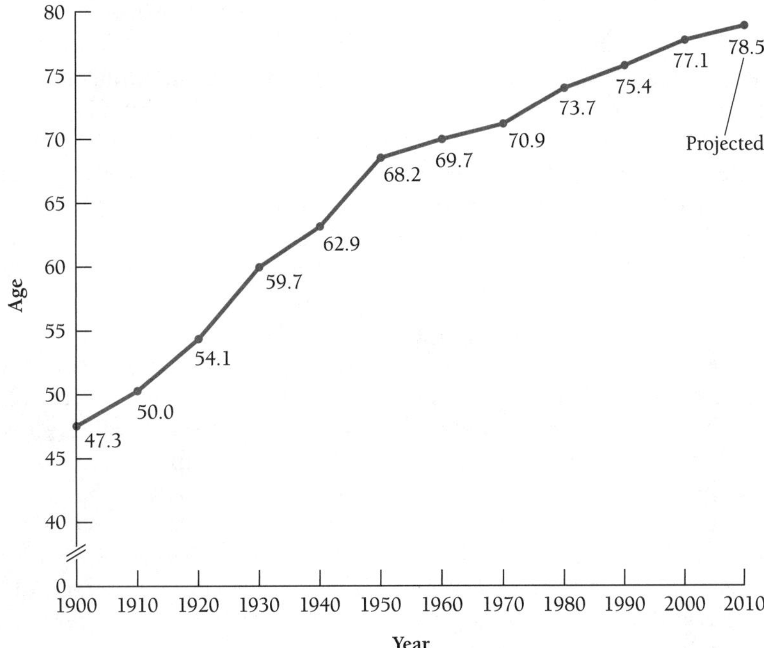

Figure 17.1 Actual and projected life expectancy, United States, 1900–2010.

Sources: Data from Historical Statistics of the United States: Colonial Times to 1970 *(p. 55) by U.S. Department of Commerce, Bureau of the Census, 1975, Washington, DC: U.S. Government Printing Office; and from* Statistical Abstracts of the United States: 2001 *(p. 73) by U.S. Bureau of the Census, 2001, Washington, DC: U.S. Government Printing Office.*

daunting task. After age 65, many people develop chronic illnesses and suffer from chronic pain.

Since 1900, the number of people in the United States 65 years old or older has increased from about 3 million to more than 34 million. In 1900, only 4% of the population was over 65, whereas in 1999, nearly 13% of U.S. citizens had reached that age. During this same period, life expectancy increased from 47 years to more than 76 years. By the year 2010, life expectancy is projected to be more than 78 years (see Figure 17.1), with more than 18 million people, or 6.2% of the total population, over age 75 (USBC, 2001).

As the population continues to age during the next few decades, psychology will play an important role in helping older people achieve and maintain healthy and productive lifestyles and adjust to the problems of chronic illness. As we have seen, health psychology has a role in preventing illness, promoting health, and helping people cope with pain. In old age, lifestyles can still be changed to help prevent illness, but health psychology's alliance with gerontology will more likely produce an emphasis on promoting and maintaining health, managing pain, and formulating health care policy.

The elimination of health disparities based on gender, ethnicity, age, income, educational level, and disability will be even more difficult. The health and life expectancy disadvantage for African Americans exists throughout the lifespan (Whitfield, Weidner, Clark, & Anderson, 2002), and Hispanic Americans and Native Americans also have shorter life and health expectancies than European Americans and Asian Americans. Many of these disparities can be traced back to economic and educational differences among ethnic groups (Crimmins & Saito, 2001). The health disparity attributable to gender is not so easy to pinpoint. However, this disparity is large: women live about

7 years longer than men do (USBC, 2001). Efforts to trace this gender difference to biology have been largely unsuccessful, but health-related behaviors, social support, and coping strategies favor women (Whitfield et al., 2002).

The Women's Health Initiative is a 16-year longitudinal study designed to investigate factors involved with the health of older women (Matthews et al., 1997). The design includes over 150,000 women and encompasses both biological and psychosocial components of disease and treatment, including prevention. One of the first findings from the Initiative was that estrogen replacement therapy presents more cardiovascular dangers than benefits to postmenopausal women (Writing Group for the Women's Health Initiative Investigators, 2002). The Initiative was designed to emphasize issues in women's health and to assure that women were included in health research. This massive research effort will not directly address the health disparities that men experience, which remain important areas of investigation for the future.

Woven throughout these issues is escalating costs—the primary challenge facing health care in the United States. The health care system is in turmoil over the rising costs of medical care. Insurance costs continue to increase, and a growing number of people have no insurance and cannot afford to pay for care (NCHS, 2001). The changes in patterns of death and disability that occurred during the 20th century also have an impact on the cost of health care because the system of providing care has not accommodated to those changes. These two problems with health care exert influences on the future of health psychology.

Controlling Health Care Costs The richest nation in the world is having trouble paying its health care bills. Health care costs in the United States have escalated at a higher rate than inflation and other costs of living (USDHHS, 2002), leaving many people unable to afford health care and others in the position of fearing that they will not be able to do so in the future.

A number of factors have contributed to the high costs, and many of those factors can be traced to the system that provides care and the economic forces within that system (Research and Policy Committee, 2002). The problems stem from proliferation of hospitals, a large proportion of physicians who are specialists, inefficient administration, and inappropriate treatments.

Figure 17.2 shows where health care dollars go. Hospitals receive 33% and physicians 22% of the dollars spent. Health care costs could be lower if the number of hospital beds matched the demand for beds, but hospitals have overbuilt, resulting in the need to fill these hospital beds. Indeed, areas of the country with more hospital beds available have higher rates of hospitalization than areas with fewer beds (Fisher et al., 2000). Some national policy to control hospital overbuilding could help control the costs added by this situation (Research and Policy Committee, 2002).

Although physicians receive less of the health care dollar than hospitals, their fees contribute significantly to the high costs of health care (Weitz, 2001). Managed care curtailed physicians' fees during the late 1980s and early 1990s, but the backlash against managed care loosened these restrictions, and physicians' fees began to increase again in the late 1990s (Research and Policy Committee, 2002). In addition, the number of specialists adds to the cost of medical care, and the scarcity of family practitioners (and the lack of incentive for going into family practice) also plays a role (Weitz, 2001). Ironically, more physicians created competition but rather than decreasing costs, this situation has contributed to higher costs.

Administrative costs contribute substantially to high health care costs in the United States (Research and Policy Committee, 2002; Weitz, 2001). The complex system of insurance, private physicians, private and public hospitals, and government-supported medical programs such as Medicare has produced different procedures, forms, payment plans, expenses allowed, maximum payments, and deductibles involved with

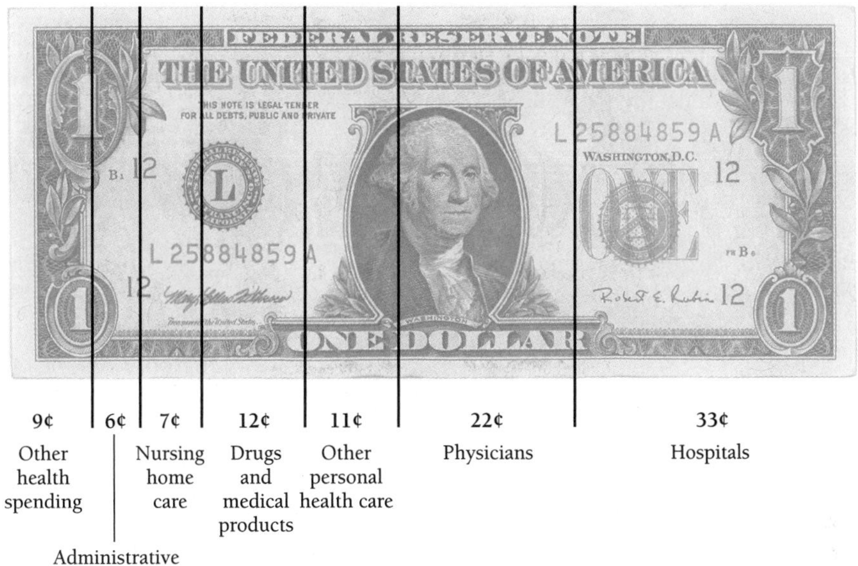

Figure 17.2 Where health care dollars go.

Source: Health, United States, 2001 *(p. 332) by National Center for Health Statistics, 2001, Hyattsville, MD: U.S. Government Printing Office.*

payment for medical services. Thus, payment is a complex matter of filling out and filing forms, not only by patients but also by health care providers. In addition to the costs of inefficiency, this over-complicated system adds to people's frustration of dealing with the health care system and creates possibilities for errors and fraud.

Health care reform has been recognized as an urgent priority for the United States, but many conflicting interests have prevented widespread changes. During the 1980s, health maintenance organizations (HMOs) proliferated as a way to control costs (Weitz, 2001). Originally, HMOs were nonprofit organizations oriented toward preventive care, but corporations entered the HMO market and profit became a motive. The growth of HMOs and the restriction of care received through these organizations contributed to slowing of the health care cost escalation. A backlash against the restrictions of care imposed by HMOs has produced patients' rights movements, which have edged the system back toward high spending.

Examining other countries that are faced with similar health problems and their solutions can give direction about ways to provide health care for people in the United States. Other industrialized countries such as Canada, Japan, Australia, the countries of western Europe, and Scandinavia share factors with the United States: high rates of cardiovascular disease and cancer as well as aging populations, which pose similar problems for their health care systems (Caragata, 1995; OECD Publications and Information Centre, 2001). Many of these countries do a better job of providing health care to a larger percentage of their residents at lower costs than does the U.S. system.

Germany, Canada, and Great Britain all have faced the problems of escalating health care costs, but these nations have found better ways to control costs than the United States (Weitz, 2001). The history of health care costs for these countries and the United States appear in Figure 17.3. These countries have managed to contain health care expenditures by controlling all of the factors that account for the rise in medical costs for the

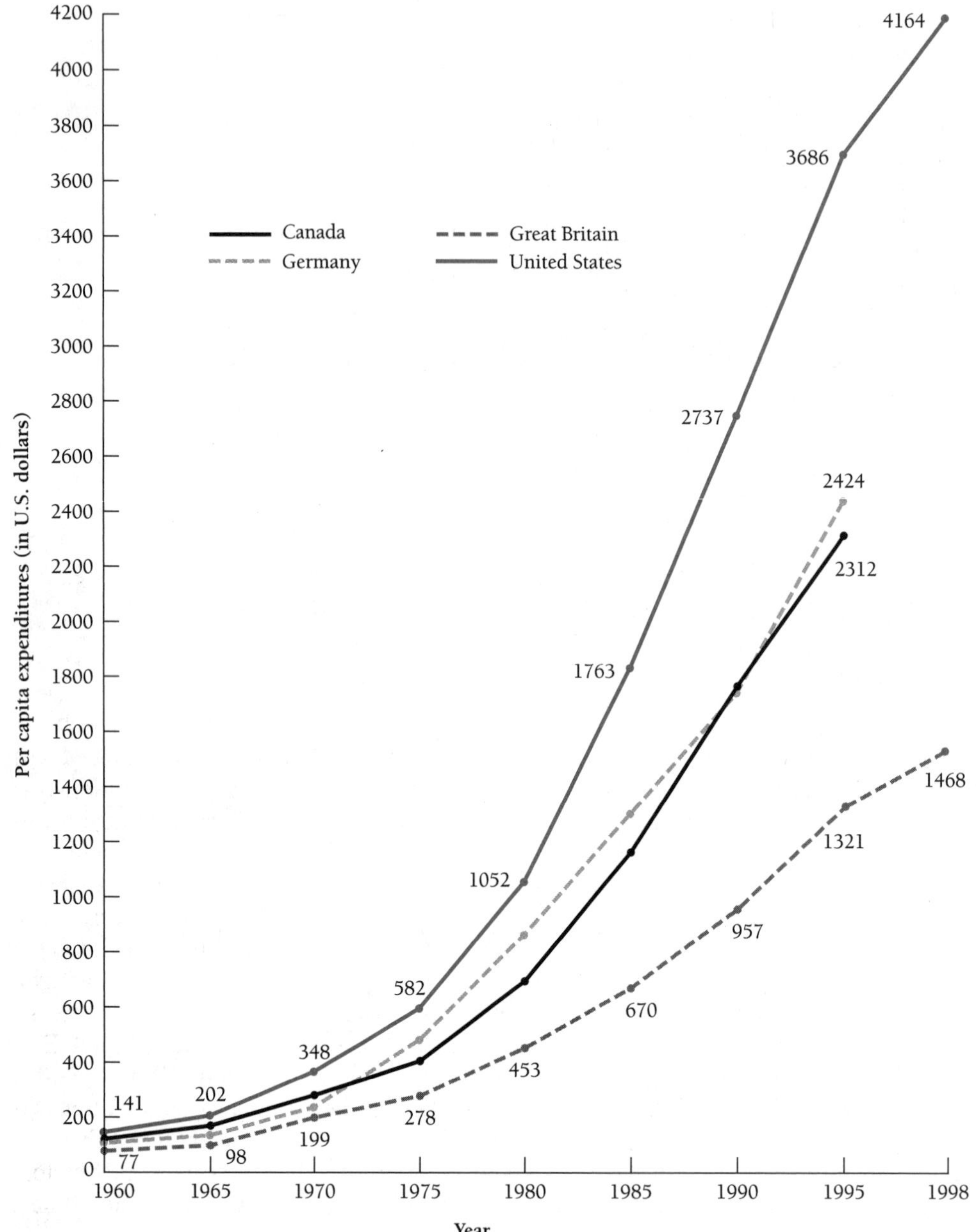

Figure 17.3 Health care expenditures in Canada, Germany, Great Britain, and United States, 1960–1998.

Source: Health, United States, 2001 *(p. 327) by National Center for Health Statistics, 2001, Hyattsville, MD: U.S. Government Printing Office.*

United States: growth of hospitals, availability of medical technology, abundance of specialists, and complex administrative requirements.

All these countries limit hospital proliferation by making the government responsible for giving money for capital expenditures to hospitals rather than allowing hospitals to overbuild. This same control process limits purchases of expensive technology. The limits on technology also decrease patients' access to this technology and technological medicine, which may be a drawback in some cases. For example, people have quicker access to medical procedures such as MRIs, mammograms, and knee replacement surgery in the United States compared to Canada, but these procedures are significantly more expensive in the United States (Bell, Crystal, Detsky, & Redelmeier, 1998). Time delays for some services may pose risks, but in other cases, patients in the United States are overtreated, and limiting access could actually boost health and life expectancy (Research and Policy Committee, 2002). Recall that Canadians have a longer life expectancy and more years of healthy life than people in the United States, which suggests that the delays they experience do not pose major threats (Michaud, Murray, & Bloom, 2001).

By devising systems in which all people have access to health care, Germany, Canada, and Great Britain have eliminated competitive profit making, which remains a central feature of the U.S. system. These three countries have different systems for paying for health care, and all have experienced cost problems, but each has universal coverage. Without the system of advertising to attract customers and the multitude of different filing procedures, forms, allowed procedures, deductibles, and other differences among insurers, administrative costs are much lower than in the United States (Weitz, 2001).

Some restrictions of costs in the United States are similar to those in Canada, Germany, and Great Britain (Weitz, 2001). For example, many physicians in the United States now have restrictions on their fees. In Canada, fees are set as a result of negotiations between government and physicians' groups, and these negotiated fees represent the limit of what physicians can charge for their services. Great Britain has limited the number of specialists trained and access to those specialists.

Other possibilities for controlling health care costs include reducing the need and the demand for services (Fries, 1998). Health psychologists can have a role in reducing health care cost because unhealthy behaviors are related to chronic diseases such as cardiovascular disease, cancer, and chronic lower respiratory disease. People with a healthy lifestyle are much less likely to develop these diseases. Those with good health habits have lifetime medical costs of about half that for people with poor health habits. Promotion of good health habits is an important way to decrease the need for medical services.

Reducing the demand for medical services is another strategy that represents a different approach to controlling health care costs. To this point, reductions of the use of medical services have occurred through limiting access to medical care, which does not affect demand and leaves patients dissatisfied with their level of care. Reducing the demand for medical services may have benefits. The availability of a wide range of medical technology has led to the widespread belief that modern medicine can cure any disease, and this belief has fostered an overreliance on medicine to heal rather than a reliance on good health habits to avoid disease. Building feelings of personal efficacy for health can help reduce the demand for medical services (Fries, 1998), and this approach has potential benefits for health in U.S. society. Several pilot programs have indicated that such training is less expensive than providing health care, making such programs a good buy. Additional research in this area may reveal that this approach can be a good strategy for containing health care costs.

Controlling health care costs will probably require substantial changes in the U.S. health care system. Insurance companies, hospitals, and physicians will all be affected. As the examination of health care systems in other countries showed, no system can provide a good quality of medical care for low costs, but some countries do a better job than the United States. The health care systems of all industrialized countries are faced with the problem of providing care to an aging population whose health concerns predominantly stem from chronic illnesses.

Changing Health Care Needs In 1900, infectious diseases were the major health concern, but that situation changed during the 20th century. By the beginning of the 21st century, chronic illnesses were the leading cause of death and disability in the United States and other industrialized countries. The health care system, however, remains oriented toward providing acute care for sick people rather than providing services that will prevent, ameliorate, or manage chronic conditions. That is, the health care system has not responded to meet the needs created by changed patterns of disease that occurred during the 20th century (Research and Policy Committee, 2002). Therefore, people need services that may not be available and may receive (and pay for) services that do not best suit their health needs (Research and Policy Committee, 2002). Controlling chronic illness can occur through two routes: management to control these disabling conditions and prevention to avoid them.

Management of chronic illness is a current need that will become more important in the future. Cardiovascular disease, cancer, chronic lower respiratory disease, and diabetes account for over 70% of deaths in the United States (Research and Policy Committee, 2002). However, treatments for these and other chronic illnesses are plagued by undertreatment, overtreatment, and mistreatment. For example, undertreatment was detected for patients with diabetes, over half of whom failed to receive an eye exam, although diabetes often causes visual problems (Chassin, 1997). Overuse occurs when patients receive unnecessary medications or procedures, such as prescriptions for antibiotics for colds. Misuse occurs when health care providers make medical errors, which occurs with alarming frequency (Kohn et al., 1999). Creating a system that will provide more effective management of chronic illnesses will demand a shift from hospital- and physician-based care to a team approach that includes access to medical care and patient education to improve monitoring and self-care.

Self-care is also a priority for prevention, which is a strategy that can reduce the need for medical services. However, primary prevention offers more savings than secondary prevention. *Primary prevention* consists of immunizations and programs that encourage lifestyle changes, and this type of prevention is usually a good bargain. Immunizations have some potential for harm but remain good choices unless the risks from side effects of the immunization are comparable to the risk of catching the disease. Programs that encourage people to quit smoking, eat properly, exercise, and moderate their drinking generally have low cost and little potential to do harm (Leutwyler, 1995). In addition, some of these behaviors, such as smoking and inactivity, are risks for many health problems, and efforts oriented toward changing these behaviors can pay off by decreasing risks for several disorders. For example, a study of people who led a life that included the recommended exercise, body mass index, eating habits, and no history of smoking (Fraser & Shavlik, 2001) showed a significant life extension that led to the conclusion that healthy lifestyle can add 10 years of life. Therefore, primary prevention efforts pose few risks and offer many potential benefits.

Most prevention efforts are aimed at young and middle-aged adults who feel the need to change their behavior for health reasons, but a broadened emphasis may be more productive. A review of health behaviors in older people (Siegler, Bastian, Steffens, Bosworth, & Costa, 2002) concluded that not only lifelong health habits but also healthy behavior begun after age 65 can add healthy years to life. Efforts to build health-promoting behaviors in adolescents would be even more advantageous, but this group has been even more neglected for lifestyle interventions (Williams, Holmbeck, & Greenley, 2002). Most of the health research and interventions for adolescents have centered on injury prevention and smoking deterrence, but adolescents build a foundation for a lifetime of health-related behaviors. Thus, primary prevention efforts tailored for people throughout the lifespan have the potential to improve health and life expectancy.

Secondary prevention consists of screening people at risk for developing a disease in order to find potential problems in their early and more treatable stages. However, such efforts can be costly because the number of people at risk may be much larger than the number who has developed the disease. Based on the economic considerations of cost-benefit analysis—that is, how much money is spent and how much is saved—secondary prevention may cost more than it saves.

However, neither hospitals nor physicians are ideally suited to provide prevention services (Research and Policy Committee, 2002). Hospitals are oriented toward acute care, and physicians' time is very expensive to be devoted to health education. Providing health education and even immunizations is more cost efficient when handled by public health agencies, health educators, and health psychologists than by hospitals and physicians. Making these changes in the health care system would provide better care.

Will Health Psychology Continue to Grow?

What do the problems in the U. S. health care system mean for health psychology? Those problems have an impact on those in clinical health psychology and behavioral medicine; these practitioners must work within that troubled system. However, health psychologists are also working to reform the system. Their commitment to the biopsychosocial model has helped to promote a more comprehensive view of health and to end the false dichotomy between mental and physical health. Clinical health psychologists have firmly established their expertise as consultants, but health psychologists may become even more prominent as health care providers. For example, Kaiser Permanente of Northern California has designated psychologists as primary health care providers in its health maintenance facilities (Bruns, 1998). These psychologists are designated Behavioral Medicine Specialists and serve as part of teams that implement an integrated care approach to health care services.

This innovation was not motivated by psychologists seeking additional roles but by the HMO seeking savings on providing care. Behavioral Medicine Specialists can decrease the number of medical visits and help to keep patients well. These goals are important in controlling health care costs and in promoting wellness, and health psychology may play a more prominent role than in the past. This type of development paints an optimistic picture for clinical health psychology.

Health psychology research has contributed to the field of health by developing a knowledge base that continues to expand. The vision from the 1976 American Psychological Association Task Force on Health Research has been fulfilled; psychologists have taken a leading role in creating a scientific knowledge of the behavioral factors in disease development and prevention. This approach was new to health care because the biomedical model dominated medicine at that time. The biomedical model is fading as health care researchers and practitioners from all backgrounds come to realize that psychological and social factors also contribute to health and disease. Promoting the biopsychosocial model is important in changing the emphasis from treatment to prevention (Belar, 1997).

The problems in the health care system present major challenges for the future of health psychology. The short history of health psychology shows that the field has developed rapidly and made substantial contributions to research and practice in health care. The rapid gains of the

1980s slowed in the 1990s, but health psychology continued with steady growth. The 21st century will likely see continued growth for health psychology.

In Summary

Health psychology has made significant contributions to health care research and practice, but health psychology must meet several challenges to continue to grow, several of which are tied to the troubled health care system in the United States. Health care costs have risen in the United States more rapidly than in other industrialized countries, but some of those countries manage to provide health care to a wider segment of their populations and with a better outcome in terms of life expectancy. The United States needs to reform its inefficient health care system so that a larger segment of the population can receive quality health care services.

The future of health care will demand better management of chronic illnesses and a greater emphasis on prevention. The aging population will increase the need for management of chronic conditions that are more common among older people. Prevention may be the key to both better health and to controlling health care costs. Health psychology has a role to play in both the management and prevention of chronic illness.

With its promotion of the biopsychosocial model, health psychology continues to grow. Clinical health psychology continues to gain recognition in providing health care as part of multidisciplinary teams. Health psychology researchers continue to build a knowledge base that will furnish information about the interconnections among psychological, social, and biological factors that relate to health.

Answers

This chapter addressed three basic questions.

1. **What role does health psychology play in contributing to the goals of *Healthy People 2010?***
Health psychology is one of several disciplines that have a role in helping the nation achieve the goals and objectives of *Healthy People 2010.* The two broad goals of this document are (1) increasing the span of healthy life and (2) eliminating health disparities among various ethnic groups. Health psychologists emphasize adding healthy years of life, not merely more years. They cooperate with other health professionals in understanding and reducing health discrepancies among different ethnic groups.

2. **What type of training do health psychologists receive and what kinds of work do they do?**
Health psychologists receive doctoral-level training in the basic core of psychology, including (1) the biological, cognitive, psychological, and social bases of behavior, health, and disease; (2) advanced research, methodology, and statistics; (3) psychology and health measurement; (4) interdisciplinary collaboration; and (4) ethics and professional issues. In addition, they often receive at least 2 years of postdoctoral work in a specialized area of health psychology.
Health psychologists are employed in a variety of settings, including universities, hospitals, clinics, private practice, and health maintenance organizations. Many work for governmental agencies such as the CDC and the National Institutes of Health.

3. **What is the outlook for the future of health psychology?**
Health psychology faces challenges in the 21st century. Finding ways to control health care

costs is a major goal for all health care providers. Health psychologists are able to contribute to that goal through their expertise in understanding and treating the chronic diseases that have become the leading causes of death in industrialized countries. Even more important, health psychologists have advocated for prevention, which has the potential to decrease the need for health care. Prevention through behavior change can help in controlling health care costs. To be included in future health care, health psychologists must continue to add to both the research and practice components of the field: build a research base and develop more effective strategies for behavior change.

Suggested Readings

Belar, C. D. (1997). Clinical health psychology: A specialty for the 21st century. *Health Psychology, 16,* 411–416. In this presidential address to Division 38 of APA, Cynthia Belar outlines goals for clinical health psychologists for the 21st century, including accumulating a scientific body of knowledge, disseminating this knowledge, using the knowledge in their practice, and providing appropriate training for future health psychologists.

Sobel, D. S. (1995). Rethinking medicine: Improving health outcomes with cost-effective psychosocial interventions. *Psychosomatic Medicine, 57,* 234–244. David Sobel makes a persuasive argument for the effectiveness and cost effectiveness of the types of interventions that health psychologists have to offer.

Whitfield, K. E., Weidner, G., Clark, R., & Anderson, N. B. (2002). Sociodemographic diversity in behavioral medicine. *Journal of Consulting and Clinical Psychology, 70,* 463–481. Keith Whitfield and his colleagues provide a comprehensive review of ethnic, gender, and economic factors that affect health and life expectancy, analyzing each into the risks and protective factors associated with each demographic group.

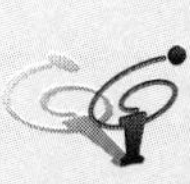

Search InfoTrac College Edition

Search these terms to learn more about topics in this chapter:

Healthy People 2010

Healthy life expectancy

Health disparities

Life expectancy and analysis

Life expectancy and models

Life expectancy and chronic disease

Life expectancy and sex differences

Disease prevention and life expectancy

Medical costs and increase

Medical care and cost increase

Models of health

Health psychologist and medical

Moderation and health

Glossary

A

A-beta fibers Large fibers in the spinal cord that inhibit the transmission of pain. (Chapter 7)

absolute risk A person's chances to developing a disease or disorder independent of any risk that other people may have for that disease or disorder. (Chapter 2)

acetylcholine A neurotransmitter in the autonomic nervous system. (Chapter 5)

acquired immune deficiency syndrome (AIDS) An immune deficiency caused by viral infection and resulting in vulnerability to a wide range of bacterial, viral, and malignant diseases. (Chapter 6)

acrolein A yellowish or colorless, pungent liquid produced as a by-product of tobacco smoke; one of the aldehydes. (Chapter 13)

action potential A discharge of the neuron's electrical potential. (Chapter 7)

acupressure The application of pressure rather than needles to the points used in acupuncture. (Chapter 7)

acupuncture An ancient Chinese form of analgesia that consists of inserting needles into specific points on the skin and continuously stimulating the needles. (Chapter 7)

acute pain Short-term pain that results from tissue damage or other trauma. (Chapter 7)

addiction Dependence on a drug such that stopping results in withdrawal symptoms. (Chapter 14)

A-delta fibers Small fibers that facilitate the transmission of pain. (Chapter 7)

adherence Patient's ability and willingness to follow recommended health practices. (Chapter 4)

adrenal cortex The outer layer of the adrenal glands; secretes glucocorticoids. (Chapter 5)

adrenal glands Endocrine glands that are located on top of each kidney and secrete hormones and affect metabolism. (Chapter 5)

adrenal medulla The inner layer of the adrenal glands; secretes epinephrine and norepinephrine. (Chapter 5)

adrenocortical response The response of the adrenal cortex, prompted by ACTH and resulting in release of cortisol. (Chapter 5)

adrenocorticotropic hormone (ACTH) A hormone produced by the anterior portion of the pituitary gland that acts on the adrenal gland and is involved in the stress response. (Chapter 5)

adrenomedullary response The response of the adrenal medullla, prompted by sympathetic nervous system activation and resulting in release of epinephrine. (Chapter 5)

aerobic exercise Exercise that requires an increased amount of oxygen consumption over an extended period of time. (Chapter 16)

afferent neurons Sensory neurons that relay information from the sense organs toward the brain. (Chapter 5)

agoraphobia An anxiety state characterized by fear about or avoidance of places or situations from which escape might be difficult. (Chapter 6)

alarm reaction The first stage of the general adaptation syndrome (GAS), in which the body's defenses are mobilized against a stressor. (Chapter 5)

alcohol dehydrogenase A liver enzyme that metabolizes alcohol into aldehyde. (Chapter 14)

aldehyde dehydrogenase An enzyme that converts aldehyde to acetic acid. (Chapter 14)

aldehydes A class of organic compounds obtained from alcohol by oxidation and also found in cigarette smoke; they cause mutations and are related to the development of cancer. (Chapter 13)

alkalosis An abnormally high level of alkaline in the body. (Chapter 15)

allergy An immune system response characterized by an abnormal reaction to a foreign substance. (Chapter 6)

allostasis The concept that different circumstances require different levels of physiological activation. (Chapter 5)
alveoli Small, saclike structures at the end of the bronchioles; the sites of oxygen and carbon dioxide exchange. (Chapter 13)
amenorrhea Cessation of the menses. (Chapter 15)
amphetamines One type of stimulant drug. (Chapter 14)
anabolic steroids Steroid drugs that increase muscle bulk and decrease body fat but also have toxic effects. (Chapter 14)
analgesic drugs Drugs that decrease the perception of pain. (Chapter 7)
anemia A low level of red blood cells, leading to generalized weakness and lack of vitality. (Chapter 15)
anesthesia Loss of sensations of temperature, touch, or pain. (Chapter 14)
angina pectoris A disorder involving a restricted blood supply to the myocardium, which results in chest pain and restricted breathing. (Chapter 9)
angiography A method of viewing cardiovascular damage through the use of X-ray pictures and the injection of dye into the circulatory system. (Chapter 9)
angioplasty Medical intervention in which a catheter with an inflatable tip is passed into an obstructed artery in order to flatten atherosclerotic deposits of plaque. (Chapter 9)
anorexia nervosa An eating disorder characterized by intentional starvation, distorted body image, excessive amounts of energy, and an intense fear of gaining weight. (Chapter 15)
antibodies Protein substances produced in response to a specific invader or antigen, marking it for destruction and thus creating immunity to that invader. (Chapter 6)
antigens Substances that provoke the immune system to produce antibodies. (Chapter 6)
anus Opening through which feces are eliminated. (Chapter 15)
arteries Vessels carrying blood away from the heart. (Chapter 9)
arterioles Small branches of an artery. (Chapter 9)
arteriosclerosis A condition marked by loss of elasticity and hardening of arteries. (Chapter 9)
asthma A chronic disease that causes constriction of the bronchial tubes, preventing air from passing freely and causing wheezing and difficulty breathing during attacks. (Chapters 6, 11)
atheromatous plaques Deposits of cholesterol and other lipids, connective tissue, and muscle tissue. (Chapter 9)
atherosclerosis The formation of plaque within the arteries. (Chapter 2, 9)
autoimmune diseases Disorders that occur as a result of the immune system's failure to differentiate between body cells and foreign cells, resulting in the body's attack and destruction of its own cells. (Chapter 6)
autonomic nervous system (ANS) The part of the peripheral nervous system that primarily serves internal organs. (Chapter 5)
aversion therapy A type of behavioral therapy based on classical conditioning technique and using some aversive stimulus to countercondition the patient's response. (Chapter 14)
avoidance coping Reacting to illness by the denial of threat and the use of such strategies as overeating, taking drugs, or hoping for a miracle. (Chapter 4)

B

barbiturates Synthetic sedative drug used medically to induce sleep. (Chapter 14)
B-cell A variety of lymphocyte that attacks invading microorganisms. (Chapter 6)
behavioral medicine An interdisciplinary field concerned with developing and integrating behavioral and biomedical sciences. (Chapter 1)
behavior modification Shaping behavior by manipulating reinforcement in order to obtain a desired behavior. (Chapter 8)
benign Limited in cell growth to a single tumor. (Chapter 10)
beta-carotene A form of vitamin A found in abundance in vegetables such as carrots and sweet potatoes. (Chapter 10)
bile salts Salts produced in the liver and stored in the gall bladder that aid in digestion of fats. (Chapter 15)
biofeedback The process of providing feedback information *about* the status of a biological system *to* that system. (Chapter 8)
biomedical model A perspective that considers disease to result from exposure to a specific a disease-causing organism. (Chapter 1)
biopsy A diagnostic procedure in which living tissue is removed from the body and examined for possible disease. (Chapter 10)
biopsychosocial model The approach to health that includes biological, psychological, and social influences. (Chapter 1)
body mass index (BMI) An estimate of obesity determined by body weight and height. (Chapter 15)
bronchitis Any inflammation of the bronchi. (Chapter 13)
bulimia An eating disorder characterized by periodic bingeing and purging, the latter usually taking the form of self-induced vomiting or laxative abuse. (Chapter 15)

C

C fibers Small-diameter nerve fibers that provide information concerning slow, diffuse, lingering pain. (Chapter 7)
cancer A group of diseases characterized by the presence of new cells that grow and spread beyond control. (Chapter 10)
capillaries Very small vessels that connect arteries and veins. (Chapter 9)
carcinogen A substance that induces cancer. (Chapter 13)
carcinogenic Substances that induce cancer. (Chapter 10)
carcinoma Cancer of the epithelial tissues. (Chapter 10)

cardiac arrhythmia Irregularity in the heartbeat rhythm. (Chapter 16)
cardiac rehabilitation A complex of approaches designed to restore heart patients to cardiovascular health. (Chapter 9)
cardiologist A medical doctor who specializes in the diagnoses and treatment of heart disease. (Chapter 9)
cardiovascular disease (CVD) Disorders of the circulatory system, including coronary artery disease and stroke. (Chapter 9)
cardiovascular reactivity (CVR) An increase in blood pressure and heart rate as a reaction to frustration or harassment. (Chapter 9)
cardiovascular system The system of the body that includes the heart, arteries, and veins. (Chapter 9)
case-control study A retrospective epidemiological study in which people affected by a given disease (cases) are compared to others not affected (controls). (Chapter 2)
catecholamines A class of chemicals containing epinephrine and norepinephrine. (Chapter 5)
catharsis The spoken or written expression of strong negative emotion, which may result in improvement in physiological or psychological health. (Chapter 8)
central control trigger A nerve impulse that descends from the brain and influences the perception of pain. (Chapter 7)
central nervous system (CNS) All those neurons within the brain and spinal cord. (Chapter 5)
cholecystokinin (CCK) A peptide hormone released by the intestines that may be involved in feelings of satiation after eating. (Chapter 15)
chronic diseases Diseases that develop or persist over a long period of time. (Chapter 1)
chronic pain Pain that endures beyond the time of normal healing; frequently experienced in the absence of detectable tissue damage. (Chapter 7)
cilia Tiny, hairlike structures lining parts of the respiratory system. (Chapter 13)
cirrhosis A liver disease resulting in the production of nonfunctional scar tissue. (Chapter 14)
cluster headache A type of severe headache that occurs in daily clusters for 4 to 16 weeks. Symptoms are similar to migraine, but duration is much briefer. (Chapter 7)
cocaine A stimulant drug extracted from the coca plant. (Chapter 14)
cognitive therapy Attempts to change behavior by altering beliefs, expectations, and personal standards. (Chapter 8)
cohort A group of subjects starting an experience at the same time. (Chapter 2)
compliance See adherence. (Chapter 4)
compulsions Persistent and pathological repetitions of behaviors. (Chapter 4)
coping Strategies that individuals use to manage the distressing problems and emotions in their lives. (Chapter 8)
coronary artery disease (CAD) A disorder of the myocardium arising from atherosclerosis and/or arteriosclerosis. (Chapter 9)
coronary heart disease (CHD) Any damage to the myocardium due to insufficient blood supply. (Chapter 9)
correlation coefficient Any positive or negative relationship between two variables. Correlational evidence cannot prove causation, but only that two variables vary together. (Chapter 2)
correlational studies Studies designed to yield information concerning the degree of relationship between two variables. (Chapter 2)
cortisol A type of glucocorticoid that provides a natural defense against inflammation and regulates carbohydrate metabolism. (Chapter 5)
cross-sectional study A type of research design in which subjects of different ages are studied at one point in time. (Chapter 2)
crowding A person's perception of discomfort due to a high-density environment. (Chapter 5)
cynical hostility Resentment and distrust of other people. (Chapter 4, 8)
cytokines Chemical messengers secreted by cells in the immune system, forming a communication system between the nervous and immune systems. (Chapter 6)

D

delirium tremens A condition induced by alcohol withdrawal and characterized by excessive trembling, sweating, anxiety, and hallucinations. (Chapter 14)
delta alcoholism A drinking pattern characterized by an inability to abstain from alcohol. (Chapter 14)
dependence A condition that occurs when a drug becomes incorporated into the functioning of the body's cells so that it is needed for "normal" functioning. (Chapter 7, 8, 14)
dependent variable A variable within an experimental setting whose value is hypothesized to change as a consequence of changes in the independent variable. (Chapter 2)
descriptive research A type of research that describes the relationship between variables rather than determining causation. (Chapter 2)
diabetes mellitus A disorder caused by insulin deficiency. (Chapter 6, 11)
diaphragm The partition separating the cavity of the chest from that of the abdomen. (Chapter 13)
diastolic pressure A measure of blood pressure between contractions of the heart. (Chapter 9)
diathesis-stress model A theory of stress that suggests that some individuals are vulnerable to stress-related illnesses because they are genetically predisposed to those illnesses. (Chapter 6)
disulfiram A drug that causes an aversive reaction when taken with alcohol; used to treat alcoholism; Antabuse. (Chapter 14)
dopamine A neurotransmitter that is especially important in mediating the reward associated with taking psychoactive drugs. (Chapter 14)

dorsal horns The part of the spinal cord away from the stomach that receives sensory input and that may play an important role in the perception of pain. (Chapter 7)

dose-response relationship A direct, consistent relationship between an independent variable, such as a behavior, and a dependent variable, such as an illness. For example, the greater the number of cigarettes one smokes, the greater the likelihood of lung cancer. (Chapter 2)

double blind An experimental design in which neither the subjects nor those who dispense the treatment condition have knowledge of who receives the treatment and who receives the placebo. (Chapter 2)

E

eating disorder Any serious and habitual disturbance in eating behavior that produces unhealthy consequences. (Chapter 15)

efferent neurons Motor neuron that conveys impulses away from the brain. (Chapter 5)

electrocardiogram (ECG) A measure of electrical signals of the heart. (Chapter 9)

electrolyte imbalance A condition caused by loss of body minerals. (Chapter 15)

electromyograph (EMG) biofeedback Feedback that reflects activity of the skeletal muscles. (Chapter 8)

emetine A drug that induces vomiting. (Chapter 14)

emotional disclosure A therapeutic technique whereby people express their strong emotions by talking or writing about them. (Chapter 8)

emotion-focused coping Coping strategies oriented toward managing the emotions that accompany the perception of stress. (Chapter 8)

emphysema A chronic lung disease in which scar tissue and mucus obstruct the respiratory passages. (Chapter 13)

endocrine system That system of the body consisting of ductless glands. (Chapter 5)

endorphins Naturally occurring neurochemicals whose effects resemble those of the opiates. (Chapter 7)

environmental tobacco smoke (ETS) The smoke of spouses, parents, or coworkers to which nonsmokers are exposed; passive smoking. (Chapter 13)

epidemiology A branch of medicine that investigates the various factors that contribute to either positive health or to the frequency and distribution of a disease or disorder. (Chapter 2)

epinephrine A chemical manufactured by the adrenal medulla that accounts for much of the hormone production of the adrenal glands; sometimes called *adrenalin*. (Chapter 5)

esophagus The tube leading from the pharynx to the stomach. (Chapter 15)

essential hypertension Elevations of blood pressure that have no known cause. (Chapter 9)

ethanol The variety of alcohol used in beverages. (Chapter 14)

ex post facto designs Scientific studies in which the values of the independent variable are not manipulated, but selected by the experimenter *after* the groups have naturally divided themselves. (Chapter 2)

exhaustion stage The final stage of the general adaptation syndrome (GAS), in which the body's ability to resist a stressor has been depleted. (Chapter 5)

exposure therapy A therapeutic technique whereby patients relive their traumatic experience in their imagination (Chapter 8)

F

feces Any materials left over after digestion. (Chapter 15)

fetal alcohol syndrome (FAS) A pattern of physical and psychological symptoms found in infants whose mothers drank heavily during pregnancy. (Chapter 14)

formaldehyde A colorless, pungent gas found in cigarette smoke; it causes irritation of the respiratory system and has been found to be carcinogenic; one of the aldehydes. (Chapter 13)

G

gall bladder A sac on the liver in which bile is stored. (Chapter 15)

gamma alcoholism A drinking pattern characterized by loss of control. (Chapter 14)

gastric juices Stomach secretions that aid in digestion. (Chapter 15)

gate control theory A theory of pain holding that structures in the spinal cord act as a gate for sensory input that is interpreted as pain. (Chapter 7)

general adaptation syndrome (GAS) The body's generalized attempt to defend itself against stress; consists of alarm reaction, resistance, and exhaustion. (Chapter 5)

glucagon A hormone secreted by the pancreas that stimulates the release of glucose, thus elevating blood sugar level. (Chapter 11)

glucocorticoids Hormones secreted by the adrenal cortex that increase the concentration of liver glycogen and blood sugar. (Chapter 5)

granulocytes A type of lymphocyte that acts rapidly to kill invading organisms. (Chapter 6)

H

hardy personality model The theory that suggests some people are buffered against the potentially harmful effects of stress due to their hardy personality. (Chapter 8)

health expectancy The period of life that a person spends free from disability. (Chapter 17)

health psychology A field of psychology that contributes to both behavioral medicine and behavioral health; the scientific study of behaviors that relate to health enhancement, disease prevention, and rehabilitation. (Chapter 1)

high-density lipoprotein (HDL) A form of lipoprotein that confers some protection against coronary artery disease. (Chapter 9)

hormones Chemical substances released into the blood and having effects on other parts of the body. (Chapter 5)

human immunodeficiency virus (HIV) A virus that attacks the human immune system, depleting the body's ability to fight infection; the infection that causes AIDS. (Chapter 11)

humoral immunity Immunity created through the process of exposure to antigens and production of antibodies in the blood stream. (Chapter 6)

hydrocyanic acid A poisonous acid produced by treating a cyanide with an acid; one of the products of cigarette smoke. (Chapter 13)

hypertension Abnormally high blood pressure, with either a systolic reading in excess of 160 or a diastolic reading in excess of 105. (Chapter 9)

hypoglycemia Deficiency of sugar in the blood. (Chapter 15)

hypothalamus A small structure beneath the thalamus, involved in the control of eating, drinking, and emotional behavior. (Chapter 15)

I

illness behavior Those activities undertaken by people who feel ill and who wish to discover their state of health, as well as suitable remedies. Illness behavior precedes formal diagnosis. (Chapter 3)

immune surveillance theory A theoretical model suggesting that cancer is the result of an immune system dysfunction. (Chapter 6)

immunity A response to foreign microorganisms that occurs with repeated exposure and results in resistance to a disease. (Chapter 6)

incidence A measure of the frequency of new cases of a disease or disorder during a specified period of time. (Chapter 2)

independent variable A variable that is manipulated by the experimenter in order to assess its possible effect on behavior; that is, on the dependent variable. (Chapter 2)

induction The process of being placed into a hypnotic state. (Chapter 8)

inflammation A general response that works to restore damaged tissue. (Chapter 6)

insulin A hormone that enhances glucose intake to the cells. (Chapter 11)

interneurons Neurons that connect sensory neurons to motor neurons; association neurons. (Chapter 5)

ischemia Restriction of blood flow to tissue or organs; often used with reference to the heart. (Chapter 9)

islet cells The part of the pancreas that produces glucagon and insulin. (Chapter 11)

isokinetic exercise Exercise requiring exertion for lifting and additional effort for returning weight to the starting position. (Chapter 16)

isotonic exercise Exercise that requires the contraction of muscles and the movement of joints, as in weight lifting. (Chapter 16)

K

Korsakoff syndrome A brain dysfunction found in some long-term heavy users of alcohol and resulting in both physiological and psychological impairment. (Chapter 14)

L

laminae Layers of cell bodies. (Chapter 7)

leptin A protein hormone produced by fat cells in the body and related to eating and weight control. (Chapter 15)

leukemia Cancer originating in blood or blood-producing cells. (Chapter 10)

lipoproteins Substances in the blood consisting of lipid and protein. (Chapter 9)

liver The largest gland in the body; it aids digestion by producing bile, regulates organic components of the blood, and acts as a detoxifier of blood. (Chapter 15)

longitudinal studies Research designs in which one group of subjects is studied over a period of time. (Chapter 2)

low-density lipoprotein (LDL) A form of lipoprotein found to be positively related to coronary artery disease. (Chapter 9)

lymph Tissue fluid that has entered a lymphatic vessel. (Chapter 6)

lymph nodes Small nodules of lymphatic tissue spaced throughout the lymphatic system that help clean lymph of debris. (Chapter 6)

lymphatic system System that transports lymph through the body. (Chapter 6)

lymphocytes White blood cells that are found in lymph and that are involved in the immune function. (Chapter 6)

lymphoma Cancer of the lymphoid tissues, including lymph nodes. (Chapter 10)

M

macrophages A type of lymphocyte that attacks invading organisms. (Chapter 6)

malignant Having the ability not only to grow but also to spread to other parts of the body. (Chapter 10)

mammography An X-ray technique for detecting breast tumors before they can be seen or felt. (Chapter 3)

medulla The structure of the hindbrain just above the spinal cord. (Chapter 7)

meta-analysis A statistical technique for combining results of several studies when these studies have similar definitions of variables. (Chapter 2)

metastasize To undergo metastasis, the spread of malignancy from one part of the body to another by way of the blood or lymph systems. (Chapter 10)

migraine headache Headache pain caused by constriction and dilation of the vascular arteries. (Chapter 7)

model A set of related principles or hypotheses constructed to explain significant relationships among concepts or observations. (Chapter 2)

mucociliary escalator The mechanism by which debris is moved toward the pharynx. (Chapter 13)

myelin A fatty substance that acts as insulation for neurons. (Chapter 7)

myocardial infarction Heart attack. (Chapter 9)

myocardium The heart muscle. (Chapter 9)

N

natural killer (NK) cells A type of lymphocyte that attacks invading organisms. (Chapter 6)

negative reinforcer Any painful or aversive condition that, when removed from a situation, strengthens the behavior it follows. (Chapters 4, 8)

neoplastic Characterized by new, abnormal growth of cells. (Chapter 10)

neuroendocrine system The system pertaining to the influence of the neural and endocrine systems and hypothesized to be the mechanism underlying the relationship between stress and illness. (Chapter 5)

neurons Nerve cells. (Chapter 5)

neurotransmitters Chemicals that are released by neurons and that affect the activity of other neurons. (Chapter 5)

nitric oxide A colorless gas prepared by the action of nitric acid on copper and also produced in cigarette smoke; it affects oxygen metabolism and may be dangerous. (Chapter 13)

nitrosamines Powerful carcinogens that may be produced by nitrites. (Chapter 10)

nocebo effect Adverse effect of a placebo. (Chapter 2)

nociceptors Sensory receptors in the skin and organs that are capable of responding to various types of stimulation that may cause tissue damage. (Chapter 7)

non-Hodgkin's lymphoma A malignancy characterized by rapidly growing tumors that are spread through the circulatory or lymphatic systems. (Chapter 10)

norepinephrine One of two major neurotransmitters of the autonomic nervous system. (Chapter 5)

O

obsessions Persistent and pathological thoughts that often lead to compulsive behaviors. (Chapter 4)

oncologist A physician who specializes in the treatment of cancer. (Chapter 10)

opiates Drugs derived from the opium poppy, including codeine, morphine, and heroin. (Chapter 14)

optimistic bias The belief that other people, but not oneself, will develop a disease, have an accident, or experience other negative events. (Chapters 3, 4, 9, 12, 13)

osteoarthritis Progressive inflammation of the joints. (Chapter 7)

osteoporosis A disease characterized by a reduction in bone density, brittleness of bones, and a loss of calcium from the bones. (Chapter 16)

P

pancreas An endocrine gland, located below the stomach, that produces digestive juices and hormones. (Chapter 11)

pancreatic juices Acid-reducing enzymes secreted by the pancreas into the small intestine. (Chapter 15)

parasympathetic nervous system A division of the autonomic nervous system that promotes relaxation and functions under normal, nonstressful conditions. (Chapter 5)

passive smoking The exposure of nonsmokers to the smoke of spouses, parents, or coworkers; environmental tobacco smoke. (Chapter 13)

pathogen Any disease-causing organism. (Chapter 1)

pepsin Enzyme that is produced by gastric mucosa and that initiates digestive activity. (Chapter 15)

periaqueductal gray An area of the midbrain that, when stimulated, decreases pain. (Chapter 7)

peripheral nervous system (PNS) The nerves that lie outside the brain and spinal cord. (Chapter 5)

peristalsis Contractions that propel food through the digestive tract. (Chapter 15)

phagocytosis The process of engulfing and killing foreign particles. (Chapter 6)

phantom limb pain The experience of chronic pain in an absent body part. (Chapter 7)

pharynx Part of the digestive tract between the mouth and the esophagus. (Chapter 15)

pituitary gland An endocrine gland that lies within the brain and whose secretions regulate many other glands. (Chapter 5)

placebo An inactive substance or condition that has the appearance of the independent variable and that may cause subjects in an experiment to improve or change behavior due to their belief in the placebo's efficacy; a treatment that is effective because of a patient's belief in the treatment. (Chapter 2)

placebo effect An effect that is due to expectation rather than to effects of the treatment. (Chapter 2)

plasma cells Cells that are derived from B-cells and that secrete antibodies. (Chapter 6)

population density A physical condition in which a high level of population is confined in a limited space. (Chapter 5)

positive reinforcer Any positively valued stimulus that, when added to a situation, strengthens the behavior it follows. (Chapters 4, 8)

posttraumatic stress disorder (PTSD) An anxiety disorder caused by experience with an extremely traumatic event and characterized by recurrent and intrusive reexperiencing of that event. (Chapters 5, 6)

prechronic pain Pain that endures beyond the acute phase but has not yet become chronic. (Chapter 7)

prevalence The proportion of a population that has a disease or disorder at a specific point in time. (Chapter 2)

primary afferents Sensory neurons that convey impulses from the skin to the spinal cord. (Chapter 7)

primary appraisal One's initial appraisal of a potentially stressful event (Lazarus and Folkman's term). (Chapter 5)

problem-focused coping Coping strategies aimed at changing the source of the stress. (Chapter 8)

prospective studies Longitudinal studies that begin with a disease-free group of subjects and follow the occurrence of disease in that population or sample. (Chapter 2)

psychoneuroimmunology A multidisciplinary field that focuses on the interactions among behavior, the nervous system, the endocrine system, and the immune system. (Chapter 6)

punishment The presentation of an aversive stimulus or the removal of a positive one. Punishment sometimes, but not always, weakens a response. (Chapter 4)

R

Raynaud's disease A vasoconstrictive disorder stemming from inadequate circulation in the extremities, especially the fingers or toes, and resulting in pain. (Chapter 8)

reappraisal One's nearly constant reevaluation of stressful events (Lazarus and Folkman's term). (Chapter 5)

reciprocal determinism Bandura's model that includes environment, behavior, and person as mutually interacting to determine conduct. (Chapter 4)

rectum The end of the digestive tract leading to the anus. (Chapter 15)

relative risk The risk a person has for a particular disease compared with the risk of other people who do not have that person's condition or lifestyle. (Chapter 2)

reliability The extent to which a test or other measuring instrument yields consistent results. (Chapter 2)

resistance stage The second stage of the general adaptation syndrome (GAS), in which the body adapts to a stressor. (Chapter 5)

retrospective studies Longitudinal studies that look back at the history of a population or sample. (Chapter 2)

rheumatoid arthritis An autoimmune disorder characterized by a dull ache within or around a joint. (Chapters 6, 7)

risk factor An characteristic or condition that occurs with greater frequency in people with a disease than it does in people free from that disease. (Chapter 2)

S

salivary glands Glands that furnish moisture that helps in tasting and digesting food. (Chapter 15)

sarcoma Cancer of the connective tissues. (Chapter 10)

secondary appraisal One's perceived ability to control or cope with harm, threat, or challenge (Lazarus and Folkman's term). (Chapter 5)

secondary hypertension Elevations in blood pressure that are triggered by other diseases. (Chapter 9)

sedatives Drugs that induce relaxation and sometimes intoxication by lowering the activity of the brain, the neurons, the muscles, the heart, and even by slowing the metabolic rate. (Chapter 14)

self-efficacy The belief that one is capable of performing the behaviors that will produce desired outcomes in any particular situation. (Chapters 3, 4, 8)

self-selection A condition of an experimental investigation in which subjects are allowed, in some manner, to determine their own placement in either the experimental or the control group. (Chapter 2)

setpoint A hypothetical ratio of fat to lean tissue at which a person's weight will tend to stabilize. (Chapter 15)

sick role behavior Those activities undertaken by people who have been diagnosed as sick and that are directed at getting well. (Chapter 3)

single-blind design A design in which the participants do not know if they are receiving the active or inactive treatment, but the providers are not blind to treatment conditions. (Chapter 2)

social contacts Number and kinds of people with whom one associates; members of one's social network. (Chapter 8)

social isolation The absence of specific role relationships. (Chapter 8)

social network Number and kinds of people with whom one associates; social contacts. (Chapter 8)

social support Both tangible and intangible support a person receives from other people. (Chapter 4, 8)

somatic nervous system The part of the PNS that serves the skin and voluntary muscles. (Chapter 5)

somatosensory cortex The part of the brain that receives and processes sensory input from the body. (Chapter 7)

somatosensory system The part of the nervous system that carries sensory information from the body to the brain. (Chapter 7)

spleen A large organ near the stomach that serves as a repository for lymphocytes and red blood cells. (Chapter 6)

spontaneous remission Disappearance of problem behavior or illness without treatment. (Chapter 14)

staleness Negative mood, fatigue, and depression as a result of overtraining in athletes. (Chapter 16)

state anxiety A temporary condition of dread or uneasiness stemming from a specific situation. (Chapter 16)

stress test An exercise test to diagnose coronary artery disease. (Chapter 9)

stress-response-dampening (SRD) Decrease in strength of responses to stress, caused by consumption of alcohol. (Chapter 14)

stroke Damage to the brain resulting from lack of oxygen; typically the result of cardiovascular disease. (Chapter 9)

subject variable A variable chosen (rather than manipulated) by a researcher to provide levels of comparison for groups of subjects. (Chapter 2)

substantia gelatinosa Two layers of the dorsal horns of the spinal cord. (Chapter 7)

sympathetic nervous system A division of the autonomic nervous system that mobilizes the body's resources in emergency, stressful, and emotional and emergency situations. (Chapter 5)

synaptic cleft The space between neurons. (Chapter 5)

syndrome A cluster of symptoms that characterize a particular condition. (Chapter 7)

synergistic effect The combined effect of two or more variables that exceeds the sum of their individual effects. (Chapter 10)

systolic pressure A measure of blood pressure generated by the heart's contraction. (Chapter 9)

T

T-cells The cells of the immune system that produce immunity. (Chapter 6)

tension headache Pain produced by sustained muscle contractions in the neck, shoulders, scalp, and face. (Chapter 7)

thalamus Structure in the forebrain that acts as a relay center for incoming sensory information and outgoing motor information. (Chapter 7)

theory A set of related assumptions from which testable hypotheses can be drawn. (Chapter 2)

thermal biofeedback Feedback concerning changes in skin temperature. (Chapter 8)

thermister A temperature-sensitive resistor used in thermal biofeedback. (Chapter 8)

thymosin A hormone produced by the thymus. (Chapter 6)

thymus An organ located near the heart that secretes thymosin and thus processes and activates T-lymphocytes. (Chapter 6)

tolerance The condition of requiring increasing levels of a drug in order to produce a constant level of effect. (Chapters 7, 8, 14)

tonsils Masses of lymphatic tissue located in the pharynx. (Chapter 6)

trait anxiety A personality characteristic that manifests itself as a more or less constant feeling of dread or uneasiness. (Chapter 16)

tranquilizers A type of sedative drug that reduces anxiety. (Chapter 14)

transcutaneous electrical nerve stimulation (TENS) Treatment for pain involving electrical stimulation of neurons from the surface of the skin. This stimulation blocks other sensory input, providing pain relief. (Chapter 7)

transmission cells Afferent neurons that connect to other neurons; also called secondary afferents. (Chapter 7)

triglycerides A group of molecules consisting of glycerol and three fatty acids; one of the components of serum lipids that has been implicated in the formation of atherosclerotic plaque. (Chapter 9)

U

urban press The many environmental stressors that affect city living, including noise, crowding, crime, and pollution. (Chapter 5)

V

vaccination A method of inducing immunity in which a weakened form of a virus or bacteria is introduced into the body. (Chapter 6)

validity Accuracy; the extent to which a test or other measuring instrument measures what it is supposed to measure. (Chapter 2)

veins Vessels that carry blood to the heart. (Chapter 9)

venules The smallest veins. (Chapter 9)

W

well-year The equivalent of a year of complete wellness. (Chapter 17)

withdrawal Adverse physiological reactions exhibited when a drug-dependent person stops using that drug; the withdrawal symptoms are typically unpleasant and opposite from the drug's effects. (Chapter 14)

References

Abbott, R. D., Rodriguez, B. L., Burchfiel, C. M., & Curb, J. D. (1994). Physical activity in older middle-aged men and reduced risk of stroke: The Honolulu Heart Program. *American Journal of Epidemiology, 139,* 881–893.

Abdel-Ghany, M., & Wang, M. Q. (2001). Factors associated with different degrees of health insurance. *Family and Consumer Sciences Research Journal, 29,* 252–266.

Achterberg, J., Kenner, C., & Lawlis, G. F. (1988). Severe burn injuries: A comparison of relaxation imagery and biofeedback for pain management. *Journal of Mental Imagery, 12,* 71–87.

Acierno, R., Resnick, H. S., & Kilpatrick, D. G. (1997). Prevalence rates, case identification, and risk factors for sexual assault, physical assault, and domestic violence in men and women, part 1 (Health impact of interpersonal violence). *Behavioral Medicine, 23,* 53–65.

Ackard, D. M., Brehm, B. J., & Steffen, J. J. (2002). Exercise and eating disorders in college-aged women: Profiling excessive exercisers. *Eating Disorders, 10,* 31–47.

Ader, R. (2001). Psychoneuroimmunology. *Current Directions in Psychological Science, 10,* 94–98.

Ader, R., & Cohen, N. (1975). Behaviorally conditioned immunosuppression. *Psychosomatic Medicine, 37,* 333–340.

Adler, N., & Matthews, K. (1994). Health psychology: Why do some people get sick and some stay well? *Annual Review of Psychology, 45,* 229–259.

Ahlbom, A., & Norell, S. (1990). *Introduction to modern epidemiology* (2nd ed.). Chestnut Hill, MA: Epidemiology Resources.

Ahluwalia, I. B., Grummer-Strawn, L., & Scanlon, K. S. (1997). Exposure to environmental tobacco smoke and birth outcome: Increased effects on pregnant women aged 30 years or older. *American Journal of Epidemiology, 146,* 42–47.

AIDS Alert. (2001). Changes in risk behaviors. *AIDS Alert, 16,* 125–126.

Aiken, L. S., West, S. G., Woodward, C. K., & Reno, R. R. (1994). Health beliefs and compliance with mammography-screening recommendations in asymptomatic women. *Health Psychology, 13,* 122–129.

Ajani, U. A., Hennekens, C. H., Spelsberg, A., & Manson, J. E. (2000). Alcohol consumption and risk of Type 2 diabetes mellitus among US male physicians. *Archives of Internal Medicine, 160,* 11025–11030.

Ajzen, I. (1985). From intentions to actions: A theory of planned behavior. In J. Kuhland & J. Beckman (Eds.), *Action-control: From cognitions to behavior* (pp. 11–39) Heidelberg, Germany: Springer.

Ajzen, I. (1988). *Attitudes, personality, and behavior.* Chicago: Dorsey Press.

Ajzen, I. (1991). The theory of planned behavior. *Organizational Behavior and Human Decision Processes, 50,* 179–211.

Ajzen, I., & Fishbein, M. (1980). *Understanding attitudes and predicting social behavior.* Englewood Cliffs, NJ: Prentice-Hall.

Albarracin, D., Fishbein, M., Johnson, B. T., & Muellerleile, P. A. (2001). Theories of reasoned action and planned behavior as models of condom use: A meta-analysis. *Psychological Bulletin, 127,* 142–161.

Albert, C. M., Hennekens, C. H., O'Donnell, C. J., Ajani, U. A., Carey, V. J., Willett, W. C., et al. (1998). Fish consumption and risk of sudden cardiac death. *Journal of the American Medical Association, 279,* 23–28.

Albert, C. M., Mittleman, M. A., Chae, C. U., Lee, I. -M., Hennekens, C. H., & Manson, J. E. (2000). Triggering of sudden death from cardiac causes by vigorous exertion. *New England Journal of Medicine, 343,* 1355–1361.

Alden, L. E. (1988). Behavioral self-management controlled-drinking strategies in a context of secondary prevention. *Journal of Consulting and Clinical Psychology, 56,* 280–286.

Alexander, F. (1950). *Psychosomatic medicine.* New York: Norton.

Allen, J., Markovitz, J., Jacobs, D. R., Jr., & Knox, S. S. (2001). Social support and health behavior in hostile Black and White men and women in CARDIA. *Psychosomatic Medicine, 63,* 609–618.

Allison, D. B., Fontaine, K. R., Manson, J. E., Stevens, J., & VanItallie, T. B. (1999). Annual deaths attributable to obesity in the United States. *Journal of the American Medical Association, 282,* 1530–1538.

Allport, G. W. (1966). Traits revisited. *American Psychologist, 21,* 1–10.

Alper, J. (1993). Ulcers as infectious diseases. *Science, 260,* 159–160.

Amanzio, M., & Benedetti, F. (1999). Neuropharmacological dissection of placebo analgesia: Expectation-activated opioid systems versus conditioning-activated specific subsystems. *Journal of Neuroscience, 19,* 484–494.

Amato, P. R. (2000). The consequences of divorce for adults and children. *Journal of Marriage and the Family, 62,* 1269–1287.

American Cancer Society. (2002). *Cancer facts & figures—2002.* Atlanta: American Cancer Society.

American Dietetic Association. (2001). Adherence to a very-low-fat diet in cardiac rehabilitation patients. *Journal of the American Dietetic Association, 101,* 709.

American Lung Association. (2002). *Trends in asthma mortality and morbidity.* Retrieved from the World Wide Web, April 29, 2002, at www.lungusa.org/data/asthma/ASTHMAdt.pdf.

American Medical Association (AMA). (2002). *AMA policies on alcohol.* Retrieved from the World Wide Web, June 24, 2002, at www.amaassn.org/ama/pub/category/3342.html.

American Psychiatric Association (APA). (2000). *Diagnostic and statistical manual of mental disorders* (4th ed., text revision). Washington, DC: Author.

American Psychological Association (APA). Task Force on Health Research. (1976). Contributions of psychology to health research: Patterns, problems, and potentials. *American Psychologist, 31,* 263–274.

American Psychological Association (APA). (1992). Ethical principles of psychologists and code of conduct. *American Psychologist, 47,* 1597–1611.

American Psychological Association (APA). (1999). *Warning signs.* Retrieved from the World Wide Web, June 14, 2002, at http://helping.apa.org/warningsigns/index.html.

Ammerman, R. T., Ott, P. J., Tarter, R. E., & Blackson, T. C. (1999). Critical issues in prevention of substance abuse. In R. T. Ammerman, P. J. Ott, & R. E. Tarter (Eds.), *Prevention and societal impact of drug and alcohol abuse* (pp. 3–20). Mahwah, NJ: Erlbaum.

Amschler, D. H. (2002). The alarming increase of Type 2 diabetes in children. *Journal of School Health, 72,* 39–41.

Andersen, B. L. (1998). Psychology's science in responding to the challenge of cancer: Biobehavioral perspectives. *Psychological Science Agenda, 11* (1), 14–15.

Andersen, R. E., Crespo, C. J., Bartlett, S. J., Cheskin, L. J., & Pratt, M. (1998). Relationship of physical activity and television watching with body weight and level of fatness among children: Results from the third National Health and Nutrition Examination Survey. *Journal of the American Medical Association, 279,* 938–942.

Andersen, R. E., Walden, T. A., Bartlett, S. J., Zemel, B., Verde, T. J., & Franckowiak, S. C. (1999). Effects of lifestyle activity vs. structured aerobic exercise in obese women: A randomized trial. *Journal of the American Medical Association, 281,* 335–240.

Anderson, K. O., Syrjala, K. L., & Cleeland, C. S. (2001). How to assess cancer pain. In D. C. Turk & R. Melzack (Eds.), *Handbook of pain assessment* (2nd ed., pp. 579–600). New York: Guilford Press.

Andrasik, F. (2001). Assessment of patients with headache. In D. C. Turk & R. Melzack (Eds.), *Handbook of pain assessment* (2nd ed., pp. 454–474). New York: Guilford Press.

Andres, R. (1995). Body weight and age. In K. D. Brownell & C. G. Fairburn. *Eating disorders and obesity: A comprehensive handbook* (pp. 65–70). New York: Guilford Press.

Apodaca, J. X., Woodruff, S. I., Candelaria, J., Elder, J. P., & Zlot, A. (1997). Hispanic health program participant and nonparticipant characteristics. *American Journal of Health Behavior 21,* 356–369.

Argyle, M. (1992). Benefits produced by supportive social relationships. In H. O. E. Veiel & U. Baumann (Eds.), *The meaning and measurement of social support* (pp. 13–32). New York: Hemisphere.

Armor, D. J., Polich, J. M., & Stambul, H. B. (1976). *Alcoholism and treatment.* Santa Monica, CA: Rand.

Aromaa, M., Sillanpaa, M., Rautava, P., & Helenius, H. (2000). Pain experience of children with headache and their families: A controlled study. *Pediatrics, 106,* 270–275.

Arriaza, C. A., & Mann, T. (2001). Ethnic differences in eating disorder symptoms among college students: The confounding role of body mass index. *Journal of American College Health, 49,* 309–315.

Arruda-Olson, A. M., Mahoney, D. W., Nehra, A., Leckel, M., & Pellikka, P. A. (2002). Cardiovascular effects of sidenafil during exercise in men with known or probable coronary artery disease: A randomized crossover trial. *Journal of the American Medical Association, 287,* 719–725.

Ary, D. V., & Biglan, A. (1988). Longitudinal changes in adolescent cigarette smoking behavior: Onset and cessation. *Journal of Behavioral Medicine, 11,* 361–382.

Ashley, M. J., Rehm, J., Bondy, S., Single, E., & Rankin, J. (2000). Beyond ischemic heart disease: Are there other health benefits from drinking alcohol? *Contemporary Drug Problems, 27,* 735–778.

Ashmore, J. P., Krewski, D., Zielinksi, J. M., Jiang, H., Semenciw, R. & Band, P. R. (1998). First analysis of mortality and occupational radiation exposure based on the National Dose Registry of Canada. *American Journal of Epidemiology, 148,* 564–574.

Ashton, W., Nanchahal, K., & Wood, D. (2001). Body mass index and metabolic risk factors for coronary heart disease in women. *European Health Journal, 22,* 46–55.

Asthma and Allergy Foundation of America. (2002). Climb 4 air. Retrieved from the World Wide Web, April 29, 2002, at http://www.aafa.org/templ/display.cfm?id=275.

Astin, J. A. (1997). Stress reduction through mindfulness meditation: Effects on psychological symptomatology, sense of control, and spiritual experiences. *Psychotherapy and Psychosomatics, 66,* 97–106.

Austin, J. A. (1998). Why patients use alternative medicine: Results of a national study. *Journal of the American Medical Association, 279,* 1548–1553.

Australian Consumers' Association. (2002, March). Painkillers: With so many painkillers on the market these days, choosing one is enough to give anyone a headache. *Choice,* 12–16.

Averbuch, M., & Katzper, M. (2000). A search for sex differences in response to analgesia. *Archives of Internal Medicine, 160,* 3424–3428.

Ayanian, J. Z., & Cleary, P. D. (1999). Perceived risks of heart disease and cancer among cigarette smokers. *Journal of the American Medical Association, 281,* 1019–1021.

Bagnardi, V., Blangiardo, M., La Vecchia, C., & Corrao, G. (2001). Alcohol consumption and the risk of cancer: A meta-analysis. *Alcohol Research & Health, 25,* 263–270.

Bahrke, M. S., & Morgan, W. P. (1978). Anxiety reduction following exercise and meditation. *Cognitive Therapy and Research, 2,* 323–334.

Baik, I., Ascherio, A., Rimm, E. B., Giovannucci, E., Spiegelman, D., Stampfer, M. J., et al. (2000). Adiposity and mortality in men. *American Journal of Epidemiology, 152,* 264–271.

Bailey, J. E., Kellerman, A. L., Somes, G. W., Banton, J. G., Rivara, F. P., & Rushforth, N. P. (1997). Risk factors for violent death of women in the home. *Archives of Internal Medicine, 157,* 777–782.

Bailis, D. S., Segall, A., Mahon, M. J., Chipperfield, J. G., & Dunn, E. M. (2001). Perceived control in relation to socioeconomic and behavioral resources for health. *Social Science & Medicine, 52,* 1661–1676.

Baker, F., Ainsworth, S. P., Dye, J. T., Crammer, C., Thun, M. J., Hoffmann, D., et al. (2000). Health risks associated with cigar smoking. *Journal of the American Medical Association, 284,* 735–740.

Ballard, J. E., Koepsell, T. D., & Rivara, F. (1992). Association of smoking and alcohol drinking with residential fire injuries. *American Journal of Epidemiology, 135,* 26–34.

Banaji, M. R., & Steele, C. M. (1989). The social cognition of alcohol use. *Social Cognition, 7,* 137–151.

Bandura, A. (1986). *Social foundations of thought and action: A social cognitive theory.* Englewood Cliffs, NJ: Prentice-Hall.

Bandura, A. (1997). *Self-efficacy: The exercise of control.* New York: Freeman.

Bandura, A. (2001). Social cognitive theory: An agentic perspective. *Annual Review of Psychology, 52,* 1–26.

Barber, G. R. (2001). Feeling the burn. *American Fitness, 19*(6), 51–53.

Barber, J. (1996). A brief introduction to hypnotic analgesia. In J. Barber (Ed.), *Hypnosis and suggestion in the treatment of pain: A clinical guide.* New York: Norton.

Barber, T. X. (1982). Hypnosuggestive procedures in the treatment of clinical pain: Implications for theories of hypnosis and suggestive therapy. In T. Millon, C. J. Green, & R. B. Meagher, Jr. (Eds.), *Handbook of clinical health psychology.* New York: Plenum.

Barber, T. X. (1984). Hypnosis, deep relaxation, and active relaxation: Data, theory, and clinical applications. In R. L. Woolfolk & P. M. Lehrer (Eds.), *Principles and practice of stress management.* New York: Guilford Press.

Barker, J. C., Morrow, J., & Mitteness, L. S. (1998). Gender, informal social support networks, and elderly urban African Americans. *Journal of Aging Studies, 12,* 199–222.

Barr, A., & MacKinnon, D. P. (1998). Designated driving among college. *Journal of Studies on Alcohol, 59,* 549–564.

Barrett, J. J., Ford, G. R., Stewart, K. E., & Haley, W. E. (1994, August). *Family caregiver appraisals of stressors in senile dementia: Gender differences?* Paper presented at the American Psychological Association, Los Angeles, CA.

Barrett, K. E., Riggar, T. F., & Flowers, C. R. (1997). Violence in the workplace: Preparing for the age of rage. *Journal of Rehabilitation Administration, 21,* 171–188.

Batty, D., & Thune, I. (2000). Does physical activity prevent cancer? *British Medical Journal, 321,* 1424–1425.

Baum, A., Gatchel, R. J., & Schaeffer, M. A. (1983). Emotional, behavioral, and physiological effects of chronic stress at Three Mile Island. *Journal of Consulting and Clinical Psychology, 51,* 565–572.

Baum, A., & Grunberg, N. (1995). Measurement of stress hormones. In S. Cohen, R. C. Kessler, & L. U. Gordon (Eds.), *Measuring stress: A guide for health and social scientists* (pp. 175–192). New York: Oxford University Press.

Baum, A., & Posluszny, D. M. (1999). Health psychology: Mapping biobehavioral contributions to health and illness. *Annual Review of Psychology, 50,* 137–164.

Beaglehole, R., Bonita, R., & Kjellström, T. (1993). *Basic epidemiology.* Geneva, Switzerland: World Health Organization.

Beaglehole, R., Stewart, A. W., Jackson, R., Dobson, A. J., McElduff, P., D'Este, K., et al. (1997). Declining rates of coronary heart disease in New Zealand and Australia, 1983–1993. *American Journal of Epidemiology, 145,* 707–713.

Beck, A. T. (1976). *Cognitive therapy and the emotional disorders.* New York: International Universities Press.

Beck, A. T., Ward, C. H., Mendelson, M., Mock, J., & Erbaugh, J. (1961). An inventory for measuring depression. *Archives of General Psychiatry, 4,* 561–571.

Becker, G. (2001). Effects of being uninsured on ethnic minorities' management of chronic illness. *Western Journal of Medicine, 175,* 19–22.

Becker, M. H. (1979). Understanding patient compliance: The contributions of attitudes and other psychosocial factors. In S. J. Cohen (Ed.), *New directions in patient compliance* (pp. 1–31). Lexington, MA: Lexington Books.

Becker, M. H., & Rosenstock, I. M. (1984). Compliance with medical advice. In A. Steptoe & A. Mathews (Eds.), *Health care and human behavior.* London: Academic Press.

Beecher, H. K. (1946). Pain of men wounded in battle. *Annals of Surgery, 123,* 96–105.

Beecher, H. K. (1955). The powerful placebo. *Journal of the American Medical Association, 149,* 1602–1607.

Beecher, H. K. (1956). Relationship of significance of wound to pain experience. *Journal of the American Medical Association, 161,* 1609–1613.

Beecher, H. K. (1957). The measurement of pain. *Pharmacological Review, 9,* 59–209.

Behrens, V., Seligman, P., Cameron, L., Mathias, C. G. T., & Fine, L. (1994). The prevalence of back pain, hand discomfort, and dermatitis in the US work population, *American Journal of Public Health, 84,* 1780–1785.

Belar, C. D. (1997). Clinical health psychology: A specialty for the 21st century. *Health Psychology, 16,* 411–416.

Bell, C. M., Crystal, M., Detsky, A. S., & Redelmeier, D. A. (1998). Shopping around for hospital services: A comparison of the United States and Canada. *Journal of the American Medical Association, 279,* 1015–1017.

Bell, R. A., Kravitz, R. L., Thom, D., Krupat, & Azari, R. (2001). Unsaid but not forgotten: Physician-patient relationship. *Archives of Internal Medicine, 161,* 1977–1983.

Belloc, N. (1973). Relationship of health practices and mortality. *Preventive Medicine, 2,* 67–81.

BenDebba, M., Torgerson, W. S., Boyd, R. J., Dawson, E. G., Hardy, R. W., Robertson, J. T., et al. (2002). Persistent low back pain and sciatica in the United States: Treatment outcomes. *Journal of Spinal Disorders & Techniques, 15,* 2–15.

Bender, R., Trautner, C., Spraul, M., & Berger, M. (1998). Assessment of excess mortality in obesity. *American Journal of Epidemiology, 147,* 42–48.

Benedetti, F., & Amanzio, M. (1997). The neurobiology of placebo analgesia: From endogenous opioids to cholescystokinin. *Progressive Neurobiology, 52,* 109–125.

Ben-Eliyahu, S., Yirmiya, R., Liebeskind, J. C., Taylor, A. N., & Gale, R. P. (1991). Stress increases metastatic spread of mammary tumor in rats: Evidence for mediation by the immune system. *Brain, Behavior, and Immunity, 5,* 193–205.

Benishek, L. A., (1996). Evaluation of the factor structure underlying two measures of hardiness. *Assessment, 3,* 423–435.

Bennett, H. L., & Disbrow, E. A. (1993). Preparing for surgery and medical procedures. In D. Goleman & J. Gurin (Eds.), *Mind/body medicine: How to use your mind for better health* (pp. 401–427). Yonkers, NY: Consumer Reports Books.

Ben-Shlomo, Y., Smith, G. D., Shipley, M. S., & Marmot, M. G. (1994). What determines mortality risk in male former cigarette smokers? *American Journal of Public Health, 84,* 1235–1242.

Benson, H. (1975). *The relaxation response.* New York: Morrow.

Benson, H., Beary, J. F., & Carol, M. P. (1974). The relaxation response. *Psychiatry, 37,* 37–46.

Benyamini, Y., Leventhal, E. A., & Leventhal, H. (1997). Attributions and health. In A. Baum, S. Newman, J. Weinman, R. West, & C. McManus (Eds.), *Cambridge handbook of psychology, health and medicine* (pp. 72–77). Cambridge, UK: Cambridge University Press.

Benyamini, Y., Leventhal, E. A., & Leventhal, H. (2000). Gender differences in processing information for making self-assessments of health. *Psychosomatic Medicine, 62,* 354–364.

Berger, K., Ajani, U. A., Kase, C. S., Gaziano, J. M., Buring, J. E., Glynn, R. J., et al. (1999). Light-to-moderate alcohol consumption and the risk of stroke among U.S. male physicians. *The New England Journal of Medicine, 341,* 1557–1564.

Berg, P., & Westerling, R. (2001). Bicycle helmet use among schoolchildren—The influence of parental involvement and children's attitudes. *Injury Prevention, 7,* 218–222.

Berkman, L. F. (1986). Social networks, support, and health: Taking the next step forward. *American Journal of Epidemiology, 123,* 559–562.

Berkman, L. F., & Breslow, L. (1983). *Health and ways of living: The Alameda County Study.* New York: Oxford University Press.

Berkman, L. F., Breslow, L., & Wingard, D. (1983). Health practices and mortality risk. In L. F. Berkman & L. Breslow (Eds.), *Health and ways of living: The Alameda County study.* New York: Oxford University Press.

Berkman, L. F., & Syme, S. L. (1979). Social networks, host resistance, and mortality: A nine-year follow-up study of Alameda County residents. *American Journal of Epidemiology, 109,* 186–204.

Berne, R. M., & Levy, M. N. (2000). *Principles of physiology* (3rd ed.). St. Louis: Mosby.

Berns, S. (2000). Startling statistics in child firearm deaths. *The Brown University Child and Adolescent Behavior Letter, 16,* 3.

Bernstein, L., Henderson, B. E., Hanisch, R., Sullivan-Halley, J., & Ross, R. K. (1994). Physical exercise and reduced risk of breast cancer in young women. *Journal of the National Cancer Institute, 86,* 1403–1408.

Biener, L., & Heaton, A. (1995). Women dieters of normal weight: Their motives, goals, and risks. *American Journal of Public Health, 85,* 714–717.

Biener, L., & Siegel, M. (2000). Tobacco marketing and adolescent smoking: More support for a causal inference. *American Journal of Public Health, 90,* 407–411.

Bird, C. E. (1999). Gender, household labor, and psychological distress: The impact of the amount and division of housework. *Journal of Health and Social Behavior, 40,* 32–45.

Bird, S. T., Harvey, S. M., Beckman, L. J., & Johnson, C. H. (2000). Getting your partner to use condoms: Interviews with men and women at risk of HIV/STDs. *Journal of Sex Research, 38,* 233–240.

Bishop, G. D., & Robinson, G. (2000). Anger, harassment, and cardiovascular reactivity among Chinese and Indian men in Singapore. *Psychosomatic Medicine, 62,* 684–692.

Bjornson, W., Rand, C., Connett, J. E., Lundgren, P., Nides, M., Pope, F., et al. (1995). Gender differences in smoking cessation after 3 years in the Lung Health Study. *American Journal of Public Health, 85,* 223–230.

Blackwell, B. (1997). From compliance to alliance: A quarter century of research. In B. Blackwell (Ed.), *Treatment compliance and the therapeutic alliance* (pp. 1–15). Amsterdam: Harwood Academic Publishers.

Blair, S. N., Cheng, Y, & Holder, J. S. (2001). Is physical activity or physical fitness more important in defining health benefits? *Medicine and Science in Sports & Exercise, 33,* S379–S399.

Blalock, S. J., DeVellis, R. F., Giorgino, K. B., DeVellis, B. M., Gold, D. T., Dooley, M. A., et al. (1996). Osteoporosis prevention in premenopausal women: Using a stage model approach to examine the predictors of behavior. *Health Psychology, 15,* 84–93.

Blanchard, E. B., & Andrasik, F. (1985). *Management of chronic headaches: A psychological approach.* New York: Pergamon Press.

Blanchard, E. B., Appelbaum, K. A., Radniz, C. L., Morrill, B., Michultka, D., Kirsch, C., et al. (1990). A controlled evaluation of thermal biofeedback and thermal biofeedback combined with cognitive therapy in the treatment of vascular headache. *Journal of Consulting and Clinical Psychology, 58,* 216–224.

Blascovich, J., Spencer, S. J., Quinn, D., & Steele, C. (2001). African Americans and high blood pressure: The role of stereotype threat. *Psychological Science, 12,* 225–229.

Blount, R. L., Smith, A. J., & Frank, N. C. (1999). Preparation to undergo medical procedures. In A. J. Goreczny & M. Hersen (Eds.), *Handbook of pediatric and adolescent health psychology* (pp. 305–326). Boston: Allyn and Bacon.

Blumstein, P., & Schwartz, P. (1983). *American couples.* New York: Pocket Books.

Bode, C., & Bode, J. C. (1997). Alcohol absorption, metabolism, and production in the gastrointestinal tract. *Alcohol Health & Research World, 21,* 82–83.

Bolger, N., Zuckerman, A., & Kessler, R. C. (2000). Invisible support and adjustment to stress. *Journal of Personality and Social Psychology, 79,* 953–961.

Bolinder, G., Alfredsson, L., England, A., & de Faire, U. (1994). Smokeless tobacco use and increased cardiovascular mortality among Swedish construction workers. *American Journal of Public Health, 84,* 399–404.

Bond, G. G., Aiken, L. S., & Somerville, S. C. (1992). The health belief model and adolescents with insulin-dependent diabetes mellitus. *Health Psychology, 11,* 190–198.

Bonham, V. L. (2001). Race, ethnicity, and pain treatment: Striving to understand the causes and solutions to the disparities in pain treatment. *Journal of Law, Medicine & Ethics, 29* (1), 52–68.

Bonica, J. J. (1990). Definitions and taxonomy of pain. In J. J. Bonica (Ed.), *The management of pain* (2nd ed., pp. 18–27). Malvern, PA: Lea & Febiger.

Bonneau, R. H., Padgett, D. A., & Sheridan, J. F. (2001). Psychoneuroimmune interactions in infectious disease: Studies in animals. In R. Ader, D. L. Felten, & N. Cohen (Eds.), *Psychoneuroimmunology* (3rd ed., Vol. 2, pp. 483–497). San Diego, CA: Academic Press.

Bosscher, R. J. (1993). Running and mixed physical exercises with depressed psychiatric patients. Special Issue: Exercise and psychological well-being. *International Journal of Sport Psychology, 24,* 170–184.

Botvin, G. J. (1999). Prevention in schools. In R. T. Ammerman, P. J. Ott, & R. E. Tarter (Eds.), *Prevention and societal impact of drug and alcohol abuse* (pp. 281–305). Mahwah, NJ: Erlbaum.

Bouchard, C. (2001). Physical activity and health: Introduction to the dose-response. *Medicine and Science in Sports and Exercise, 33,* S347–S350.

Boult, C., Kane, R. L., & Brown, R. (2000). Managed care of chronically ill older people: The U.S. experience. *British Medical Journal, 321,* 1011–1014.

Bovbjerg, V. E., McCann, B. S., Brief, D. J., Follette, W. C., Retzlaff, B. M., Dowdy, A. A., et al. (1995). Spouse support and long-term adherence to lipid-lowering diets. *American Journal of Epidemiology, 141,* 451–460.

Bower, P. J., Rubik, B., Weiss, S. J., & Starr, C. (1997). Manual therapy: Hands-on healing. *Patient Care, 31,* 69–81.

Bowles, L, & Kopelman, P. (2001). Leptin: Of mice and men? *Journal of Clinical Pathology, 54,* 1–3.

Brace, M. J., Smith, M. S., McCauley, E., & Sherry, D. D. (2000). Family reinforcement of illness behavior: A comparison of adolescents with chronic fatigue syndrome, juvenile arthritis, and healthy controls. *Journal of Developmental & Behavioral Pediatrics, 21,* 332–339.

Bradley, L. A., Prokop, C. K., Gentry, W. D., Van der Heide, L. H., & Prieto, E. J. (1981). Assessment of chronic pain. In C. K. Prokop & L. A. Bradley (Eds.), *Medical psychology: Contributions to behavioral medicine.* New York: Academic Press.

Bradley, L. A., & Van der Heide, L. H. (1984). Pain-related correlates of MMPI profile subgroups among back pain patients. *Health Psychology, 3,* 157–174.

Brain, K., Norman, P., Gray, J, & Mansel, R. (1999). Anxiety and adherence to breast self-examination in women with a family history of breast cancer. *Psychosomatic Medicine, 61,* 161–167.

Brandon, T. H., Collins, B. N., Juliano, L. M., & Lazev, A. B. (2000). Preventing relapse among former smokers: A comparison of minimal interventions through telephone and mail. *Journal of Consulting and Clinical Psychology, 68,* 103–113.

Braun, B. L., Murray, D., & Sidney, S. (1997). Lifetime cocaine use and cardiovascular characteristics among young adults: The CARDIA study. *American Journal of Public Health, 87,* 629–634.

Braver, E. R., Ferguson, S. A., Greene, M. A., & Lund, A. K. (1997). Reductions in deaths in frontal crashes among right front passengers in vehicles equipped with passenger air bags. *Journal of the American Medical Association, 278,* 1437–1439.

Bray, G. A. (1992). Pathophysiology of obesity. *American Journal of Clinical Nutrition, 55,* 488S–494S.

Brecher, E. M. (1972). *Licit and illicit drugs.* Boston: Little, Brown.

Breibart, W., & Payne, D. (2001). Psychiatric aspects of pain management in patients with advanced cancer. In H. Chochinov & W. Breibart (Eds.), *Handbook of psychiatry in palliative medicine* (pp. 131–199). New York: Oxford University Press.

Brennan, T. A., Leape, L. L., Laird, N. M., Hebert, L., Localio, A. R., Lawthers, A. G., et al. (1991). Incidence of adverse events and negligence in hospitalized patients: Results of the Harvard Medical Practice Study I. *New England Journal of Medicine, 324,* 370–366.

Breslau, N., Peterson, E., Schultz, L., Andreski, P., & Chilcoat, H. (1996). Are smokers with alcohol disorders less likely to quit? *American Journal of Public Health, 86,* 985–990.

Breuer, J., & Freud, S. (1955). *Studies on hysteria.* In J. Strachey (Ed. and Trans.), *The standard edition of the complete psychological works of Sigmund Freud* (Vol. 2). London: Hogarth Press. (Original work published 1895)

Brink, S. (2001, May 7). Your brain on alcohol. *U.S. News & World Report, 130,* 50+.

Brock, D. W., & Wartman, S. A. (1990). When competent patients make irrational choices. *New England Journal of Medicine, 322,* 1595–1599.

Brookmeyer, R., Gray, S., & Kawas, C. (1998). Projections of Alzheimer's disease in the United States and the public health impact of delaying disease onset. *American Journal of Public Health, 88,* 1337–1342.

Brown, B. (1970). Recognition of aspects of consciousness through association with EEG alpha activity represented by a light signal. *Psychophysics, 6,* 442–446.

Brown, J. M., Mehler, P. S., Harris, R. H. (2000). Medical complications occurring in adolescents with anorexia nervosa. *Western Journal of Medicine, 172,* 189–193.

Brown, L. R. (2001). Obesity is a threat to world health. *American Fitness, 19*(3), 62–64.

Brown, R. A., Kahler, C. W., Zvolensky, M. J., Lejuez, C. W., & Ransey, S. E. (2001). Anxiety sensitivity: Relationship to negative affect smoking and smoking cessation in smokers with past major depressive disorder. *Addictive Behaviors, 26,* 887–898.

Brown, S. A., Tate, S. R., Vik, P. W., Haas, A. L., & Aarons, G. A. (1999). Modeling of alcohol use mediates the effect of family history of alcoholism on adolescent alcohol expectancies. *Experimental and Clinical Psychopharmacology, 7,* 20–27.

Brownell, K. D., & Rodin, J. (1994). Medical, metabolic, and psychological effects of weight cycling. *Archives of Internal Medicine, 154,* 1325–1330.

Brownell, P. (1996). Domestic violence in the workplace: An emergent issue. *Crisis Intervention, 3,* 129–141.

Brownlee-Duffeck, M., Peterson, L., Simonds, J. F., Goldstein, D., Kilo, C., & Hoette, S. (1987). The role of health beliefs in the regimen adherence and metabolic control of adolescents and adults with diabetes mellitus. *Journal of Consulting and Clinical Psychology, 55,* 139–144.

Bruch, H. (1973). *Eating disorders. Obesity, anorexia nervosa and the person within.* New York: Basic Books.

Bruch, H. (1978). *The golden cage: The enigma of anorexia nervosa.* Cambridge, MA: Harvard University Press.

Bruch, H. (1982). Anorexia nervosa: Therapy and theory. *American Journal of Psychiatry, 139,* 1531–1538.

Brummett, B. H., Barefoot, J. C., Siegler, S. I. C., Clapp-Channing, N. E., Lytle, B. L., Bosworth, H. B., et al. (2001). Characteristics of socially isolated patients with coronary artery disease who are at elevated risk for mortality. *Psychosomatic Medicine, 63,* 267–272.

Brunner, E., White, I., Thorogood, M., Bristow, A., Curle, D., & Marmot, M. (1997). Can dietary interventions change diet and cardiovascular risk factors? A meta-analysis of randomized controlled trials. *American Journal of Public Health, 87,* 1415–1422.

Bruns, D. (1998). Psychologists as primary care providers: A paradigm shift. *Health Psychologist, 20* (4), 19.

Bryant, L. (2001). Asthma management. *Practice Nurse, 22*(4), 35–36, 38–39, 42–44.

Bryant, R. A. (1993). Beliefs about hypnosis: A survey of acute and chronic pain therapists. *Contemporary Hypnosis, 10,* 89–98.

Budney, A. J., Hughes, J. R., Moore, B. A., & Novy, P. L. (2001). Marijuana abstinence effects in marijuana smokers maintained in their home environment. *Archives of General Psychiatry, 58,* 917–924.

Buka, S. L., Stichick, T. L., Birdthistle, I., & Earls, F. J. (2001). Youth exposure to violence: Prevalence, risks, and consequences. *American Journal of Orthopsychiatry, 71,* 298–310.

Bullock, J. R. (2002). Bullying among children. *Childhood Education, 78,* 130–133.

Burish, T. G., Meyerowitz, B. E., Carey, M. P., & Morrow, G. R. (1987). The stressful effects of cancer in adults. In A. Baum & J. E. Singer (Eds.), *Handbook of psychology and health: Vol. 5. Stress* (pp. 137–173). Hillsdale, NJ: Erlbaum.

Burling, T. A., Burling, A. S., Latini, D. (2001). A controlled smoking cessation trial for substance-dependent inpatients. *Journal of Consulting and Clinical Psychology, 69,* 295–304.

Burns, J. W., Kubilus, A., Bruehl, S., & Harden, R. N. (2001). A fourth empirically derived cluster of chronic pain patients based on the Multidimensional Pain Inventory: Evidence for repression within the dysfunctional group. *Journal of Consulting and Clinical Psychology, 69,* 663–673.

Burte, J. M., Burte, W. D., & Araoz, D. L. (1994). Hypnosis in the treatment of back pain. *Australian Journal of Clinical Hypnotherapy and Hypnosis, 15,* 93–115.

Burtscher, M., Pachinger, O., Mittleman, M. A., & Ulmer, H. (2000). Prior myocardial infarction is the major risk factor associated with sudden cardiac death during downhill skiing. *International Journal of Sports Medicine, 21,* 613–615.

Bush, C., Ditto., B., & Feuerstein, M. (1985). A controlled evaluation of paraspinal EMG biofeedback in the treatment of chronic low back pain. *Health Psychology, 4,* 307–321.

Bush, J. P., Melamed, B. G., Sheras, P. L., & Greenbaum, P. E. (1986). Mother-child patterns of coping with anticipatory medical stress. *Health Psychology, 5,* 137–157.

Bybee, D. I., & Sullivan, C. M. (2002). The process through which an advocacy intervention resulted in positive change for battered women over time. *American Journal of Community Psychology, 30,* 103–132.

Cacioppo, J. T., Poehlmann, K. M., Kiecolt-Glaser, J. K., Malarkey, W. B., Burleson, M. H., Berntson, G. G., et al. (1998). Cellular immune responses to acute stress in female caregivers of dementia patients and matched controls. *Health Psychology, 17,* 182–189.

Calhoun, J. B. (1956). A comparative study of the social behavior of two inbred strains of house mice. *Ecological Monogram, 26,* 81.

Calhoun, J. B. (1962, February). Population density and social pathology. *Scientific American, 206,* 139–148.

Calle, E. E., Miracle-McMahill, H. L., Thun, M. J., & Heath, C. W., Jr. (1994). Cigarette smoking and risk of fatal breast cancer. *American Journal of Epidemiology, 139,* 1001–1007.

Calle, E. E., Thun, M. J., Petrelli, J. M., Rodriguez, C., & Heath, C. W., Jr. (1999). Body-mass index and mortality in a prospective cohort of U.S. adults. *New England Journal of Medicine, 341,* 1097–1105.

Camacho, T. C., & Wiley, J. A. (1983). Health practices, social networks, and change in physical health. In L. F. Berkman & L. Breslow (Eds.), *Health and ways of living: The Alameda County Study.* New York: Oxford University Press.

Cameron, L., Leventhal, E. A., & Leventhal, H. (1995). Seeking medical care in response to symptoms and life stress. *Psychosomatic Medicine, 57,* 37–47.

Campbell, F. A., Tramer, M. R., Carroll, D., Reynolds, D. J. M., Moore, R. A., & McQuay, H. J. (2001). Are cannabinoids an effective and safe treatment option in the management of pain? A qualitative systematic review. *British Medical Journal, 323,* 13–15.

Campbell, J. A. (1999). Health insurance coverage, 1998. *Current Population Reports,* Series P60–208.

Campfield, L. A., Smith, F. J., Guisez, Y., Devos, R., & Burn, P. (1995). Recombinant mouse OB protein: Evidence for a peripheral signal linking adiposity and central neural networks. *Science, 269,* 546–549.

Campion, E. W. (1997). Power lines, cancer, and fear. *New England Journal of Medicine, 337,* 44–46.

Cancian, F. M., & Oliker, S. J. (2000). *Caring and gender.* Thousand Oaks, CA: Pine Forge Press.

Cannon, W. (1932). *The wisdom of the body.* New York: Norton.

Capaldi, E. D. (1996). Conditioned food preferences. In E. D. Capaldi (Ed.), *Why we eat what we eat: The psychology of eating* (pp. 53–80). Washington, DC: American Psychological Association.

Caragata, W. (1995, April 3). Medicare wars: Canada's health care cuts. *Maclean's, 108,* 14–15.

Carden, A. D. (1994). Wife abuse and the wife abuser: Review and recommendations. *Counseling Psychologist, 22,* 539–582.

Carlat, D. J., Camargo, C. A., &, Herzog, D. B. (1997). Eating disorders in males: A report on 135 patients. *American Journal of Psychiatry, 154,* 1127–1132.

Carlson, C. R., & Hoyle, R. H. (1993). Efficacy of abbreviated progressive muscle relaxation training: A quantitative review of behavioral medicine research. *Journal of Consulting and Clinical Psychology, 61,* 1059–1067.

Carmack, C. L., Boudreaux, E., Amaral, M. M., Brantley, P. J., & de Moor, C. (1999). Aerobic fitness and leisure physical activity as moderators of the stress-illness relation. *Annals of Behavioral Medicine, 21,* 251–257.

Carpenter, R. L. (1997). Optimizing postoperative pain management. *American Family Physician, 56,* 835–858.

Carson, B. S. (1987). Neurologic and neurosurgical approaches to cancer pain. In D. B. McGuire & C. H. Yarbro (Eds.), *Cancer pain management* (pp. 223–243). Philadelphia: Saunders.

Cash, T. F., & Deagle, E. A, III. (1997). The nature and extent of body-image disturbances in anorexia nervosa and bulimia nervosa: A meta-analysis. *International Journal of Eating Disorders, 22,* 107–125.

Castro, C. M., Wilcox, S., O'Sullivan, P., Bauman, K., & King, A. C. (2002). An exercise program for women who are caring for relatives with dementia. *Psychosomatic Medicine, 64,* 458–468.

Catz, S. L., Kelly, J. A., Bogart, L. M., Genosch, E. G., & McAuliffe, T. L. (2000). Patterns, correlates, and barriers to medication adherence among persons prescribed new treatments for HIV disease. *Health Psychology, 19,* 124–133.

Caudron, S. (1998). Target: HR. *Workforce, 77* (8), 44–50.

Cecil, H., Evans, R. I., & Stanley, M. (1996). Perceived believability among adolescents of health warning labels on cigarette packs. *Journal of Applied Social Psychology, 26,* 502–519.

Cell phones save lives. (2000, October). *Association Management, 52,* 22.

Centers for Disease Control and Prevention (CDC). (1992). 1993 revised classification system for HIV infection and expanded surveillance case definition for AIDS among adolescents and adults. *Morbidity and Mortality Weekly Report, 41,* No. RR-17.

Centers for Disease Control and Prevention (CDC). (1993). Cigarette smoking—attributable mortality and years of potential life lost—United States, 1990. *Morbidity and Mortality Weekly Report, 42,* 645–649.

Centers for Disease Control and Prevention (CDC). (1994). Reasons for tobacco use and symptoms of nicotine withdrawal among adolescent and young adult tobacco users—United States, 1993. *Morbidity and Mortality Weekly Report, 43,* 745–750.

Centers for Disease Control and Prevention (CDC). (1998a). AIDS among persons aged ≥50 years—United States, 1991–1996. *Morbidity and Mortality Weekly Report, 47,* 21–27.

Centers for Disease Control and Prevention (CDC). (1998b). Deaths resulting from residential fires and the prevalence of smoke alarms—United States, 1991–1995. *Morbidity and Mortality Weekly Report. 47,* 803–906.

Centers for Disease Control and Prevention (CDC). (1999a). Decline in deaths from heart disease and stroke—United States, 1900–1999. *Morbidity and Mortality Weekly Report, 148,* 649.

Centers for Disease Control and Prevention (CDC). (1999b). Improvements in workplace safety—United States, 1900–1999. *Morbidity and Morality Weekly Report, 48,* 461–469.

Centers for Disease Control and Prevention (CDC). (2001a). Cigarette smoking among adults—United States, 1999. *Morbidity and Mortality Weekly Report, 50,* 869, 873.

Centers for Disease Control and Prevention (CDC). (2001b). *HIV/AIDS Surveillance Report, 13*(1).

Centers for Disease Control and Prevention (CDC). (2001c). *HIV prevention strategic planning through 2005.* Retrieved from the World Wide Web, August 5, 2002, at www.cdc.gov/hiv/pubs/prev-strat-plan.pdf.

Centers for Disease Control and Prevention (CDC). (2001d). Major cardiovascular disease (CVD) during 1997–1999 and major CVD hospital discharge rates in 1997 among women with diabetes—United States. *Morbidity smf Mortality Weekly Report, 50,* 948–954.

Centers for Disease Control and Prevention (CDC). (2001e). Tobacco information and prevention source (TIPS) at http://www.cdc.gov/tobacco/research_data/adults_prev/tab_3.htm.

Centers for Disease Control and Prevention (CDC). (2002). Annual smoking-attributable mortality, year of potential life lost, and economic costs—United States, 1995–1000. *Mortality and Morbidity Weekly Report, 51,* 300–303.

Chalk, R., & King, P. A. (Eds.). (1998). *Violence in families: Assessing prevention and treatment programs.* Washington, D.C.: National Academy Press.

Champion, V. L., & Miller, A. (1997). Adherence to mammography and breast self-examination regimen. In D. S. Gochman (Ed.), *Handbook of health behavior research II: Provider determinants* (pp. 245–267). New York: Plenum Press.

Chapman, C. R., Nakamura, Y., & Flores, L. Y. (1999). Chronic pain and consciousness: A constructivist perspective. In R. J. Gatchel & D. C. Turk (Eds.), *Psychosocial factors in pain: Critical perspectives* (pp. 35–55). New York; Guilford Press.

Chapman, S., Wong, W. L., & Smith, W. (1993). Self-exempting beliefs about smoking and health: Differences between smokers and ex-smokers. *American Journal of Public Health, 83,* 215–219.

Charlee, C., Goldsmith, L. J., Chambers, L, & Haynes, R. B. (1996). Provider-patient communication among elderly and nonelderly patients in Canadian hospitals: A national survey. *Health Communication, 8,* 281–302.

Chassin, M. R. (1997). Assessing strategies for qualilty improvement. *Health Affairs, 16,* 151–161.

Cheadle, A., Pearson, D., Wagner, E., Psaty, B. M., Diehr, P., & Koepsell, T. (1994). Relationship between socioeconomic status, health status, and lifestyle practices of American Indians: Evidence from a Plains reservation population. *Public Health Reports, 109,* 405–413.

Chen, E., Bloomberg, G. R., Fisher, E. B., Jr., Strunk, R. C. (2003). Predictors of repeat hospitalizations in children with asthma: The role of psychosocial and socioenvironmental factors. *Health Psychology, 22,* 12–18.

Chen, Y., Horne, S. L., & Dosman, J. A. (1993). The influence of smoking cessation on body weight may be temporary. *American Journal of Public Health, 83,* 1330–1332.

Chen, Z., Xu, Z., Collins, R., Li, W., & Peto, R. (1997). Early health effects of the emerging tobacco epidemic in China: A 16-year prospective study. *Journal of the American Medical Association, 278,* 1500–1504.

Cheng, T. Y. L., & Boey, K. W. (2002). The effectiveness of a cardiac rehabilitation program on self-efficacy and exercise. *Clinical Nursing Research, 11,* 10–19.

Cheng, Y., Kawachi, I., Coakley, E. H., Schwartz, J., & Colditz, G. (2000). Association between psychosocial work characeristics and health functioning in American women: Prospective study. *British Medical Journal, 320,* 1432–1436.

Cherkin, D. C., Eisenberg, D., Sherman, K. J., Barlow, W., Kaptchuk, T. J., Street, J., et al. (2001). Randomized trial comparing traditional Chinese medical acupuncture, therapeutic massage, and self-care education for chronic low back pain. *Archives of Internal Medicine, 161,* 1081–1088.

Cherner, R. (2001). Diabetes therapy: How to enlist patient compliance. *Consultant, 41,* 1259–1261.

Chesney, M., & Darbes, L. (1998). Social support and heart disease in women: Implications for intervention. In K. Orth-Gomér, M. Chesney, & N. K. Wenger (Eds.), *Women, stress, and heart disease* (pp. 165–182). Mahwah, NJ: Erlbaum.

Chilcoat, H. D., Deshion, T. J., & Anthony, J. C. (1995). Parent monitoring and the incidence of drug sampling in urban elementary school children. *American Journal of Epidemiology, 141,* 25–31.

Ching, P. L. Y. H., Willett, W. C., Rimm, E. B., Colditz. G. A., Gortmaker, S. L., & Stampfer, M. J. (1996). Activity level and risk of overweight in male health professionals. *American Journal of Public Health, 86,* 25–30.

Christ, G. H., Siegel, K., Freund, B., Langosch, D., Hendersen, S., Sperber, D., et al. (1993). Impact of parental terminal cancer on latency-age children. *American Journal of Orthopsychiatry, 63,* 417–425.

Christen, W., Glynn, R. J., Manson, J. E., Ajani, U., & Buring, J. E. (1997). A prospective study of cigarette smoking and risk of age-related macular degeneration in men. *Journal of the American Medical Association, 276,* 1147–1151.

Christenfeld, N., Glynn, L. M., Phillips, D. P., & Shrira, I. (1999). Exposure to New York City as a risk factor for heart attack mortality. *Psychosomatic Medicine, 61,* 740–743.

Christensen, A. J., Moran, P. J., & Wiebe, J. S. (1999). Assessment of irrational health beliefs: Relation to health practices and medical regimen adherence. *Health Psychology, 18,* 169–176.

Christensen, A. J., Wiebe, J. S., & Lawton, W. J. (1997). Cynical hostility, powerful others control expectancies, and patient adherence in hemodialysis. *Psychosomatic Medicine, 59,* 307–312.

Christensen, D. (2001). Medicinal mimicry: Sometimes, placebos work—but how? *Science News, 159,* 74–76.

Ciechanowski, P. S., Katon, W. J., Russo, J. E., & Walker, E. A. (2001). The patient-provider relationship: Attachment theory and adherence to treatment for diabetes. *American Journal of Psychiatry, 158,* 29–35.

Clarke, V. A., Lovegrove, H., Williams, A., & Machperson, M. (2000). Unrealistic optimism and the health belief model. *Journal of Behavior Medicine, 23,* 367–376.

Clay, R. A. (2002, April). Overcoming barriers to pain relief. *Monitor on Psychology, 33,* 58–60.

Cochran, S. D. (1984). Preventing medical noncompliance in the outpatient treatment of bipolar affective disorders. *Journal of Consulting and Clinical Psychology, 52,* 873–878.

Cohen, A., & Colligan, M. J. (1997). Accepting occupational safety and health regimens. In D. S. Gochman (Ed.), *Handbook of health behavior research II: Provider determinants* (pp. 379–394). New York: Plenum Press.

Cohen, S. (1996). Psychological stress, immunity, and upper respiratory infections. *Current Directions in Psychological Science, 5,* 86–90.

Cohen, S., Doyle, W. J., Skoner, D. P., Fireman, P., Gwaltney, J. M., Jr., & Newson, J. T. (1995). State and trait negative affect as predictors of objective and subjective symptoms of respiratory viral infections. *Journal of Personality and Social Psychology, 68,* 159–169.

Cohen, S., Frank, E., Doyle, W. J., Skoner, D. P., Rabin, B. S., & Gwaltney, J. M., Jr. (1998). Types of stressors that increase susceptibility to the common cold in healthy adults. *Health Psychology, 17,* 214–223.

Cohen, S., & Herbert, T. B. (1996). Health psychology: Psychological factors and physical disease from the perspective of human psychoneuroimmunology. *Annual Review of Psychology, 47,* 113–132.

Cohen, S., Kamarck, T., & Mermelstein, R. (1983). A global measure of perceived stress. *Journal of Health and Social Behavior, 24,* 385–396.

Cohen, S., Tyrrell, D. A. J., Russell, M. A. H., Jarvis, M. J., & Smith, A. P. (1993). Smoking, alcohol consumption, and susceptibility to the common cold. *American Journal of Public Health, 83,* 1277–1283.

Cohen, S., Tyrrell, D. A. J., & Smith, A. P. (1991). Psychological stress and susceptibility to the common cold. *New England Journal of Medicine, 325,* 606–612.

Cohen, S., Tyrrell, D. A. J., & Smith, A. P. (1993). Negative life events, perceived stress, negative affect, and susceptibility to the common cold. *Journal of Personality and Social Psychology, 64,* 131–140.

Cohen, Y., Spirito, A., & Brown, L. K. (1996). Suicide and suicidal behavior. In R. J. Di Clemente, W. B. Hansen, & L. E. Ponton (Eds.), *Handbook of adolescent health risk behavior* (pp. 193–224). New York: Plenum Press.

Cohler, B. J., Groves, L., Borden, W., & Lazarus, L. (1989). Caring for family members with Alzheimer's disease. In E. Light & B. D. Lebowitz (Eds.), *Alzheimer's disease treatment and family stress: Direction for research* (pp. 50–105). (DHHS Publication No. ADM 89–1569). Washington, DC: U.S. Government Printing Office.

Colditz, G. A. (1995). Weight gain as a risk factor for clinical diabetes mellitus in women. *Annals of Internal Medicine, 122,* 481–486.

Colditz, G. A., Bonita, R., Stampfer, M. J., Willett, W. C., Rosner, B., Speizer, F. E., et al. (1988). Cigarette smoking and risk of stroke in middle-aged women. *New England Journal of Medicine, 318,* 937–941.

Colditz, G. A., Willett, W. C., Hunter, D. J., Stampfer, M. J., Manson, J. E., Hennekens, C. H., et al. (1993). Family history, age, and risk of breast cancer. *Journal of the American Medical Association, 270,* 338–343.

Cole, S. W., Kemeny, M. E., & Taylor, S. E. (1997). Social identity and physical health: Accelerated HIV progression in rejection-sensitive gay men. *Journal of Personality and Social Psychology, 72,* 320–335.

Cole, S. W., Kemeny, M. E., Taylor, S. E., Visscher, B. R., & Fahey, J. L. (1996). Accelerated course of human immunodeficiency virus infection in gay men who conceal their homosexual identity. *Psychosomatic Medicine, 58,* 219–231.

Cole, S. W., Naliboff, B. D., Kemeny, M. E., Griswold, M. P., Fahey, J. L., & Zack, J. A. (2001). Impaired response to HAART in HIV-infected individuals with high autonomic nervous system activity. *Proceedings of the National Academy of Sciences of the United States of America, 98,* 12695–12700.

Cole, T. B., & Flanagin, A. (1999). What can we do about violence? *Journal of the American Medical Association, 282,* 481–483.

Colhoun, H. M., Rubbens, M. B., Underwood, S. R., & Fuller, J. H. (2000). Cross sectional study of differences in coronary artery calcification by socioeconomic status. *British Medical Journal, 321,* 1262–1263.

Collins, J., Robin, L., Wooley, S., Fenley, D., Hun, P., Taylor, J., et al. (2002). Programs-That-Work: CDC's guide to effective programs that reduce health-risk behavior of youth. *Journal of School Health, 72,* 93–99.

Compas, B. E., Haaga, D. A., Keefe, F. J., Leitenberg, H., & Williams, D. A. (1998). Sampling of empirically supported psychological treatments from health psychology: Smoking, chronic pain, cancer, and bulimia nervosa. *Journal of Consulting and Clinical Psychology, 66,* 89–112.

Concato, J., Shah, N., & Horwitz, R. I. (2000). Randomized, controlled trials, observational studies, and the hierarchy of research. *New England Journal of Medicine, 342,* 1887–1872.

Conger, J. (1956). Reinforcement theory and the dynamics of alcoholism. *Quarterly Journal of Studies on Alcohol, 17,* 296–305.

Conner, M., & Flesch, D., (2001). Having casual sex: Additive and interactive effects of alcohol and condom availability on the determinants of intentions. *Journal of Applied Social Psychology, 31,* 89–112.

Connor, W. E., & Connor, S. L. (1997). The case for a low-fat, high-carbohydrate diet. *New England Journal of Medicine, 337,* 562–563.

Constantini, A., Solano, L., Di-Napoli, R., & Bosco, A. (1997). Relationship between hardiness and risk of burnout in a sample of 92 nurses working in oncology and AIDS wards. *Psychotherapy and Psychosomatics, 66,* 78–82.

Consumer Reports. (2002, June). The truth about dieting. *Consumer Reports, 67*(6), 26–31.

Cook, W., & Medley, D. (1954). Proposed hostility and pharisaic-virtue scales for the MMPI. *Journal of Applied Psychology, 38,* 414–418.

Cooper, B. (2001, March). Long may you run. *Runner's World, 36*(3), 64–67.

Cooper, K. H. (1968). *Aerobics.* New York: Evans.

Cooper, K. H. (1982). *The aerobics program for total well-being.* New York: Evans.

Cooper, K. H. (1985). *Running without fear: How to reduce the risks of heart attack and sudden death during aerobic exercise.* New York: Evans.

Corbitt, G., Bailey, A., & Williams, G. (1990). HIV infection in Manchester, 1959. *Lancet, 336,* 51.

Cottington, E. M., & House, J. S. (1987). Occupational stress and health: A multivariate relationship. In A. Baum & J. E. Singer (Eds.), *Handbook of psychology and health: Vol. 5. Stress* (pp. 41–62). Hillsdale, NJ: Erlbaum.

Cotton, D. H. G. (1990). *Stress management: An integrated approach to therapy.* New York: Brunner/Mazel.

Cousins, S. O. (2000). "My heart couldn't take it": Older women's beliefs about exercise benefits and risks. *Journals of Gerontology, Series B,* 283–287.

Covington, E. C. (2000). The biological basis of pain. *International Review of Psychiatry, 12,* 128–147.

Cowley, G. (1998, November 30). Cancer and diet. *Newsweek, 132,* 60–66.

Cowley, G., King, P., Hager, M., & Rosenberg, D. (1995, June 26). Going mainstream. *Newsweek, 125,* 56–57.

Cox, D. J., & Gonder-Frederick. L. (1992). Major developments in behavioral diabetes research. *Journal of Consulting and Clinical Psychology, 60,* 628–638.

Coyne, J. C., & Racioppo, M. W. (2000). Never the twain shall meet? Closing the gap between coping research and clinical intervention reserach. *American Psychologist, 55,* 655–664.

Cramer, J. A., Mattson, R. H., Prevey, M. L., Scheyer, R. D., & Ouellette, V. L. (1989). How often is medication taken as prescribed? *Journal of the American Medical Association, 261,* 3273–3277.

Crandall, C. S., Preisler, J. J., & Aussprung, J. (1992). Measuring life event stress in the lives of college students: The Undergraduate Stress Questionnaire (USQ). *Journal of Behavioral Medicine, 15,* 627–662.

Creer, T. L., & Bender, B. G. (1993). Asthma. In R. J. Gatchel & E. B. Blanchard (Eds.), *Psychophysiological disorders: Research and clinical applications* (pp. 151–203). Washington, DC: American Psychological Association.

Crimmins, E. M., & Saito, Y. (2001). Trends in healthy life expectancy in the United States, 1970–1990: Gender, racial, and educational differences. *Social Science & Medicine, 52,* 1629–1642.

Crosscope-Happel, C., Hutchins, D. E., Getz, H. G., & Hayes, G. L. (2000). Male anorexia nervosa: A new focus. *Journal of Mental Health Counseling, 22,* 365–370.

Crowell, T. L., & Emmers-Sommer, T. M. (2001). "If I knew then what I know now": Seropositive individuals' perceptions of partner trust, safety and risk prior to HIV infection. *Communication Studies, 52,* 302–323.

Cruickshanks, K. J., Klein, R., Klein, B. E. K., Wiley, T. L., Nondahl, D. M., & Tweed, T. S. (1998). Cigarette smoking and hearing loss: The Epidemiology of Hearing Loss Study. *Journal of the American Medical Association, 279,* 1715–1719.

Cullen, K. J., Knuimon, M. W., & Ward, N. J. (1993). Alcohol and mortality in Busselton, Western Australia. *American Journal of Epidemiology, 137,* 242–248.

Cummings, D. E., Purnell, J. Q., Frayo, R. S., Schmidova, K., Wisse, B. E., & Weigle, D. S. (2001). A preprandial rise in plasma ghrelin levels suggests a role in meal initiation in humans. *Diabetes, 50,* 1714–1719.

Cummings, P., & Psaty, B. M. (1994). The association between cholesterol and death from injury. *Annals of Internal Medicine, 120,* 848–855.

Cummings, P., Koepsell, T. D., Moffat, J. M., & Rivara, F. P. (2001). Drowsiness, counter-measures to drowsiness, and the risk of a motor vehicle crash. *Injury Prevention, 7,* 194–199.

Cunningham, J. A., & Breslin, F. C. (2001). Exploring patterns of remission from alcohol dependence with and without Alcoholics Anonymous in a population sample. *Contemporary Drug Problems, 28,* 559–567.

Cunningham, P. B., Henggeler, S. W., Limber, S. P., Melton, G. B., & Nation, M. A. (2000). Patterns and correlates of gun ownership among nonmetropolitan and rural middle school students. *Journal of Clinical Child Psychology, 29,* 432–442.

Curtis, A. B., James, S. A., Strogatz, D. S., Raghunathan, T. E., & Harlow, S. (1997). Alcohol consumption and changes in blood pressure among African Americans: The Pitt County Study. *American Journal of Epidemiology, 146,* 727–733.

Cvijanovich, N. Z., Cook, L. J., Mann, C., & Dean, J. M. (2001). A population-based study of crashes involving 16- and 17-year-old drivers: The potential benefit of graduated driver licensing restrictions. *Pediatrics, 107,* 632–637.

Daly, M. J. (1998). Untangling the genetics of a complex disease. *Journal of the American Medical Association, 280,* 652–653.

Dattore, P. J., Shontz, F. C., & Coyne, L. (1980). Premorbid personality differentiation of cancer and noncancer groups: A list of the hypotheses of cancer proneness. *Journal of Consulting and Clinical Psychology, 48,* 388–394.

Davidson, K., MacGregor, M. W., Stuhr, J., Dixon, K., & MacLean, D. (2000). Constructive anger verbal behavior predicts blood pressure in a population-based sample. *Health Psychology 19,* 55–64.

Davidson, L. L., Durkin, M. S., Kuhn, L., O'Connor, P., Barlow, B., & Heagarity, M. C. (1994). The impact of the Safe Kids/Healthy Neighborhoods Injury Prevention Program in Harlem, 1988–1991. *American Journal of Public Health, 84,* 580–586.

Davies, D. L. (1962). Normal drinking in recovered alcohol addicts. *Quarterly Journal of Studies on Alcohol, 24,* 321–332.

Daviglus, M. L., Stamler, J., Orencia, A. J., Dyer, A. R, Liu, K., Greenland, P., et al. (1997). Fish consumption and the 30-year risk of fatal myocardial infarction. *New England Journal of Medicine, 336,* 1046–1053.

Davis, C., Kennedy, S. H., Ravelski, E., & Dionne, M. (1994). The role of physical activity in the development and maintenance of eating disorders. *Psychological Medicine, 24,* 957–964.

Davis, C. E., Williams, D. H., Oganov, R. G., Tao, S-C, Rywiik, S. L., Stein, Y., et al. (1996). Sex differences in high-density lipoprotein cholesterol in six countries. *American Journal of Epidemiology, 143,* 1100–1106.

Davis, K. D. (2000). Studies of pain using functional magnetic resonance imaging. In K. L. Casey & M. C. Bushnell (Eds.), *Pain imaging: Progress in pain research and management* (pp. 195–210). Seattle, WA: IASP Press.

Davis, M. K., & Gidycz, C. A. (2000). Child sexual abuse prevention programs: A meta-analysis. *Journal of Clinical Child Psychology, 29,* 257–265.

Davis, R. C., Smith, B. E., & Nickles, L. B. (1998). The deterrent effect of prosecuting domestic violence misdemeanors. *Crime and Delinquency, 44,* 434–443.

Dawber, T. R. (1980). *The Framingham study: The epidemiology of atherosclerotic disease.* Cambridge, MA: Harvard University Press.

DeBaggio, T. (2002). *Losing my mind: An intimate look at life with Alzheimer's.* New York: Free Press.

Dehle, C., Larsen, D., & Landers, J. E. (2001). Social support in marriage. *American Journal of Family Therapy, 29,* 307–324.

DeJong, W., & Wallack, L. (1992). The role of designated driver programs in the prevention of alcohol-impaired driving: A critical reassessment. *Health Education Quarterly, 19,* 429–442.

DeJong, W. & Winsten, J. A. (1999). The use of designated drivers by US collage students: A national study. *Journal of American College Health, 47,* 151.

De Lew, N., & Weinick, R. M. (2000). An overview: Eliminating racial, ethnic, and SES disparities in health care. *Health Care Financing Review, 21*(4), 1–7.

Dellinger, A. M., Langlois, J. A., & Li, G. (2002). Fatal crashes among older drivers: Decomposition of rates into contributing factors. *American Journal of Epidemiology, 155,* 234–241.

DeLongis, A., Folkman, S., & Lazarus, R. S. (1988). The impact of daily stress on health and mood: Psychological and social resources as mediators. *Journal of Personality and Social Psychology, 54,* 486–495.

Dembroski, T. M., MacDougall, J. M., Williams, R. B., Haney, T. L., & Blumenthal, J. A. (1985). Components of Type A, hostility, and anger-in: Relationship to angiographic findings. *Psychosomatic Medicine, 47,* 219–233.

DeNitto, E. (1993, September 29). 100 leaders monopolize pain relievers. *Advertising Age, 64,* 2.

Dermen, K. H., Cooper, M. L., & Agocha, V. B. (1998). Sex-related alcohol expectancies as moderators of the relationship between alcohol use and risky sex in adolescents. *Journal of Studies on Alcohol, 59,* 71–77.

Derogatis, L. R. (1977). *Manual for the Symptom Checklist-90, revised.* Baltimore, MD: John Hopkins University School of Medicine.

Des Jarlais, D. C., Marmor, M., Friedmann, P., Titus, S., Avles, E., Deren, S., et al. (2000). HIV incidence among injection drug users in New York City, 1992–1997. *American Journal of Public Health, 90,* 352–359.

Dew, M. A., Bromet, E. J., Brent, D., & Greenhouse, J. B. (1987). A quantitative literature review of the effectiveness of suicide prevention centers. *Journal of Consulting and Clinical Psychology, 55,* 239–244.

Deyo, R. A. (1998, August). Low-back pain. *Scientific American, 279,* 48–53.

Diehr, P., Bild, D. E., Harris, T. B., Duxbury, A., Siscovick, D., & Rossi, M. (1998). Body mass index and mortality in nonsmoking older adults: The Cardiovascular Health Study. *American Journal of Public Health, 88,* 623–629.

DiMatteo, M. R. (1994). Enhancing patient adherence to medical recommendations. *Journal of the American Medical Association, 271,* 79, 83.

DiMatteo, M. R. (1997). Health behaviors and care decisions: An overview of professional-patient communication. In D. S. Gochman (Ed.), *Handbook of health behavior research II: Provider determinants* (pp. 5–22). New York: Plenum Press.

DiMatteo, M. R., & DiNicola, D. D. (1982). *Achieving patient compliance: The psychology of the medical practitioner's role.* New York: Pergamon Press.

Dinges, D. F, Whitehouse, W. G., Orne, E. C., Bloom, P. B., Carlin, M. M., Bauer, N. K., et al. (1997). Self-hypnosis training as an adjunctive treatment in the management of pain associated with sickle cell disease. *International Journal of Clinical and Experimental Hypnosis, 45,* 417–432.

DiNicola, D. D., & DiMatteo, M. R. (1984). Practitioners, patients, and compliance with medical regimens: A social psychological perspective. In A. Baum, S. E. Taylor, & J. E. Singer (Eds.), *Handbook of psychology and health: Vol. 4. Social psychological aspects of health* (pp. 55–84). Hillsdale, NJ: Erlbaum.

Dishman, R. K., & Buckworth, J. (1997). Adherence to physical activity. In W. P. Morgan (Ed.), *Physical activity and mental health* (pp. 63–80). Washington, DC: Taylor & Francis.

Dixon, J., Dixon, M., & O'Brien, P. (2001). Quality of life after lap-band placement: Influence of time, weight loss, and comorbidities. *Obesity Research, 9,* 713–721.

Dolbier, C. L., Cocke, R. R., Leiferman, J. A., Steinhardt, M. A., Schapiro, S. J., Nehete, P. N., et al. (2001). Differences in functional immune responses of high vs. low hardy healthy individuals. *Journal of Behavioral Medicine, 24,* 219–229.

Doll, R., & Hill, A. B. (1956). Lung cancer and other causes of death in relation to smoking: A second report on the mortality of British doctors. *British Medical Journal,* 1071–1081.

Dollard, M. F., Winefield, H. R., Winefield, A. H., & de Jonge, J. (2000). Psychosocial job strain and productivity in human service workers: A test of the demand-control-support model. *Journal of Occupational and Organizational Psychology, 73,* 501–510.

Domar, A. D., Clapp, D., Slawsby, E., Kessel, B., Orav, J., & Freizinger, M. (2000). The impact of group psychological interventions on distress in infertile women. *Health Psychology, 19,* 568–575.

Donaldson, C. S., Stanger, L. M., Donaldson, M. W., Cram, J., & Skubick, D. L. (1993). A randomized crossover investigation of a back pain and disability prevention program: Possible mechanisms of change. *Journal of Occupational Rehabilitation, 3,* 83–94.

Donaldson, S. I., Graham, J. W., Piccinin, A. M., & Hansen, W. B. (1995). Resistance-skills training and onset of alcohol use: Evidence for beneficial and potentially harmful effects in public schools and in private Catholic schools. *Health Psychology, 14,* 291–300.

Donovan, M. I. (1989). Relieving pain: The current basis for practice. In S. G. Funk, E. M. Tornquist, M. T. Champagne, L. A. Copp, & R. A. Wiese (Eds.), *Key aspects of comfort: Management of pain, fatigue, and nausea* (pp. 25–31). New York: Springer.

Dougall, A. L., & Baum, A. (2001). Stress, health, and illness. In A. Baum, T. A. Revenson, & J. E. Singer (Eds.), *Handbook of health psychology* (pp. 321–337). Mahwah, NJ: Erlbaum.

Droomers, M., Schrijvers, C. T. M., & Mackenbach, J. P. (2002). Why do lower educated people continue smoking? Explanations from the longitudinal GLOBE study. *Health Psychology, 21,* 263–272.

Dubbert, P. (2002). Physical activity and exercise: Recent advances and current challenges. *Journal of Consulting and Clinical Psychology, 70,* 525–536.

Dube, S. R., Anda, R. F., Felitti, V. J., Chapman, D. P., Williamson, D. F., & Giles, W. H. (2001). Childhood abuse, household dysfunction, and the risk of attempted suicide throughout the life span: Findings from the Adverse Childhood Experiences Study. *Journal of the American Medical Association, 286,* 3089–3094.

Dunbar, H. F. (1943). *Psychomatic diagnosis.* New York: Hoeber.

Dunbar, P. J. (1995). Use of patient-controlled analgesia for pain control for children receiving bone marrow transplant. *Journal of Pain and Symptom Management. 10,* 604–611.

Dunkel-Schetter, C., Feinstein, L. G., Taylor, S. E., & Falke, R. L. (1992). Patterns of coping with cancer. *Health Psychology, 11,* 79–87.

Dunkel-Schetter, C., & Lobel, M. (1998). Pregnancy and childbirth. In E. A. Blechman & K. D. Brownell (Eds.), *Behavioral medicine and women: A comprehensive handbook* (pp. 475–482). New York: Guilford.

Dunn, A. L., Marcus, B. H., Kampert, J. B., Garcia, M. E., Kohl, H. W., III, & Blair, S. N. (1999). Comparison of lifestyle and structured interventions to increase physical activity and cardiorespiratory fitness. *Journal of the American Medical Association, 281,* 327–334.

Dunn, A. L., Trivedi, M. H., & O'Neal, H. A. (2001). Physical activity dose-response effects on outcomes of depression and anxiety. *Medicine and Science in Sports and Exercise, 33,* S587–S597.

Duquette, A., Kerouac, S., Sandhu, B. K., Ducharme, F., & Saulnier, P. (1995). Psychosocial determinants of burnout in geriatric nursing. *International Journal of Nursing Studies, 32,* 443–456.

DuRant, R. H., Smith, J. A., Kreiter, S. R., & Krowchuk, D. P. (1999). The relationship between early age and onset of initial substance use and engaging in multiple health risk behaviors among young adolescents. *Archives of Pediatric & Adolescent Medicine, 153,* 286–291.

Durkheim, E. (1954). *Elementary forms of religious life* (J. W. Swain, Trans.). Glencoe, IL: Free Press. (Original work published n 1912)

Durlak, J. A. (1997). *Successful prevention programs for children and adolescents.* New York: Plenum Press.

Dusseldrop, E., van Elderen, T., Maes, S., Meulman, J., & Kraaj, V. (1999). A meta-analysis of psychoeducational programs for coronary heart disease patients. *Health Psychology, 18,* 506–519.

Dwyer, J. H. (1995). Genes, blood pressure, and African heritage. *Lancet, 346,* 392.

Dyer, A. R., Stamler, J., & Greenland, P. (2000). Associations of weight change and weight variability with cardiovascular and all-cause mortality in the Chicago Western Electric Company Study. *American Journal of Epidemiology, 152,* 324–333.

Eaker, E. D., Pinsky, J., & Castelli, W. P. (1992). Myocardial infarction and coronary death among women: Psychosocial predictors from a 20-year follow-up of women in the Framingham Study. *American Journal of Epidemiology, 135,* 854–864.

Eakin, J. M. (1997). Work-related determinants of health behavior. In D. S. Gochman (Ed.), *Handbook of health behavior research I: Personal and social determinants* (pp. 337–357). New York: Plenum Press.

Eckenrode, J., Ganzel, B., Henderson, C. R., Smith, E., Olds, D. L., Powers, J., et al. (2000). Preventing child abuse and neglect with a program of nurse home visitation: The limiting effects of domestic violence. *Journal of the American Medical Association, 284,* 1385–1391.

Eckholm, E. (1977). *The picture of health: Environmental sources of disease.* New York: Norton.

Edwards, C. L., Fillingim, R. B., & Keefe, F. (2001). Race, ethnicity and pain. *Pain, 94,* 133–137.

Edwards, G. (1977). The alcohol dependence syndrome: Usefulness of an idea. In G. Edwards & M. Grant (Eds.), *Alcoholism: New knowledge and new responses.* London: Croom Helm.

Edwards, G. (2000). *Alcohol: The world's favorite drug.* New York: Thomas Dunne Books.

Edwards, G., & Gross, M. M. (1976). Alcohol dependence: Provisional description of a clinical syndrome. *British Medical Journal,* 1058–1061.

Edwards, G., Gross, M. M., Keller, M., Moser, J., & Room, R. (1977). *Alcohol-related disabilities* (WHO Offset Pub. No. 32). Geneva, Switzerland: World Health Organization.

Egger, G., Cameron-Smith, D., & Stanton, R. (1999). The effectiveness of popular, non-prescription weight loss supplements. *Medical Journal of Australia, 171,* 604–608.

Eigenbrodt, M., Mosley, T. H., Jr., Hutchinson, R. G., Watson, R. L., Chambless, L. E., & Szklo, M. (2001). Alcohol consumption with age: A cross-sectional and longitudinal study of the Atherosclerosis Risk in Communities (ARIC) Study, 1987–1995. *American Journal of Epidemiology, 153,* 1102–1111.

Ellestad, M. H. (1996). *Stress testing* (4th ed.). Philadelphia: Davis.

Ellickson, P., Saner, H., & McGuigan, K. A. (1997). Profiles of violent youth: Substance use and other concurrent problems. *American Journal of Public Health, 87,* 985–991.

Ellis, A. (1962). *Reason and emotion in psychotherapy.* New York: Stuart.

Ellis, E. M. (2000). *Divorce wars: Interventions with families in conflict.* Washington, DC: American Psychological Association.

Ennett, S. T., Tobler, N. S., Ringwalt, C. L., & Flewelling, R. L. (1994). How effective is drug abuse resistance education? A meta-analysis of Project DARE outcome evaluations. *American Journal of Public Health, 84,* 1394–1401.

Enqvist, B. & Fischer, K. (1997). Preoperative hypnotic techniques reduce consumption of analgesics after surgical removal of third mandibular molars: A brief communication. *International Journal of Clinical and Experimental Hypnosis, 45,* 102–108.

Epstein, L. H. (1996). Family-based behavioural intervention for obese children. *International Journal of Obesity, 20*(Suppl. 1), S14–S21.

Epstein, L. H., Paluch, R. A., Gordy, C. C., & Dorn, J. (2000). Decreasing sedentary behaviors in treating pediatric obesity. *Archives of Pediatrics & Adolescent Medicine, 154,* 220–226.

Epstein, L. H., Valoski, A., Wing, R. R., & McCurley, J. (1994). Ten-year outcomes of behavioral family-based treatment for childhood obesity. *Health Psychology, 13,* 373–383.

Ernster, V. L., Grady, D., Müke, R., Black, D., Selby, J., & Kerlikowske, K. (1995). Facial wrinkling in men and women by smoking status. *American Journal of Public Health, 85,* 78–82.

Escamilla, G., Cradock, A. L., & Kawachi, I. (2000). Women and smoking in Hollywood movies: A content analysis. *American Journal of Public Health, 90,* 412–414.

Esplen, M. J., Toner, B., Hunter, J., Glendon, G., Butler, K., & Field, B. (1998). A group therapy approach to facilitate integration of risk information for women at risk for breast cancer. *Canadian Journal of Psychiatry, 43,* 375–380.

Ettner, S. L., & Grzywacz, J. G. (2001). Workers' perceptions of how jobs affect health: A social ecological perspective. *Journal of Occupational Health Psychology, 6,* 101–113.

Evans, D. A., Funkenstein, H., Albert, M. S., Scherr, P. A., Cook, N. R., Chown, M. J., et al. (1989). Prevalence of Alzheimer's disease in a community population of older persons: Higher than previously reported. *Journal of the American Medical Association, 262,* 2551–2556.

Evans, G. W., Hygge, S., & Bullinger, M. (1995). Chronic noise and psychhological stress. *Psychological Science, 6,* 333–338.

Evans, G. W., & Johnson, D. (2000). Stress and open-office noise. *Journal of Applied Psychology, 85,* 779–783.

Evans, G. W., Lercher, P., Meis, M., Ising, H., & Kifler, W. W. (2001). Community noise exposure and stress in children. *Journal of the Acoustical Society of America, 109,* 1023–1027.

Evans, G. W., Rhee, E., Forbes, C., Allen, K. M., & Lepore, S. J. (2000). The meaning and efficacy of social withdrawal as a strategy for coping with chronic residential crowding. *Journal of Environmental Psychology, 20,* 335–342.

Evans, G. W., & Saegert, S. (2000). Residential crowding in the context of inner-city poverty. In S. Wapner, J. Demick, T. Tamamoto, & H. Minami (Eds.), *Theoretical perspectives in environment-behavior research: Underlying assumptions, research problems, and methdologies* (pp. 247–267). New York: Kluwer Academic/Plenum.

Evans, R. I., Rozelle, R. M., Maxwell, S. E., Raines, B. E., Dill, C. A., Guthrie, T. J., et al. (1981). Social modeling films to deter smoking in adolescents: Results of a three-year field investigation. *Journal of Applied Psychology, 66,* 399–414.

Evans, R. I., Smith, C. K., & Raines, B. E. (1984). Deterring cigarette smoking in adolescents: A psychosocial-behavioral analysis of an intervention strategy. In A. Baum, S. E. Taylor, & J. E. Singer (Eds.), *Handbook of psychology and health: Vol. 4. Social psychological aspects of health* (pp. 301–318). Hillsdale, NJ: Erlbaum.

Everhart, J., & Wright, D. (1995). Diabetes mellitus as a risk factor for pancreatic cancer: A meta-analysis. *Journal of the American Medical Association, 273,* 1605–1609.

Everson, S. A., Kauhanen, J., Kaplan, G. A., Goldberg, D. E., Julkunen, J., Tuomilehto, J., et al. (1997). Hostility and increased risk of mortality and acute myocardial infarction: The mediating role of behavioral risk factors. *American Journal of Epidemiology, 146,* 142–152.

Everson, S. A., Lynch, J. W., Kaplan, G. A., Lakka, T. A., Sivenius, J., & Salonen, J. T. (2001). Stress-induced blood pressure reactivity and incident stroke in middle-aged men. *Stroke, 32,* 1263–1270.

Everson, S. A., Roberts, R. E., Goldberg, D. E., & Kaplan, G. A. (1998). Depressive symptoms and increased risk of stroke mortality over a 29-year period. *Archives of Internal Medicine, 158,* 1133–1138.

Ezekiel, J. E., & Miller, F. G. (2001). The ethics of placebo-controlled trials; A middle ground. *New England Journal of Medicine, 345,* 915–920.

Faden, R. R. (1987). Ethical issues in government-sponsored public health campaigns. *Health Education Quarterly, 14,* 27–37.

Fairburn, C. G., Hay, P. J., & Welch, S. L. (1993). Binge eating and bulimia nervosa: Distribution and determinants. In C. G. Fairburn & G. T. Wilson (Eds.), *Binge eating: Nature, assessment, and treatment* (pp. 123–143). New York: Guilford Press.

Fang, C. V., & Myers, H. F. (2001). The effects of racial stressors and hostility on cardiovascular reactivity in African American and Caucasian men. *Health Psychology, 20,* 64–70.

Farley, C., Haddad, S., & Brown, B. (1996). The effects of a 4-year program promoting bicycle helmet use among children in Quebec. *American Journal of Public Health, 86,* 46–51.

Farrer, L. A., Cupples, A., Haines, J. L., Hyman, B., Kukull, W. A, Mayeaux, R., et al. (1998). Effects of age, sex, and ethnicity on association between apolipoprotein E genotype and Alzheimer disease: A meta-analysis. *Journal of the American Medical Association, 278,* 1349–1356.

Fauvel, J. P. (2001). Perceived job stress but not individual cardiovascular reactivity to stress is related to higher blood pressure at work. *Journal of the American Medical Association, 286,* 1814. (Abstract only).

Feist, J., & Feist, G. J. (2002). *Theories of personality* (5th ed.). Boston: McGraw-Hill.

Feldman, P. J., Cohen, S., Gwaltney, J. M., Jr., Doyle, W. J., & Skoner, D. P. (1999). The impact of personality on the reporting of unfounded symptoms and illness. *Journal of Personality and Social Psychology, 77,* 370–378.

Fernandez, E., & Sheffield, J. (1996). Relative contributions of life events versus daily hassles to the frequency and intensity of headaches. *Headache, 36,* 595–602.

Fernandez-Checa, J. C., Kaplowitz, N., Colell, A., & Garcia-Ruiz, C. (1997). Oxidative stress and alcoholic liver disease. *Alcohol Health & Research World, 21,* 321–324.

Fichtenberg, C. M., & Glantz, S. A. (2000). Association of the California Tobacco Control Program with declines in cigarette consumption and mortality from heart disease. *New England Journal of Medicine, 343,* 1772–1777.

Field, A. E., Byers, T., Hunter, D. J., Laird, N. M., Manson, J. E., Williamson, D. F., et al. (1999). Weight cycling, weight gain, and risk of hypertension in women. *American Journal of Epidemiology, 150,* 573–579.

Field, T. M. (1998). Massage therapy effects. *American Psychologist, 53,* 1270–1281.

Fielding, J. E. (1985). Smoking: Health effects and control. *New England Journal of Medicine, 313,* 491–498.

Fife, B. L. (1994). The conceptualization of meaning in illness. *Social Science in Medicine, 38,* 309–316.

Fife, B. L., Irick, N., & Painter, J. D. (1993). A comparative study of the attitudes of physicians and nurses toward the management of cancer pain. *Journal of Pain Symptom Management, 8,* 132–139.

Finley, J. W., Davis, C. D., & Feng, Y. (2000). Selenium from high-selenium broccoli protects rats from colon cancer. *Journal of Nutrition, 130,* 2384–2389.

Fiore, M. C., Bailey, W. C., Cohen, S. J., Dorfman, S. F., Goldstein, M. G., Gritz, E. R., et al. (1996). *Smoking Cessation: Clinical Practice Guideline No. 18.* AHCPR Publication No. 69–0692. Rockville, MD: U.S. Department of Health and Human Services. Public Health Service, Agency for Health Care Police and Research.

Fishbein, M., & Ajzen, I. (1975). *Belief, attitude, intention, and behavior: An introduction to theory and research.* Reading, MA: Addison-Wesley.

Fisher, E. S., Wennberg, J. E., Stukel, T. A., Skinner, J. S., Sharp, S. M., Freeman, J. L., et al. (2000). Associations among hospital capacity, utilization, and mortality of U.S. Medicare beneficiaries, controlling for sociodemographic factors. *Health Services Research, 34,* 1351–1362.

Fixx, J. F. (1977). *The complete book of running.* New York: Random House.

Fixx, J. F. (1980). *Jim Fixx's second book of running.* New York: Random House.

Flanders, W. D., & Rothman, K. J. (1982). Interaction of alcohol and tobacco in laryngeal cancer. *American Journal of Epidemiology, 115,* 371–379.

Flay, B. R., Koepke, D., Thomson, S. J., Santi, S., Best, A., & Brown, S. (1989). Six-year follow-up of the first Waterloo school smoking prevention trial. *American Journal of Public Health, 79,* 1371–1376.

Fleishman, J. A., & Fogel, B. (1994). Coping and depressive symptoms among people with AIDS. *Health Psychology, 13,* 156–169.

Fleury, J. (1992). The application of motivational theory to cardiovascular risk reduction. *Image: Journal of Nursing Scholarship, 24,* 229–239.

Flor, H. (2001). Psychophysiological assessment of the patient with chronic pain. In D. C. Turk & R. Melzack (Eds.), *Handbook of pain assessment* (2nd ed., pp. 70–96). New York: Guilford Press.

Flor, H., & Birbaumer, N. (1993). Comparison of the efficacy of electromyographic biofeedback, cognitive-behavioral therapy, and conservative medical interventions in the treatment of chronic musculoskeletal pain. *Journal of Consulting and Clinical Psychology, 61,* 653–658.

Foa, E. B., Dancu, C. V., Hembree, E. A., Jaycox, L. H., Meadows, E.A., & Street, G. P. (1999). A comparison of exposure therapy stress inoculation training, and their combination for reducing posttraumatic stress disorder in female assault victims. *Journal of Counseling and Clinical Psychology, 67,* 194–200.

Foa, E. B., & Meadows, E. A. (1997). Psychosocial treatments for posttraumatic stress disorder: A critical review. *Annual Review of Psychology, 48,* 449–460.

Folkman, S. (1993). Psychosocial effects of HIV infection. In L. Goldberger & S. Breznitz (Eds.), *Handbook of stress: Theoretical and clinical aspects* (2nd ed., pp. 658–681). New York: Free Press.

Folkman, S., & Lazarus, R. S. (1980). An analysis of coping in a middle-aged community sample. *Journal of Health and Social Behavior, 21,* 219–239.

Folkman, S., & Moskowitz, J. T. (2000). Positive affect and the other side of coping. *American Psychologist, 55,* 647–654.

Folsom, A. R., Kushi, L. H., Anderson, K. E., Mink, P. J., Olson, J. E., Hong, C. P., et al. (2000). Associations of general and abdominal obesity with multiple health outcomes in older women. *Archives of Internal Medicine, 160,* 2117–2128.

Fontham, E. T. H., Correa, P., Reynolds, P., Wu-Williams, A., Buffler, P. A., Greenberg, R. S., et al. (1994). Environmental tobacco smoke and lung cancer in nonsmoking women: A multicenter study. *Journal of the American Medical Association, 271,* 1952–1759.

Forbes, G. B. (1992). Exercise and lean weight: The influence of body weight. *Nutrition Reviews, 50,* 147–161.

Ford, E. S. (1999). Body mass index and colon cancer in a national sample of adult US men. *American Journal of Epidemiology, 150,* 390–398.

Forde, D. R. (1993). Perceived crime, fear of crime, and walking alone at night. *Psychological Reports, 73,* 403–407.

Fordyce, W. E. (1974). Pain viewed as learned behavior. In J. J. Bonica (Ed.), *Advances in neurology* (Vol. 4). New York: Raven Press.

Fordyce, W. E. (1976). *Behavioral methods for chronic pain and illness.* St. Louis: Mosby.

Fordyce, W. E. (1990). Contingency management. In J. J. Bonica (Ed.), *The management of pain* (2nd ed., pp. 1702–1710). Malvern, PA: Lea & Febiger.

Fordyce, W. E., Brockway, J. A., Bergman, J. A., & Spengler, D. (1986). Acute back pain: A control-group comparison of behavioral vs. traditional management methods. *Journal of Behavioral Medicine, 9,* 127–140.

Fordyce, W. E., Shelton, J. L., & Dundore, D. E. (1982). The modification of avoidance learning pain behavior. *Journal of Behavioral Medicine, 5,* 405–414.

Forrest, K. Y. Z., Bunker, C. H., Kriska, A. M., Ukoli, F. A. M., Huston, S. L, & Markovic, N. (2001). Physical activity and cardiovascular risk factors in a developing population. *Medicine and Science in Sports and Exercise, 33,* 598–604.

Fortmann, S. P., & Killen, J. D. (1994). Who shall quit? Comparisons of volunteer and population-based recruitment in two minimal-contact smoking cessation studies. *American Journal of Epidemiology, 140,* 39–51.

Francis, M. E., & Pennebaker, J. W. (1992). Putting stress into words: The impact of writing on physiological, absentee, and self-reported emotional well-being measures. *Americal Journal of Health Promotion, 6,* 280–287.

Frank, R. G., Bouman, D. E., Cain, K., & Watts, C. (1992). A preliminary study of a traumatic injury program. *Psychology and Health, 8,* 129–140.

Franz, I. D. (1913). On psychology and medical education. *Science, 38,* 555–566.

Fraser, G. E., & Shavlik, D. J. (2001). Ten years of life: Is it a matter of choice? *Archives of Internal Medicine, 161,* 1645–1652.

Frasure-Smith, N., Lesperance, F., & Talajic, M. (2000). In P. M. McCabe, N. Schneiderman, T. Field, & A. R. Wollens (Eds.). *Stress, coping, and cardiovascular disease: Stress and coping* (pp. 203–228). Mahwah, NJ: Erlbaum.

Fredrickson, B. L., Maynard, K. E., Helms, M. J., Hanney, T. L., Siegler, I. C., & Barefoot, J. C. (2000). Hostility predicts magnitude and duration of blood pressure response to anger. *Journal of Behavioral Medicine, 23,* 229–243.

Freedman, D. S., Williamson, D. F., Croft, J. B., Ballew, C., & Byers, T. (1995). Relationship of body fat distribution to ischemic heart disease: The National Health and Nutrition Examination Survey I (NHANES I): Epidemiologic Follow-up Study. *American Journal of Epidemiology, 142,* 53–63.

Freeman, V. L., Meydani, M., Yong, S., Pyle, J., Wan, Y., Arvizu-Durazo, R., et al. (2000). Prostatic levels of tocopherols, carotenoids, and retinol in relation to plasma levels and self-reported usual dietary intake. *American Journal of Epidemiology, 151,* 109–118.

French, S. A., Perry, C. L., Leon, G. R., & Fulkerson, J. A. (1994). Weight concerns, dieting behavior and smoking initiation among adolescents: A prospective study. *American Journal of Public Health, 84,* 1818–1820.

Fried, L. P., Kronmal, R. A., Newman, A. B., Bild, D. E., Mittelmark, M. B., Polak, J. F., et al. (1998). Risk factors for 5-year mortality in older adults: The Cardiovascular Health Study. *Journal of the American Medical Association, 279,* 585–592.

Friedenreich, C. M., Bryant, H. E., & Courneya, K. S. (2001). Case-control study of lifetime physical activity and breast cancer risk. *American Journal of Epidemiology, 154,* 336–347.

Friedländer, L. (1968). *Roman life and manners under the early empire.* New York: Barnes & Noble.

Friedman, E. S., Clark, D. B., & Gershon, S. (1992). Stress, anxiety, and depression: Review of biological, diagnostic, and nosologic issues. *Journal of Anxiety Disorders, 6,* 337–363.

Friedman, L. A., & Kimball, A. W. (1986). Coronary heart disease mortality and alcohol consumption in Framingham. *American Journal of Epidemiology, 124,* 481–489.

Friedman, M., & Rosenman, R. H. (1974). *Type A behavior and your heart.* New York: Knopf.

Friedman, S. L. (1997). Scarring in alcoholic liver disease: New insights and emerging therapies. *Alcohol Health & Research World, 21,* 310–316.

Fries, J. F. (1998). Reducing the need and demand for medical services. *Psychosomatic Medicine, 60,* 140–142.

Fritz, G. K. (2000). The evolution of psychosomatic medicine. *Brown University Child and Adolescent Behavior Letter, 16*(4), 8.

Froland, S. S., Jenum, P., Lendboe, C. F., Wefring, K. W., Linnestad, P. J., & Bohmer, T. (1988). HIV-1 infection in a Norwegian family before 1970. *Lancet, i,* 1344–1345.

Fromme, K., & D'Amico, E. J. (1999). Neurobiological bases of alcohol's psychological effects. In K. E. Leonard & H. T. Blane (Eds)., *Psychological theories of drinking and alcoholism* (2nd ed., pp. 422–455). New York: Guilford Press.

Froom, P., Kristal-Boneh, E., Melamed, S., Gofer, D., Benbassat, J., & Ribak, J. (1999). Smoking cessation and body mass index of occupationally active men: The Israeli CORDIS Study. *American Journal of Public Health, 89,* 718–722.

Fu, C. K., & Shaffer, M. A. (2001). The tug of work and family: Direct and indirect domain-specific determinants of work-family conflict. *Personnel Review, 30,* 502–522.

Fuchs, C. S., Stampfer, M. J., Colditz, G. A., Giovannucci, E. L., Manson, J. E., Kawachi, I., et al. (1995). Alcohol consumption and mortality among women. *New England Journal of Medicine, 332,* 1245–1250.

Fuente-Fernández, R. de la, Ruth, T. J., Sossi, V., Schluzer, M., Calne, D. B., & Stoessl, A. J. (2001). Expectation and dopamine release: Mechanism of the placebo effect in Parkinson's disease. *Science, 293,* 1164–1166.

Fuller, T. D., Edwards, J. N., Vorakitphokatorn, S., & Sermsri, S. (1996). Chronic stress and psychological well-being: Evidence from Thailand on household crowding. *Social Science and Medicine, 42,* 265–280.

Funk, S. C. (1992). Hardiness: A review of theory and research. *Health Psychology, 11,* 335–345.

Futterman, A. D., Kemeny, M. E., Shapiro, D., & Fahey, J. L. (1994). Immunological and physiological changes associated with induced positive and negative mood. *Psychosomatic Medicine, 56,* 499–511.

Galea, S., Ahern, J., Resnick, H., Kilpatrick, D., Bucuvalas, M., Gold, J., & Vlahov, D. (2002). Psychological sequelae of the September 11 terrorist attacks in New York City. *New England Journal of Medicine, 346,* 982–987.

Gallagher, E. J., Viscoli, C. M., & Horwitz, R. I. (1993). The relationship of treatment adherence to the risk of death after myocardial infarction in women. *Journal of the American Medical Association, 270,* 742–743.

Galton, F. (1879). Psychometric experiments. *Brain, 2,* 149–162.

Galton, F. (1883). *Inquiries into human faculty and its development.* London: Macmillan.

Gao, F., Bailes, E., Robertson, D. L., Chen, Y., Rodenburg, C. M., Michael, S. F., et al. (1999). Origin of HIV-1 in the chimpanzee Pan troglodytes troglodytes. *Nature, 397,* 436–441.

Garbarino, J., & Kostelny, K. (1997). What children can tell us about living in a war zone. In J. D. Osofsky (Ed.), *Children in a violent society* (pp. 32–41). New York: Guilford Press.

Gardea, M. A., Gatchel, R. J., & Mishra, K. D. (2001). Long-term efficacy of behavioral treatment of temporomandibular disorders. *Journal of Behavoral Medicine, 24,* 341–359.

Garland, A. F., & Zigler, E. F. (1994). Psychological correlates of help-seeking attitudes among children and adolescents. *American Journal of Orthopsychiatry, 64,* 586–593.

Garner, D. M., & Garfinkel, P. E. (1980). Social-cultural factors in the development of anorexia nervosa. *Psychological Medicine, 10,* 647–656.

Garner, D. M., Garfinkel, P. E., Schwartz, D., & Thompson, M. (1980). Cultural expectations of thinness in women. *Psychological Reports, 47,* 483–491.

Gatchel, R. J., & Epker, J. (1999). Psychosocial predictors of chronic pain and response to treatment. In R. J. Gatchel & D. C. Turk (Eds.), *Psychosocial factors in pain: Critical perspectives* (pp. 412–434). New York: Guilford Press.

Genuis, M. L. (1995). The use of hypnosis in helping cancer patients control anxiety, pain, and emesis: A review of recent empirical studies. *American Journal of Clinical Hypnosis, 37,* 316–326.

Gerbert, B., Caspers, N., Milliken, N., Berlin, M., Bronstone, A., & Moe, J. (2000). Interventions that help victims of domestic violence. *Journal of Family Practice, 49,* 889–895.

Ghoname, E. A., Craig, W. F., White, P. F., Ahmed, H. E., Hamza, M. A., Henderson, B. N., et al. (1999). Percutaneous electrical nerve stimulation for low back pain: A randomized crossover study. *Journal of the American Medical Association, 281,* 818–823.

Gibbons, F. X., Eggleston, T. J., & Benthin, A. C. (1997). Cognitive reactions to smoking relapse: The reciprocal relation between dissonance and self-esteem. *Journal of Personality and Social Psychology, 72,* 184–195.

Gibson, L. E., & Leitenberg, H. (2000). Child sexual abuse prevention programs: Do they decrease the occurrence of child sexual abuse? *Child Abuse and Neglect, 24,* 1115–1125.

Gielen, A. C., McDonald, E. M., Wilson, M. P. H., Hwang, W. T., Serwint, J. R., Andrews, J. S., et al. (2002). Effects of improved access to safety counseling, products, and home visits on parents' safety practices: Results of a randomized trial. *Archives of Pediatrics & Adolescent Medicine, 156,* 33–40.

Gilbar, O. (1989). Who refuses chemotherapy: A profile. *Psychological Reports, 64,* 1291–1297.

Gilliland, F. D., Li, Y. F., Baumgartner, K., Crumley, D., & Samet, G. M. (2001). Physical activity and breast cancer risks in Hispanic and non-Hispanic white women. *American Journal of Epidemiology, 154,* 442–450.

Gillum, R. F., Mussolino, M. E., & Ingram, D. D. (1996). Physical activity and stroke incidence in women and men: The NHANES Epidemiologic Follow-Up Study. *American Journal of Epidemiology, 143,* 660–869.

Gillum, R. F., Mussolino, M. E., & Madans, J. H. (1998). Coronary heart disease risk factors and attributable risks in African-American women and men: NHANES I Epidemiologic Follow-Up Study. *American Journal of Public Health, 88,* 913–917.

Giovannucci, E. (1999). Tomatoes, tomato-based products, lycopene, and cancer: Review of the epidemiologic litertture. *Journal of the National Cancer Institute, 91,* 317–331.

Glasgow, R. E., & Anderson, R. M. (1999). In diabetes care, moving from compliance to adherence is not enough. *Diabetes Care, 22,* 2090–2091.

Glinder, J. G. & Compas, B. E. (1999). Self-blame attributions in women with newly diagnosed breast cancer: A prospective study of psychological adjustment. *Health Psychology, 18,* 475–481.

Goff, K. G. (2000, September 18). Breathtaking. *Insight on the News, 16,* 33.

Gold, D. R., Wang, X., Wypij, D., Speizer, F. E., Ware, J. H., & Dockery, D. W. (1996). Effects of cigarette smoking on lung function in adolescent boys and girls. *New England Journal of Medicine, 335,* 931–937.

Goldberg, L., Elliot, D., Clarke, G. N., MacKinnon, D. P., Moe, E., Zoref, L., et al. (1996). Effects of a multidimensional anabolic steroid prevention intervention: The Adolescents Training and Learning to Avoid Steroids (ATLAS) program. *Journal of the American Medical Association, 276,* 1555–1562.

Golding, J. M. (1999). Intimate partner violence as a risk factor for mental disorders: A meta-analysis. *Journal of Family Violence, 14,* 99–101.

Goldner, E. M., & Birmingham, C. L. (1994). Anorexia nervosa: methods of treatment. In L. Alexander-Mott & D. B. Lumsden (Eds.), *Understanding eating disorders: Anorexia nervosa, bulimia nervosa, and obesity* (pp. 135–157). Washington, DC: Taylor & Francis.

Goldstein, A. (1976). Opioid peptides (endorphins) in pituitary and brain. *Science, 193,* 1081–1086.

Goldston, D. B., Kovacs, M., Obrosky, D. S., & Iyengar, S. (1995). A longitudinal study of life events and metabolic control among youths with insulin-dependent diabetes mellitus. *Health Psychology, 14,* 409–414.

Gonder-Frederick, L. A., Cox, D. J., Bobbitt, S. A., & Pennebaker, J. W. (1986). Blood glucose symptom beliefs of diabetic patients: Accuracy and implications. *Health Psychology, 5,* 327–341.

Gonder-Frederick, L. A., Cox, D. J., & Ritterband, L. M. (2002). Diabetes and behavioral medicine: The second decade. *Journal of Consulting and Clinical Psychology, 70,* 611–625.

Gonzalez, L. P. (1998). Electrophysiological changes after repeated alcohol withdrawal. *Alcohol Health & Research World, 22,* 34–37.

Goodwin, D. G. (1976). *Is alcoholism hereditary?* New York: Oxford University Press.

Goodwin, P. J., Leszcz, M., Ennis, M., Koopmans, J., Vincent, L., Guther, H., et al. (2001). The effect of group psychosocial support on survival in metastatic breast cancer. *New England Journal of Medicine, 345,* 719–726.

Gorin, A. A., & Stone, A. A. (2001). Recall biases and cognitive errors in retrospective self-reports: A call for momentary assessments. In A. Baum, T. A. Revenson, & J. E. Singer (Eds.), *Handbook of health psychology* (pp. 405–413). Mahwah, NJ: Erlbaum.

Gottlieb, B. H. (1996). Theories and practices of mobilizing support in stressful circumstances. In C. L. Cooper (Ed.), *Handbook of stress, medicine, and health* (pp. 339–356). Boca Raton, FL: CRC Press.

Gottman, J. M. (1991). Predicting the longitudinal course of marriages. *Journal of Marital and Family Therapy, 17,* 3–7.

Gottman, J. M. (1998). Psychology and the study of marital processes, *Annual Review of Psychology, 49,* 169–187.

Grady, D., & Ernster, V. (1992). Does cigarette smoking make you ugly and old? *American Journal of Epidemiology, 135,* 839–842.

Graig, E. (1993). Stress as a consequence of the urban physical environment. In L. Goldberger & S. Breznitz (Eds.), *Handbook of stress: Theoretical and clinical aspects* (2nd ed., pp. 316–332). New York: Free Press.

Greaves, C. J., Eiser, C., Seamark, D., & Halpin, D. M. G. (2002). Attack context: An important mediator of the relationship between psychological status and asthma outcomes. *Thorax, 57,* 217–221.

Greeley, J., & Oei, T. (1999). Alcohol and tension reduction. In K. E. Leonard & H. T. Blane (Eds.), *Psychological theories of drinking and alcoholism* (2nd ed., pp. 14–53). New York: Guilford Press.

Green, R. C., Cupples, A., Go, R., Benke, K. S., Edeki, T., Griffith, P. A., et al. (2002). Risk of dementia among White and African American relatives of patients with Alzheimer disease. *Journal of the American Medical Association, 287,* 329–336.

Greenberg, M. R., & Schneider, D. (1994). Violence in American cities: Young Black males is the answer, but what was the question? *Social Science and Medicine, 39,* 179–187.

Greendale, G. A., Barrett-Connor, E., Edelstein, S., Ingles, S., & Halle, R. (1995). Lifetime leisure exercise and osteoporosis: The Rancho Bernardo Study. *American Journal of Epidemiology, 141,* 951–959.

Greer, S., & Morris, T. (1978). The study of psychological factors in breast cancer: Problems of method. *Social Science and Medicine, 12,* 129–134.

Greist, J. H. (1984). Exercise in the treatment of depression. *Coping with mental stress: The potential and limits of exercise intervention.* Washington, DC: National Institute of Mental Health.

Greist, J. H., Eischens, R. R., Klein, M. H., & Linn, D. (1981). Addendum to "Running through your mind." In M. H. Sacks & M. L. Sachs (Eds.), *Psychology of running.* Champaign, IL: Human Kinetics Publishers.

Greist, J. H., & Greist, T. H. (1979). *Antidepressant treatment: The essentials.* Baltimore: Williams & Wilkins.

Greist, J. H., Klein, M. H., Eischens, R. R., Faris, J., Gurman, A. S., & Morgan, W. P. (1978). Running through your mind. *Journal of Psychosomatic Research, 22,* 259–294.

Greist, J. H., Klein, M. H., Eischens, R. R., Faris, J., Gurman, A. S., & Morgan, W. P. (1979). Running as treatment of depression. *Comprehensive Psychiatry, 20,* 41–54.

Grinspoon, L., & Bakalar, J. B. (1995). Marihuana as medicine: A plea for reconsideration. *Journal of the American Medical Association, 273,* 1875–1876.

Grover, S. A., Gray-Donald, K., Joseph, L., Abrahamowicz, M., & Coupal, L. (1994). Life expectancy following dietary modification or smoking cessation. *Archives of Internal Medicine, 154,* 1697–1704.

Grunbaum, J. A., Kann, L., Kinchen, S. A., Williams, B., Ross, J. G., Lowry, R., et al. (2002). Youth Risk Behavior Surveilance—Unites States, 2001. *Morbidity and Mortality Weekly Report, 51.* No. ss-4.

Guck, T. P., Kavan, M. G., Elsasser, G. N., & Barone, E. J. (2001). Assessment and treatment of depression following myocardial infarction. *American Family Physician, 64,* 641–656.

Guendelman, S., Meade, K., Benson, M., Chen, Y. Q., & Samuels, S. (2002). Improving asthma outcomes and self-management behaviors of inner-city children: A randomized trial of the health buddy interactive device and an asthma diary. *Archives of Pediatrics & Adolescent Medicine, 156,* 114–120.

Guerra, S., Ribeiro, J., Duarte, J., & Mota, J. (2002). Physical activity and blood pressure patterns: A cross-sectional study on Portuguese school children aged 8 through 13 years old. *Children's Health Care, 31,* 119–130.

Gull, W. W. (1874). Anorexia nervosa (apepsia hysterica, anorexia hysterica). *Transactions of the Clinical Society of London, 7,* 22–28. (Reprinted in R. M. Kaufman & M. Heiman [Eds.], *Evolution of psychosomatic concepts: Anorexia nervosa, a paradigm.* New York: International University Press, 1964.)

Gullette, E. C. D., Blumenthal, J. A., Babyak, M., Jiang, W., Waugh, R. A., Frid, D. J., et al. (1997). Effects of mental stress on myocardial ischemia during daily life. *Journal of the American Medical Association, 277,* 1521–1526.

Gump, B. B., Matthews, K. A., Scheier, M. F., Schulz, R., Bridges, M. W., & Magovern, G. J. (2001). Illness representations according to age and effects on health behaviors following coronary artery bypass graft surgery. *Journal of the American Geriatrics Society, 49,* 284–289.

Gunthert, K. C., Cohen, L. H., & Armeli, S. (1999). The role of neuroticism in daily stress and coping. *Journal of Personality and Social Psychology, 77,* 1087–1100.

Gureje, O., Von Korff, M., Simon, G. E., & Gater, R. (1996). Persistent pain and well-being: A World Health Organization study in primary care. *Journal of the American Medical Association, 280,* 147–151.

Gustavsson, P., Jakobsson, R., Nyberg, F., Pershagen, G., Järup, L., & Schéele, P. (2000). Occupational exposure and lung cancer risk: A population-based case-referent study in Sweden. *American Journal of Epidemiology, 152,* 32–40.

Guyll, M., Matthews, K. A., Bromberger, J. T. (2001). Discrimination and unfair treatment: Relationship to cardiovascular reactivity among African American and European American women. *Health Psychology, 20,* 315–325.

Haddon, W. H., Jr. (1970). On the escape of tigers: An ecologic note. *Technology Reviews, 72,* 3–7.

Haddon, W. H., Jr. (1972). A logical framework for categorizing highway safety phenomena and activity. *Journal of Trauma, 12,* 193–207.

Haddon, W. H., Jr. (1980, September–October). The basic strategies for reducing damage from hazards of all kinds. *Hazard Prevention, 6,* 16–22.

Hader, S. L., Smith, D. K., Moore, J. S., & Holmberg, S. D. (2001). HIV infection in women in the United States: Status at the millennium. *Journal of the American Medical Association, 285,* 1186–1192.

Hagedoorn, M., Kujer, R. G., Buuk, B. P., DeJong, G. M., Wobbes, T., & Sanderman, R. (2000). Marital satisfaction in patients with cancer: Does support from intimate partners benefit those who need it the most? *Health Psychology, 19,* 274–282.

Hakim, A. A., Petrovitch, H., Burchfiel, C. M., Ross, G. W., Rodriguez, B. L., White, L. R., et al. (1998). Effects of walking on mortality among nonsmoking retired men. *New England Journal of Medicine, 338,* 94–99.

Hale-Carlsson, G., Hutton, B., Fuhrman, J., Morse, D., McNutt, L., & Clifford, A. (1996). Physical violence and injuries in intimate relationships—New York, Behavioral Risk Factor Surveillance System, 1994. *Morbidity and Mortality Weekly Report, 45,* 765–767.

Hales, D. (1997). *An invitation to health* (7th ed.). Pacific Grove, CA: Brooks/Cole.

Hall, H. I., May, D. S., Lew, R. A., Koh, H. K., & Nadel, M. (1997). Sun protection behaviors in the U.S. White population. *Preventive Medicine, 26,* 401–407.

Hall, J. A., Irish, J. T., Roter, D. L., Ehrlich, C. M., & Miller, L. H. (1994). Gender in medical encounters: An analysis of physician and patient communication in a primary care setting. *Health Psychology, 13,* 384–392.

Hambidge, S. J., Davidson, A. J., Gonzales, R., Steiner, J. F. (2002). Epidemiology of pediatric injury-related primary care office visits in the Unites States. *Pediatrics, 109,* 559–565.

Hansen, C. J., Stevens, L. C., & Coast, J. R. (2001). Exercise duration and mood state: How much is enough to feel better? *Health Psychology, 20,* 267–275.

Hanvik, L. J. (1951). MMPI profiles in patients with low back pain. *Journal of Consulting and Clinical Psychology, 15,* 350–353.

Harrell, E. H., Kelly, K., & Stutts, W. A. (1996). Situational determinants of correlations between serum cortisol and self-reported stress measures. *Psychology: A Journal of Human Behavior, 33,* 22–25.

Harris, M. A., & Lustman, P. J. (1998). The psychologist in diabetes care. *Clinical Diabetes, 16* (2), 91–93.

Harris, M. I. (2001). Racial and ethnic differences in health care access and health outcomes for adults with Type 2 diabetes. *Diabetes Care, 24,* 454–459.

Harris, S. S., Caspersen, C. J., DeFriese, G. H., & Estes, H. (1989). Physical activity counseling for healthy adults as a primary preventive intervention in the clinical setting: Report for the US Preventive Services Task Force. *Journal of the American Medical Association, 261,* 3590–3598.

Harris, T. B., Ballard-Barbasch, R., Madans, J., Makuc, D. M., & Feldman, J. J. (1993). Overweight, weight loss and risk of coronary heart disease in older women: The NHANES I Epidemiologic Follow-up Study. *American Journal of Epidemiology, 137,* 1318–1327.

Hartz, A. J., Rupley, D. C., & Rimm, A. A. (1984). The association of girth measurements with disease in 32,856 women. *American Journal of Epidemiology, 119,* 71–80.

Harvard Mental Health Letter. (2000, May). Treatment of alcoholism, part 2. *Harvard Mental Health Letter, 16*(12).

Harvey-Berino, J., Pintauro, S. J., & Gold, E. C. (2002). The feasibility of using Internet support for the maintenance of weight loss. *Behavior Modification, 26,* 103–116.

Hashima, P. Y., & Finkelhor, D. (1999). Violent victimization of youth versus adults in the National Crime Victimization Survey. *Journal of Interpersonal Violence, 14,* 799–800.

Hatfield, J., & Job, R. F. S. (2001). Optimism bias about environmental degradation: The role of the range of impact of precautions. *Journal of Environmental Psychology, 21,* 17–30.

Hausenblas, H. A., Carron, A. V., & Mack, D E. (1997). Application of the theories of reasoned action and planned behavior to exercise behavior: A meta-analysis. *Journal of Sport and Exercise Psychology, 19,* 36–51.

Hausenblas, H. A., & Symons Downs, D. (2002a). Exercise dependence: A systematic review. *Psychology of Sport and Exercise, 3,* 89–123.

Hausenblas, H. A., & Symons Downs, D. (2002b). Relationship among sex, imagery, and exercise dependence symptoms. *Psychology of Addictive Behaviors, 16,* 169–172.

Hayes, S., Bulow, C., Clarke, R., Vega, E., Vega-Perez, E., Ellison, L., et al. (2000). Incidence of low back pain in women who are pregnant. *Physical Therapy, 80,* 34.

Hayes-Bautista, D. E., Hsu, P., Hayes-Bautista, M., Iniguez, D., Chamberlin, C. L., Rico, C., et al. (2002). An anomaly within the Latino epidemiological paradoz: The Latino adolescent male mortality peak. *Archives of Pediatrics & Adolescent Medicine, 156,* 480–484.

Haynes, R. B. (1976). Strategies for improving compliance: A methodologic analysis and review. In D. L. Sackett & R. B. Haynes (Eds.), *Compliance with therapeutic regimens* (pp. 69–82). Baltimore: Johns Hopkins University Press.

Haynes, R. B. (1979). Introduction. In R. B. Haynes, D. W. Taylor, & D. L. Sackett (Eds.), *Compliance in health care* (pp. 1–7). Baltimore: Johns Hopkins University Press.

Haynes, R. B., McKibbon, K. A., & Kanani, R. (1996). Systematic review of randomized trials of interventions to assist patients to follow prescriptions for medications. *Lancet, 348,* 383–386.

Haynes, R. B., Wang, E., & da Mota Gomes, M. (1987). A critical review of interventions to improve compliance with prescribed medications. *Patient Education and Counseling, 10,* 155–166.

He, J., Ogden, L. G., Vupputuri, S., Bazzano, L. A., Loria, C., & Whelton, P. K. (1999). Dietary sodium intake and subsequent risk of cardiovascular disease in overweight adults. *Journal of the American Medical Association, 282,* 2027–2034.

He, J., Vupputuri, S., Allen, K., Prerost, M. R., Hughes, J., & Whelton, P. K. (1999). Passive smoking and the risk of coronary heart disease—a meta-analysis of epidemiologic studies. *New England Journal of Medicine, 340,* 920–926.

Hearn, W. L., Flynn, D. D., Hime, G. W., Rose, S., Cofino, J. C., Mantero-Atienza, E., et al. (1991). Cocaethylene: A unique cocaine metabolite displays high affinity for the dopamine transporter. *Journal of Neurochemistry, 56,* 698–701.

Hebert, P. R., Gaziano, J. M., Chan, K. S., & Hennekens, C. H. (1997). Cholesterol lowering with statin dugs, risk of stroke, and total mortality: An overview of randomized trials. *Journal of the American Medical Association, 278,* 313–321.

Heck, A., Collins, J., & Peterson, L. (2001). Decreasing children's risk taking on the playground. *Journal of Applied Behavior Analysis, 34,* 349.

Hegel, M. T., Ayllon, T., Thiel, G., & Oulton, B. (1992). Improving adherence to fluid restrictions in male hemodialysis patients: A comparison of cognitive and behavioral approaches. *Health Psychology, 11,* 324–330.

Heise, L., Ellsberg, M., & Gottemoeller, M. (1999). Ending violence against women. *Population Reports,* Series L, No. 11. Baltimore, MD: Johns Hopkins University School of Public Health, Population Information Program.

Helby, E. M., Gafarian, C. T., & McCann, S. C. (1989). Situational and behavioral correlates of compliance to a diabetic regimen. *Journal of Compliance in Health Care, 4,* 101–116.

Helgeson, V. S. (2003). Cognitive adaptation, psychological adjustment, and disease progression among angioplasty patients: 4 years later. *Health Psychology, 22,* 30–38.

Helgeson, V. S., Cohen, S., & Fritz, H. L. (1998). Social ties and cancer. In J. C. Holland (Ed.), *Psycho-oncology* (pp. 99–109). New York: Oxford University Press.

Helgeson, V. S., Cohen, S., Schulz, R., & Yasko, J. (2000). Group support interventions for women with breast cancer: Who benefits from what? *Health Psychology. 19,* 107–114.

Hemingway, H., & Marmot, M. (1999). Psychosocial factors in the etiology and prognosis of coronary heart disease: Systematic review of prospective cohort studies. *British Medical Journal, 318,* 1460–1467.

Hennekens, C. H., Buring, J. E., Manson, J. E., Stampfer, M. J., Rosner, B., Cook, N. F., et al. (1996). Lack of long-term supplementations with beta-carotene on the the incidence of malignant neoplasms and cardiovascular disease. *New England Journal of Medicine, 394,* 1145–1149.

Hennrikus D. J., Jeffery, R. W., Lando, H. A., Murray, D. M., Brelje, K., Davidann, B., et al. (2002). The SUCCESS project: The effect of program format and incentives on participation and cessation in worksite smoking cessation programs. *American Journal of Public Health, 92,* 274–279.

Hepler, R. S., & Frank, I. M. (1971). Marijuana smoking and intraocular pressure. *Journal of the American Medical Association, 217,* 1392.

Herbert, T. B., & Cohen, S. (1993a). Depression and immunity: A meta-analytic review. *Psychological Bulletin, 113,* 472–486.

Herbert, T. B., & Cohen, S. (1993b). Stress and immunity in humans: A meta-analytic review. *Psychosomatic Medicine, 55,* 364–379.

Herbert, T. B., & Cohen, S. (1994). Stress and illness. In V. S. Ramachandran (Ed.), *Encyclopedia of human behavior, Vol. 4* (pp. 325–332). San Diego, CA: Academic Press.

Hermann, C., Kim M., & Blanchard, E. B. (1995). Behavioral and prophylactic pharmacological intervention studies of pediatric migraine: A exploratory meta-analysis. *Pain, 60,* 139–255.

Hernán, M. A., Olek, M. J., & Ascherio, A. (2001). Cigarette smoking and incidence of multiple sclerosis, *American Journal of Epidemiology, 154,* 69–74.

Herning, R. I., Jones, R. T., Bachman, J., & Mines, A. H. (1981). Puff volume increases when low-nicotine cigarettes are smoked. *British Medical Journal, 283,* 187–189.

Herschbach, P., Duran, G., Waadt, S., Zettler, A., Amm, C., Marten-Mittag, B., et al. (1997). Psychometric properties of the Questionnaire on Stress in Patients with Diabetes—Revised (QSD—R). *Health Psychology, 16,* 171–174.

Hetherington, M. M., & Rolls, B. J. (1996). Sensory-specific satiety: Theoretical frameworks and central characteristics. In E. D. Capaldi (Ed.), *Why we eat what we eat: The psychology of eating* (pp. 267–290). Washington, DC: American Psychological Association.

Heymsfield, S. B., Greenberg, A. S., Fujioka, K., Dixon, R. M., Kushner, R., Hunt, T., et al. (1999). Recombinant leptin for weight loss in obese and lean adults: A randomized, controlled, dose-escalation trial. *Journal of the American Medical Association, 282,* 1568–1575.

Hilgard, E. R. (1978). Hypnosis and pain. In R. A. Sternbach (Ed.), *The psychology of pain.* New York: Raven Press.

Hilgard, E. R., & Hilgard, J. R. (1994). *Hypnosis in the relief of pain* (Rev. ed.). Los Altos, CA: Kaufmann.

Hill, A. J., & Franklin, J. A. (1998). Mothers, daughters and dieting: Investigating the transmission of weight control. *British Journal of Clinical Psychology, 37,* 3–13.

Hingson, R. W., Heeren, T., Jamanka, A., & Howland, J. (2000). Age of drinking onset and unintentional injure involvement after drinking. *Journal of the American Medical Association, 284,* 1527–1533.

Hochbaum, G. (1958). *Public participation in medical screening programs* (DHEW Publication No. 572, Public Health Service). Washington, DC: U.S. Government Printing Office.

Høldrup, S., Sørensen, T. I. A., Strøger. U., Lauritzen, J. B., Schroll, M., & Grønbaak, M. (2001). Leisure-time physical activity levels and changes in relation to risk of hip fracture in men and women. *American Journal of Epidemiology, 154,* 60–68.

Holme, I. (1990). An analysis of randomized trials evaluating the effect of cholesterol reduction on total mortality and coronary heart disease incidence. *Circulation, 82,* 1916–1924.

Holmes, M. D., Hunter, D. J., Colditz, G. A., Stampfer, M. J., Hankinson, S. E., Speizer, F. E., et al. (1999). Association of dietary intake of fat and fatty acids with risk of breast cancer. *Journal of the American Medical Association, 281,* 914–920.

Holmes, T. H., & Rahe, R. H. (1967). The Social Readjustment Rating Scale. *Journal of Psychosomatic Research, 11,* 213–218.

Holmes, W. C., Bix, B., Meritz, M., Turner, J., & Hutelmyer, C. (1997). Human immunodeficiency virus (HIV) infection and quality of life: The potential impact of Axis I psychiatric disorders in a sample of 95 HIV seropositive men. *Psychosomatic Medicine, 59,* 187–192.

Holroyd, K. A. (2002). Assessment and psychological management of recurrent headache disorders. *Journal of Consulting and Clinical Psychology, 70,* 656–677.

Holroyd, K. A., & Lipchik, G. L. (1999). Psychological management of recurrent headache disorders: Progress and prospects. In R. J. Gatchel & D. C. Turk (Eds.), *Psychosocial factors in pain: Critical perspectives* (pp. 193–212). New York: Guilford Press.

Holroyd, K. A., & Penzien, D. B. (1990). Pharmacological versus non-pharmacological prophylaxis of recurrent migraine headache: A meta-analytic review of clinical trials. *Pain, 42,* 1–13.

Holt, N. L., Daling, J. R., McKnight, B., Moore, D. E., Stergachis, A., & Weiss, N. S. (1994). Cigarette smoking and functional ovarian cysts. *American Journal of Epidemiology, 139,* 781–786.

Holtzman, D., Bland, S. D., Lansky, A., & Mack, K. A. (2001). HIV-related behaviors and perceptions among adults in 25 states: 1997 Behavioral Risk Factor Surveillance System. *American Journal of Public Health, 91,* 1882–1888.

Hootman, J. M., Macera, C. A., Ainsworth, B. E., Addy, C. L., Martin, M., & Blair, S. N. (2002). Epidemiology of musculoskeletal injuries among sedentary and physically active adults. *Medicine and Science in Sports and Exercise, 34,* 838–844.

Hopper, J. L., & Seeman E. (1994). The bone density of female twins discordant for tobacco use. *New England Journal of Medicine, 330,* 387–392.

Hornbrook, M. C., Stevens, V. J., Wingfield, D. J., Hollis, J. F., Greenlick, M. R., & Ory, M. G. (1994). Preventing falls among community-dwelling older persons: Results from a randomized trial. *Gerontologist, 34,* 16–23.

Horng, S., & Miller, F. G. (2002). Is placebo surgery unethical? *New England Journal of Medicine, 347,* 137–139.

Horwitz, R. I., Viscoli, C. M., Berkman, L., Donaldson, R. M., Horwitz, S. M., Murray, C. J., et al. (1990). Treatment adherence and risk of death after myocardial infarction. *Lancet, 336,* 542–545.

House, J. S., Landis, K. R., & Umberson, D. (1988). Social relationships and health. *Science, 241,* 540–545.

Howard, G., Wagenknecht, L. E., Burk, G. L., Diez-Roux, A., Evans, G. W., McGovern, P., et al. (1998). Cigarette smoking and progression of atherosclerosis: The Atherosclerosis Risk in Communities (ARIC) Study. *Journal of the American Medical Society, 279,* 119–124.

Howard, M. O. (2001). Production and prediction of conditioned alcohol aversion (pharmacological aversion treatment of alcohol dependence, part 1). *American Journal of Drug and Alcohol Abuse, 27,* 561–585.

Howe, H. L., Wingo, P. A., Thun, M. J., Ries, L. A., Rosenberg, H. M., Feigal, E. G., et al. (2001). Annual report to the nation on the status of cancer (1973 through 1998), featuring cancers with recent increasing trends. *Journal of the National Cancer Institute, 93,* 824–842.

Hoyert, D. L., Freedman, M. A., Strobino, D. M., & Guyer, B. (2001). Annual summary of vital statistics: 2000. *Pediatrics, 108,* 124–138.

Hrøbjartsson, A., & Gøtzsche, P. C. (2001). An analysis of clinical trials comparing placebo with no treatment. *New England Journal of Medicine, 344,* 1594–1602.

Hu, F. B., Leitzmann, M. F., Stampfer, M. J., Colditz, G. A., Willett, W. C., & Rimm, E. B. (2001). Physical activity and television watching in relation to risk for Type 2 diabetes mellitus in men. *Archives of Internal Medicine, 161,* 1542–1549.

Hu, F. B., Stampfer, M. J., Colditz, G. A., Ascherio, A., Rexrode, K. M., Willett, W. C., et al. (2000). Physical activity and risk of stroke in women. *Journal of the American Medical Association, 283,* 7961–7967.

Hu, F. B., Stampfer, M. J., Manson, J. E., Goldstein, F., Colditz, G. A., Speizer, F. E., et al. (2000). Trends in the incidence of coronary heart disease and changes in diet and lifestyle in women. *New England Journal of Medicine, 343,* 530–537.

Hu, F. B., Stampfer, M. J., Rimm, E. B., Manson, J. E., Ascherio, A., Colditz, G. A., et al. (1999). A prospective study of egg consumption and risk of cardiovascular disease in men and women. *Journal of the American Medical Association, 281,* 1387–1394.

Hu, F. B., Stampfer, M. J., Solomon, C. G., Liu, S., Willett, W. C., Speizer, F. E., et al. (2001). The impact of diabetes mellitus on mortality from all causes and coronary heart disease in women: 20 years of follow-up. *Archives of Internal Medicine, 161,* 1717–1723.

Huang, J. Q., Sridhar, S., & Hunt, R. H. (2002). Role of *Helicobacter pylori* infection and non-steroidal anti-inflammatory drugs in peptic-ulcer disease: A meta-analysis. *Lancet, 359,* 14–21.

Huang, Z, Hankinson, S. E., Colditz, G. A., Stampfer, M. J., Hunter, D. J., Manson, J. E., et al. (1997). Dual effects of weight and weight gain on breast cancer risk. *Journal of the American Medical Association, 278,* 1407–1411.

Hughes, J. (1975). Isolation of an endogenous compound from the brain with pharmacological properties similar to morphine. *Brain Research, 88,* 295–308.

Hughes, J. R., Gulliver, S. B., Fenwick, J. W., Valliere, W. A., Cruser, K., Pepper, S., et al. (1992). Smoking cessation among self-quitters. *Health Psychology, 11,* 331–334.

Hughes, J. R., Gust, S. W., Keenan, R. M., Fenwick, J. W., & Healey, M. L. (1989). Nicotine vs placebo gum in general medical practice. *Journal of the American Medical Association, 261,* 1300–1305.

Hull, J. G. (1981). A self-awareness model of the causes and effects of alcohol consumption. *Journal of Abnormal Psychology, 90,* 586–600.

Hull, J. G. (1987). Self-awareness model. In H. T. Blane & K. E. Leonard (Eds.), *Psychological theories of drinking and alcoholism* (pp. 272–304). New York: Guilford Press.

Hull, J. G., & Bond, C. F. (1986). Social and behavioral consequences of alcohol consumption and expectancy: A meta-analysis. *Psychological Bulletin, 99,* 347–360.

Hulley, S., Grady, D., Bush, T., Furberg, C., Herrington, D., Riggs, B., et al. (1998). Randomized trial of estrogen plus progestin for secondary prevention of coronary heart disease in postmenopausal women. *Journal of the American Medical Association, 280,* 605–613.

Hunink, M. G., Goldman, L., Tosteson, N. A., Mittlemen, M. A., Goldman, P. A., Williams, L. W., et al. (1997). The recent decline in mortality from coronary heart disease, 1980–1990: The effect of secular trends in risk factors and treatment. *Journal of the American Medical Association, 277,* 535–542.

Hunt, L. M., Jordan, B., Irwin, S., & Browner, C. H. (1989). Compliance and the patient's perspective: Controlling symptoms in everyday life. *Culture, Medicine, and Psychiatry, 13,* 315–334.

Hunt, W. A., Barnett, L. W., & Branch, L. G. (1971). Relapse rates in addiction programs. *Journal of Clinical Psychology, 27,* 455–456.

Hunter, D. J., Manson, J. E., Colditz, G. A., Stampfer, M. J., Rosner, B., Hennekens, C. H., et al. (1993). A prospective study of the intake of vitamins C, E, and A and the risk of breast cancer. *New England Journal of Medicine, 329,* 234–240.

Hwang, M. Y. (1999). Living with asthma. *Journal of the American Medical Association, 281,* 2160.

Hyman, R. B., Baker, S., Ephraim, R., Moadel, A., & Philip, J. (1994). Health Belief Model variables as predictors of screening mammography utilization. *Journal of Behavior Medicine, 17,* 391–406.

Iacono, W. G., & Lykken, D. T. (1997). The validity of the lie detector: Two surveys of scientific opinion. *Journal of Applied Psychology, 82,* 426–433.

Ickovics, J. R., Druley, J. A., Grigorenko, E. L., Morrill, A. C., Beren, S. E., & Rodin, J. (1998). Long-term effects of HIV counseling and testing for women: Behavioral and psychological consequences are limited at 18 months posttest. *Health Psychology, 17,* 395–402.

Ilacqua, G. E. (1994). Migraine headaches: Coping efficacy of guided imagery training. *Headache, 34,* 99–102.

Ingraham, J. L., & Ingraham, C. A. (1995). Introduction to microbiology. Belmont, CA: Wadsworth.

Institute of Medicine. (2002). *Unequal treatment: Confronting racial and ethnic disparities in health care.* Washington, DC: Author.

International Association for the Study of Pain (IASP), Subcommittee on Taxonomy. (1979). Pain terms: A list with definitions and notes on usage. *Pain, 6,* 249–252.

International Society of Sport Psychology. (1992). Physical activity and psychological benefits: A position statement from the International Society of Sport Psychology. *Journal of Applied Sport Psychology, 4,* 94–98.

In'tveld, B. A., Ruitenberg, A., Hofman, A., Launer, L. J., van Duijn, C. M., Stijnen, T., et al. (2001). Nonsteroidal anti-inflammatory drugs and the risk of Alzheimer's disease. *New England Journal of Medicine, 345,* 1515–1521.

Irbarren, C., Tekawa, S., Sidney, S., & Friedman, G. D. (1999). Effect of cigar smoking on the risk of cardiovascular disease, chronic obstructive pulmonary disease, and cancer in men. *New England Journal of Medicine, 340,* 1773–1781.

Ismail, A. I., Burt, B. A., & Eklund, S. A. (1983). Epidemiologic patterns of smoking and peridontal disease in the United States. *Journal of the American Dental Association, 106,* 617–621.

Iso, H., Jacobs, D. R., Jr., Wentworth, P., Neaton, J. D., & Cohen, J. D. (1989). Serum cholesterol levels and six-year mortality from stroke in 350,977 men screened for the Multiple Risk Factor Intervention Trial. *New England Journal of Medicine, 320,* 904–910.

Iso, H., Rexrode, K. M., Stampfer, M. J., Manson, J. E., Colditz. G. A., Speizer, F. E., et al. (2001). Intake of fish and omega-3 fatty acids and risk of stroke in women. *Journal of the American Medical Association, 285,* 304–312.

Jablon, S., Hrubec, Z., & Boise, J. D. (1991). Cancer in populations living near nuclear facilities. *Journal of the American Medical Association, 265,* 1403–1408.

Jackson, K. M., Sher, K. J., Gotham, H. J., & Wood, P. K. (2001). Transitioning into and out of large-effect drinking in young adulthood. *Journal of Abnormal Psychology, 110,* 378–391.

Jacobs, A. L., Kurtz, R. M., & Strube, M. J. (1995). Hypnotic analgesia, expectancy effects, and choice of a design: A reexamination. *International Journal of Clinical and Experimental Hypnosis, 43,* 55–68.

Jacobs, E., Thun, M. J., & Appicella, L. F. (1999). Cigar smoking and death from coronary heart disease in a prospective study of U.S. men. *Archives of Internal Medicine, 159,* 2413–2421.

Jacobsen, P. B., & Hann, D. M. (1998). Cognitive-behavioral interventions. In J. C. Holland (Ed.), *Psycho-oncology* (pp. 717–729). New York: Oxford University Press.

Jacobson, E. (1938). *Progressive relaxation: A physiological and clinical investigation of muscle states and their significance in psychology and medical practice* (2nd ed.). Chicago: University of Chicago Press.

Jagal, S. B., Kreiger, N., & Darlington, G. (1993). Past and recent physical activity and risk of hip fractrue. *American Journal of Epidemiology, 138,* 107–118.

Jakicic, J. M., Winters, C., Lang, W., & Wing, R. R. (1999). Effects of intermittent exercise and use of home exercise equipment on adherence, weight loss, and fitness in overweight women: A randomized trial. *Journal of the American Medical Association, 282,* 1554–1560.

Jamieson, P., & Romer, D. (2001). What do young people think they know about the risks of smoking? In P. Slovic (Ed.), *Smoking: Risk, perception & policy* (pp. 51–63). Twin Oaks, CA: Sage.

Jay, S. M., Elliott, C. H., Woody, P. D., & Siegel, S. (1991). An investigation of cognitive-behavior therapy combined with oral valium for children undergoing painful medical procedures. *Health Psychology, 10,* 317–322.

Jeffery, P. K. (2000). Comparison of the structural and inflammatory features of COPD and asthma. *Chest, 117*(5 Suppl 1), 251S–260S.

Jeffery, R. W., & French, S. A. (1998). Epidemic obesity in the United States: Are fast foods and television viewing contributing? *American Journal of Public Health, 88,* 277–280.

Jellinek, E. M. (1960). *The disease concept of alcoholism.* New Haven, CT: College and University Press.

Jenkins, C. D. (1998). Cardiovascular disease. In E. A. Blechman & K. D. Brownell (Eds.), *Behavioral medicine and women: A comprehensive handbook* (pp. 604–614). New York: Guilford Press.

Jensen, M. P., & Karoly, P. (2001). Self-report scales and procedures for assessing pain in adults. In D. C. Turk & R. Melzack (Eds.), *Handbook of pain assessment* (2nd ed., pp. 15–34). New York: Guilford Press.

Jensen, T. K., Hjollund, N. H. I., Henriksen, T. B., Scheike, T., Kolstad, H., Giwercman, A., et al. (1998). Does moderate alcohol consumption affect fertility? Follow up study among couples planning first pregnancy. *British Medical Journal, 317,* 505–510.

Jewkes, R. (2002). Intimate partner violence: Causes and prevention. *Lancet, 359,* 1423–1429.

John, E. M., Savitz, D. A., & Sandler, D. P. (1991). Prenatal exposure to parents' smoking and childhood cancer. *American Journal of Epidemiology, 133,* 123–132.

Johnson, C. C., Li, D., Perry, C. L., Elder, J. P., Feldman, H. A., Kelder, S. H., et al. (2002). Fifth through eighth grade longitudinal predictors of tobacco use among a racially diverse cohort: CATCH. *Journal of School Health, 72,* 58–64.

Johnson, D. W., & Johnson, R. T. (2002). Teaching students to resolve their own and their schoolmates' conflicts. *Counseling and Human Development, 34,* 1–11.

Johnson, J. V., & Hall, E. M. (1988). Job strain, work place social support, and cardiovascular disease: A cross-sectional study of a random sample of the Swedish working population. *American Journal of Public Health, 78,* 1336–1342.

Johnson, M. P. (1995). Patriarchal terrorism and common couple violence: Two forms of violence against women. *Journal of Marriage and the Family, 57,* 283–294.

Johnson, R. A., & Gerstein, D. R. (1998). Initiation of use of alcohol, cigarettes, marijuana, cocaine, and other substances in US birth cohorts since 1919. *American Journal of Public Health, 88,* 27–33.

Johnson, S. B. (1993). Chronic diseases of childhood: Assessing compliance with complex medical regimens. In N. A. Krasnegor, L. Epstein, S. B. Johnson, & S. J. Yaffe (Eds.), *Developmental aspects of health compliance behavior* (pp. 167–184). Hillsdale, NJ: Erlbaum.

Johnson, S. B., Freund, A., Silverstein, J., Hansen, C. A., & Malone, J. (1990). Adherence-health status relationships in childhood diabetes. *Health Psychology, 9,* 606–631.

Johnston, L. D., O'Malley, P. M., & Bachman, J. G. (2001). *Monitoring the future national survey results on drug use, 1975–2000. Volume II: College students and adults ages 19–40.* (NIH Publication No. 01-4925). Bethesda, MD: National Institute on Drug Abuse.

Johnston, L. D., O'Malley, P. M., & Bachman, J. G. (2002). *The Monitoring the Future national survey results on adolescent drug use: Overview of key findings.* Bethesda, MD: National Institute on Drug Abuse.

Jonas, B. S., & Mussolino, M. E. (2000). Symptoms of depression as a prospective risk factor for stroke. *Psychosomatic Medicine, 62,* 463–471.

Jones, J. A., Eckhardt, L. E., Mayer, J. A., Bartholomew, S., Malcarne, V. L., Hovell, M. F., et al. (1993). The effects of an instructional audiotape on breast self-examination proficiency. *Journal of Behavioral Medicine, 16,* 225–235.

Joranson, D. E., Ryan, K. M., Gilson, A. M., & Dahl, J. L. (2000). Trends in medical use and abuse of opioid analgesics. *Journal of the American Medical Association, 283,* 1710–1714.

Jung, W., & Irwin, M. (1999). Reduction of natural killer cytotoxic activity in major depression: Interaction between depression and cigarette smoking. *Psychosomatic Medicine, 61,* 263–270.

Kabat, G. C., Stellman, S. D., & Wynder, E. L. (1995). Relation between exposure to environmental tobacco smoke and lung cancer in lifetime nonsmokers. *American Journal of Epidemiology, 142,* 141–148.

Kabat-Zinn, J. (1993). Mindfulness meditation: Health benefits of an ancient Buddhist practice. In D. Goleman & J. Gurin (Eds.), *Mind/body medicine: How to use your mind for better health* (pp. 259–275). Yonkers, NY: Consumer Reports Books.

Kabat-Zinn, J., & Chapman-Waldrop, A. (1988). Compliance with an outpatient stress reduction program: Rates and predictors of program completion. *Journal of Behavioral Medicine, 11,* 333–352.

Kabat-Zinn, J., Massion, A. O., Kristeller, J., Peterson, L. G., Fletcher, K. E., Pbert, L., et al. (1992). Effectiveness of a meditation-based stress reduction program in the treatment of anxiety disorders. *American Journal of Psychiatry, 149,* 936–943.

Kahn, H. A. (1963). The relationship of reported coronary heart disease mortality to physical activity of work. *American Journal of Public Health, 53,* 1058–1067.

Kahn, H. S., Tatham, L. M., Rodriquez, C., Calle, E. E., Thun, M. J., & Heath, C. W., Jr. (1997). Stable behaviors associated with adults' 10-year change in body mass index and likelihood of gain at the waist. *American Journal of Public Health, 87,* 747–754.

Kalafat, J. (1997). Prevention of youth suicide. In R. P. Weissberg, T. P. Gullotta, R. L. Hampton, B. A. Ryan, & G. R. Adams (Eds.), *Enhancing children's wellness* (pp. 175–213). Thousand Oaks, CA: Sage.

Kalafat, J., & Elias, M. (1994). An evaluation of a school-based suicide awareness intervention. *Suicide and Life Threatening Behavior, 24,* 224–233.

Kalb, C. (1998, April 27). When drugs do harm, *Newsweek 131,* 8.

Kamarck, T. W., Jennings, R., Pogue-Geile, M., & Manuck, S. B. (1994). A multidimensional measurement model for cardiovascular reactivity: Stability and cross-validation in two adult samples. *Health Psychology, 13,* 471–478.

Kaminski, P. L., & McNamara, K. (1996). A treatment for college women at risk for bulimia: A controlled evaluation. *Journal of Counseling & Development, 74,* 288–294.

Kamiya, J. (1969). Operant control of the EEG alpha rhythm and some of its reported effects on consciousness. In C. Tart (Ed.), *Altered states of consciousness.* New York: Wiley.

Kann, L., Kinchen, S. A., Williams, B. I., Ross, J. G. Lowry, R., Grunbaum, J. A., et al. (2000). Yourth Risk Behavior Surveilance—Unites States, 1999. *Morbidity and Mortality Weekly Report, 49.* No. ss-5.

Kann, L., Kinchen, S. A., Williams, B. I., Ross, J. G. Lowry, R., Hill, C. V., et al. (1998). Youth Risk Behavior Surveillance—United States, 1997. *Morbidity and Mortality Weekly Report, 47,* No. ss-3.

Kann, L., Warren, C. W., Harris, W. A., Collins, J. L., Douglas, K. A., Collins, M. E., et al. (1995). Youth Risk Behavior Surveillance—United States, 1993. *Morbidity and Mortality Weekly Report 44,* No. ss-1.

Kanner, A. D., Coyne, J. C., Schaefer, C., & Lazarus, R. S. (1981). Comparison of two modes of stress measurement: Daily hassles and uplifts versus major life events. *Journal of Behavioral Medicine, 4,* 1–39.

Kanny, D., Schieber, R. A., Pryor, V., & Kresnow, M. J. (2001). Effectiveness of a state law mandating use of bicycle helmets among children: An observational evaluation. *American Journal of Epidemiology, 154,* 172–176.

Kaplan, J. R., Fontenot, M. B., Manuck, S. B., & Muldoon, M. F. (1996). Influence of dietary lipids on agonistic and affirmative behavior in macaca fascicularis. *American Journal of Primatology, 38,* 333–347.

Kaplan, R. M., & Bush, J. W. (1982). Health-related quality of life measurement for evaluation research and policy analysis. *Health Psychology, 1,* 61–80.

Karani, R., McLaughlin, M. A., & Cassel, C. K. (2001). Exercise in the healthy older adult. *American Journal of Geriatric Cardiology, 10,* 269–273.

Karasek, R. A., & Theorell, T. (1990). *Healthy work: Stress, productivity, and the reconstruction of working life.* New York: Basic Books.

Kasl, S. V. (1996). Theory of stress and health. In C. L. Cooper (Ed.), *Handbook of stress, medicine, and health* (pp. 13–26). Boca Raton, FL: CRC Press.

Kasl, S. V., & Cobb, S. (1966a). Health behavior, illness behavior, and sick role behavior I. Health and illness behavior. *Archives of Environmental Health, 12,* 246–266.

Kasl, S. V., & Cobb, S. (1966b). Health behavior, illness behavior, and sick role behavior II. Sick role behavior. *Archives of Environmental Health, 12,* 531–541.

Katan, M. B., Grundy, S. M., & Willett, W. C. (1997). Should a low-fat, high-carbohydrate diet be recommended for everyone? Beyond low-fat diets. *New England Journal of Medicine, 337,* 563–567.

Kawachi, I., Colditz, G. A., Ascherio, A., Rimm, E. B., Giovannucci, E., Stampfer, M. J., et al. (1994). Prospective study of phobic anxiety and risk of coronary heart disease in men. *Circulation, 89,* 1992–1997.

Kawachi, I., Colditz, G. A., Stampfer, M. J., Willett, W. C., Manson, J. E., Rosner, B., et al. (1993). Smoking cessation and decreased risk of stroke in women. *Journal of the American Medical Association, 269,* 232–236.

Kawachi, I., Troist, R. J., Robnitzky, A. G., Coakley, E. H., & Colditz, G. A. (1996). Can physical activity minimize weight gain in women after smoking cessation? *American Journal of Public Health, 86,* 999–1004.

Kawamura, N., Kim, Y., & Asukai, N. (2001). Suppression of cellular immunity in men with a past history of post-traumatic stress disorder. *American Journal of Psychiatry, 158,* 484–486.

Kaye, W. H., Nagata, T., Weltzin, T. E., Hsu, L. K., Sokol, M. S., McConaha, C., Plotnicov, K. H., Weise, J., & Deep, D. (2001). Double-blind placebo-controlled administration of fluoxetine in restricting- and restricting-purging-type anorexia nervosa. *Biological Psychiatry, 49,* 644–652.

Keefe, F. J. (1982). Behavioral assessment and treatment of chronic pain: Current status and future directions. *Journal of Consulting and Clinical Psychology, 50,* 896–911.

Keefe, F. J., & Block, A. R. (1982). Development of an observation method for assessing pain behavior in chronic low back pain patients. *Behavior Therapy, 13,* 363–375.

Keefe, F. J., Brown, G. K., Wallston, K. A., & Caldwell, D. S. (1989). Coping with rheumatoid arthritis pain: Catastrophizing as a maladaptive strategy. *Pain, 37,* 51–56.

Keefe, F. J., Smith, S. J., Buffington, A. L. H., Gibson, J., Studts, J. L., & Caldwell, D. S. (2002). Recent advances and future directions in the biopsychosocial assessment and treatment of arthritis. *Journal of Consulting and Clinical Psychology, 70,* 640–655.

Keefe, F. J., & Van Horn, Y. (1993). Cognitive-behavioral treatment of rheumatoid arthritis pain: Maintaining treatment gains. Special Issue: The challenges of pain in arthritis. *Arthritis Care and Research, 6,* 213–222.

Keller, S. E., Shiflett, S. C., Schleifer, S. J., & Bartlett, J. A. (1994). Stress, immunity, and health. In R. Glaser & J. K. Kiecolt-Glaser (Eds.), *Handbook of human stress and immunity* (pp. 217–244). San Diego, CA: Academic Press.

Kelly, J. A., & Kalichman, S. C. (1998). Reinforcement value of unsafe sex as a predictor of condom use and continued HIV/AIDS risk behavior among gay and bisexual men. *Health Psychology, 17,* 328–335.

Kelly, J. A., & Kalichman, S. C. (2002). Behavioral research in HIV/AIDS primary and secondary prevention: Recent advances and future directions. *Journal of Consulting and Clinical Psychology, 70,* 626–639.

Kelly, M. A., McKinty, H. R., & Carr, R. (1988). Utilization of hypnosis to promote compliance with routine dental flossing. *American Journal of Clinical Hypnosis, 31,* 57–60.

Kempe, R. S. (1997). A developmental approach to the treatment of abused children. In M E. Helfer, R. S. Kempe, & R. D. Krugman (Eds.), *The battered child* (5th ed., pp. 543–565). Chicago: University of Chicago Press.

Kendler, K. S., Thornton, L. M., & Gardner, C. O. (2001). Genetic risk, number of previous depressive episodes, and stressful life events in predicting onset of major depression. *American Journal of Psychiatry, 158,* 582–586.

Kenford, S. L., Fiore, M. C., Jorenby, D. E., Smith, S. S., Wetter, D., & Baker, T. B. (1994). Predicting smoking cessation: Who will quit with and without the nicotine patch. *Journal of the American Medical Association, 271,* 589–604.

Kerns, R. D., Turk, D. C., & Rudy, T. E. (1985). The West Haven-Yale Multidimensional Pain Inventory. *Pain, 23,* 345–356.

Kesaniemi, Y. A, Danforth, E., Jr., Jensen, M. D., Kopelman, P. G., Lefebvre, P., & Reader, B. A. (2001). Dose-response issues concerning physical activity and health: An evidence-based symposium. *Medicine and Science in Sports and Exercise, 33,* S351–S358.

Kesmodel, U., Wisborg, K., Olsen, S. F., Henriksen, T. B., & Secher, N. J. (2002). Moderate alcohol intake during pregnancy and the risk of stillbirth and death in the first year of life. *American Journal of Epidemiology, 155,* 305–312.

Kessler, R. C. (1997). The effects of stressful life events on depression. *Annual Review of Psychology, 48,* 191–214.

Keys, A., Brozek, J., Henschel, A., Mickelsen, O., & Taylor, H. L. (1950). *The biology of human starvation.* 2 vols. Minneapolis: University of Minnesota Press.

Khattak, A. J., Pawlovich, M. D., Souleyrette, R. R., & Hallmark, S. L. (2002). Factors related to more severe older driver traffic crash injuries. *Journal of Transportation Engineering, 128,* 243–249.

Kiecolt-Glaser, J. K. (1999). Stress, personal relationships, and immune function: Health implications. *Brain, Behavior, and Immunity, 13,* 61–72.

Kiecolt-Glaser, J. K., Dura, J. R., Speicher, C. E., Trask, J., & Glaser, R. (1991). Spousal caregivers of dementia victims: Longitudinal changes in immunity and health. *Psychosomatic Medicine, 53,* 345–362.

Kiecolt-Glaser, J. K., Fisher, L., Ogrocki, P., Stout, J. C., Speicher, C. E., & Glaser, R. (1987). Marital quality, marital disruption, and immune function. *Psychosomatic Medicine, 49,* 13–35.

Kiecolt-Glaser, J. K., & Glaser, R. (1989). Psychoneuroimmunology: Past, present, and future. *Health Psychology, 8,* 677–682.

Kiecolt-Glaser, J, K., Glaser, R., Cacioppo, J. T., MacCallum, R. C., Snydersmith, M., Cheongtag, K., et al. (1996). Marital conflict in older adults: Endocrinal and immunological correlates. *Psychosomatic Medicine, 59,* 339–349.

Kiecolt-Glaser, J. K., Glaser, R., Dyer, C., Shuttleworth, E. C., Ogrocki, P., & Speicher, C. E. (1987). Chronic stress and immune function in family caregivers of Alzheimer's disease victims. *Psychosomatic Medicine, 49,* 523–535.

Kiecolt-Glaser, J. K., Malarkey, W. B., Cacioppo, J. T., & Glaser, R. (1994). Stressful personal relationships: Immune and endocrine function. In R. Glaser & J. K. Kiecolt-Glaser (Eds.), *Handbook of human stress and immunity* (pp. 321–339). San Diego, CA: Academic Press.

Kiecolt-Glaser, J. K., Marucha, P. T., Atkinson, C., & Glaser, R. (2001). Hypnosis as a modulator of cellular immune dysregulation during acute stress. *Journal of Consulting and Clinical Psychology, 69,* 674–682.

Kiecolt-Glaser, J. K., Marucha, P. T., Malarkey, W. B., Mercado, A. M., & Glaser, R. (1995). Slowing of wound healing by psychological stress. *Lancet, 346,* 1194–1196.

Kiecolt-Glaser, J. K., & Newton, T. L. (2001). Marriage and health: His and hers. *Psychological Bulletin, 127,* 472–503.

Kiecolt-Glaser, J. K., Newton, T. L., Cacioppo, J. T., MacCallum, R. C., Glaser, R., & Malarkey, W. B. (1997). Marital conflict and endocrine function: Are men really more physiologically affected than women? *Journal of Consulting and Clinical Psychology, 64,* 324–332.

Kiely, D. K., Wolf, P. A., Cupples, L. A., Beiser, A. S., & Kannel, W. B. (1994). Physical activity and stroke risk: The Framingham Study. *American Journal of Epidemiology, 140,* 608–620.

Kimball, C. P. (1981). *The biopsychosocial approach to the patient.* Baltimore: Williams & Wilkins.

King, A. C., Oman, R. F., Brassington, G. S., Bliwise, D. L., & Haskell, W. L. (1997). Moderate-intensity exercise and self-rated quality of sleep in older adults: A randomized controlled trial. *Journal of the American Medical Association, 277,* 32–37.

King, K. A. (2001). Developing a comprehensive school suicide prevention program. *Journal of School Health, 71,* 132–137.

King, K. M., Humen, D. P., Smith, H. L., Phan, C. L., & Teo, K. K. (2001). Psychosocial components of cardiac recovery and rehabilitation attendance. *Heart, 85,* 290–293.

King, L. A., & Miner, K. N. (2000). Writing about the perceived benefits of traumatic events: Implications for physical health. *Personality and Social Psychology Bulletin, 26,* 220–230.

King, N., Touyz, S., & Charles, M. (2000). The effect of body dissatisfaction on women's perceptions of female celebrities. *International Journal of Eating Disorders, 27,* 341–346.

Kirsch, I., Moore, T. J., Scoboria, A., & Nicholls, S. S. (2002). The emperor's new drugs: An analysis of antidepressant medication data submitted to the U.S. Food and Drug Administration. *Prevention & Treatment, 5,* Article 23. Available on the World Wide Web at http://www.journals.apa.org/prevention/volume5/pre0050023a.html.

Kitamura, A., Hiroyasu, I., Sankai, T., Naito, Y., Sato, S., Klyama, M., et al. (1998). Alcohol intake and premature coronary heart disease in urban Japanese men. *American Journal of Epidemiology, 147,* 59–65.

Klein, R., Klein, B. E. K., & Moss, S. E. (1998). Relation of smoking to the incidence of age-related maculopathy: The Beaver Dam Eye Study. *American Journal of Epidemiology, 147,* 103–110.

Klohn, L. S., & Rogers, R. W. (1991). Dimensions of the severity of a health threat: The persuasive effects of visibility, time of onset, and rate of onset on young women's intentions to prevent osteoporosis. *Health Psychology, 10,* 323–329.

Klonoff, E. A., & Landrine, H. (1993). Cognitive representations of bodily parts and products: Implications for health behavior. *Journal of Behavioral Medicine, 16,* 497–508.

Klonoff, E. A., & Landrine, H. (1994). Culture and gender diversity in commonsense beliefs about the causes of six illnesses. *Journal of Behavioral Medicine, 17,* 407–418.

Klonoff, E. A., & Landrine, H. (1999). Acculturation and cigarette smoking among African Americans: Replication and implications for prevention and cessation programs. *Journal of Behavioral Medicine, 22,* 195–204.

Klonoff, E. A., & Landrine, H. (2000). Is skin color a marker for racial discrimination? Explaining the skin color–hypertension relationship. *Journal of Behavioral Medicine, 23,* 329–338.

Kluger, R. (1996). *Ashes to ashes; America's hundred-year cigarette war, the public health and the unabashed triumph of Philip Morris.* New York: Knopf.

Knafl, K. A., & Deatrick, J. A. (2002). The challenge of normalization for families of children with chronic conditions. *Pediatric Nursing, 28,* 49–54.

Knekt, P., Järvinen, R., Seppänen, R., Hellövaara, M., Teppo, L., Pukkala, E., et al. (1997). Dietary flavonoids and the risk of lung cancer and other malignant neoplasms. *American Journal of Epidemiology, 146,* 223–230.

Knopp, R. H., Walden, C. E., Retzlaff, B. M., McCann, B. S., Dowdy, A. A., Albers, J. J., et al. (1997). Long-term cholesterol-lowering effects of 4 fat-restricted diets in hypercholesterolemic and combined hyperlipidemic men. *Journal of the American Medical Association, 278,* 1509–1515.

Kobasa, S. C. (1979). Stressful life events, personality, and health: An inquiry into hardiness. *Journal of Personality and Social Psychology, 37,* 1–11.

Kobasa, S. C. O., & Maddi, S. R. (1977). Existential personality theory. In R. Corsini (Ed.), *Current personality theories* (pp. 242–276). Itasca, IL: Peacock.

Kobasa, S. C., Maddi, S. R., & Kahn, S. (1982). Hardiness and health: A prospective study. *Journal of Personality and Social Psychology, 42,* 168–177.

Koh, H. K., Bak, S. M., Geller, A. C., Mangione, T. W., Hingson, R. W., Levenson, S. M., et al. (1997). Sunbathing habits and sunscreen use among White adults: Results of a national survey. *American Journal of Public Health, 87,* 1214–1217.

Kohl, H. W., III. (2001). Physical activity and cardiovascular disease: Evidence for a dose response. *Medicine and Science in Sports and Exercise, 33,* S472–S483.

Kohn, L. T., Corrigan, J. M., & Donaldson, M. (Eds.). (1999). *To err is human: Building a safer health system.* Washington, DC: Institute of Medicine.

Kole-Snijders, A. M. J., Vlaeyen, J. W. S., Goossens, M. E. J. B., Rutten-van Mölken, M. P. M. H., Heuts, P. H. T. G., van Breukelen, G., et al. (1999). Chronic low-back pain: What does cognitive coping skills training add to operant behavioral treatment? Results of a randomized clinical trial. *Journal of Consulting and Clinical Psychology, 67,* 931–944.

Koomen, W., Visser, M., & Stapel, D. A. (2000). The credibility of newspapers and fear of crime. *Journal of Applied Social Psychology, 30,* 921–934.

Koss, M. P., & Kilpatrick, D. G. (2001). Rape and sexual assault. In L. Gerrity, T. M. Keane, & F. Tuma (Eds.), *The mental health consequences of torture* (pp. 177–193). New York: Kluwer Academic/Plenum.

Kostanski, M., & Gullone, E. (1999). Dieting and body image in the child's world: Conceptualization and behavior. *Journal of Genetic Psychology, 160,* 488–499.

Kovacs, M., Iyengar, S., Goldston, D., Obrosky, D. S., Stewart, J., & Marsh, J. (1990). Psychological functioning among mothers of children with insulin-dependent diabetes mellitus: A longitudinal study. *Journal of Consulting and Clinical Psychology, 58,* 189–195.

Kozlowski, L. T., Wilkinson, A., Skinner, W., Kent, C., Franklin, T., & Pope, M. (1989). Comparing tobacco cigarette dependence with other drug dependences. *Journal of the American Medical Association, 261,* 898–901.

Kramer, A. M. (1995). Health care for elderly persons—myths and realities. *New England Journal of Medicine, 332,* 1027–1029.

Kramsch, D. M., Aspen, A. J., Abramowitz, B. M., Kreimendahl, T., & Hood, W. B., Jr. (1981). Reduction of coronary atherosclerosis by moderate conditioning exercise in monkeys on an atherogenic diet. *New England Journal of Medicine, 305,* 1483–1489.

Krantz, D. S., Sheps, D. S., Carney, R. M., & Natelson, B. H. (2000). Effects of mental stress in patients with coronary artery disease: Evidence and clinical implications. *Journal of the American Medical Association, 283,* 1800–1802.

Kreuzer, M., Krauss, M., Kreienbrock, L., Jóckel, K. H., & Wichmann, H. E. (2000). Environmental tobacco smoke and lung cancer: A case-control study in Germany. *American Journal of Epidemiology, 151,* 241–250.

Krieger, N., Sidney, S., & Coakley, E. (1998). Racial discrimination and skin color in the CARDIA study: Implications for public health research. *American Journal of Public Health, 88,* 1308–1313.

Krokosky, N. J., & Reardon, R. C. (1989). The accuracy of nurses' and doctors' perception of patient pain. In S. G. Funk, E. M. Tornquist, M. T. Champagne, L. A. Copp, & R. A. Wiese (Eds.), *Key aspects of comfort: Management of pain, fatigue, and nausea* (pp. 127–140). New York: Springer.

Kronmal, R. A., Cain, K. C., Ye, Z., & Omenn, G. (1993). Total serum cholesterol levels and mortality risk as a function of age: A report based on the Framingham data. *Archives of Internal Medicine, 153,* 1065–1073.

Krystal, J. H., Cramer, J. A., Krol, W. F., Kirk, G. F., & Rosenheck, R. A. (2001). Naltrexone in the treatment of alcohol dependence. *New England Journal of Medicine, 345,* 1734–1739.

Kubetin, S. K. (2001). Weight-loss maintenance requires long-term management. *Family Practice News, 31*(4), 6–7.

Kulik, J. A., & Carlino, P. (1987). The effect of verbal commitment and treatment choice on medication compliance in a pediatric setting. *Journal of Behavioral Medicine, 10,* 367–376.

Kulik, J. A., & Mahler, H. I. M. (1993). Emotional support as a moderator of adjustment and compliance after coronary artery bypass surgery: A longitudinal study. *Journal of Behavioral Medicine, 16,* 48–63.

Kurz, D. (1997). Physical assaults by male partners: A major social problem. In M. R. Walsh (Ed.), *Men, women, and gender: Ongoing debates* (pp. 222–231). New Haven, CT: Yale University Press.

Kushi, L., Fee, R. M., Folsom, A. R., Mink, P. J., Anderson, K. E., & Sellers, T. A. (1997). Physical activity and mortality in postmenopausal women. *Journal of the American Medical Association, 227,* 1287–1292.

LaBrie, J. W., & Earleywine, M. (2000). Sexual risk behaviors and alcohol: Higher base rates revealed using the unmatched-count technique. *Journal of Sex Research, 37,* 321–326.

Lacey, K., Zaharia, M. D., Griffiths, J., Ravindran, A. V., Merali, Z., & Anisman, H. (2000). A prospective study of neuroendocrine and immune alterations associated with the stress of an oral academic examination among graduate students. *Psychoneuroendocrinology, 25,* 339–356.

Laden, F., Neas, L. M., Tolbert, P. E., Holmes, M. D., Hankinson, S. E., Spiegelman, D., et al. (2000). Electric blanket use and breast cancer in the Nurses' Health Study. *American Journal of Epidemiology, 152,* 41–49.

Laforge, R. G., Greene, G. W., & Prochaska, J. O. (1994). Psychosocial factors influencing low fruit and vegetable consumption. *Journal of Behavioral Medicine, 17,* 361–374.

Lahelma, E., Arber, S., Martikainen, P., & Silventoinen, K. (2001). The myth of gender differences in health: Social structural determinants across adult ages in Britain and Finland. *Current Sociology, 49,* 31–54.

Lakka, T. A., Venäläinen, J. M., Rauramaa, R., Salonen, R., Tuomilehto, J., & Salonen, J. T. (1994). Relations of leisure-time physical activity and cardiorespiratory fitness to the risk of acute myocardial infarction in men. *New England Journal of Medicine, 330,* 1549–1554.

Lambert, S. A. (1996). The effects of hypnosis/guided imagery on the postoperative course of children. *Journal of Developmental and Behavioral Pediatrics, 17,* 307–310.

Lamptey, P. R. (2002). Reducing heterosexual transmission of HIV in poor countries. *British Medical Journal, 324,* 207–211.

Landrine, H. & Klonoff, E. A. (2001). Cultural diversity and health psychology. In A. Baum, T. A. Revenson, & J. E. Singer (Eds.), *Handbook of Health Psychology* (pp. 851–891). Mahwah, NJ: Erlbaum.

Landsberg, G., & Wattam, C. (2001). Differing approaches to combating child abuse: United States vs. United Kingdom. *Journal of International Affairs, 55,* 111–123.

Lang, E. V., Benotsch, E. G., Fick, L. J., Lutgendorf, S., Berbaum, M. L., Berbaum, K. S., et al. (2000). Adjunctive non-pharmacological analgesia for invasive medical procedures: A randomised trial. *Lancet, 355,* 1486–1490.

Langer, E. J., & Rodin, J. (1976). The effects of choice and enhanced personal responsibility for the aged: A field experiment in an institutional setting. *Journal of Personality and Social Psychology, 34,* 191–198.

Langlais, P. J. (1995). Alcohol-related thiamin deficiency. *Alcohol Health & Research World, 19,* 113–121.

Lantz, P. M., House, J. S., Lepkowsi, J. M., Williams, D. R., Mero, R. P., & Chen, J. (1998). Socioeconomic factors, health behaviors, and mortality: Results from a nationally representative prospective study of US adults. *Journal of the American Medical Association, 279,* 1703–1708.

Larroque, B., Kaminski, M., Dehaene, P., Subtil, D., Delfosse, M. J., & Querleu, D. (1995). Moderate prenatal alcohol exposure and psychomotor development at preschool age. *American Journal of Public Health, 85,* 1654–1661.

Larsson, M. L. Frisk, M., Hallstrom, J., Kiviloog, J., & Lundback, B. (2001). Environmental tobacco smoke exposure during childhood is associated with increased prevalence of asthma in adults. *Chest, 120,* 711–717.

Lasser, K., Boyd, J. W., Woolhandler, S., Himmelstein, D. U., McCormick, D., & Bor, D. H. (2000). Smoking and mental illness: A population-based prevalence study. *Journal of the American Medical Association, 284,* 2606–2610.

Lau, R. R. (1997). Cognitive representations of health and illness. In D. S. Gochman (Ed.), *Handbook of health behavior research I: Personal and social determinants* (pp. 51–69). New York: Plenum Press.

Launer, L. J., Feskens, E. J. M., Kalmjin, S., & Kromhout, D. (1996). Smoking, drinking, and thinking: The Zuphen Elderly Study. *American Journal of Epidemiology, 143,* 219–227.

LaVeist, T. A., Bowie, J. V., & Cooley-Quille, M. (2000). Minority health status in adulthood: The middle years of life. *Health Care Financing Review, 21* (4), 9–21.

Lavie, C. J., Milani, R. V., & Mehra, M. R. (2000). Choosing a stress test. *Patient Care, 34*(3), 81–82, 91–92, 94.

Lawrence, J. (2000). The Indian Health Service and the sterilization of Native American women. *American Indian Quarterly, 24,* 400–419.

Lazarou, J., Pomeranz, B. H., & Corey, P. N. (1998). Incidence of adverse drug reactions in hospitalized patients: A meta-analysis of prospective studies. *Journal of the American Medical Association, 278,* 1200–1205.

Lazarus, R. S. (1984). Puzzles in the study of daily hassles. *Journal of Behavioral Medicine, 7,* 375–389.

Lazarus, R. S. (1993). From psychological stress to the emotions: A history of changing outlooks. *Annual Review of Psychology, 44,* 1–21.

Lazarus, R. S. (2000). Toward better research on stress and coping. *American Psychologist, 55,* 665–673.

Lazarus, R. S., & DeLongis, A. (1983). Psychological stress and coping in aging. *American Psychologist, 38,* 245–254.

Lazarus, R. S., DeLongis, A., Folkman, S., & Gruen, R. (1985). Stress and adaptational outcomes. *American Psychologist, 40,* 770–779.

Lazarus, R. S., & Folkman, S. (1984). *Stress, appraisal, and coping.* New York: Springer.

Lee, D. M., & Weinblatt, M. E. (2001). Rheumatoid arthritis. *The Lancet, 358,* 903–911.

Lee, I-M., Hsieh, C-c., & Paffenbarger, R. S., Jr. (1995). Exercise intensity and longevity in men. *Journal of the American Medical Association, 273,* 1179–1184.

Lee, I-M., & Paffenbarger, R. S., Jr. (1998a). Life is sweet: Candy consumption and longevity. *British Medical Journal, 317,* 1683–1684.

Lee, I-M., Paffenbarger, R. S., Jr., & Hsieh, C-c. (1992). Physical activity and risk of prostatic cancer among college alumni. *American Journal of Epidemiology, 135,* 169–179.

Lee, I-M., Rexrode, K. M., Cook, N. R., Manson, J. E., & Buring, J. E. (2001). Physical activity and coronary heart disease in women: Is "no pain, no gain" passé? *Journal of the American Medical Association, 285,* 1447–1454.

Lee, I-M., & Skerrett, P. J. (2001). Physical activity and all-cause mortality. What is the dose-response relation? *Medicine and Science in Sports and Exercise, 33,* S459–D471.

Lee, J. A. H. (1997). Declining effect of latitude on melanoma mortality rates in the United States: A preliminary study. *American Journal of Epidemiology, 146,* 413–417.

Lee, L. M., Karon, J. M., Selik, R., Neal, J. J., & Fleming, P. L. (2001). Survival after AIDS diagnosis in adolescents and adults during the treatment era, United States, 1984–1997. *Journal of the American Medical Association, 285,* 1308–1315.

Leevy, C. M., Gellene, R., & Ning, M. (1964). Primary liver cancer in cirrhosis of the alcoholic. *Annals of the New York Academy of Science, 114,* 1026–1040.

Lehrer, P. M., Carr, R., Sargunaraj, D., & Woolfolk, R. L. (1994). Stress management techniques: Are they all equivalent, or do they have specific effects? *Biofeedback and Self-Regulation, 19,* 353–401.

Leibel, R. L., Rosenbaum, M., & Hirsch, J. (1995). Changes in energy expenditure resulting from altered body weight. *New England Journal of Medicine, 332,* 621–629.

Le Marchand, L., Kolonel, L. N., & Yoshizawa, C. N. (1991). Lifetime occupational physical activity and prostate cancer risk. *American Journal of Epidemiology, 133,* 103–111.

Leon, A. S., & Sanchez, O. A., (2001). response of blood lipids to exercise training alone or combined with dietary intervention. *Medicine and Science in Sports and Exercise, 33,* S502–S515.

Lerman, C., Caporaso, N. E., Audrain, J., Main, D., Bowman, E. D., Lockshin, B., et al. (1999). Evidence suggesting the role of specific genetic factors in cigarette smoking. *Health Psychology, 18,* 14–20.

LeRoy, P. L., & Filasky, R. (1990). Thermography. In J. J. Bonica (Ed.), *The management of pain* (2nd ed., pp. 610–621). Malvern, PA: Lea & Febiger.

Lescohier, L., & Gallagher, S. S. (1996). Unintentional injury. In R. J. DiClemente, W. B. Hansen, & L. E. Ponton (Eds.), *Handbook of adolescent health risk behavior* (pp. 225–258). New York: Plenum Press.

Lester, D. (1994). Are there unique features of suicide in adults of different ages and developmental stages? *Omega Journal of Death and Dying, 29,* 337–348.

Leutwyler, K. (1995, April). The price of prevention. *Scientific American, 272,* 124–129.

Levenson, R. L., & Mellins, C. A. (1992). Pediatric HIV disease: What psychologists need to know. *Professional Psychology Research and Practice, 23,* 410–415.

Levenson, R. W., Sher, K. J., Grossman, L. M., Newman, J., & Newlin, D. B. (1980). Alcohol and stress response dampening: Pharmacological effects, expectancy, and tension reduction. *Journal of Abnormal Psychology, 89,* 528–538.

Levenstein, S. (2000). The very model of a modern etiology: A biopsychosocial view of peptic ulcer. *Psychosomatic Medicine, 62,* 176–185.

Leventhal, H., & Avis, N. (1976). Pleasure, addiction, and habit: Factors in verbal report or factors in smoking behavior? *Journal of Abnormal Psychology, 85,* 478–488.

Leventhal, H., & Diefenbach, M. (1991). The active side of illness cognition. In J. A. Skelton & R. T. Croyle (Eds.), *Mental representation in health and illness* (pp. 247–272). New York: Springer-Verlag.

Leventhal, H., Leventhal, E. A., & Cameron, L. (2001). Representations, procedures, and affect in illness self-regulation: A perceptual-cognitive model. In A. Baum, T. A. Revenson, & J. E. Singer (Eds.), *Handbook of health psychology* (pp. 19–47). Mahwah, NJ: Erlbaum.

Levi, L. (1974). Psychosocial stress and disease: A conceptual model. In E. K. E. Gunderson & R. H. Rahe (Eds.), *Life stress and illness* (pp. 8–33). Springfield, IL: Thomas.

Levy, S. M. (1985). *Behavior and cancer: Life-style and psychosocial factors in the initiation and progression of cancer.* San Francisco: Jossey-Bass.

Lewinsohn, P. M., Rohde, P., & Joiner, T. E., Jr. (2001). Evaluation of cognitive diathesis-stress models in predicting major depressive disorders in adolescents. *Journal of Abnormal Psychology, 110,* 203–215.

Lewis, P. C., Harrell, J. S., Deng, S., & Bradley, C. (1999). Smokeless tobacco use in adolescents: The Cardiovascular Health in Children (CHIC II) study. *Journal of School Health, 69,* 320–325.

Ley, P. (1997). Compliance among patients. In A. Baum, S. Newman, J. Weinman, R. West, & C. McManus (Eds.), *Cambridge handbook of psychology, health and medicine* (pp. 281–284). Cambridge, UK: Cambridge University Press.

Li, A. J., Cass, I., & Karlan, B. Y. (2001). BRCA 1 and BRCA 2: Genetic testing and intervention strategies. *Contemporary OB/GYN, 46*(7), 83–95.

Li, G., Baker, S P., Smialek, J. F., & Soderstrom, C. A. (2001). Use of alcohol as a risk factor for bicycling injury. *Journal of the American Medical Association, 285,* 893–896.

Lichtenstein, A. H., Ausman, L. M., Jalbert, S. M., & Schaefer, E. J. (1999). Effects of different forms of dietary hydrogenated fats on serum lipoprotein cholesterol levels. *New England Journal of Medicine, 340,* 1933–1940.

Light, K. C., Kopke, J. P., Obrist, P. A., & Willis, P. W. (1983). Psychological stress induces sodium fluid retention in men at high risk for hypertension. *Science, 220,* 429–431.

Ligier, S., & Sternberg, E. M. (2001). The neuroendocrine system and rheumatoid arthritis: Focus on the hypothalamo-pituitary-adrenal axis. In R. Ader, D. L. Felten, & N. Cohen (Eds.), *Psychoneuroimmunology* (3rd ed., Vol. 2, pp. 449–469). San Diego, CA: Academic Press.

Lilienfeld, A. M., & Lilienfeld, D. E. (1980). *Foundations of epidemiology* (2nd ed.). New York: Oxford University Press.

Linden, W. (1988). Biopsychological barriers to the behavioral treatment of hypertension. In W. Linden (Ed.), *Biological barriers in behavioral medicine* (pp. 163–191). New York: Plenum Press.

Linden, W. (2000). Psychological treatments in cardiac rehabilitation: Review of rationales and outcomes. *Journal of Psychosomatic Research, 48,* 443–454.

Lindstrom, I., Ohlund, C., Eek, C., Wallin, L., Peterson, L. E., Fordyce, W. E., et al. (1992). The effect of graded activity on patients with subacute low back pain: A randomized prospective clinical study with an operant-conditioning behavioral approach. *Physical Therapy, 72,* 297–311.

Linn, S., Carroll, M., Johnson, C., Fulwood, R., Kalsbeek, W., & Briefel, R. (1993). High-density lipoprotein cholesterol and alcohol consumption in US White and Black adults: Data from NHANES II. *American Journal of Public Health, 83,* 811–816.

Linton, S. J. (1999). Prevention with special reference to chronic musculoskeletal disorders. In R. J. Gatchel & D. C. Turk (Eds.). *Psychosocial factors in pain: Critical perspectives* (pp. 374–389). New York: Guilford Press.

Liu, H., Golin, C. E., Miller, L. G., Hays, R. D., Beck, C. K., Sanandji, S., et al. (2001). A comparison study of multiple measures of adherence to HIV protease inhibitors. *Annals of Internal Medicine, 134,* 968–977.

Liu, S., Manson, J. E., Stampfer, M. J., Rexrode, K. M., Hu, F. B., Rimm, E. B., et al. (2000). Whole grain consumption and risk of ischemic stroke in women. *Journal of the American Medical Association, 284,* 1534–1540.

Liu, S., Siegel, P. Z., Brewer, R. D., Mokdad, A. H., Sleet, D. A., & Serdula, M. (1997). Prevalence of alcohol-impaired driving: Results from a national self-reported survey of health behaviors. *Journal of the American Medical Association, 277,* 122–125.

Livneh, H. (2000). Psychosocial adaptation to cancer. *Journal of Rehabilitation, 66,* 40–49.

Livneh, H. (2001). Psychosocial adaptation to chronic illness and disability: A conceptual framework. *Rehabilitation Counseling Bulletin, 44,* 151–160.

Locke, J., Le Grange, D., Agras, W. S., & Dare, C. (2001). *Treatment manual for anorexia nervosa: A family-based approach.* New York: Guilford Press.

Loitman, J. E. (2000). Pain management: Beyond pharmacology to acupuncture and hypnosis. *Journal of the American Medical Association, 283,* 118–120.

Lonn, J. H. (1999). Active Back School: Prophylactic management for low back pain: A randomized, controlled, 1-year follow-up study. *Journal of the American Medical Association, 282,* 410n.

Loomis, D., Marshall, S. W., Wolf, S. H., Runyan, C. W., & Butts, J. D. (2002). Effectiveness of safety measures recommended for prevention of workplace homicide. *Journal of the American Medical Association, 287,* 1011–1017.

Loomis, D., & Richardson, D. (1998). Race and the risk of fatal injury at work. *American Journal of Public Health, 88,* 40–44.

Lotufo, P. A., Chae, C. U., Ajani, U. A., Hennekens, C. H., & Manson, J. E. (2000). Male pattern baldness and coronary heart disease. *Archives of Internal Medicine, 160,* 165–171.

Lotufo, P. A., Gaziano, J. M., Chae, C. U., Ajani, U. A., Moreno-John, G., Buring, J. E., et al. (2001). Diabetes and all-cause and coronary heart disease mortality among US male physicians. *Archives of Internal Medicine, 161,* 242–247.

Lovallo, W. R. (1997). *Stress & health: Biological and psychological interactions.* Thousand Oaks, CA: Sage.

Lubin, J. H., Blot, W. J., Berrino, F., Flamant, R., Gillis, C. R., Kunzer, M., et al. (1984). Patterns of lung cancer according to type of cigarette smokers. *International Journal of Cancer, 33,* 569–576.

Lubin, J. H., Richter, B. S., & Blot, W. J. (1984). Lung cancer risk with cigar and pipe use. *Journal of the National Cancer Institute, 73,* 377–381.

Lucchesi, B. R., Schuster, C. R., & Emley, G. S. (1967). The role of nicotine as a determinant of cigarette smoking frequency in man with observations of certain cardiovascular effects associated with the tobacco alkaloid. *Clinical Pharmacology and Therapeutics, 8,* 791.

Luce, D., Bugel, I., Goldberg, P., Goldberg, M., Salomon, C., Billon-Galland, M. A., et al. (2000). Environmental exposure to tremolite and respiratory cancer in New Caledonia: A case-control study. *American Journal of Epidemiology, 151,* 259–266.

Ludwig, D. S., & Ebbeling, C. B. (2001). Type 2 diabetes mellitus in children: Primary care and public health considerations. *Journal of the American Medical Association, 286,* 1427–1430.

Luecken, L. J., Suarez, E. C., Kuhn, C. M., Barefoot, J. C., Blumenthal, J. A., Siegler, I. C., et al. (1997). Stress in employed women: Impact of marital status and children at home on neurohormone output and home strain. *Psychosomatic Medicine, 59,* 352–359.

Lundberg, U. (1998). Work and stress in women. In K. Orth-Gomér, M. Chesney, & N. K. Wenger (Eds.), *Women, stress, and heart disease* (pp. 41–56). Mahwah, NJ: Erlbaum.

Lutgendorf, S. K., Antoni, M. H., Ironson, G., Starr, K., Costello, N., Zuckerman, M., et al. (1998). Changes in cognitive coping skills and social support during cognitive behavioral stress management intervention and distress outcomes in symptomatic human immunodeficiency virus (HIV)-seropositive gay men. *Psychosomatic Medicine, 60,* 204–214.

Lutz, R. W., Silbret, M., & Olshan, W. (1983). Treatment outcome and compliance with therapeutic regimens: Long-term follow-up of a multidisciplinary pain program. *Pain, 17,* 301–308.

Lyles, J. N., Burish, T. G., Krozely, M. G., & Oldham, R. K. (1982). Efficacy of relaxation training and guided imagery in reducing the aversiveness of cancer chemotherapy. *Journal of Consulting and Clinical Psychology, 50,* 509–524.

Lynch, D. J., Birk, T. J., Weaver, M. T., Gohara, A. F., Leighton, R. F., Repka, F. J., et al. (1992). Adherence to exercise interventions in the treatment of hypercholesterolemia. *Journal of Behavior Medicine, 15,* 365–377.

MacDonald, T. K., MacDonald, G., Zanna, M. P., & Fong, G. T. (2000). Alcohol, sexual arousal, and intentions to use condoms in young men: Applying alcohol myopia theory to risky sexual behavior. *Health Psychology, 19,* 290–298.

MacDonald, T. K., Fong, G. T., Zanna, M. P., & Martineau, A. M. (2000). Alcohol myopia and condom use: Can alcohol intoxication be associated with more prudent behavior? *Journal of Personality and Social Psychology, 78,* 605–619.

MacDonald, T. K., Zanna, M. P., & Fong, G. T. (1995). Decision making in altered states: Effects of alcohol on attitudes toward drinking and driving. *Journal of Personality and Social Psychology, 68,* 973–985.

MacDorman, M. F., Cnattingius, S., Hoffman, H. J., Kramer, M. S., & Haglund, B. (1997). Sudden infant death syndrome and smoking in the United States and Sweden. *American Journal of Epidemiology, 146,* 249–257.

MacDougall, J. M., Dembroski, T. M., Dimsdale, J. E., & Hackett, T. P. (1985). Components of Type A, hostility, and anger-in: Further relationships to angiographic findings. *Health Psychology, 4,* 137–142.

Macharia, W. M., Leon, G., Rowe, B. H., Stephenson, B. J., & Haynes, R. B. (1992). An overview of interventions to improve compliance with appointment keeping for medical services. *Journal of the American Medical Association, 267,* 1813–1817.

MacLean, M. G., & Lecci, L. (2000). A comparison of models of drinking motives in a university sample. *Psychology of Addictive Behaviors, 14,* 83–87.

Macrodimitris, S. D., & Endler, N. S. (2001). Coping, control, and adjustment in Type 2 diabetes. *Health Psychology, 20,* 208–216.

Maddi, S. R. (1990). Issues and interventions in stress mastery. In H S. Friedman (Ed.). *Personality and disease* (pp. 121–154). New York: Wiley.

Maes, M., Hendricks, D., Van Gastel, A., Demedts, P., Wauters, A., Neels, H., et al. (1997). Effects of psychological stress on serum immunoglobulin, complement and acute phase protein concentrations in normal volunteers. *Psychoneuroendocrinology, 22,* 397–410.

Maes, S., Leventhal, H., & de Ridder, D. T. D. (1996). Coping with chronic diseases. In M. Zeidner & N. Endler (Eds.), *Handbook of coping: Theory, research, application* (pp. 221–251). New York: Wiley.

Magdol, L., Moffitt, T. E., Caspi, A., Newman, D. L., Fagan, J., & Silva, P. A. (1997). Gender differences in partner violence in a birth cohort of 21-year-olds bridging the gap between clinical and epidemiological approaches. *Journal of Consulting and Clinical Psychology, 65,* 68–78.

Maher, R. A., & Rickwood, D. (1997). The theory of planned behavior, domain specific self-efficacy and adolescent smoking. *Journal of Child and Adolescent Substance Abuse, 6,* 57–76.

Maier, S. F., & Watkins, L. R. (1998). Cytokines for psychologists: Implications of bidirectional immune-to-brain communications for understanding behavior, mood, and cognition. *Psychological Review, 105,* 83–107.

Maier, S. F., Watkins, L. R., & Fleshner, M. (1994). Psychoneuroimmunology: The interface between behavior, brain, and immunity. *American Psychologist, 49,* 1004–1017.

Mairs, D. A. E. (1995). Hypnosis and pain in childbirth. *Contemporary Hypnosis, 12,* 111–118.

Malmivaara, A., Hakkinen, U., Aro, T., Heinrichs, M., Koskenniemi, L., Klosma, E., et al. (1995). The treatment of acute low back pain—bed rest, exercise, or ordinary activity. *New England Journal of Medicine, 332,* 351–355.

Manne, S. L., Bakeman, R., Jacobsen, P. B., Gorfinkle, K., Bernstein, D., & Redd, W. H. (1992). Adult-child interaction during invasive medical procedures. *Health Psychology, 11,* 241–249.

Mannino, D. M., Klevens, R. M., & Flanders, W. D. (1994). Cigarette smoking: An independent risk factor for impotence? *American Journal of Epidemiology, 140,* 1003–1008.

Mannino, D. M., Moorman, J. E., Kingsley, B., Rose, D., & Repace, J. (2001). Health effects related to environmental tobacco smoke exposure in children in the United States: Data from the Third National Health and Nutrition Examination Survey. *Archives of Pediatrics & Adolescent Medicine, 155,* 36–41.

Manson, J. E., Hu, F. B., Rich-Edwards, J. W., Coldiz, G. A., Stampfer, M. J., Willett, W. C., et al. (1999). A prospective study of walking as compared with vigorous exercise in the prevention of coronary heart disease in women. *New England Journal of Medicine, 341,* 650–668.

Marcus, D. A. (2001). Gender differences in treatment-seeking chronic headache sufferers. *Headache, 41,* 698–703.

Marcus, H. H., Aabrecht, A. E., King, T. K., Parisi, A. F., Pinto, B. M., Roberts, M., et al. (1999). The efficacy of exercise as an aid for smoking cessation in women. *Archives of Internal Medicine, 159,* 1229.

Margolin, G., & Gordis, E. B. (2000). The effects of family and community violence on children. *Annual Review of Psychology, 51,* 445–479.

Margolis, L. H., Foss, R. D., & Tolbert, W. G. (2000). Alcohol and motor vehicle-related deaths of children as passengers, pedestrians, and bicyclists. *Journal of the American Medical Association, 283,* 2245–2248.

Markovitz, J. H., Matthews, K. A., Kannel, W. B., Cobb, J. L., & D'Agostino, R. B. (1993). Psychological predictors of hypertension in the Framingham study: Is there tension in hypertension? *Journal of the American Medical Association, 270,* 2439–2443.

Marlatt, G. A. (1987). Alcohol, the magic elixir: Stress, expectancy, and the transformation of emotional states. In E. Gottheil, K. A. Druly, S. Pashko, & S. P. Weinstein (Eds.), *Stress and addiction* (pp. 302–322). New York: Brunner/ Mazel.

Marlatt, G. A., Demming, B., & Reid, J. (1973). Loss of control drinking in alcoholics: An experimental analogue. *Journal of Abnormal Psychology, 81,* 233–241.

Marlatt, G. A., & Gordon, J. R. (1980). Determinants of relapse: Implication for the maintenance of behavior change. In P. O. Davidson & S. M. Davidson (Eds.), *Behavioral medicine: Changing health lifestyles* (pp. 410–452). New York: Brunner/Mazel.

Marlatt, G. A., & Rohsenow, D. J. (1980). Cognitive processes in alcohol use: Expectancy and the balanced placebo design. In N. Mello (Ed.), *Advances in substance abuse: Behavioral and biological research.* Greenwich, CT: JAI Press.

Marlowe, N. (1998). Stressful events, appraisal, coping and recurrent headache. *Journal of Clinical Psychology, 54,* 247–256.

Maron, D. J., & Fortmann, S. P. (1987). Nicotine yield and measures of cigarette smoke exposure in a large population: Are lower-yield cigarettes safer? *American Journal of Public Health, 77,* 546–549.

Marshall, B. J. (1995). Helicobacter pylori: The etiologic agent for peptic ulcers. *Journal of the American Medical Association, 274,* 1064–1066.

Marsland, A. L., Bachen, E. A., Cohen, S., & Manuck, S. B. (2001). Stress, immunity, and susceptibility to infectious disease. In A. Baum, T. A. Revenson, & J. E. Singer (Eds.), *Handbook of health psychology* (pp. 683–695). Mahwah, NJ: Erlbaum.

Martikainen, P., & Valkonen, T. (1996). Mortality after the death of a spouse: Rates and causes of death in a large Finnish cohort. *American Journal of Public Health, 86,* 1087–1093.

Martikainen, P., Valkonen, T., & Martelin, T. (2001). Change in male and female life expectancy by social class: Decomposition by age and cause of death in Finland 1971–95. *Journal of Epidemiology & Community Health, 55,* 494–499.

Martin, I. (1998). Dispelling myths about heart disease. *World Health, 51*(5), 6–7.

Martin, R., & Lemos, K. (2002). From heart attacks to melanoma: Do common sense models of somatization influence symptom intepretation for female victims? *Health Psychology, 21,* 25–32.

Martindale, D. (2001, May 26). Needlework: Whether it's controlling the flow of vital energy or releasing painkilling chemicals, acupuncture seems plausible enough. But does it really work? *New Scientist, 170,* 42–45.

Martindale, D. (2002, May). Peeling plaque: Researchers remain optimistic about a vaccine against Alzheimer's. *Scientific American, 286,* 18–19.

Martinsen, E. W., & Morgan, W. P. (1997). Antidepressant effects of physical activity. In W. P. Morgan (Ed.), *Physical activity and mental health* (pp. 93–106). Washington, DC: Taylor & Francis.

Marucha, P. T., Kiecolt-Glaser, J. K., & Favagehi, M. (1998). Mucosal wound healing is impaired by examination stress. *Psychosomatic Medicine, 60,* 362–365.

Mason, J. W. (1971). A reevaluation of the concept of "nonspecificity" in stress theory. *Journal of Psychiatric Research, 8,* 323–333.

Mason, J. W. (1975). A historical view of the stress field. Pt. 2. *Journal of Human Stress, 1,* 22–36.

Masur, F. T., III. (1981). Adherence to health care regimens. In C. K. Prokop & L. A. Bradley (Eds.), *Medical psychology: Contributions to behavioral medicine.* New York: Academic Press.

Matarazzo, J. D. (1987a). Postdoctoral education and training of service providers in health psychology. In G. C. Stone, S. M. Weiss, J. D. Matarazzo, N. E. Miller, J. Rodin, C. D. Belar, et al. (Eds.), *Health psychology: A discipline and a profession* (pp. 371–388). Chicago: University of Chicago Press.

Matarazzo, J. D. (1987b). Relationships of health psychology to other segments of psychology. In G. C. Stone, S. M. Weiss, J. D. Matarazzo, N. E. Miller, J. Rodin, C. D. Belar, et al. (Eds.), *Health psychology: A discipline and a profession* (pp. 41–59). Chicago: University of Chicago Press.

Matarazzo, J. D. (1994). Health and behavior: The coming together of science and practice in psychology and medicine after a century of benign neglect. *Journal of Clinical Psychology in Medical Settings, 1,* 7–39.

Mathers, C. D., Sadana, R., Salomon, J. A., Murray, C. J. L., & Lopez, A. D. (2001). Healthy life expectancy in 191 countries. *Lancet, 357,* 1685–1690.

Matlin, S., & Spence, N. (2001). The gender aspects of the HIV/AIDS pandemic. *WIN News, 27*(1), 11–13.

Matthews, K. A., Shumaker, S. A., Bowen, D. J., Langer, R. D., Hunt, J. R., Kaplan, R. M., et al. (1997). Women's health initiative: Why now? What is it? What's new? *American Psychologist, 52,* 101–116.

Matthies, E., Hoeger, R., & Guski, R. (2000). Living on polluted soil: Determinants of stress symptoms. *Environment and Behavior, 32,* 270–286.

May, P. A., & Gossage, J. P. (2001). Estimating the prevalence of fetal alcohol syndrome : A summary. *Alcohol Research & Health, 25,* 159–167.

Mayeux, R., & Schupf, N. (1995). Apolipoprotein E and Alzheimer's disease; The implications of progress in molecular medicine. *American Journal of Public Health, 85,* 1280–1284.

Mayfield, D. (1976). Alcoholism, alcohol intoxication, and assaultive behavior. *Diseases of the Nervous System, 37,* 228–291.

McAuley, E. (1993). Self-efficacy and the maintenance of exercise participation in older adults. *Journal of Behavioral Medicine, 16,* 103–113.

McAuley, E. (1994). Physical activity and psychosocial outcomes. In C. Bouchard, R. J. Shephard, & T. Stephens (Eds.), *Physical activity, fitness, and health: International proceedings and consensus statement* (pp. 551–568). Champaign, IL: Human Kinetics.

McBride, C. M., Curry, S. J., Grothaus, L. C., Nelson, J. C., Lando, H., & Pirie, P. L. (1998). Partner smoking status and pregnant smoker's perceptions of support for the likelihood of smoking cessation. *Health Psychology, 17,* 63–69.

McCabe, M. P., & Ricciardelli, L. A. (2003). Body image and strategies to lose weight and increase muscle among boys and girls. *Health Psychology, 22,* 39–46.

McCaughey, M. (1999). Fleshing out the discomforts of femininity: The parallel cases of female anorexia and male compulsive bodybuilding. In J. Sobal & D. Maurer (Eds.), *Weighty issues: Fatness and thinness as social problems* (pp. 133–155). New York: Aldine de Gruyter.

McCaul, K. D., Sandgren, A. K., O'Neill, H. K., & Hinsz, V. B. (1993). The value of the theory of planned behavior, perceived control, and self-efficacy for predicting health-protective behaviors. *Basic and Applied Social Psychology, 14,* 231–252.

McCracken, L. M. (1997). "Attention" to pain in persons with chronic pain: A behavioral approach. *Behavior Therapy, 28,* 271–284.

McCrady, B. S. (1994). Alcoholics Anonymous and behavior therapy: Can habits be treated as diseases? Can diseases be treated as habits? *Journal of Consulting and Clinical Psychology, 62,* 1159–1166.

McCullough, M. E., Hoyt, W. T., Larson, D. S., Koenig, H. G., & Thoresen, C. (2000). Religious involvement and mortality: A meta-analytic review. *Health Psychology, 19,* 211–222.

McCutchan, J. A. (1990). Virology, immunology, and clinical course of HIV infection. *Journal of Consulting and Clinical Psychology, 58,* 5–12.

McGilley, B. M., & Pryor, T. L. (1998). Assessment and treatment of bulimia nervosa. *American Family Physician, 57,* 2743–2750.

McGrady, A. (1994). Effects of group relaxation training and thermal biofeedback on blood pressure and related physiological and psychological variables in essential hypertension. *Biofeedback and Self Relaxation, 19,* 51–66.

McGue, M. (1999). Behavioral genetic models of alcoholism and drinking. In K. E. Leonard & H. T. Blane (Eds.), *Psychological theories of drinking and alcoholism* (2nd ed., pp. 372–421). New York: Guilford Press.

McGwin, G., Jr. (2000). Fire fatalities in older people. *Journal of the American Medical Association, 283,* 312.

McKinnon, W., Weisse, C. S., Reynolds, C. P., Bowles, C. A., & Baum, A. (1989). Chronic stress, leucocyte subpopulations, and humoral response to latent viruses. *Health Psychology, 8,* 389–402.

McLaughlin, L. A., & Braun, K. L. (1998). Asian and Pacific islander cultural values: Considerations for health care decision making. *Health and Social Work, 23,* 116–126.

McLean, S., Skirboll, L. R., & Pert, C. B. (1985). Comparison of substance P and enkephalin distribution in rat brain: An overview using radioimmunocytochemistry. *Neuroscience, 14,* 837–852.

McLellan, A. T., Arndt, I. O., Metzger, D. S., Woody, G. E., & O'Brien, C. P. (1993). The effects of psychosocial services in substance abuse treatment. *Journal of the American Medical Association, 269,* 1953–1959.

McLellan, A. T., Lewis, D. C., O'Brien, C. P., & Kleber, H. D. (2000). Drug dependence, a chronic medical illness: Implications for treatment, insurance, and outcomes. *Journal of the American Medical Association, 284,* 1689–1695.

McMurran, M. (1994). *The psychology of addiction.* London: Taylor & Francis.

Mechanic, D. (1978). *Medical sociology* (2nd ed.). New York: Free Press.

Medical Update. (2000, August). Liposuction is not a benign procedure. *Medical Update, 24*(2), 3.

Meichenbaum, D., & Cameron, R. (1983). Stress inoculation training: Toward a general paradigm for training coping skills. In D. Meichenbaum & M. E. Jaremko (Ed.), *Stress reduction and prevention* (pp. 115–154). New York: Plenum Press.

Meichenbaum, D., & Turk, D. C. (1976). The cognitive-behavioral management of anxiety, anger and pain. In P. O. Davidson (Ed.), *The behavioral management of anxiety, depression, and pain.* New York: Brunner/Mazel.

Melamed, B. G., Kaplan, B., & Fogel, J. (2001). Childhood health issues across the life span. In A. Baum, T. A. Revenson, & J. E. Singer (Eds.), *Handbook of health psychology* (pp. 449–457). Mahwah, NJ: Erlbaum.

Melamed, S., Fried, Y., & Froom, P. (2001). The interactive effect of chronic exposure to noise and job complexity on changes in blood pressure and job satisfaction: A longitudinal study of industrial employees. *Journal of Occupational Health Psychology, 6,* 182–195.

Melnyk, B. M., & Feinstein, N. F. (2001). Mediating functions of maternal anxiety and participation in care on young children's posthospital adjustment. *Research in Nursing and Health, 24,* 18–26.

Melzack, R. (1973). *The puzzle of pain.* New York: Basic Books.

Melzack, R. (1975). The McGill Pain Questionnaire: Major properties and scoring methods. *Pain, 1,* 277–299.

Melzack, R. (1987). The short-form McGill Pain Questionnaire. *Pain, 30,* 191–197.

Melzack, R. (1992, April). Phantom limbs. *Scientific American, 266,* 120–126.

Melzack, R. (1993). Pain: Past, present and future. *Canadian Journal of Experimental Psychology, 47,* 615–629.

Melzack, R. (1999). Pain and stress: A new perspective. In R. J. Gatchel & D. C. Turk (Eds.), *Psychosocial factors in pain: Critical perspectives* (pp. 89–106). New York; Guilford Press.

Melzack, R., & Katz, J. (2001). The McGill Pain Questionnaire: Apprasial and current status. In D. C. Turk & R. Melzack (Eds.), *Handbook of pain assessment* (2nd ed., pp. 35–52). New York: Guilford Press.

Melzack, R., & Wall, P. D. (1965). Pain mechanisms: A new theory. *Science, 150,* 971–979.

Melzack, R., & Wall, P. D. (1982). *The challenge of pain.* New York: Basic Books.

Melzack, R., & Wall, P. D. (1988). *The challenge of pain* (rev. ed.). London: Penguin.

Metropolitan Life Insurance Company. (1959). New weight standards for men and women. *Statistical Bulletin, 40,* 1.

Metropolitan Life Foundation. (1983). Metropolitan height and weight tables. *Statistical Bulletin, 64* (1), 2–9.

Meyer, D., Leventhal, H., & Gutman, M. (1985). Common-sense models of illness: The example of hypertension. *Health Psychology, 4,* 115–135.

Meyer, T. J., & Mark, M. M. (1995). Effects of psychosocial interventions with adult cancer patients: A meta-analysis of randomized experiments. *Health Psychology, 14,* 101–108.

Meyerowitz, B. E., Richardson, J., Hudson, S., & Leedham, B. (1998). Ethnicity and cancer outcomes: Behavioral and psychosocial considerations. *Psychological Bulletin, 123,* 47–70.

Miaskowski, C. (1999). The role of sex and gender in pain perception and responses to treatment. In R. J. Gatchel & D. C. Turk (Eds.). *Psychosocial factors in pain: Critical perspectives* (pp. 401–411). New York: Guilford Press.

Michaud, C. M., Murray, C. J. L., & Bloom, B. R. (2001). Burden of disease—Implications for future research. *Journal of the American Medical Association, 285,* 535–539.

Michaud, D. S., Spiegelman, D., Clinton, S. K., Rimm, E. B., Curhan, G. C., Willett, W. C., et al. (1999). Fluid intake and the risk of bladder cancer in men. *New England Journal of Medicine, 340,* 1390–1397.

Mikail, S. F., DuBreuil, S. C., & D'Eon, J. L. (1993). A comparative analysis of measures used in the assessment of chronic pain patients. *Psychological Assessment, 5,* 117–120.

Miller, B. A., Kolonel, L. N., Bernstein, L., Young, J. L., Swanson, G. M., West, D., et al. (Eds). (1996). *Racial/ethnic patterns of cancer in the United States 1988–1992.* (National Institutes of Health Publication No. 96-4104). Bethesda, MD: U.S. Department of Health and Human Services, Public Health Service, and National Institutes of Health. National Cancer Institute.

Miller, G. E., & Cohen, S. (2001). Psychological interventions and the immune system: A meta-analytic review and critique. *Health Psychology, 20,* 47–63.

Miller, G. E., Dopp, J. M., Myers, H. F., Stevens, S. Y., & Fahey, J. L. (1999). Psychosocial predictors of natural killer cell mobilization during marital conflict. *Health Psychology, 18,* 262–271.

Miller, J. J., Fletcher, K., & Kabat-Zinn, J. (1995). Three-year follow-up and clinical implications of a mindfulness meditation-based stress reduction intervention in the treatment of anxiety disorders. *General Hospital Psychiatry, 17,* 192–200.

Miller, M., Hemenway, D., & Rimm, E. (2000). Cigarettes and succeed: A prospective study of 50,000 men. *American Journal of Public Health, 90,* 768–773.

Miller, M. F., Barabasz, A. F., & Barabasz, M. (1991). Effects of active alert and relaxation hypnotic inductions on cold pressor pain. *Journal of Abnormal Psychology, 100,* 223–226.

Miller, N. E. (1969). Learning of visceral and glandular responses. *Science, 163,* 434–445.

Miller, S. B., Friese, M., Dolgoy, L., Sita, A., Lavoie, K., & Campbell, T. (1998). Hostility, sodium consumption, and cardiovascular response to interpersonal stress. *Psychosomatic Medicine, 60,* 71–77.

Miller, W. R. (1993). Alcoholism: Toward a better disease model. *Psychology of Addictive Behaviors, 7,* 129–163.

Miller, W. R., Walters, S. T., & Bennett, M. E. (2001). How effective is alcoholism treatment in the United States? *Journal of Studies on Alcohol, 62,* 211–220.

Mills, L. G. (1998). Mandatory arrest and prosecution policies for domestic violence: A critical literature review and the case for more research to test victim empowerment approaches. *Criminal Justice and Behavior, 25,* 306–318.

Minino, A. M., & Smith, B. L. (2001). Deaths: Preliminary data for 2000. *National Vital Statistics Reports, 49*(12). Hyattsville, MD: National Center for Health Statistics.

Mishra, K. D., Gatchel, R. J., & Gardea, M. A. (2000). The relative efficacy of three cognitive-behavioral treatment approaches to temporomandibular disorders. *Journal of Behavioral Medicine, 23,* 293–309.

Mittelmark, M. B., Murray, D. M., Luepker, R. V., Pechacek, T. F., Pirie, P. L., & Pallonen, U. E. (1987). Predicting experimentation with cigarettes: The Childhood Antecedents of Smoking Study (CASS). *American Journal of Public Health, 77,* 206–208.

Modesti, D. G., & Tryon, W. W. (1994, August). *Emotional strain on adult children of a parent with Alzheimer's disease.* Paper presented at the American Psychological Association convention, Los Angeles, CA.

Moen, P., & Yu, Y. (2000). Effective work/life strategies: Working couples, work conditions, gender, and life quality. *Social Problems, 47,* 291–326.

Moerman, D. E. (2002). "The loaves and the fishes": A comment on "The emperor's new drugs: An analysis of antideprssant medication data submitted to the U.S. Food and Drug Administration." *Prevention & Treatment, 5,* Article 29. Available on the World Wide Web at http://www.journals.apa.org/prevention/volume5/pre0050029c.html.

Moffatt, S., Phillimore, P., Bhopal, J., & Foy, C. (1995). "If this is what it is doing to our washing, what is it doing to our lungs?" Industrial pollution and public understanding in North East England. *Social Science and Medicine, 41,* 883–891.

Mokdad, A. H., Serdula, M. K., Dietz, W. H., Bowman, B. A., Marks, J. S., & Koplan, J. P. (1999). The spread of the obesity epidemic in the United States, 1991–1998. *Journal of the American Medical Association, 282,* 1519–1522.

Molarius, A., Seidell, J. C., Sans, S., Tuomilehto, J., & Kuulasmaa, K. (2000). Educational level, relative body weight, and changes in their association over 10 years: An international perspective from the WHO MONICA project. *American Journal of Public Health, 90,* 1260–1268.

Moller, J., Ahlbom, A., Hulting, J., Diderichsen, F., de Faire, U., Reuterwall, C., et al. (2001). Sexual activity as a trigger of myocardial infarction: A case-crossover analysis in the Stockholm Heart Epidemiology Programme. *Heart, 86,* 387–390.

Monane, M., Bohn, R. L., Gurwitz, J. H., Glynn, R. J., Levin, R., & Avorn, J. (1996). Compliance with antihypertensive therapy among elderly Medicaid enrollees: The rates of age, gender, and race. *American Journal of Public Health, 86,* 1805–1808.

Monroe, S. M. (1982). The assessment of life events: Event-symptom associations and the cause of disorder. *Journal of Abnormal Psychology, 91,* 14–24.

Montano, D. E., Thompson, B., Taylor, V. M., & Mahloch, J. (1997). Understanding mammography intention and utilization among women in an inner city public hospital clinic. *Preventive Medicine, 26,* 817–824.

Montgomery, G. H., DuHamel, K. N., & Redd, W. H. (2000). A meta-analysis of hypnotically induced analgesia: How effective is hypnosis? *International Journal of Clinical and Experimental Hypnosis, 48,* 138–153.

Moos, R. H., & Schaefer, J. A. (1984). The crisis of physical illness: An overview and conceptual analysis. In R. H. Moos (Ed.), *Coping with physical illness 2: New perspectives* (pp. 3–25). New York: Plenum Press.

Moraska, A., & Fleshner, M. (2001). Voluntary physical activity prevents stress-induced behavioral depression and anti-KLH antibody suppression. *American Journal of Physiology, 281,* 484–485.

Morey, S. S. (1998). NIH issues consensus statement on acupuncture. *American Family Physician, 57,* 2545–2546.

Morgan, R. E., Palinkas, L. A., Barrett-Connor, E. L., & Wingard, D. L. (1993). Plasma cholesterol and depressive symptoms in older men. *Lancet, 341,* 75–79.

Morgan, W. P. (1979, February). Negative addiction in runners. *The Physician and Sportsmedicine, 7,* pp. 56–63, 67–70.

Morgan, W. P. (1981). Psychological benefits of physical activity. In F. J. Nagle & H. J. Montoye (Eds.), *Exercise in health and disease.* Springfield, IL: Thomas.

Morgan, W. P. (1997). Methodological considerations. In W. P. Morgan (Ed.), *Physical activity and mental health* (pp. 3–32). Washington, DC: Taylor & Francis.

Morris, D. L., Kritchevsky, S. B., & Davis, C. E. (1994). Serum carotenoids and coronary heart disease: The Lipid Research Clinics Coronary Primary Prevention Trial and Follow-up Study. *Journal of the American Medical Association, 272,* 1439–1441.

Morris, J. C., Storandt, M., Miller, J. P., McKeel, D. W., Price, J. L., Rubin, E. H., & Berg, L. (2001). Mild cognitive impairment represents early-stage Alzheimer disease. *Archives of Neurology, 58,* 397–405. (This reference may be on the original list, or it may have been omitted.)

Morris, J. N., Heady, J. A., Raffle, P. A. B., Roberts, C. G., & Parks, J. W. (1953). Coronary heart-disease and physical activity of work. *Lancet, ii,* 1053–1057, 1111–1120.

Mosbach, P., & Leventhal, H. (1988). Peer group identification and smoking: Implications for intervention. *Journal of Abnormal Psychology, 97,* 238–245.

Moseley, J. B., O'Malley, K. P., Petersen, N. J., Menke, T. J., Brody, B. A., Kuykendall, D. H., et al. (2002). A controlled trial of arthroscopic surgery for osteoarthritis of the knee. *New England Journal of Medicine, 347,* 81–88.

Moser, D. K., & Dracup, K. (1996). Is anxiety early after myocardial infarction associated with subsequent ischemic and arrhythmic events? *Psychosomatic Medicine, 58,* 395–401.

Moskowitz, H., Griffith, J. L., DiScala, C., & Sege, R. D. (2001). Serious injuries and deaths of adolescent girls resulting from interpersonal violence: Characteristics and trends from the United States, 1989–1998. *Archives of Pediatrics & Adolescent Medicine, 155,* 903–908.

Moss, M., Bucher, B., Moore, F. A., Moore, E. E., & Parsons, P. E. (1996). The role of chronic alcohol abuse in the development of acute respiratory distress syndrome. *Journal of the American Medical Association, 275,* 50–54.

Mouzakes, J., Koltai, P. J., Kuhar, S., Bernstein, D. S., Wing, P., & Salsberg, E. (2001). The impact of airbags and seatbelts on the incidence and severity of maxillofacial injuries in automobile accidents in New York State *Archives of Otolaryngology—Head & Neck Surgery, 127,* 1189–1193.

Moy, C. S., Songer, T. J., LaPorte, R. E., Dorman, J. S., Kriska, A. M., Orchard, T. J., et al. (1993). Insulin-dependent diabetes mellitus, physical activity, and death. *American Journal of Epidemiology, 137,* 74–81.

Mufti, R. M., Balon, R., & Arfken, C. L. (1998). Low cholesterol and violence. *Psychiatric Services, 49,* 221–224.

Mukamal, K. J., Conigrave, K. M., Mittleman, M. A., Camargo, C. A., Jr., Stampfer, M. J., Willett, W. C., & Rimm, E. B. (2003). Roles of drinking pattern and type of alcohol consumed in coronary heart disease in men. *New England Journal of Medicine, 348,* 109–118.

Mulder, C. L., van Griensven, G. J. P., Sandfort, T. G. M., de Vroome, E. M. M., & Antoni, M. H. (1999). Avoidance as a predictor of the biological course of HIV infection over a 7-year period in gay men. *Health Psychology, 18,* 107–113.

Muldoon, M. F., Manuck, S. B., & Matthews, K. A. (1992). Lowering cholesterol concentrations and mortality: A quantitative review of primary prevention trials. *British Medical Journal, 301,* 309–314.

Muldoon, N. F., Manuck, S. B., Mendelsohn, A. B., Kaplan, J. R., & Belle, S. H. (2001). Cholesterol reduction and non-illness mortality: Meta-analysis of randomised clinical trials. *British Medical Journal, 322,* 11–14.

Mulsant, B. H., Pollock, B. G., Nebes, R. D., Hoch, C. C., & Reynolds, C. F., III. (1997). Depression in Alzheimer's dementia. In L. L. Heston (Ed.), *Progress in Alzheimer's disease and similar conditions* (pp. 161–175). Washington, DC: American Psychiatric Press.

Murphy, D. A., Mann, T., O'Keefe, Z., & Rotherram-Borus, M. J. (1998). Number of pregnancies, outcome expectancies, and social norms among HIV-infected young women. *Health Psychology, 17,* 470–475.

Murphy, J. K., Stoney, C. M., Alpert, B. S., & Walker, S. S. (1995). Gender and ethnicity in children's cardiovascular reactivity: 7 years of study. *Health Psychology, 14,* 48–55.

Murray, M. E., Guerra, N. G., & Williams, K. R. (1997). Violence prevention for the 21st century. In R. P. Weissberg, T. P. Gullotta, R. L. Hampton, B. A. Ryan, & G. R. Adams (Eds.), *Enhancing children's wellness* (pp. 105–128). Thousand Oaks, CA: Sage.

Murray, R. P., Connett, J. E., Tyas, S. L., Bond, R., Ekuma, O., Silversides, C. K., et al. (2002). Alcohol volume, drinking pattern, and cardiovascular disease morbidity and mortality: Is there a U-shaped function? *American Journal of Epidemiology, 155,* 242–248.

Mussel, M. P., Crosby, R. D., Crow, S. J., Knopke, A. J., Peterson, C. B., Wonderlich, S. A., et al. (2000). Utilization of empirically supported psychotherapy treatments for individuals with eating disorders: A survey of psychologists. *International Journal of Eating Disorders, 27,* 230–237.

Mussolino, A. E., Looker, A. C., & Orwoll, E. S. (2001). Jogging and bone mineral density in men: Results from NHANES III. *American Journal of Public Health, 91,* 1056–1059.

Must, A., Spadano, J., Coakley, E. H., Field, A. E., Colditz, G., & Dietz, W. H. (1999). The disease burden associated with overweight and obesity. *Journal of the American Medical Association, 282,* 1523–1529.

Mustard, T. R., & Harris, A. V. E. (1989). Problems in understanding prescription labels. *Perceptual and Motor Skills, 69,* 291–299.

Muthen, B. O., & Muthen, L. K. (2000). The development of heavy drinking and alcohol-related problems from ages 18 to 37 in a U.S. national sample. *Journal of Studies on Alcohol., 61,* 290–300.

Myers, J. (2000). Physical activity and cardiovascular disease. *IDEA Health & Fitness Source, 18,* 38–45.

Nakao, M., Nomura, S., Shimosawa, T., Yoshiuchi, K., Kumano, H., Kuboki, T., et al. (1997). Clinical effects of blood pressure biofeedback treatment on hypertension by auto-shaping. *Psychosomatic Medicine, 59,* 331–338.

Nash, M. R. (2001, July). The truth and the hype of hypnosis. *Scientific American, 285,* 47–55.

National Association for Sport and Physical Education. (2002). *Guidelines for infants and toddlers.* Retrieved from the World Wide Web, August 5, 2002, at www.aahperd.org/naspe/template.cfm?template =toddlers.html.

National Center for Health Statistics (NCHS). (1994). *Health, United States.* Hyattsville, MD: U.S. Government Printing Office.

National Center for Health Statistics (NCHS). (2001). *Health, United States, 2001.* Hyattsville, MD. U.S. Government Printing Office.

National Center for Injury Prevention and Control. (1998). 10 leading causes of deaths by age group—1995. Retrieved from the World Wide Web, June 16, 2002, at http://www.cdc.gov/ncipc/images.

National Center on Elder Abuse. (1998). *National Elder Abuse Incidence Study: Final report.* Washington, DC: American Public Human Services Association. Retrieved from the World Wide Web, June 14, 2002, at http://www.aoa.gov/abuse/report/default.htm.

National Education Association. (1998). What can we do about school violence? *NEA Today, 17,* 19.

National Heart, Lung, and Blood Institute. (1998). *Guidelines on the identification, evaluation, and treatment of overweight and obesity in adults: The evidence report.* Bethesda, MD: National Institutes of Health.

National Highway Traffic Safety Administration. (1993–1996). *Fatality analysis reporting system, 1992–1995.* Washington, DC: U.S. Department of Transportation.

National Highway Traffic Safety Administration. (1998). Presidential initiative for increasing seat belt use nationwide. http://www.nhtsa.dot.gov/people/injury.

National Safe Kids Campaign. (1997). The National Safe Kids Campaign motor vehicle occupant injury fact sheet. http://www.safekids.org/fact97/.

National Task Force on the Prevention and Treatment of Obesity. (2000). Overweight, obesity, and health risk. *Archives of Internal Medicine, 160,* 898–904.

Neighbors, H. W. (1997). Husbands, wives, family, and friends: Sources of stress, sources of support. In R. J. Taylor, J. S. Jackson, & L. M. Chatters (Eds.), *Family life in Black America* (pp. 277–292). Thousand Oaks, CA: Sage.

Nelson, C. C., & Allen, J. (1999). Reduction of healthy children's fears related to hospitalization and medical procedures: The effectiveness of multimedia computer instruction in pediatric psychology. *Children's Health Care, 28,* 1–13.

Nelson, H. D., Nevitt, M. C., Scott, J. C., Stone, K. L., & Cummings, S. R. (1994). Smoking, alcohol, and neuromuscular and physical functioning of older women. *Journal of the American Medical Association, 272,* 1825–1831.

Nelson, M. E., Fiatarone, M. A., Marganti, C. M., Trice, I., Greenberg, R. A., & Evans, W. J. (1994). Effects of high-intensity strength training on multiple risk factors for osteoporotic fractures. *Journal of the American Medical Association, 272,* 1909–1914.

Nelson, W. L., Hughes, H. M., Katz, B., & Searight, H. R. (1999). Anorexic eating attitudes and behaviors of male and female college students. *Adolescence, 34,* 621–634.

Nemeroff, C. J. (1995). Magical thinking about illness virulence: Conceptions of germs from "safe" versus "dangerous" others. *Health Psychology, 14,* 147–151.

Nestle, M. (1997). Alcohol guidelines for chronic disease prevention: From Prohibition to moderation. *Nutrition Today, 32* (2), 86–92.

Neumark-Sztainer, D., Wall, M. M., Story, M., & Perry, C. L. (2003). Correlates of unhealthy weight-control behaviors among adolescents: Implications for prevention programs. *Health Psychology, 22,* 88–98.

Niaura, R., & Abrams, D. B. (2002). Smoking cessation: Progress, priorities, and prospectus. *Journal of Consulting and Clinical Psychology, 70,* 494–509.

Nicholas, M. K., Wilson, P. H., & Goyen, J. (1991). Operant-behavioral and cognitive-behavioral treatment for chronic low back pain. *Behavior Research and Therapy, 29,* 235–238.

Nichols, M. L., Allen, B. J., Rogers, S. D., Ghilardi, J. R., Honore, P., Luger, N. M., et al. (1999). Transmission of chronic nociception by spinal neurons expressing the substance P receptor. *Science, 286,* 1558–1560.

NIDA Research Report. (1999). *Cocaine abuse and addiction.* NIH Publication No. 99-4343. Washington, DC: U.S. Department of Health and Human Services.

NIDA Research Report. (2000). *Anabolic steroid abuse.* Publication No. 00-3721. Washington, DC: Department of Health and Human Services.

Nides, M., Rand, C., Dolce, J., Murray, R., O'Hara, P., Voelker, H., et al. (1994). Weight gain as a function of smoking cessation and 2-mg nicotine gum use among middle-aged smokers with mild lung impairment in the first 2 years of the Lung Health Study. *Health Psychology, 13,* 354–361.

Nied, R. J., & Franklin, B. (2002). Promoting and prescribing exercise for the elderly. *American Family Physician, 65,* 419–426, 427–428.

Nieto, F. J. (1999). Cardiovascular disease and risk factor epidemiology: A look back at the epidemic of the 20th century. *American Journal of Public Health, 89,* 291–294.

Nikiforov, S. V., & Mamaev, V. B. (1998). The development of sex differences in cardiovascular disease mortality: A historical perspective. *American Journal of Public Health, 88,* 1345–1353.

Nivision, M. E., & Endresen, I. M. (1993). An analysis of relationships among environmental noise, annoyance and sensitivity to noise, and the consequences for health and sleep. *Journal of Behavior Medicine, 16,* 257–276.

Noble, R. E. (2001). Waist-to-hip ratio versus BMI as predictors of cardiac risk in obese adult women. *Western Journal of Medicine, 174,* 240.

Nolen-Hoeksema, S. (2000). The role of rumination in depressive disorders and mixed anxiety/depressive symptoms. *Journal of Abnormal Psychology, 109,* 504–511.

Nordstrom, B. L., Kinnunen. T., Utman, C. H., Krall, E. A., Vokanas, P. S., & Garvey, A. J. (2000). Predictors of continued smoking over 25 years of follow-up in the Normative Aging Study. *American Journal of Public Health, 90,* 404–406.

Norris, F. H., Byrne, C. M., Diaz, E., & Kaniasty, K. (2001). *The range, magnitude, and duration of effects of natural and human-caused disasters: A review of the empirical literature.* Boston: National Center for PTSD.

Norrish, A. E., Jackson, R. T., Sharpe, S. J., & Skeaff, C. M. (2000). Prostate cancer and dietary carotenoids. *American Journal of Epidemiology 151,* 119–123.

North, C. S., Nixon, S. J., Shariat, S., Mallonee, S., McMillen, J. C., Spitznagel, E. L., & Smith, E. M. (1999). Psychiatric disorders among survivors of the Oklahoma City bombing. *Journal of the American Medical Association, 282,* 755–762.

Occupational Safety and Health Administration. (1996). *Guidelines for preventing workplace violence for health care and social service workers.* Washington, DC: OSHA Publications Office.

Occupational Safety and Health Administration. (1998). OSHA facts: Common sense at work. http://www.osha-slc.gov/OshDoc/OSHFacts.

O'Connor, P. J. (1997). Overtraining and staleness. In W. P. Morgan (Ed.), *Physical activity and mental health* (pp. 145–160). Washington, DC: Taylor & Francis.

O'Donnell, C. R. (1995). Firearm deaths among children and youth. *American Psychologist, 50,* 771–776.

OECD Publications and Information Centre. (2001, December). Economic surveys—Japan. Healthcare reform. *OECD Economic Surveys,* 141–164.

Oguma, Y., Sesso, H. D., Paffenbarger, R. S., Jr., & Lee, I-M. (2002). Physical activity and all cause mortality in women: A review of the evidence. *British Journal of Sports Medicine, 36,* 162–172.

Ohannessian, C. M., Stabenau, J. R., & Hesselbrock, V. M. (1995). Childhood and adulthood temperament and problem behaviors and adulthood substance use. *Addictive Behaviors, 20,* 77–86.

O'Hara, P., Connett, J. E., Wee, W. W., Nides, M., Murray, R., & Wise, R. (1998). Early and late weight gain following smoking cessation in the Lung Health Study. *American Journal of Epidemiology, 148,* 821–830.

O'Leary, A. (1990). Stress, emotion, and human immune function. *Psychological Bulletin, 108,* 363–382.

Olesen, J. (1988). Classification and diagnostic criteria for headache disorders, cranial neuralgias, and facial pain: Headache Classification Committee of the International Headache Society [Special issue]. *Cephalalgia, 8*(Suppl. 7).

Olkkonen, S., & Honkanen, R. (1990). The role of alcohol in nonfatal bicycle injuries. *Accident Analysis and Prevention, 22,* 89–96.

Olsen, R., & Sutton, J. (1998). More hassle, more alone: Adolescents with diabetes and the role of formal and informal support. *Child Care, Health and Development, 24,* 31–39.

Olson, J., & Wilson, R. (2000). Subclinical artheroseclerosis markers as predictors of coronary artery disease in Type I diabetes. *Diabetes, 49,* 145–146.

Oman, R. F., & King, A. C. (2000). The effect of life events and exercise program on the adoption and maintenance of exercise behavior. *Health Psychology, 19,* 605–612.

Oomen, C. M., Feskens, E. J. M., Räsänen, L., Fidanza, F., Nissinen, A. M., Menotti, A., et al. (2000). Fish consumption and coronary heart disease mortality in Finland, Italy, the Netherlands. *American Journal of Epidemiology, 151,* 999–1006.

Orbell, S., Blair, C., Sherlock, K., & Conner, M. (2001). The theory of planned behavior and ecstasy use: Roles for habit and perceived control over taking versus obtaining substances. *Journal of Applied Social Psychology, 31,* 31–47.

Orme, C. M., & Binik, Y. M. (1989). Consistency of adherence across regimen demands. *Health Psychology, 8,* 27–43.

Ornish, D. (1993). *Eat more, weigh less.* New York: Harper Collins.

Ornish, D. (1995, May). *Reversing heart disease.* Presented by St. Patrick's Hospital, Lake Charles, LA.

Ornish, D., Brown, S. E., Scherwitz, L. W., Billings, J. H., Armstrong, W. T., Ports, T., et al. (1990). Can lifestyle changes reverse coronary heart disease? The Lifestyle Heart Trial. *Lancet, 336,* 129–133.

Ornish, D., Scherwitz, L. W., Billings, J. H., Gould, L., Merritt, T. A., Sparler, S., et al. (1998). Intensive lifestyle changes for reversal of coronary heart disease. *Journal of the American Medical Association, 280,* 2001–2007.

Orth-Gomér, K. (1998). Psychosocial risk factor profile in women with coronary heart disease. In K. Orth-Gomér, M. Chesney, & N. K. Wenger (Eds.), *Women, stress, and heart disease* (pp. 25–38). Mahwah, NJ: Erlbaum.

Orth-Gomér, K., Wamala, S. P., Horsten, M., Schenck-Gustafsson, K., Scheiderman, N., & Mittleman, M. A. (2000). Marital stress worsens prognosis in women with coronary heart disease: The Stockholm Female Coronary Risk Study. *Journal of the American Medical Association, 284,* 3008–3014.

Osofsky, J. D. (1997). Prevention and policy: Directions for the future. In J. D. Osofsky (Ed.), *Children in a violent society* (pp. 323–328). New York: Guilford Press.

Oster, G., Thompson, D., Edelsberg, J., Bird, A. P., & Colditz, G. A. (1999). Lifetime health and economic benefits of weight loss among obese persons. *American Journal of Public Health, 89,* 1536–1542.

Ouellette, S. C. (1993). Inquiries into hardiness. In L. Goldberger & S. Breznitz (Eds.), *Handbook of stress: Theoretical and clinical aspects* (2nd ed., pp. 77–100). New York: Free Press.

Ouellette, S. C., & DiPlacido, J. (2001). Personality's role in the protection and enhancement of health: Where the research has been, where it is stuck, how it might move. In A. Baum, T. A. Revenson, & J. E. Singer (Eds.), *Handbook of health psychology* (pp. 175–193). Mahwah, NJ: Erlbaum.

Oxman, T. E., Berkman, L. F., Kasl, S., Freeman, D. H., Jr., & Barrett, J. (1992). Social support and depressive symptoms in the elderly. *American Journal of Epidemiology, 135,* 356–368.

Padian, N. S., Shiboski, S. C., Glass, S. O., & Vittinghoff, E. (1997). Heterosexual transmission of human immunodeficiency virus (HIV) in northern California: Results from a ten-year study. *American Journal of Epidemiology, 146,* 350–357.

Paffenbarger, R. S., Jr., Gima, A. S., Laughlin, M. E., & Black, R. A. (1971). Characteristics of longshoremen related to fatal coronary heart disease and stroke. *American Journal of Public Health, 61,* 1362–1370.

Paffenbarger, R. S., Jr., Laughlin, M. E., Gima, A. S., & Black, R. A. (1970). Work activity of longshoremen as related to death from coronary heart disease and stroke. *New England Journal of Medicine, 282,* 1109–1114.

Paffenbarger, R. S., Jr., Wing, A. L., & Hyde, R. T. (1978). Physical activity as an index of heart attack risk in college alumni. *American Journal of Epidemiology, 108,* 161–175.

Palmer, S. E., Canzona, L., & Wai, L. (1984). Helping families respond effectively to chronic illness: Home dialysis as a case example. In R. H. Moos (Ed.), *Coping with physical illness 2: New perspectives* (pp. 283–294). New York: Plenum Press.

Pancer, S. M., Pratt, M., Hunsberger, B., & Gallant, M. (2000). Thinking ahead: Complexity of expectations and the transition to parenthood. *Journal of Personality, 68,* 253–280.

Pandey, S. (1999). Role of perceived control in coping with crowding. *Psychological Studies, 44,* 86–91.

Paran, E., Amir, M., & Yaniv, N. (1996). Evaluating the response of mild hypertensives to biofeedback-assisted relaxation using a mental stress test. *Journal of Behavior Therapy and Experimental Psychiatry, 27,* 157–167.

Parascandola, M. (2001). Cigarettes and the US Public Health Service in the 1950s. *American Journal of Public Health, 91,* 196–205.

Parrott, A. C. (1999). Does cigarette smoking cause stress? *American Psychologist, 54,* 817–820.

Parrott, D. J., & Zeichner, A. (2002). Effects of alcohol and trait anger on physical aggression in men. *Journal of Studies on Alcohol, 63,* 196–204.

Pate, R. R., Heath, G. W., Dowda, M., & Trost, S. G. (1996). Associations between physical activity and other health behaviors in a representative sample of US adolescents. *American Journal of Public Health, 86,* 1477–1581.

Pate, R. R., Pratt, M., Blair, S. N., Haskell, W. L., Macera, C. A., Bouchard, C., et al. (1995). Physical activity and public health: A recommendation from the Centers for Disease Control and Prevention and the American College of Sports Medicine. *Journal of the American Medical Association, 273,* 402–407.

Pattishall, E. G. (1989). The development of behavioral medicine: Historical models. *Annals of Behavioral Medicine, 11,* 43–48.

Paul, C. L., Sanson-Fisher, R. W., Redman, S., & Carter, S. (1994). Preventing accidental injury to young children in the home using volunteers. *Health Promotion International, 9,* 241–249.

Paul, D. P., & Clarke, I. (2001). Satisfaction with HMO coverage: An empirical study of a medical school's faculty, staff, and administrators. *Hospital Topics, 79,* 14–20.

Pauling, L. (1980). Vitamin C therapy of advanced cancer. *New England Journal of Medicine, 302,* 694–698.

Paull, T. T., Cortez, D., Bowers, B., Elledge, S. J., & Gellert, M. (2001). Direct DNA binding by Brca 1. *Proceedings of the National Academy of Sciences for the United States of America, 98,* 6086–6091.

Pearce, J. M. S. (1994). Headache. *Journal of Neurology, Neurosurgery and Psychiatry, 57,* 134–143.

Peay, M. Y., & Peay, E. R. (1998). The evaluation of medical symptoms by patients and doctors. *Journal of Behavioral Medicine, 21,* 57–81.

Peele, S. (1993). The conflict between public health goals and the temperance mentality. *American Journal of Public Health, 83,* 805–810.

Peele, S., & Brodsky, A. (1996). The antidote to alcohol abuse: Sensible drinking messages. In *Wine in context: Nutrition, physiology, policy* (pp. 66–70). Davis, CA: Society for Enology and Viticulture.

Peila, R., Rodriguez, B. L., Launer, L. J. (2002). Type 2 diabetes, APOE gene, and the risk for dementia and related pathologies. *Diabetes, 51,* 1256–1262.

Pelleymounter, M. A., Cullen, M. J., Baker, M. B., Hecht, R., Winters, D., Boone, T., et al. (1995). Effects of *obese* gene production body weight regulation in *ob/ob* mice. *Science, 269,* 540–543.

Penley, J. A., Tomaka, J., & Wiebe, J. S. (2002). The association of coping to physical and psychological health outcomes: A meta-analytic review. *Journal of Behavioral Medicine, 25,* 551–603.

Pennebaker, J. W. (1982). *The psychology of physical symptoms.* New York: Springer-Verlag.

Pennebaker, J. W., Barger, S. D., & Tiebout, J. (1989). Disclosure of traumas and health among Holocaust survivors. *Psychosomatic Medicine, 51,* 577–589.

Pennebaker, J. W., Colder, M., & Sharp, L. K. (1990). Accelerating the coping process. *Journal of Personality and Social Psychology, 58,* 528–537.

Pennebaker, J. W., & Graybeal, A. (2001). Patterns of natural language use: Disclosure, personality, and social integration. *Current Directions in Psychological Science, 10,* 90–93.

Perera, F. P. (1997). Environment and cancer: Who are susceptible? *Science, 278,* 1068–1073.

Perkins, K. A., Dubbert, P. M., Martin, J. E., Faulstich, M. E., & Harris, J. K. (1986). Cardiovascular reactivity to psychological stress in aerobically trained versus untrained mild hypertensives and normotensives. *Health Psychology, 5,* 407–421.

Perkins, K. A., Epstein, L. H., Marks, B. L., Stiller, R. L., & Jacob, R. G. (1989). The effect of nicotine on energy expenditure during light physical activity. *New England Journal of Medicine, 320,* 898–903.

Perkins, K. A., Marcus, M. D., Levine, M. D., D'Amico, D., Miller, A., Broge, M., Ashcom, J., & Shiffman, S. (2001). Cognitive-behavioral therapy to reduce weight concerns improves smoking cessation outcome in weight-concerned women. *Journal of Consulting and Clinical Psychology, 69,* 604–613.

Perri, M. G., McKelvey, W. E., Renjilian, D. A., Nezu, A. M., Shermer, R. L., & Viegener, B. J. (2001). Relapse prevention training and problem-solving therapy in the long-term management of obesity. *Journal of Consulting and Clinical Psychology, 69,* 722–726.

Persky, V. W., Kempthrone-Rawson, J., & Shekelle, R. B. (1987). Personality and risk of cancer: 20-year follow-up of the Western Electric Study. *Psychosomatic Medicine, 49,* 435–439.

Pert, C. B., & Snyder, S. H. (1973). Opiate receptor: Demonstration in nervous tissue. *Science, 179,* 1011–1014.

Peterson, C. B., & Mitchell, J. E. (1999). Psychosocial and pharmacological treatment of eating disorders: A review of research findings. *Journal of Clinical Psychology, 55,* 685–698.

Peterson, L., DiLillo, D., Lewis, T., & Sher, K. (2002). Improvement in quaintly and quality of prevention measurement of toddler injuries and parental interventions. *Behavior Therapy, 35,* 271–297.

Peterson, L., & Gable, S. (1997). Holistic injury prevention. In J. R. Lutzker (Ed.), *Handbook of child abuse research and treatment* (pp. 291–316).

Peterson, L., & Schick, B. (1993). Empirically derived injury prevention rules. Special section: Behavioral pediatrics. *Journal of Applied Behavior Analysis, 26,* 451–460.

Peterson, L., & Tremblay, G. (1999). Self-monitoring in behavioral medicine: Children. *Psychological Assessment, 11,* 458–465.

Pettinati, H. M., Meyers, K., Evans, B. D., Ruetsch, C. R., Kaplan, F. N., Jensen, J. M., & Hadley, T. R. (1999). Inpatient alcohol treatment in a private healthcare setting: Which patients benefit and at what cost? *American Journal on Addictions, 8,* 220–233.

Pettingale, K. W., Morris, T., Greer, S., & Haybittle, J. L. (1985). Mental attitudes to cancer: An additional prognostic factor. *Lancet, i,* 750.

Phillips, D. P., Liu, G. C., Kwok, K., Jarvinen, J. R., Zhang, W., & Abramson, I. S. (2001). The Hound of the Baskervilles effect: Natural experiment on the influence of psychological stress of timing of death. *British Medical Journal, 323,* 1443–1446.

Phillips, L. R., Torres de Ardon, E., Komnenich, P., Killeen, M., & Rusinak, R. (2000). The Mexican American caregiving experience. *Hispanic Journal of Behavioral Sciences, 22,* 296–313.

Picard, C. L. (1999). The level of competition as a factor for the development of eating disorders in female collegiate athletes. *Journal of Youth and Adolescence, 28,* 583–594.

Pierce, J. P., Choi, W. S., Gilpin, E. A., Farkas, A. J., & Berry, C. C. (1998). Tobacco industry promotion of cigarettes and adolescent smoking. *Journal of the American Medical Association, 279,* 511–515.

Pike, J. L., Smith, T. L., Hauger, R. L., Nicassio, P. M., & Irwin, M. R. (1994, August). *Immunologic effects of acute stress: Chronic life stress as a moderator.* Presented at the American Psychological Association convention, Los Angeles, CA.

Pinel, J. P. J. (2003). *Biopsychology* (5th ed.). Boston: Allyn and Bacon.

Pinel, J. P. J., Assanand, S., & Lehman, D. R. (2000). Hunger, eating, and ill health. *American Psychologist, 55,* 1105–1116.

Pingitore, D., Scheffler, R., Haley, M., Seniell, T., & Schwalm, D. (2001). Professional psychology in a new era: Practice-based evidence from California. *Professional Psychology, Research and Practice, 32,* 585–596.

Pinto, R. P., & Hollandsworth, J. G., Jr. (1989). Using videotape modeling to prepare children psychologically for surgery: Influence of parents and costs versus benefits of providing preparation services. *Health Psychology, 8,* 79–95.

Pinsky, L. E., Burke, W., & Bird, T. D. (2001). Why should primary care physicians know about the genetics of dementia? *Western Journal of Medicine, 175,* 412–416.

Piotrowski, C. (1998). Assessment of pain: A survey of practicing clinicians. *Perceptual and Motor Skills, 86,* 181–182.

Pipho, C. (1998). Living with zero tolerance. *Phi Delta Kappan, 79,* 725–726.

Pirie, P. L., Murray, D. M., & Luepker, R. V. (1991). Gender differences in cigarette smoking and quitting in a cohort of young adults. *American Journal of Public Health, 81,* 324–327.

Plaud, J. J., Mosley, T. H., & Moberg, M. (1998). Alzheimer's disease and behavioral gerontology. In J. J. Plaud & G. H. Eifert (Eds.), *From behavior theory to behavior therapy* (pp. 223–245). Boston: Allyn and Bacon.

Plaut, S. M., & Friedman, S. B. (1981). Psychosocial factors in infectious disease. In R. Ader (Ed.), *Psychoneuroimmunology* (pp. 3–30). New York: Academic Press.

Polatin, P. B. (1996). Integration of pharmacotherapy with psychological treatment of chronic pain. In R. J. Gatchel & D. C. Turk (Eds.), *Psychological approaches to pain management: A practitioner's handbook* (pp. 305–328). New York: Guilford Press.

Polich, J. M., Armor, D. J., & Braiker, H. B. (1980). *The course of alcoholism: Four years after treatment.* Santa Monica, CA: Rand.

Polivy, J., & Herman, C. P. (1995). Dieting and its relation to eating disorders. In K. D. Brownell & C. G. Fairburn. *Eating disorders and obesity: A comprehensive handbook* (pp. 83–92). New York: Guilford Press.

Polivy, J., & Herman, C. P. (2000). The false-hope syndrome: Unfulfilled expectations of self-change. *Current Directions in Psychological Science, 9,* 128–131.

Polivy, J., & Herman, C. P. (2002). Causes of eating disorders. *Annual Review of Psychology, 53,* 187–214.

Pollock, M. L., Wilmore, J. H., & Fox, S. M., III. (1978). *Health and fitness through physical activity.* New York: Wiley.

Pomerleau, C. S., Brouwer, R. J. N., & Jones, L. T. (2000). Weight concerns in women smokers during pregnancy and postpartum. *Addictive Behaviors, 25,* 759–767.

Pomerleau, C. S., Zucker, A. N., Brouwer, R. J. N., Pomerleau, O. F., & Stewart, A. J. (2001). Race differences in weight concerns among women smokers: Results from two independent samples. *Addictive Behaviors, 26,* 651–663.

Pomerleau, O. F., & Kardia, S. L. R. (1999). Introduction to the features section: Genetic research on smoking. *Health Psychology, 18,* 3–6.

Pope, H. G., Jr., Hudson, J. I., & Yurgelun-Todd, D. (1984). Anorexia nervosa and bulimia among 300 suburban women shoppers. *American Journal of Psychiatry, 141,* 292–293.

Popham, R. E. (1978). The social history of the tavern. In Y. Israel, F. B. Glaser, H. Kalant, R. E. Popham, W. Schmidt, & R. G. Smart (Eds.), *Research advances in alcohol and drug problems* (Vol. 2, pp. 225–302). New York: Plenum Press.

Popkin, B. M., & Udry, J. R. (1998). Adolescent obesity increases significantly in second and third generation U.S. immigrants: The national longitudinal study of adolescent health. *Journal of Nutrition, 128,* 701–706.

Population Reports. (2001). Can we avoid catastrophe? *Population Reports, 29* (3), 1–38.

Porter, J., & Jick, H. (1980). Addiction rate in patients treated with narcotics. *New England Journal of Medicine, 302,* 123.

Poss, J. E. (2000). Developing a new model for cross-cultural research: Synthesizing the health belief model and the theory of reasoned action. *Advances in Nursing Science, 23,* 1–15.

Power, C., Frank, J., Hertzman, C., Schierhout, G., & Li, L. (2001). Predictors of low back pain onset in a prospective British study. *American Journal of Public Health, 91,* 1671–1678.

Pratt, M. (1999). Benefits of lifestyle activity vs structured exercise. *Journal of the American Medical Association, 281,* 375–376.

Preventing fatal medical errors. (1999, December 1). *The New York Times,* p. A22.

Price, R. A., Li, W. D., & Kilker, R. (2002). An X-chromosome scan reveals a locus for fat distribution in chromosome region Xp21-22. *Diabetes, 51,* 1989–1991.

Prochaska, J. O., DiClemente, C. C., & Norcross, J. C. (1992). In search of how people change: Applications to addictive behaviors. *American Psychologist, 47,* 1102–1114.

Prochaska, J. O., Norcross, J. C., & DiClemente, C. C. (1994). *Changing for good.* New York: Avon Books.

Prochaska, J. O., Velicer, W. F., Rossi, J. S., Goldstein, M. G., Marcus, B. H., Rakowski, W., et al. (1994). Stages of change and decisional balance for 12 problem behaviors. *Health Psychology, 13,* 39–46.

Pugliese, K., & Shook, S. L. (1998). Gender, ethnicity, and network characteristics: Variation in social support resources. *Sex Roles, 38,* 215–238.

Pukish, M. M., & Tucker, J. A. (1994, August). *Natural recovery from alcoholism: Contexts surrounding abstinent and moderation outcomes.* Paper presented at the 102nd convention of the American Psychological Association, Los Angeles, CA.

Puska, P., Vartiainen, E., Tuomilehto, J., Salomaa, V., & Nissinen, A. (1998). Changes in premature death in Finland: Successful long-term prevention of cardiovascular diseases. *Bulletin of the World Health Organization, 76,* 419–425.

Pyle, R. L., Mitchell, J. E., Eckert, E. D., Halvorson, P. A., Neuman, P. A., & Goff, G. M. (1983). The incidence of bulimia in freshman college students. *International Journal of Eating Disorders, 2,* 75–85.

Quinlan, K. B., & McCaul, K. D. (2000). Matched and mismatched interventions with young adult smokers: Testing a stage theory. *Health Psychology 19,* 165–171.

Rabins, P. V. (1989). Behavior problems in the demented. In E. Light & B. D. Lebowitz (Eds.), *Alzheimer's disease treatment and family stress: Directions for research* (pp. 322–339). (USDHHS Publication No. ADM 89–1569). Washington, DC: US Government Printing Office.

Rabins, P. V. (1996). Developing treatment guidelines for Alzheimer's disease and other dementias. *Journal of Clinical Psychiatry, 57,* 37–38.

Rabkin, J. G. (1993). Stress and psychiatric disorders. In L. Goldberger & S. Breznitz (Eds.), *Handbook of stress: Theoretical and clinical aspects* (2nd ed., pp. 477–495). New York: Free Press.

Rabkin, J. G., & Struening, E. L. (1976). Life events, stress, and illness. *Science, 194,* 1013–1020.

Raglin, J. S. (1997). Anxiolytic effects of physical activity. In W. P. Morgan (Ed.), *Physical activity and mental health* (pp. 107–126). Washington, DC: Taylor & Francis.

Rainville, P., Bushnell, M. C., & Duncan, G. H. (2000). PET studies of the subjective experience of pain. In K. L. Casey & M. C. Bushnell (Eds.), *Pain imaging: Progress in pain research and management* (pp. 123–156). Seattle, WA: IASP Press.

Rainwater, D. L., Mitchell, B. D., Gomuzzie, A. G., Vandeberg, J. L., Stein, M. P., & MacCluer, J. W. (2000). Associations among 5-year changes in weight, physical activity, and cardiovascular disease risk factors in Mexican Americans. *American Journal of Epidemiology, 152,* 974–982.

Raitakari, O. T., Porkka, V. K., Taimela, S., Telama, R., Räsänen, L., & Vükai, J. S. A. (1994). Effects of persistent physical activity and inactivity on coronary risk factors in children and young adults: The Cardiovascular Risk in Young Finns study. *American Journal of Epidemiology, 140,* 195–205.

Ramsay, D. S., Seeley, R. J., Bolles, R. C., & Woods, S. C. (1996). Ingestive homeostasis: The primacy of learning. In E. D. Capaldi (Ed.), *Why we eat what we eat: The psychology of eating* (pp. 11–27). Washington, DC: American Psychological Association.

Ratner, H., Gross, L., Casas, J., & Castells, S. (1990). A hypnotherapeutic approach to improvement of compliance in adolescent diabetics. *American Journal of Clinical Hypnosis, 32,* 154–159.

Raymond, J., Pierce, E., Smith, S., Wagner, J. P., Gordon-Thomas, J, & Wirzbicki, A. (2001, April 9). Playing with pain killers. *Newsweek,* 44–47.

Raynor, H. A., & Epstein, L. H. (2001). Dietary variety: Energy regulation and obesity. *Psychological Bulletin, 127,* 325–341.

Reese, D. (2002). Alternatives for Alzheimer's: Three basic approaches offer help and hope. *Contemporary Long Term Care, 25* (2), 8–9.

Rehm, J., Greenfield, T. K., & Rogers, J. D. (2001). Average volume of alcohol consumption, patterns of drinking, and all-cause mortality: Results from the US National Alcohol Survey. *American Journal of Epidemiology, 153,* 64–71.

Rehm, J. T., Bondy, S. J., Sempos, C. T., & Vuong, C. V. (1997). Alcohol consumption and coronary heart disease morbidity and mortality. *American Journal of Epidemiology, 146,* 495–501.

Remafedi, G., French, S., Story, M., Resnick, M. D., & Blum, R. (1998). The relationship between suicide risk and sexual orientation: Results of a population-based study. *American Journal of Public Health, 88,* 57–60.

Reneman, L., Booij, J., de Bruin, K., Reitsma, J. B., de Wolff, F. A., Gunning, W. B., et al. (2001). Effects of dose, sex, and long-term abstention from use on toxic effects of MDMA (ecstasy) on brain serotonin neurons. *Lancet, 358,* 1864–1869.

Reppucci, J. D., Revenson, T. A., Aber, M., & Reppucci, N. D. (1991). Unrealistic optimism among adolescent smokers and nonsmokers. *Journal of Primary Prevention, 11,* 227–236.

Research and Policy Committee. (2002). *A new vision for healthcare: A leadership role for business.* New York: Committee for Economic Development.

Resnick, H. S., Kilpatrick, D. G., Best, C. L., & Kramer, T. L. (1992). Vulnerability-stress factors in development of posttraumatic stress disorder. *Journal of Nervous and Mental Disease, 180,* 424–430.

Resnick, M. D., Bearman, P. S., Blum, R. W., Bauman, K. E., Harris, K. M., Jones, J., et al. (1997). Protecting adolescents from harm: Findings from the National Longitudinal Study on Adolescent Health. *Journal of the American Medical Association, 278,* 823–832.

Rexrode, K. M., Carey, V. J., Hennekens, C. H., Walters, E. E., Colditz, G. A., Stampher, M. J., et al. (1998). Abdominal adiposity and coronary heart disease in women. *Journal of the American Medical Association, 280,* 1843–1948.

Ricciuti, C. G. (1997). Cardiac catheterization. In S. VanRiper & J. VanRiper (Eds.), *Cardiac diagnostic tests: A guide for nurses* (pp. 265–296). Philadelphia: Saunders.

Rigotti, N. A., Lee, J. E., & Wechsler, H. (2000). US college students' use of tobacco products: Results of a national survey. *Journal of the American Medical Association, 264,* 699–705.

Rimm, E. B., Stampfer, M. J., Ascherio, A., Giovannucci, E., Colditz, G. A., & Willett, W. C. (1993). Vitamin E consumption and risk of coronary heart disease in men. *New England Journal of Medicine, 328,* 1450–1456.

Rimm, E. B., Williams, P., Fosher, K., Criqui, M., & Stampfer, M. J. (1999). Moderate alcohol intake and lower risk of coronary heart disease: Meta-analysis of effects on lipids and haemostatic factors. *British Medical Journal, 319,* 1523–1528.

Ritchie, K., & Kildea, D. (1995). Is senile dementia "age-related" or "ageing-related"?—Evidence from meta-analysis of dementia prevalence in the oldest old. *Lancet, 346,* 931–934.

Rivara, F., Mueller, B. A., Somes, G., Mendoza, C. T., Rushforth, N. B., & Kellermann, A. L. (1997). Alcohol and illicit drug abuse and the risk of violent death in the home. *Journal of the American Medical Association, 278,* 569–575.

Robbins, A. S., Whittemore, A. S., & Thom, D. H. (2000). Differences in socioeconomic status and survival among white and black men with prostate cancer. *American Journal of Epidemiology, 151,* 409–416.

Roberts, S. O. (2002). A strong start: Strength and resistance training guidelines for children and adolescents. *American Fitness, 20*(1), 34–38.

Roberts, S. S. (1998). Working toward a world without Type I diabetes. *Diabetes Forecast, 51* (7), 85–87.

Robine, J. -M., & Ritchie, K. (1991). Healthy life expectancy: Evaluation of global indicator of change in population health. *British Medical Journal, 302,* 457–460.

Robins, L. N. (1995). The natural history of substance use as a guide to setting drug policy. *American Journal of Public Health, 85,* 12–13.

Robinson-Whelen, S., Tada, Y., MacCallum, R. C., McGuire, L., & Kiecolt-Glaser, J. K. (2001). Long-term caregiving: What happens when it ends? *Journal of Abnormal Psychology, 110,* 573–584.

Rockhill, B., Willett, W. C., Manson, J. E., Leitzmann, M. F., Stampfer, M. J., Hunter, D. J., et al. (2001). Physical activity and mortality: A prospective study among women. *American Journal of Public Health, 91,* 578–583.

Rodgers, W. M., Hall, C. R., Blanchard, C. M., & Munroe, K. J. (2001). Prediction of obligatory exercise by exercise-related imagery. *Psychology of Addictive Behaviors, 15,* 152–154.

Rodin, J., & Langer, E. J. (1977). Long-term effects of a control-relevant intervention with the institutionalized aged. *Journal of Personality and Social Psychology, 35,* 897–902.

Rodin, J., Silberstein, L., & Striegel-Moore, R. (1985). Women and weight: A normative discontent. In T. B. Sonderegger (Ed.), *Psychology and gender* (267–307). Lincoln, NE: University of Nebraska Press.

Romano, J. M., Jensen, M. P., Turner, J. A., Good, A. B., & Hops, H. (2000). Chronic pain patient-partner interactions: Further support for a behavioral model of chronic pain. *Behavior Therapy, 31,* 415–440.

Rondeau, V., Commenges, D., Jacqmin-Gadda, H., & Dartigues, J. F. (2000). Relation between aluminum concentrations in drinking water and Alzheimer's disease: An 8-year follow-up study. *American Journal of Epidemiology, 152,* 59–66.

Room, R., & Day, N. (1974). Alcohol and mortality. In M. Keller (Ed.), *Second special report to the U.S. Congress: Alcohol and health.* Washington, DC: U.S. Government Printing Office.

Room, R., & Greenfield, T. (1993). Alcoholics Anonymous, other 12-step movements and psychotherapy in the US population, 1990. *Addiction, 88,* 555–562.

Rosario, M., Hunter, J., Maguen, S., Gwadz, M., & Smith, R. (2001). The coming-out process and its adaptational and health-related associations among gay, lesbian, and bisexual youths: Stipulation and exploration of a model. *American Journal of Community Psychology, 29,* 113–160.

Rosen, C. S. (2000a). Integrating stage continuum models to explain processing of exercise messages and exercise initiation among sedentary college students. *Health Psychology, 19,* 172–180.

Rosen, C. S. (2000b). Is the sequencing of change processes by stage consistent across health problems? A meta-analysis. *Health Psychology, 19,* 593–604.

Rosenberg, E. L., Ekman, P., Jiang, W., Babyak, M., Coleman, R. E., Hanson, M., et al. (2001). Linkages between facial expressions of anger and transient mycardial ischemia in men with coronary artery disease. *Emotion, 1,* 107–115.

Rosenberg, H. (1993). Prediction of controlled drinking by alcoholics and problem drinkers. *Psychological Bulletin, 113,* 129–139.

Rosenblatt, K. A., Wicklund, K. G., & Stanford, J. L. (2000). Sexual factors and the risk of prostate cancer. *American Journal of Epidemiology, 152,* 1152–1158.

Rosenfeld, I. (1998, August 16). Acupuncture goes mainstream (Almost). *Parade,* 10–11.

Rosengren, A., Tibblin, G., & Wilhelmsen, L. (1991). Self-perceived psychological stress and incidence of coronary artery disease in middle-aged men. *American Journal of Cardiology, 68,* 1171–1175.

Rosenman, R. H., Brand, R. J., Jenkins, C. D., Friedman, M., Straus, R., & Wurm, M. (1975). Coronary heart disease in the Western Collaborative Group Study: Final follow-up of 8 1/2 years. *Journal of the American Medical Association, 233,* 872–877.

Rosenstock, I. M. (1990). The health belief model: Explaining health behavior through expectancies. In K. Glanz, F. M. Lewis, & B. K. Rimer (Eds.), *Health behavior and health education: Theory, research, and practice* (pp. 39–62). San Francisco: Jossey-Bass.

Ross, C. E. (1993). Fear of victimization and health. *Journal of Quantitative Criminology, 9,* 159–175.

Ross, M. J., & Berger, R. S. (1996). Effects of stress inoculation training on athletes' postsurgical pain and rehabilitation after orthopedic injury. *Journal of Consulting and Clinical Psychology, 64,* 406–410.

Roth, S., Newman, E., Pelcovitz, D., van der Kolk, B., & Mandel, F. S. (1997). Complex PTSD in victims exposed to sexual and physical abuse: Results from the DSM-IV field trial for posttraumatic stress disorder. *Journal of Traumatic Stress, 101,* 539–555.

Rotter, J. B. (1966). Generalized expectancies for internal versus external control of reinforcement. *Psychological Monographs, 80* (Whole No. 609).

Rouse, B. A. (Ed.). (1998). *Substance abuse and mental health statistics source book.* Rockville, MD: Department of Health and Human Services: Substance Abuse and Mental Health Services Administration.

Rowe, M. M. (1997). Hardiness, stress, temperament, coping, and burnout in health professionals. *American Journal of Health Behavior, 21,* 163–171.

Rozin, P. (1996). Sociocultural influences on human food selection. In E. D. Capaldi (Ed.), *Why we eat what we eat: The psychology of eating* (pp. 233–263). Washington, DC: American Psychological Association.

Rozin, P. (1999). Food is fundamental, fun, frightening, and far-reaching. *Social Research, 66,* 9–30.

Ruback, R. B., & Pandey, J. (1996). Gender differences in perceptions of household crowding: Stress, affiliation, and role obligations in rural India. *Journal of Applied Social Psychology, 26,* 417–436.

Ruback, R. B., Pandey, J., & Begum, H. A. (1997). Urban stressors in South Asia: Impact on male and female pedestrians in Delhi and Dhaka. *Journal of Cross-Cultural Psychology, 28,* 23–43.

Ruitenberg, A., van Swieten, J. C., Wittman, J. C. M., Mehta, K. M., van Duijn, C. M., Hofman, A., et al. (2002). Alcohol consumption and the risk of dementia: The Rotterdam study. *Lancet, 359,* 281–286.

Ruiz, P., & Ruiz, P. P. (1983). Treatment compliance among Hispanics. *Journal of Operational Psychiatry, 14,* 112–114.

Russell, N. K., & Roter, D. L. (1993). Health promotion counseling of chronic-disease patients during primary care visits. *American Journal of Public Health, 83,* 979–982.

Ruzicka, L. T. (1995). Suicide mortality in developed countries. In A. D. Lopez, G. Caselli, & T. Valkonen (Eds.), *Adult mortality in developed countries: From description to explanation* (pp. 83–110). Oxford, UK: Clarendon Press.

Sabol, S. Z., Nelson, M. L., Fisher, C., Gunzerath, L., Brody, C. L., Hu, S., et al. (1999). A genetic association for cigarette smoking behavior. *Health Psychology, 18,* 7–13.

Sacco, R. L., Benson, R. T., Kargman, D. E., Boden-Albala, B., Tuck, C., Lin, I-F., et al. (2001). High-density lipoprotein cholesterol and ischemic stroke in the elderly: The Northern Manhattan Stroke Study. *Journal of the American Medical Association, 285,* 2720, 2735.

Sacker, A., Bartley, M. J., Frith, D., Fitzpatrick, R. M., & Marmot, M. G. (2001). The relationship between job strain and coronary heart disease: Evidence from an English sample of the working male population. *Psychological Medicine, 31,* 279–290.

Sackett, D. L., & Snow, J. C. (1979). The magnitude of compliance and noncompliance. In R. B. Haynes, D. W. Taylor, & D. L. Sackett (Eds.), *Compliance in health care* (pp. 11–22). Baltimore: Johns Hopkins University Press.

Sadovsky, R. (2001). Driving impairment from marijuana and alcohol. *American Family Physician, 62,* 1652.

Saldana, L., & Peterson, L. (1997). Preventing injury in children: The need for parental involvement. In T. S. Watson & F. M. Gresham (Eds.), *Handbook of child behavior therapy* (pp. 221–238). New York: Plenum Press.

Samanta, A., & Beardsley, J. (1999). Low back pain: Which is the best way forward? *British Medical Journal, 318,* 1122–1123.

Sandberg, S., Paton, J. Y., Ahola, S., McCann, D. C., McGuinness, D., Hillary, C. R., et al. (2000). The role of acute and chronic stress in asthma attacks in children. *Lancet, 356,* 982–987.

Sanders, M. R., Shepherd, R. W., Cleghorn, G., & Woolford, H. (1994). The treatment of recurrent abdominal pain in children: A controlled comparison of cognitive-behavioral family intervention and standard pediatric care. *Journal of Consulting and Clinical Psychology, 62,* 306–314.

Sapolsky, R. M. (1998). *Why zebras don't get ulcers: An updated guide to stress, stress-related diseases, and coping.* New York: Freeman.

Sartory, G., Muller, B., & Pothmann, R. (1998). A comparison of psychological and pharmacological treatment of pediatric migraine. *Behaviour Research and Therapy, 36,* 155–170.

Saunders, T., Driskell, J. E., Johnston, J. H., & Sales, E. (1996). The effects of stress inoculation training on anxiety and performance. *Journal of Occupational Health Psychology, 1,* 170–186.

Sayette, M. A. (1999). Cognitive theory and research. In K. E. Leonard & H. T. Blane (Eds)., *Psychological theories of drinking and alcoholism* (2nd ed., pp. 247–291). New York: Guilford Press.

Schachter, S. (1980). Urinary pH and the psychology of nicotine addiction. In P. O. Davidson & S. M. Davidson (Eds.), *Behavioral medicine: Changing health lifestyles* (pp. 70–93). New York: Brunner/Mazel.

Schachter, S. (1982). Recidivism and self-cure of smoking and obesity. *American Psychologist, 37,* 436–444.

Schapiro, I. R., Ross-Petersen, L., Sælan, H., Garde, K., Olsen, J. H., & Johansen, C. (2001). Extroversion and neuroticism and the associated risk of cancer: A Danish cohort study. *American Journal of Epidemiology, 153,* 757–763.

Schenker, S. (2001, September). The truth about fad diets. *Student BMJ,* 318–319.

Scheufele, P. M. (2000). Effects of progressive relaxation and classical music on measurements of attention, relaxation, and stress responses. *Journal of Behavioral Medicine, 23,* 207–228.

Schindler, L., Kerrigan, D., & Kelly, J. (2002). *Understanding the immune system.* Retrieved from the World Wide Web, January 29, 2002, at newscenter.cancer.gov/sciencebehind/immune.

Schlenger, W. E., Caddell, J. M., Ebert, L., Jordan, B. K., Rourke, K. M., Wilson, D., Thalji, L., Dennis, J. M., Fairbank, J. A., & Kulka, R. A. (2002). Psychological reactions to terrorist attacks: Findings from the National Study of Americans' Reactions to September 11. *Journal of the American Medical Association, 288,* 581–588.

Schmaling, K. B. (1998). Asthma. In E. A. Blechman & K. D. Brownell (Eds.), *Behavioral medicine and women: A comprehensive handbook* (pp. 566–569). New York: Guilford.

Schneider, E. C., Zaslavsky, A. M., & Epstein, A. M. (2002). Racial disparities in the quality of care for enrollees in Medicare managed care. *Journal of the American Medical Association, 287,* 1288–1294.

Schnittker, J. (2001). When is faith enough?: The effects of religious involvement on depression. *Journal for the Scientific Study of Religion, 40,* 393–412.

Schoenbaum, M. (1997). Do smokers understand the mortality effects of smoking? Evidence from the Health Retirement Survey. *American Journal of Public Health, 87,* 755–759.

Schofield, W. (1969). The role of psychology in the delivery of health services. *American Psychologist, 24,* 568–584.

Schrijvers, C. T., Stronks, K., van de Mheen, H. D., & Mackenbach, J. P. (1999). Explaining educational differences in mortality: The role of behavioral and material factors. *American Journal of Public Health, 89,* 535–540.

Schuckit, M. A. (2000). Keep it simple. *Journal of Studies on Alcohol, 61,* 781–782.

Schulman, J. J., Sacks, J., & Provenzano, G. (2002). State level estimates of the incidence and economic burden of head injuries stemming from non-universal use of bicycle helmets. *Injury Prevention, 8,* 47–52.

Schulz, T. F., Boshoff, C. H., & Weiss, R. A. (1996). HIV infection and neoplasia. *Lancet, 348,* 587–591.

Schuster, M. A., Stein, B. D., Jaycox, L. H., Collins, R. L., Marshall, G. N., Elliott, M. N., et al. (2001). A national survey of stress reactions after the September 11, 2001, terrorist attacks. *New England Journal of Medicine, 345,* 1507–1512.

Schwarcz, S. K., Hsu, L. C., Vittinghoff, E., & Katz, M. H. (2000). Impact of protease inhibitors and other antiretroviral treatments on acquired immunodeficiency syndrome survival in San Francisco, California, 1987–1996. *American Journal of Epidemiology, 152,* 178–185.

Schwartz, B. S., Stewart, W. F., Simon, D., & Lipton, R. B. (1998). Epidemiology of tension-type headache. *Journal of the American Medical Association, 279,* 381–383.

Schwartz, G. E., & Weiss, S. M. (1978). Behavioral medicine revisited: An amended definition. *Journal of Behavioral Medicine, 1,* 249–251.

Schwarz, D. F., Grisso, J. A., Miles, C., Holmes, J. H., & Sutton, R. L. (1993). An injury prevention program in an urban African-American community. *American Journal of Public Health, 83,* 675–680.

Sciacchitano, M., Goldstein, M. B., & DiPlacido, J. (2001). Stress, burnout and hardiness in R. T.s. *Radiologic Technology, 72,* 321–328.

Sclafani, A., & Springer, D. (1976). Dietary obesity in adult rats: Similarities to hypothalamic and human obesity. *Physiology and Behavior, 17,* 461–471.

Searle, A., & Bennett, P. (2001). Psychological factors and inflammatory bowel disease: A review of a decade of literature. *Psychology and Health Medicine, 6,* 121–135.

Sears, S. R., & Stanton, A. L. (2001). Expectancy-value constructs and expectancy violation as predictors of exercise adherence in previously sedentary women. *Health Psychology, 20,* 326–333.

Secker-Walker, R. H., Flynn, B. S., Solomon, L. J., Skelly, J. M., Dorwaldt, A. L., & Ashikaga, T. (2000). Helping women quit smoking: Results of a community intervention program. *American Journal of Public Health, 90,* 940–946.

Sedlacek, K., & Taub, E. (1996). Biofeedback treatment of Raynaud's disease. *Professional Psychology: Research and Practice, 27,* 549–553.

Segall, A. (1997). Sick role concepts and health behavior. In D. S. Gochman (Ed.), *Handbook of health behavior research I: Personal and social determinants* (pp. 289–301). New York: Plenum Press.

Sellwood, W., & Tarrier, N. (1994). Demographic factors associated with extreme non-compliance in schizophrenia. *Social Psychiatry and Psychiatric Epidemiology, 29,* 172–177.

Selye, H. (1956). *The stress of life.* New York: McGraw-Hill.

Selye, H. (1976). *Stress in health and disease.* Reading, MA: Butterworths.

Selye, H. (1982). History and present status of the stress concept. In L. Goldberger & S. Breznitz (Eds.), *Handbook of stress: Theoretical and clinical aspects* (pp. 7–17). New York: Free Press.

Senécal, C., Nouwen, A., & White, D. (2000). Motivation and dietary self-care in adults with diabetes: Are self-efficacy and autonomous self-regulation complementary or competing constructs? *Health Psychology, 19,* 452–457.

Serdula, M. K., Mokdad, A. H., Williamson, D. F., Galuska, D. A., Mendlein, J. M., & Heath, G. W. (1999). Prevalence of attempting weight loss and strategies for controlling weight. *Journal of the American Medical Association, 282,* 1353–1358.

Seshadri, S., Beiser, A., Selhub, J., Jacques, P. F., Rosenberg, I. H., D'Agostino, R. B., et al. (2002). Plasma homocysteine as a risk factor for dementia and Alzheimer's disease. *New England Journal of Medicine, 346,* 476–483.

Sesso, H. D., Paffenbarger, R. S., Jr., Ha, T., & Lee, I-M. (1999). Physical activity and cardiovascular disease risk in middle-age and older women. *American Journal of Epidemiology, 150,* 408–416.

Shaffer, J. W., Graves, P. L., Swank, R. T., & Pearson, T. A. (1987). Clustering of personality traits in youth and the subsequent development of cancer among physicians. *Journal of Behavioral Medicine, 10,* 441–447.

Shapiro, A. K. (1970). Placebo effects in psychotherapy and psychoanalysis. *Journal of Clinical Pharmacology, 10,* 73–78.

Sharpe, L., Sensky, T., Timberlake, N., Ryan, B., Brewin, C. R., & Allard, S. (2001). A blind, randomized controlled trial of cognitive-behavioral intervention for patients with recent onset rheumatoid arthritis: Preventing psychological and physical mobility. *Pain, 89,* 275–283.

Shavelson, L. (2001). *Hooked: Five addicts challenge our misguided drug rehab system.* New York: New Press.

Sheeran, P., Conner, M., & Norman, P. (2001). Can the theory of planned behavior explain patterns of health behavior change? *Health Psychology, 20,* 12–19.

Sheeran, P., & Taylor, S. (1999). Predicting intentions to use condoms: A meta-analysis and comparison of the theories of reasoned action and planned behavior. *Journal of Applied Social Psychology, 29,* 1624–1675.

Sheffield, D., Biles, P. L., Orom, H., Maixner, W., & Sheps, D. S. (2000). Race and sex differences in cutaneous pain perception. *Psychosomatic Medicine, 62,* 517–523.

Shekelle, R. B., Raynar, W. J., Ostfield, A. M., Garron, D. C., Bieliauskas, L. A., Liu, S. C., et al. (1981). Psychological depression and 17-year risk of death from cancer. *Psychosomatic Medicine, 43,* 117–125.

Shekelle, R. B., Rossof, A. H., & Stamler, J. (1991). Dietary cholesterol and incidence of lung cancer: The Western Electric study. *American Journal of Epidemiology, 134,* 480–484.

Shell, E. R. (2000, May). Does civilization cause asthma? *Atlantic Monthly, 285,* 90–92, 94, 96–98, 100.

Sher, K. J. (1987). Stress response dampening. In H. T. Blane & K. E. Leonard (Eds.), *Psychological theories of drinking and alcoholism* (pp. 227–271). New York: Guilford Press.

Sher, K. J., & Levenson, R. W. (1982). Risk for alcoholism and individual differences in the stress-response-dampening effect of alcohol. *Journal of Abnormal Psychology, 91,* 350–367.

Sherbourne, C. D., Hays, R. D., Ordway, L., DiMatteo, M. R., & Kravitz, R. L. (1992). Antecedents of adherence to medical recommendations: Results from the Medical Outcomes Study. *Journal of Behavioral Medicine, 15,* 447–468.

Sherrill, D. L., Kotchou, D., & Quan, S. F. (1998). Association of physical activity and human sleep disorders. *Archives of Internal Medicine, 158,* 1894–1898.

Sherwood, R. J. (1983). Compliance behavior of hemodialysis patients and the role of the family. *Family Systems Medicine, 1,* 60–72.

Sherwood, L. (2001). *Human physiology: From cells to systems* (4th ed.). Pacific Grove, CA: Brooks/Cole.

Shi, L. (2001). The convergence of vulnerable characteristics and health insurance in the US. *Social Science and Medicine, 53,* 519–530.

Shiffman, S., Balabanis, M. H., Paty, J. A., Engberg, J., Gwaltney, C. J., Liu, K. S., et al. (2000). Dynamic effects of self-efficacy on smoking lapse and relapse. *Health Psychology, 19,* 315–323.

Sidney, S., Beck, J. E., Tekawa, I. S., Quesenberry, C. P., & Friedman, G. D. (1997). Marijuana use and mortality. *American Journal of Public Health, 87,* 585–590.

Siegel, M., & Biener, L. (2000). The impact of an antismoking media campaign on progression to established smoking: Results of a longitudinal youth study. *American Journal of Public Health, 90,* 380–386.

Siegler, I. C., Bastian, L. A., Steffens, D. C., Bosworth, H. B., & Costa, P. T. (2002). Behavioral medicine and aging. *Journal of Consulting and Clinical Psychology, 70,* 843–851.

Siegler, I. C., Peterson, B. L., Barefoot, J. C., & Williams, R. B. (1992). Hostility during late adolescence predicts coronary risk factors at mid-life. *American Journal of Epidemiology, 136,* 146–154.

Siegman, A. W. (1994). From Type A to hostility to anger: Reflections on the history of coronary-prone behavior. In A. W. Siegman & T. W. Smith (Eds.), *Anger, hostility, and the heart* (pp. 1–21). Hillsdale, NJ: Erlbaum.

Siegman, A. W., Anderson, R., Herbst, J., Boyle, S., & Wilkinson, J. (1992). Dimensions of anger-hostility and cardiovascular reactivity in provoked and angered men. *Journal of Behavioral Medicine, 15,* 257–272.

Siegman, A. W., Dembroski, T. M., & Ringel, N. (1987). Components of hostility and the severity of coronary artery disease. *Psychosomatic Medicine, 49,* 127–135.

Siegman, A. W., & Snow, S. C. (1997). The outward expression of anger, the inward experience of anger and CVR: The role of vocal expression. *Journal of Behavioral Medicine, 20,* 29–45.

Sigmon, S. T., Stanton, A. L., & Snyder, C. R. (1995). Gender differences in coping: A further test of socialization and role constraint theories. *Sex Roles, 33,* 565–587.

Silva, R. P., Alpert, M., Munoz, D. M., Singh, S., Matzner, F., & Dummit, S. (2000). Stress and vulnerability to posttraumatic stress disorder in children and adolescents. *Journal of Psychiatry, 157,* 1229–1235.

Silvert, M. (2000). Acupuncture wins BMA approval. *British Medical Journal, 321,* 11.

Simone, C. B. (1983). *Cancer and nutrition.* New York: McGraw-Hill.

Sims, E. A. H. (1974). Studies in human hyperphagia. In G. Bray & J. Bethune (Eds.), *Treatment and management of obesity.* New York: Harper & Row.

Sims, E. A. H. (1976). Experimental obesity, dietary-induced thermogenesis, and their clinical implications. *Clinics in Endocrinology and Metabolism, 5,* 377–395.

Sims, E. A. H., Danforth, E., Jr., Horton, E. S., Bray, G. A., Glennon, J. A., & Salans, L. B. (1973). Endocrine and metabolic effects of experimental obesity in man. *Recent Progress in Hormonal Research, 29,* 457–496.

Sims, E. A. H., & Horton, E. S. (1968). Endocrine and metabolic adaptation to obesity and starvation. *American Journal of Clinical Nutrition, 21,* 1455–1470.

Singh, N. A., Clements, K. M., & Singh, M. A. F. (2001). The efficacy of exercise as a long-term antidepressant in elderly subjects: A randomized, controlled trial. *Journals of Gerontology, Series A, 56,* 497–505.

Singletary, K. W., & Gapstur, S. M. (2001). Alcohol and breast cancer: Review of epidemiologic and experimental evidence and potential mechanisms. *Journal of the American Medical Association, 286,* 2143–2151.

Siwek, J. (1997). Twelve pitfalls of adequate pain control. *American Family Physician, 56,* 726–728.

Sjöström, L. V. (1992a). Morbidity of severely obese subjects. *American Journal of Clinical Nutrition, 55,* 508S–515S.

Sjöström, L. V. (1992b). Mortality of severely obese subjects. *American Journal of Clinical Nutrition, 55,* 516S–523S.

Skinner, B. F. (1953). *Science and human behavior.* New York: Macmillan.

Skinner, B. F. (1987). *Upon further reflection.* Englewood Cliffs, NJ: Prentice-Hall.

Skinner, T. C., Hampson, S. E., & Fife-Schaw, C. (2002). Personality, personal model beliefs, and self-care in adolescents and young adults with Type 1 diabetes. *Health Psychology, 21,* 61–70.

Slater, J., & Depue, R. A. (1981). The contribution of environmental events and social support to serious suicide attempts in primary depressive disorder. *Journal of Abnormal Psychology, 90,* 275–285.

Slattery, M. L., Boucher, K. M., Caan, B. J., Potter, J. D., & Ma, K. -N. (1998). Eating patterns and risk of colon cancer. *American Journal of Epidemiology, 148,* 4–16.

Slattery, M. L., & Kerber, R. A. (1993). A comprehensive evaluation of family history and breast cancer risk. *Journal of the American Medical Association, 270,* 1563–1568.

Slugg, R. M., Meyer, R. A., & Campbell, J. N. (2000). Response of cutaneous A- and C-fiber nociceptors in the monkey to controlled-force stimuli. *Journal of Neurophysiology, 83,* 2179–2191.

Smetana, G. W., (2000). The diagnostic value of historical features in primary headache syndromes: A comprehensive review. *Archives of Internal Medicine, 160,* 2729–2740.

Smiles, R. V. (2002). Race matters in health care: Experts say eliminating racial and ethnic health disparities is the civil rights issue of our day. *Black Issues in Higher Education, 19*(7), 22–29.

Smith, B. N., & Stasson, M. F., (2000). A comparison of health behavior constructs: Social psychological predictors of AIDS-preventive behavioral intentions. *Journal of Applied Social Psychology, 30,* 443–462.

Smith, G. S. (1999). Epidemiology of intentional and unintentional injuries. *Report of a Subcommittee of the National Advisory Council on Alcohol Abuse and Alcoholism on the Review of the Extramural Research Portfolio for Epidemiology.* Retrieved from the World Wide Web, June 20, 2002, at www.niaaa.nih.gov/extramural/epireport2.htm#consumptin.

Smith, J. T., Barabasz, A., & Barabasz, M. (1996). Comparison of hypnosis and distraction in severely ill children undergoing painful medical procedures. *Journal of Counseling Psychology, 43,* 187–195.

Smith, S. M. (1997). Alcohol-induced cell death in the embryo. *Alcohol Health & Research World, 21,* 287–297.

Smith, T. W. (1994). Concepts and methods in the study of anger, hostility, and health. In A. W. Siegman & T. W. Smith (Eds.), *Anger, hostility, and the heart* (pp. 23–42). Hillsdale, NJ: Erlbaum.

Smith, T. W., & Brown, P. C. (1991). Cynical hostility, attempts to exert social control, and cardiovascular reactivity in married couples. *Journal of Behavioral Medicine, 14,* 581–592.

Smith, T. W., & Ruiz, J. M. (2002). Psychosocial influences on the development and course of coronary heart disease: Current status and implications for research and practice. *Journal of Consulting and Clinical Psychology, 70,* 548–568.

Smith-Warner, S. A., Spiegelman, D., Shaw-Shyuan, Y., van den Brandt, P. A., Folsom, A. R., Goldbohm, R. A., et al. (1998). Alcohol and breast cancer in women: A pooled analysis of cohort studies. *Journal of the American Medical Association, 279,* 535–540.

Smoking Cessation Clinical Practice Guideline Panel and Staff. (1996). The Agency for Health Care Policy and Research: Smoking cessation clinical practice guideline. *Journal of the American Medical Association, 275,* 1270–1280.

Smyth, J. M., & Pennebaker, J. W. (2001). What are the health effects of disclosure? In A. Baum, T. A. Revenson, & J. E. Singer (Eds.), *Handbook of Health Psychology* (pp. 339–348). Mahwah, NJ: Erlbaum.

Smyth, J. M., Stone, A. A., Hurewitz, A., & Kaell, A. (1999). Effects of writing about stressful experiences on symptom reduction in patients with asthma or rheumatoid arthritis: A randomized trial. *Journal of the American Medical Association, 281,* 1304–1309.

Snyder, S. H. (1977, March). Opiate receptors and internal opiates. *Scientific American, 236,* 44–56.

Sobel, D. S. (1995). Rethinking medicine: Improving health outcomes with cost-effective psychosocial interventions. *Psychosomatic Medicine, 57,* 234–244.

Sobell, L. C., Cunningham, J. A., & Sobell, M. B. (1996). Recovery from alcohol problems with and without treatment: Prevalence in two population surveys. *American Journal of Public Health, 86,* 966–972.

Soderstrom, M., Dolbier, C., Leiferman, J., & Steinhardt, M. (2000). The relationship of hardiness, coping strategies, and perceived stress to symptoms of illness. *Journal of Behavioral Medicine, 23,* 311–328.

Solomon, C. M. (1998). Picture this: A safer workplace. Polaroid addresses family violence to combat workplace violence. *Workforce, 77* (2), 82–86.

Solomon, G. F., & Moos, R. H. (1964). Emotions, immunity, and disease: A speculative theoretical integration. *Archives of General Psychiatry, 11,* 657–674.

Solowij, N., Stephens, R. S., Roffman, R. A., Babor, T., Kadden, R., Miller, M., et al. (2002). Cognitive functioning of long-term heavy cannabis users seeking treatment. *Journal of the American Medical Association, 287,* 1123–1131.

Song, Y. -M., Sung, J., & Kim, J. S. (2000). Which cholesterol level is related to the lowest mortality in a population with low mean cholesterol level: A 6.4-year follow-up study of 482,472 Korean men. *American Journal of Epidemiology, 151,* 739–747.

Sonnentag, S. (2001). Work, recovery activities, and individual well-being. *Journal of Occupational Health Psychology, 6,* 196–310.

Sonstroem, R. J. (1984). Exercise and self-esteem. *Exercise and Sport Sciences Reviews, 12,* 123–155.

Sonstroem, R. J. (1997). Physical activity and self-esteem. In W. P. Morgan (Ed.), *Physical activity and mental health* (pp. 127–143). Washington, DC: Taylor & Francis.

Sont, W. N., Zielinski, J. M., Ashmore, J. P., Jiang, H., Krewski, D., Fair, M. E., et al. (2001). First analysis of cancer incidence and occupational radiation exposure based on the National Dose Registry of Canada. *American Journal of Epidemiology, 153,* 309–318.

Sorenson, S. B., Upchurch, D. M., & Shen, H. (1996). Violence and injury in marital arguments: Risk patterns and gender differences. *American Journal of Public Health, 86,* 35–40.

Soukup, J. E. (1996). *Alzheimer's disease: A guide to diagnosis, treatment, and management.* Westport, CT: Praeger.

Sours, J. A. (1980). *Starving to death in a sea of objects: The anorexia nervosa syndrome.* New York: Aronson.

Spanagel, R., & Weiss, F. (1999). The dopamine hypothesis of reward: Past and current status. *Trends in Neuroscience, 22,* 521–527.

Spiegel, D. (2001). Mind matters: Group therapy and survival in breast cancer. *New England Journal of Medicine, 345,* 1767–1768.

Spiegel, D., & Kato, P. (1996). Psychosocial influences on cancer incidence and progression. *Harvard Review of Psychiatry, 4,* 10–26.

Spiegel, D., Kraemer, H. C., Bloom, J. R., & Gottheil, E. (1989). Effect of psychosocial treatment on survival of patients with metastatic breast cancer. *Lancet, ii,* 888–891.

Spierings, E. L. H., Ranke, A. H., & Honkoop, P. C. (2001). Precipitating and aggravating factors of migraine versus tension-type headache. *Headache, 41,* 554–558.

Spillane, J. F. (1999). Regulation of sale and distribution. In R. T. Ammerman, P. J. Ott, & R. E Tarter (Eds.), *Prevention and societal impact of drug and alcohol abuse* (pp. 221–234). Mahwah, NJ: Erlbaum.

Spillman, B. C., & Lubitz, J. (2000). The effect of longevity on spending for acute and long-term care. *New England Journal of Medicine, 342,* 1409–1415.

Spitzer, B. L., Henderson, K. A., & Zivian, M. T. (1999). Gender differences in population versus media body size: A comparison over four decades. *Sex Roles, 40,* 545–566.

Stamler, J., Daviglus, M. L., Garside, D., Dyer, A. R., Greenland, P., & Neaton, J. D. (2000). Relationship of baseline serum cholesterol levels in 3 large cohorts of younger men to long-term coronary, cardiovascular, and all-cause mortality and to longevity. *Journal of the American Medical Association, 284,* 311–318.

Stamler, J., Stamler, R., Neaton, J. D., Wentworth, D., Daviglus, M. L., Garside, D., et al. (1999). Low risk-factor profile and long-term cardiovascular and noncardiovascular mortality and life expectancy: Findings for 5 large cohorts of young adult and middle-aged men and women. *Journal of the American Medical Association, 282,* 2012–2018.

Stampfer, M. J., Hennekens, C. H., Manson, J. E., Colditz, G. A., Rosner, D., & Willett, W. C. (1993). Vitamin E consumption and the risk of coronary heart disease in women. *New England Journal of Medicine, 328,* 1444–1449.

Stampfer, M. J., Hu, F. B., Manson, J. E., Rimm, E. B., & Willett, W. C. (2000). Primary prevention of coronary heart disease in women through diet and lifestyle. *New England Journal of Medicine, 343,* 16–22.

Stanner, S. A., Bulmer, K., Andres, C., Lantseva, O. E., Borodina, V., Poteen, V. V., et al. (1997). Does malnutrition in utero determine diabetes and coronary heart disease in adulthood? Results from the Leningrad siege study, a cross-sectional study. *British Medical Journal, 315,* 1342–1348.

Stanton, A. L. (1987). Determinants of adherence to medical regimens by hypertensive patients. *Journal of Behavioral Medicine, 10,* 377–394.

Stanton, A. L., Collins, C. A., & Sworowski, L. A. (2001). Adjustment to chronic illness: Theory and research. In A. Baum, T. A. Revenson, & J. E. Singer (Eds.), *Handbook of health psychology* (pp. 387–403). Mahwah, NJ: Erlbaum.

Stanton, W. R., Mahalski, P. A., McGee, R., & Silva, P. A. (1993). Reasons for smoking or not smoking in early adolescence. *Addictive Behaviors, 18,* 321–329.

Stason, W., Neff, R., Miettinen, O., & Jick, H. (1976). Alcohol consumption and nonfatal myocardial infarction. *American Journal of Epidemiology, 104,* 603–608.

Steele, C. (1997). A threat in the air: How stereotypes shape intellectual identity and performance. *American Psychologist, 52,* 613–629.

Steele, C. M., & Josephs, R. A. (1990). Alcohol myopia: Its prized and dangerous effects. *American Psychologist, 45,* 921–933.

Steele, C. M., Southwick, L., & Pagano, R. (1986). Drinking your troubles away: The role of activity in mediating alcohol's reduction of psychological stress. *Journal of Abnormal Psychology, 95,* 173–180.

Stein, M. B., Walker, J. R., & Forde, D. R. (2000). Gender differences in susceptibility to posttraumatic stress disorder. *Behaviour Research and Therapy, 38,* 619–628.

Steinhausen, H. C., Winkler, C., & Meier, M. (1997). Eating disorders in adolescence in a Swiss epidemiological study. *International Journal of Eating Disorders, 22,* 147–151.

Steinmaus, C. M., Nuñez, S., & Smith, A. H. (2000). Diet and bladder cancer: A meta-analysis of six dietary variables. *American Journal of Epidemiology, 151,* 693–702.

Steptoe, A., Doherty, S., Kerry, S., Rink, E., & Hilton, S. (2000). Sociodemographic and psychological predictors of change in dietary fat consumption in adults with high blood cholesterol following counseling in primary. *Health Psychology, 19,* 411–419.

Steptoe, A., Kerry, S., Rink, E., & Hilton, S. (2001). The impact of behavioral counseling on stage of change in fat intake, physical activity, and cigarette smoking in adults at increased risk of coronary heart disease. *American Journal of Public Health, 91,* 265–269.

Stevens, J., Cai, J., Pamuk, E. R., Williamson, D. F., Thun, M., & Wood, J. L. (1998). The effect of age on the association between body-mass index and mortality. *New England Journal of Medicine, 338,* 1–7.

Stewart, A., Greenfield, S., Hays, R. D., Wells, K., Rogers, W. H., Berry, S. D., et al. (1989). Functional status and well-being of patients with chronic conditions. *Journal of the American Medical Association, 262,* 907–913.

Stewart, W. F., Lipton, R. B., Celentano, D. D., & Reed, M. L. (1992). Prevalence of migraine headache in the United States. *Journal of the American Medical Association, 267,* 64–69.

Stice, E., & Bearman, S. K. (2001). Body-image and eating disturbances prospectively predict increases in depressive symptoms in adolescent girls: A growth curve analysis. *Developmental Psychology, 37,* 597–607.

Stice, E., Presnell, K., & Spangler, D. (2002). Risk factors for binge eating onset in adolescent girls: A 2-year prospective investigation. *Health Psychology, 21,* 131–138.

Stiffman, A. R., Earls, F., Dore, P., Cunningham, R., & Farber, S. (1996). Adolescent violence. In R. J. Di Clemente, W. B. Hansen, & L. E. Ponton (Eds.), *Handbook of adolescent health risk behavior* (pp. 289–312). New York: Plenum Press.

Stofan, J. R., DiPietro, L., Davis, D., Kohl, H. W., III, & Blair, S. N. (1998). Physical activity patterns associated with cardiorespiratory fitness and reduced mortality: The Aerobics Center Longitudinal Study. *American Journal of Public Health, 88,* 1807–1813.

Stohs, J. H. (2000). Multicultural women's experience of household labor, conflicts, and equity. *Sex Roles, 42,* 339–362.

Stojanovic, M. P. (2001). Stimulation methods for neuropathic pain control. *Current Pain and Headache Reports, 5,* 130–137.

Stokols, D. (1972). On the distinction between density and crowding: Some implications for future research. *Psychological Review, 79,* 275–277.

Stone, A. A., Reed, B. R., & Neale, J. M. (1987). Changes in daily event frequency precedes episodes of physical symptoms. *Journal of Human Stress, 13,* 70–74.

Stone, G. C. (1987). The scope of health psychology. In G. C. Stone, S. M. Weiss, J. D. Matarazzo, N. E. Miller, J. Rodin, C. D. Belar, et al. (Eds.), *Health psychology: A discipline and a profession* (pp. 27–40). Chicago: University of Chicago Press.

Stone, R. (2000). Stress: The invisible hand in eastern Europe's death rates. *Science, 288,* 1732–1733.

Stone, R., Cafferata, G. L., & Sangl, J. (1987). Caregivers of the frail elderly: A national profile. *Gerontologist, 27,* 616–626.

Straif, K., Keil, U., Taeger, D., Holthenrich, D., Sun, Y., Bungers, M., et al. (2000). Exposure to nitrosamines, carbon black, asbestos, and talc and mortality from stomach, lung, and laryngeal cancer in a cohort of rubber workers. *American Journal of Epidemiology, 152,* 297–306.

Strain, E. C., Mumford, G. K., Silverman, K., & Griffiths, R. R. (1994). Caffeine dependence syndrome: Evidence from case histories and experimental evaluation. *Journal of the American Medical Association, 272,* 1043–1047.

Straus, M. A., Gelles, R. J., & Steinmetz, S. K. (1980). *Behind closed doors: Violence in the American family.* Garden City, NY: Anchor.

Strauss, R. S., & Pollack, H. A. (2001). Epidemic increase in childhood overweight, 1986–1998. *Journal of the American Medical Association, 286,* 2845–2848.

Streisand, R., Rodrigue, J. R., Houck, C., Graham-Pole, J., & Berlant, N. (2000). Brief report: Parents of children undergoing bone marrow transplantation: Documenting stress and piloting a psychological intervention program. *Journal of Pediatric Psychology, 25,* 331–337.

Streissguth, A. P., Barr, H. M., Kogan, J., & Bookstein, F. L. (1996). *Understanding the occurrence of secondary disabilities in clients with fetal alcohol syndrome (FAS) and fetal alcohol effects (FAE).* Seattle, WA: University of Washington Publication Services.

Streltzer, J. (1997). Pain. In W. S. Tseng & J. Streltzer (Eds.), *Culture and psychopathology: A guide to clinical assessment* (pp. 87–100). New York: Brunner/Mazel.

Strong, C. A. (1895). The psychology of pain. *Psychological Review, 2,* 329–347.

Stuart, R. B. (1967). Behavioral control of overeating. *Behavior Research and Therapy, 5,* 357–365.

Stunkard, A. J., Harris, J. R., Pedersen, N. L., & McClean, G. E. (1990). The body-mass index of twins who have been reared apart. *New England Journal of Medicine, 322,* 1483–1487.

Stunkard, A. J., Sørensen, T. I. A., Hanis, C., Teasdale, T. W., Chakraborty, R., Schull, W. J., et al. (1986). An adoption study of human obesity. *New England Journal of Medicine, 314,* 193, 198.

Suarez, E. C., Kuhn, C. M., Schanberg, S. M., Williams, R. B., Jr., & Zimmermann, E. A. (1998). Neuroendocrine, cardiovascular, and emotional responses of hostile men: The role of interpersonal challenge. *Psychosomatic Medicine, 60,* 78–88.

Substance Abuse and Mental Health Services Administration (SAMHSA). (2001). *Summary of findings from the 2000 National Household Survey on Drug Abuse.* (DHHS Publication No. 01-3549) Rockville, MD: U.S. Government Printing Office.

Suchman, E. A. (1965). Social patterns of illness and medical care. *Journal of Health and Human Behavior, 6,* 2–16.

Sullum, J., Clark, M. M., & King, T. K. (2000). Predictors of exercise relapse in a college population. *Journal of American College Health, 48,* 175–180.

Sundquist, J., & Winkleby, M. A., (1999). Cardiovascular risk factors in Mexican American adults: A transcultural analysis of NHANES III, 1988–1994. *American Journal of Public Health, 89,* 723–730.

Surwit, R. S., Van Tilburg, M. A. L., Zucker, N., McCaskill, C. C., Parekh, P., Feinglos, M. N., et al. (2002). Stress management improves long-term glycemic control in type 2 diabetes. *Diabetes Care, 25,* 30–34.

Susser, M. (1991). What is a cause and how do we know one? A grammar for pragmatic epidemiology. *American Journal of Epidemiology, 133,* 635–648.

Sutton, S., McVey, D., & Glanz, A. (1999). A comparative test of the theory of reasoned action and the theory of planned behavior in the prediction of condom use intentions in a national sample of English young people. *Health Psychology, 18,* 72–81.

Syrjala, K. L., & Abrams, J. (1999). Cancer pain. In R. J. Gatchel & D. C. Turk (Eds.) *Psychosocial factors in pain: Critical perspectives* (pp. 301–314). New York: Guilford Press.

Syrjala, K. L., & Chapman, C. R. (1984). Measurement of clinical pain: A review and integration of research findings. In C. Benedetti, C. R. Chapman, & G. Moricca (Eds.), *Advances in pain research and therapy: Vol. 7. Recent advances in the management of pain.* New York: Raven Press.

Takkouche, B., Regueira, C., & Gestal-Otero, J. J. (2001). A cohort study of stress and the common cold. *Epidemiology, 12,* 345–349.

Tang, J. -L., Morris, J. K., Wald, N. J., Hole, D., Shipley, M., & Tunstall-Pedoe, H. (1995). Mortality in relation to tar yield of cigarettes: A prospective study of four cohorts. *British Medical Journal, 311,* 1530–1533.

Tang, M. -X., Stem, Y., Marder, K., Bell, K., Gurland, B., Lantigua, R., et al. (1998). The APOE-e4 allele and the risk of Alzheimer disease among African Americans, whites, and Hispanics. *Journal of the American Medical Association, 279,* 751–755.

Tanji, J. L. (1997). Sports medicine. *Journal of the American Medical Association, 277,* 1901–1902.

Tanner, E. K. W., & Feldman, R. H. L. (1997). Strategies for enhancing appointment keeping in low-income chronically ill clients. *Nursing Research, 46,* 342–344.

Taylor, E., Briner, R. B., & Folkard, S. (1997). Models of shiftwork and health: An examination of the influence of stress on shiftwork theory. *Human Factors, 39,* 67–82.

Taylor, S. E., Klein, L. C., Lewis, B. P., Gruenewald, T. L., Gurung, R. A. R., & Updegraff, J. A. (2000). Biobehavioral responses to stress in females: Tend-and-befriend, not fight-or-flight. *Psychological Review, 107,* 411–429.

Taylor, S. E., Repetti, R. L., & Seeman, T. (1997). Health psychology: What is an unhealthy environment and how does it get under the skin? *Annual Review of Psychology, 48,* 411–447.

Taylor, S. P., & Leonard, K. E. (1983). Alcohol and human physical aggression. In R. G. Geen & E. I. Donnerstein (Eds.), *Aggression: Theoretical and empirical reviews* (Vol. 2, pp. 77–101). New York: Academic Press.

ten Bensel, R. W., Rheinberger, M. M., & Radbill, S. X. (1997). Children in a world of violence: The roots of child maltreatment. In M. E. Helfer, R. S. Kempe, & R. D. Krugman (Eds.), *The battered child* (5th ed., pp. 3–28). Chicago: University of Chicago Press.

Tennant, C. (2001). Work-related stress and depressive disorders. *Journal of Psychosomatic Research, 51,* 697–704.

Tennen, H., Affleck, G., Armeli, S., & Carney, M. A. (2000). A daily process approach to coping: Linking theory, research, and practice. *American Psychologist, 55,* 626–636.

ter-Kuile, M. M., Spinhoven, P., Linssen, A., Corry, G., Zitman, F. G., & Rooijmans, H. G. M. (1994). Autogenic training and cognitive self-hypnosis for the treatment of recurrent headaches in three different subject groups. *Pain, 58,* 331–340.

Terry, P., Hu, F. B., Hansen, H., & Wolk, A. (2001). Prospective study of major dietary patterns and colorectal cancer risk in women. *American Journal of Epidemiology, 154,* 1143–1149.

Testa, M., & Leonard, K. E. (2001). The impact of marital aggression on women's psychological and marital functioning in a newlywed sample. *Journal of Family Violence, 16,* 115–130.

Thayer, R. E., Newman, J. R., & McClain, T. M. (1994). Self-regulation of mood: Strategies for changing a bad mood, raising energy, and reducing tension. *Journal of Personality and Social Psychology, 67,* 910–925.

Thomas, E. J., Studdert, M., Newhouse, J. P., Zbar, B. I. W., Howard, M., Williams, E. J., et al. (1999). Costs of medical injuries in Utah and Colorado. *Inquiry, 36,* 255–264.

Thomas, V., Gruen, R., & Shu, S. (2001). Cognitive-behavioral therapy for the management of sickle cell disease pain: Identification and assessment of costs. *Ethnicity and Health, 6,* 59–67.

Thomas, W., White, C. M., Mah, J., Geisser, M. S., Church, T. R., & Mandel, J. S. (1995). Longitudinal compliance with annual screening for fecal occult blood. *American Journal of Epidemiology, 142,* 176–182.

Thompson, D. C., Rivara, F. P., & Thompson, R. S. (1996). Effectiveness of bicycle safety helmets in preventing head injuries: A case-control study. *Journal of the American Medical Association, 276,* 1968–1973.

Thompson, M. J., & Rivara, F. P. (2001). Bicycle-related injuries. *American Family Physician, 63,* 2007–2016.

Thompson, P. D. (2001, January). Exercise rehabilitation for cardiac patients: A beneficial but underused therapy. *The Physician and Sportsmedicine, 29,* 69–75.

Thompson, R. A., & Sherman, R. T. (1993). *Helping athletes with eating disorders.* Champaign, IL: Human Kinetics Publishers.

Thorn, B., & Saab, P. (2001). Notes from the APS Council of Representatives (CoR) Meeting. *Health Psychologist, 23*(3), 5, 8.

Thorndike, A. N., Biener, L., & Rigotti, N. A., (2002). Effect on smoking cessation of switching nicotine replacement therapy to over-the-counter status. *American Journal of Public Health, 92,* 437–442.

Thun, M. J., Day-Lally, C. A., Calle, E. E., Flanders, W. D., & Heath, C. W., Jr. (1995). Excess mortality among cigarette smokers: Changes in a 20-year interval. *American Journal of Public Health, 85,* 1223–1230.

Thune, I., Brenn, T., Lund, E., & Gaard, M. (1997). Physical activity and the risk of breast cancer. *New England Journal of Medicine, 336,* 1269–1275.

Thune, I., & Furberg, A. S. (2001). Physical activity and cancer risk: Dose-response and cancer, all sites and site-specific. *Medicine and Science in Sports and Exercise, 33,* S530–S550.

Tice, D. M., Bratslavsky, E., & Baumeister, R. F. (2001). Emotional distress regulation takes precedence over impulse control: If you feel bad, do it! *Journal of Personality and Social Psychology, 80,* 53–67.

Tomar, S. L., & Giovino, G. A. (1998). Incidence and predictors of smokeless tobacco use among U.S. youth. *American Journal of Public Health, 88,* 20–26.

Tomeo, C. A., Field, A. E., Berkey, C. S., Colditz, G. A., & Frazier, A. L. (1999). Weight concerns, weight control behaviors, and smoking initiation. *Pediatrics, 104,* 918–924.

Toniolo, P., Riboli, E., Protta, F., Charrel, M., & Coppa, A. P. (1989). Calorie-providing nutrients and risk of breast cancer. *Journal of the National Cancer Institute, 81,* 278–286.

Toobert, D. J., & Glasgow, R. E. (1991). Problem solving and diabetes self-care. *Journal of Behavioral Medicine, 14,* 71–86.

Towner, E., Dowswell, T., & Jarvis, S. (2001). Updating the evidence: A systematic review of what works in preventing childhood unintentional injuries: Part 2. *Injury Prevention, 7,* 249–253.

Tracey, E. (2001). Prostate cancer trial to test preventive agents. *Family Practice News, 13,* 8–9.

Tramer, M. R., Carroll, D., Campbell, F. A., Reynolds, D. J. M., Moore, R. A., & McQuay, H. J. (2001). Cannabinoids for control of chemotherapy induced nausea and vomiting: Quantitative systematic review. *British Medical Journal, 323,* 16–20.

Travis, L. (2001). Training for interdisciplinary healthcare. *Health Psychologist, 23* (1), 4–5.

Treiber, F. A., Davis, H., Musante, L., Raunikar, R. A., Strong. W. G., McCaffrey, F., et al. (1993). Ethnicity, gender, family history of myocardial infarction, and menodynamic responses to laboratory stressors in children. *Health Psychology, 12,* 6–15.

Tsoh, J. Y., McClure, J. B., Skaar, K. L., Wetter, D. W., Cinciripini, P. M., Prokhorov, A. V., et al. (1997).

Smoking cessation 2: Components of effective intervention, *Behavioral Medicine, 23,* 15–27.

Tucker, J. S., Orlando, M., & Ellickson, P. L. (2003). Patterns and correlates of binge drinking trajectories form early adolescence to young adulthood. *Health Psychology, 22,* 79–87.

Tucker, L. A. (1989). Use of smokeless tobacco, cigarette smoking, and hypercholesterolemia. *American Journal of Public Health, 79,* 1048–1050.

Turk, D. C. (1978). Cognitive behavioral techniques in the management of pain. In J. P. Foreyt & D. P. Rathjen (Eds.), *Cognitive behavior therapy.* New York: Plenum Press.

Turk, D. C. (2001). Physiological and psychological bases of pain. In A. Baum, T. A. Revenson, & J. E. Singer (Eds.), *Handbook of health psychology* (pp. 117–131). Mahwah, NJ: Erlbaum.

Turk, D. C., & Feldman, C. S. (2001). A cognitive-behavioral approach to symptom management in palliative care: Augmenting somatic interventions. In H. Chochinov & W. Breibart (Eds.), *Handbook of psychiatry in palliative medicine* (pp. 223–239). New York: Oxford University Press.

Turk, D. C., Meichenbaum, D., & Genest, M. (1983). *Pain and behavioral medicine: A cognitive behavioral perspective.* New York: Guilford Press.

Turk, D. C., & Melzack, R. (2001). The measurement of pain and the assessment of people experiencing pain. In D. C. Turk & R. Melzack (Eds.), *Handbook of pain assessment* (2nd ed., pp. 3–11). New York: Guilford Press.

Turk, D. C., & Rudy, T. E. (1988). Toward an empirically derived taxonomy of chronic pain patients: Integration of psychological assessment data. *Journal of Consulting and Counseling Psychology, 56,* 233–238.

Turk, D. C., Sist, T. C., Okifuji, A., Miner, M. F., Florio, G., Harrison, P., et al. (1998). Adaptation to metastatic cancer pain, regional/local cancer pain and non-cancer pain: Role of psychological and behavioral factors. *Pain, 74,* 247–256.

Turner, J., & Kelly, B. (2000). Emotional dimensions of chronic disease. *Western Journal of Medicine, 172,* 124–128.

Turner, J. A., & Chapman, C. R. (1982). Psychological interventions for chronic pain: A critical review. II: Operant conditioning, hypnosis, and cognitive-behavior therapy. *Pain, 12,* 23–46.

Turner, J. A., & Clancy, S. (1988). Comparison of operant behavioral and cognitive-behavioral group treatment for chronic low back pain. *Journal of Consulting and Clinical Psychology, 56,* 261–266.

Turner, J. A., Deyo, R. A., Loeser, J. D., Von Korff, M., & Fordyce, W. E. (1994). The importance of placebo effects in pain treatment and research. *Journal of the American Medical Association, 271,* 1609–1614.

Turner, R. J., & Wheaton, B. (1995). Checklist measurement of stressful life events. In S., Cohen, R. C. Kessler, & L. U. Gordon (Eds.), *Measuring stress: A guide for health and social scientists* (pp. 29–58). New York: Oxford University Press.

Tusek, D., Church, J. M., & Fazio, V. W. (1997). Guided imagery as a coping strategy for preoperative patients. *AORN, 66,* 644–649.

Twisk, J. W. R., Kemper, H. C. G., van Mechelen, W., & Post, G. B. (1997). Tracking of risk factors for coronary heart disease over a 14-year period: A comparison between lifestyle and biologic risk factors with data from the Amsterdam Growth and Health Study. *American Journal of Epidemiology, 145,* 688–696.

Tylka, T. L., & Subich, L. M. (2002). Exploring young women's perceptions of the effectiveness and safety of maladaptive weight control techniques. *Journal of Counseling and Development, 80,* 101–110.

Uchino, B. N., & Garvey, T. S. (1997). The availability of social support reduces cardiovascular reactivity to acute psychological stress. *Journal of Behavioral Medicine, 20,* 15–27.

Unger, J. B., Boley Cruz, T., Rohrbach, L. A., Ribisl, K. M., Baezconde-Garbanati, L., Chen, X., et al. (2000). English language use as a risk factor for smoking initiation among Hispanic and Asian American adolescents: Evidence for mediation by tobacco-related beliefs and social norms. *Health Psychology, 19,* 403–410.

Uryu, K., Laurer, H., McIntosh, T., Pratico, D., Martinez, D., Leight, S., et al. (2002). Repetitive mild brain trauma accelerates Ab deposition, lipid peroxidation and cognitive impairment in a transgenic mouse model of Alzheimer amyloidosis. *Journal of Neuroscience, 22,* 446–454.

U.S. Bureau of the Census (USBC). (1975). *Historical statistics of the United States: Colonial times to 1970, Part 1.* Washington, DC: U.S. Government Printing Office.

U.S. Bureau of the Census (USBC). (1997). *Statistical abstracts of the United States: 1997* (117th ed.). Washington, DC: U.S. Government Printing Office.

U.S. Bureau of the Census (USBC). (2001). *Statistical abstracts of the United States: 2001* (122nd ed.). Washington, DC: U.S. Government Printing Office.

U.S. Department of Health and Human Services (USDHHS). (1989). *Reducing the health consequences of smoking: 25 years of progress. A report of the Surgeon General* (DHHS Publication No. CDC 89-8411). Rockville, MD: U.S. Government Printing Office.

U.S. Department of Health and Human Services (USDHHS). (1990). *The health benefits of smoking cessation: A report of the Surgeon General* (DHHS Publication No. CDC 90-8416). Washington, DC: U.S. Government Printing Office.

U.S. Department of Health and Human Services (USDHHS). (1991). *Healthy people 2000: National health promotion and disease prevention objectives.* (PHS Publication No. 91-50212). Washington, DC: Author.

U.S. Department of Health and Human Services (USDHHS). (1995). *Healthy People 2000 review, 1994* (DHHS Publication No. PHS 95–1256–1). Washington, DC: U.S. Government Printing Office.

U.S. Department of Health and Human Services (USDHHS). (1996). *Physical activity and health: A report of the Surgeon General.* Atlanta, GA: Centers for Disease Control and Prevention.

U.S. Department of Health and Human Services (USDHHS). (2000). *Healthy People 2010: Understanding and improving health (2nd ed.).* Washington, DC: U.S. Government Printing Office.

U.S. Department of Health and Human Services (USDHHS). (2001). *National strategy for suicide prevention: Goals and objectives for action.* Rockville, MD: U.S. Department of Health and Human Services.

U.S. Department of Health and Human Services (USDHHS) Administration on Children, Youth, and Families. (2001). *Child maltreatment 1999.* Washington, DC: U.S. Government Printing Office.

U.S. Department of Health and Human Services (USDHHS). (2002). Report details national health care spending increases in 2000. *Health Care Financing Review, 23,* 165–166.

U.S. Public Health Service (USPHS). (1964). *Smoking and health: Public Health Service report of the Advisory Committee to the Surgeon General of the Public Health Service* (PHS Publication No. 1103). Washington, DC: U.S. Government Printing Office.

Vaccarino, V., Parsons, P., Every, N. R., Barron, H. V., & Krumholz, H. M. (1999). Sex-based differences in early mortality after myocardial infarction. *New England Journal of Medicine, 341,* 217–225.

van Assema, P., Pieterse, M., Kok, G., Eriksen, M., & de Vries, H. (1993). The determinants of four cancer-related risk behaviours. *Health Education Research, 8,* 461–472.

Van Buyten, J. P., Van Zundert, J., Vueghs, P., & Vanduffel, L. (2001). Efficacy of spinal cord stimulation: 10 years of experience in a pain centre in Belgium. *European Journal of Pain, 5,* 299–307.

van den Hoogen, P. C. W., Feskens, E. J. M., Nagelkerke, N. J. D., Menotti, A., Nissinen, A., & Krombout, D. (2000). The relation between blood pressure and mortality due to coronary heart disease among men in different parts of the world. *New England Journal of Medicine, 342,* 1–7.

van der Doef, M., & Maes, S. (1999). The job demand-control (support) model and psychological well-being: A review of 20 years of empirical research. *Work and Stress, 13,* 87–114.

Van der Does, A. J., & Van Dyck, R. (1989). Does hypnosis contribute to the care of burn patients? Review of evidence. *General Hospital Psychiatry, 11,* 119–124.

Van der Kooy, K., Rookus, M. A., Verloop, J., Van Leeuwen, F. E., & Peterse, H. (2001). Physical activity and breast cancer risk. *American Journal of Epidemiology, 153,* S110.

van Lenthe, F. J., van Mechelen, W., Kemper, H. C. G., & Twisk, J. W. R. (1998). Association of a central pattern of body fat with blood pressure and lipoproteins from adolescence into adulthood. *American Journal of Epidemiology, 147,* 686–693.

van Ryn, M., & Burke, J. (2000). The effect of patient race and socio-economic status on physicians' perception of patients. *Social Science and Medicine, 50,* 813–828.

Vartiainen, E., Paavola, M., McAlister, A., & Puska, P. (1998). Fifteen-year follow-up of smoking prevention effects in the North Karelia Youth Project. *American Journal of Public Health, 88,* 81–85.

Vastag, B. (2001). Quitting smoking harder for women. *Journal of the American Medical Association, 285,* 2966.

Veldtman, G. R., Matley, S. L., Kendall, L., Quirk, J., Gibbs, J. L., Parsons, J. M., et al. (2001). Illness understanding in children and adolescents with heart disease. *Western Journal of Medicine, 174,* 171–173.

Vendrig, A. A. (1999). Prognostic factors and treatment-related changes associated with return to work in the multimodal treatment of chronic back pain. *Journal of Behavioral Medicine, 22,* 217–232.

Vendrig, A. A., Derksen, J. J., & de Mey, H. R. (1999). Utility of selected MMPI-2 scales in the outcome prediction for patients with chronic back pain. *Psychological Assessment, 11,* 381–385.

Vermeulen, M., & Mustard, C. (2000). Gender differences in job strain, social support at work, and psychological distress. *Journal of Occupational Health Psychology, 5,* 428–440.

Vervialle, P. F., Le Breton, P., Taillard, J., & Home, J. A. (2001). Fatigue, alcohol, and serious road crashes in France: Factorial study of national data. *British Medical Journal, 322,* 829–830.

Vincent, P. (1971). Factors influencing patient noncompliance: A theoretical approach. *Nursing Research, 20,* 509–516.

Vineis, P., Schulte, P., & McMichael, A. J. (2001). Misconceptions about the use of genetic tests in populations. *Lancet, 357,* 709–712.

Virmani, R., Burke, A. P., & Farb, A. (2001). Sudden cardiac death. *Cardiovascular Pathology, 10,* 211–218.

Visscher, T. L. S., Seidell, J. C., Menotti, A., Blackburn, H., Nissinen, A., Feskens, E. J. M., et al. (2000). Underweight and overweight in relation to mortality among men aged 40–59 and 50–69. *American Journal of Epidemiology, 151,* 660–666.

Visser, M. (1999). Food and culture: Interconnections. *Social Research, 66,* 117–132.

Vita, A. J., Terry, R. B., Hubert, H. B., & Fries, J. F. (1998). Aging, health risks, and cumulative disability. *New England Journal of Medicine, 338,* 1035–1041.

Voegele, C., Jarvis, A., & Cheeseman, K. (1997). Anger suppression, reactivity, and hypertension risk: Gender makes a difference. *Annals of Behavioral Medicine, 19,* 61–69.

Voelker, R. (1998). A "family heirloom" turns 50. *Journal of the American Medical Association, 279,* 1241–1245.

Von Korff, M., Barlow, W., Cherkin, D., & Deyo, R. A. (1994). Effects of practice style in managing back pain. *Annals of Internal Medicine, 121,* 187–195.

Wadden, T. A., Brownell, K. D., & Foster, G. D. (2002). Obesity: Responding to the global epidemic. *Journal of Consulting and Clinical Psychology, 70,* 510–525.

Wagenaar, A. C., O'Malley, P. M., & LaFond, C. (2001). Lowered legal blood alcohol limits for young drivers: Effects on drinking, driving, and driving-after-drinking behaviors in 30 states. *American Journal of Public Health, 91,* 801–803.

Waldstein, S. R., Burns, H. O., Toth, M. J., & Poehlman, E. T. (1999). Cardiovascular reactivity and central adiposity in older African Americans. *Health Psychology, 18,* 221–228.

Walen, H. R., & Lachman, M. E. (2000). Social support and strain from partner, family, and friends: Costs and benefits for men and women in adulthood. *Journal of Social and Personal Relationships, 17,* 5–30.

Wall, P. (2000). *Pain: The science of suffering.* New York: Columbia University Press.

Walsh, D. M. (1997). *TENS: Clinical applications and related theory.* New York: Churchill Livingstone.

Walsh, J. M. E., & Grady, D. (1995). Treatment of hyperlipidemia in women. *Journal of the American Medical Association, 274,* 1152–1158.

Walter, L., & Brannon, L. (1991). A cluster analysis of the Multidimensional Pain Inventory. *Headache, 31,* 476–479.

Walters, G. D. (2000). Spontaneous remission from alcohol, tobacco, and other drug abuse: Seeking quantitative answers to qualitative questions. *American Journal of Drug and Alcohol Abuse, 26,* 443–460.

Wamala, S. P., Mittleman, M. A., Horsten, M., Schenck-Gustafsson, K., & Orth-Gomér, K. (2000). Job stress and the occupational gradient in coronary heart disease risk in women: The Stockholm Female Coronary Risk study. *Social Science and Medicine, 51,* 481–489.

Wang, H., & Amato, P. R. (2000). Predictors of divorce adjustment: Stressors, resources, and definitions. *Journal of Marriage and the Family, 62,* 655–668.

Wang, X., Gao, L., Shinfuku, N., Zhang, H., Zhao, C., & Shen, Y. (2000). Longitudinal study of earthquake-related PTSD in a randomly selected community sample in North China. *American Journal of Psychiatry, 157,* 1260–1266.

Wannamethee, S. G., Shaper, A. G., & Alberti, G.M.M. (2000). Physical activity protects against diabetes and heart disease. *Geriatrics, 35,* 78.

Wannamethee, S. G., Shaper, A. G., Whincup, P. H., & Walker, M. (2000). Characteristics of older men who lose weight intentionally and unintentionally. *American Journal of Epidemiology, 151,* 667–675.

Warnecke, R. B., Morera, O., Turner, L., Mermelstein, R., Johnson, T. P., Parsons, J., et al. (2001). Changes in self-efficacy and readiness for smoking cessation among women with high school or less education. *Journal of Health and Social Behavior, 42,* 97–110.

Wartenberg, D., Calle, E. E., Thun, M. J., Heath, C. W., Jr., Lally, C., & Woodruff, T. (2000). Passive smoking exposure and female breast cancer mortality. *Journal of the National Cancer Institute, 92,* 1666–1673.

Washington, D. L. (2001). Charting the path from lack of insurance to poor health outcomes. *Western Journal of Medicine, 175,* 23.

Watanabe, M. E. (2002, April). Genes do play a role in obesity for some people, overeating is not the only culprit. *The Scientist, 16*(9), 22–23.

Watkins, L. R., & Maier, S. F. (2000). The pain of being sick: Implications of immune-to-brain communication for understanding pain. *Annual Review of Psychology, 51,* 29–59.

Watkins, L. R., Milligan, E. D., & Maier, S. F. (2001). Glial activation: A driving force for pathological pain. *Trends in Neurosciences, 24,* 450–455.

Watson, T. L., Bowers, W. A., & Andersen, A. E. (2000). Involuntary treatment of eating disorders. *American Journal of Psychiatry, 157,* 1806–1810.

Webster, D. W., Gainer, P. S., & Champion, H. P. (1993). Weapon carrying among inner-city junior high school students: Defensive behavior vs aggressive delinquency. *American Journal of Public Health, 83,* 1604–1608.

Webster, D. W., & Starnes, M. (2000). Reexamining the association between child access prevention gun laws and unintentional shooting deaths of children. *Pediatrics, 106,* 1466–1469.

Wechsler, H., Lee, J. E., Kuo, M., Seibring, M., Nelson, T. F., & Lee, H. (2002). Trends in college binge drinking during a period of increased prevention efforts: Findings for 4 Harvard School of Public Health College Alcohol Study surveys: 1993–2001. *Journal of American College Health, 50,* 203–217.

Wee, C. C., Rigotti, N. A., Davis, R. B., & Phillips, R. S. (2001). Relationship between smoking and weight control efforts among adults in the United States. *Archives of Internal Medicine, 161,* 546–550.

Weidner, G. (2000). Why do men get more heart disease than women? An international perspective. *Journal of American College Health, 48,* 291–296.

Weil, C. M., Wade, S. L., Bauman, L. J., Lynn, H., Mitchell. H., & Lavigne, J. (1999). The relationship between psychosocial factors and asthma morbidity in inner-city children with asthma. *Pediatrics, 104,* 1274–1280.

Weiner, H., & Shapiro, A. P. (2001). *Helicobacter pylori,* immune function, and gastric lesions. In R. Ader, D. L. Felten, & N. Cohen (Eds.), *Psychoneuroimmunology* (3rd ed., Vol. 2, pp. 671–686). San Diego, CA: Academic Press.

Weinstein, N. D. (1980). Unrealistic optimism about future life events. *Journal of Personality and Social Psychology, 39,* 806–820.

Weinstein, N. D. (1983). Reducing unrealistic optimism about illness susceptibility. *Health Psychology, 2,* 11–20.

Weinstein, N. D. (1984). Why it won't happen to me: Perceptions of risk factors and susceptibility. *Health Psychology, 3,* 431–457.

Weinstein, N. D. (1988). The precaution adoption process. *Health Psychology, 7,* 355–386.

Weinstein, N. D. (2000). Perceived probability, perceived severity, and health-protective behavior. *Health Psychology, 19,* 65–74.

Weinstein, N. D. (2001). Smokers' recognition of their vulnerability to harm. In P. Slovic (Ed.), *Smoking: Risk, perception & policy* (pp. 81–96). Twin Oaks, CA: Sage.

Weisner, C., Greenfield, T., & Room, R. (1995). Trends in the treatment of alcohol problems in the US general population, 1979 through 1990. *American Journal of Public Health, 85,* 55–60.

Weisner, C., & Schmidt, L. (1992). Gender disparities in treatment for alcohol problems. *Journal of the American Medical Association, 228,* 1872–1876.

Weiss, R. (1999, November 30). Medical errors blamed for many deaths; as many as 98,00 a year in US linked to mistakes. *The Washington Post,* p. A1.

Weitz, R. (2001). *The sociology of health, illness, and health care: A critical approach* (2nd ed.). Belmont, CA: Wadsworth.

Welch, S. L., Doll, H. A., & Fairburn, C. G. (1997). Life events and the onset of bulimia nervosa: A controlled study. *Psychological Medicine, 27,* 515–522.

Werner, R. M., & Pearson, T. A. (1998). What's so passive about passive smoking? Secondhand smoke as a cause of atherosclerotic disease. *Journal of the American Medical Association, 179,* 157–158.

Wertlieb, D. L., Jacobson, A., & Hauser, S. (1990). The child with diabetes: A developmental stress and coping perspective. In *Psychological aspects of serious illness: Chronic conditions, fatal diseases, and clinical care* (pp. 61–101). Washington, DC: American Psychological Association.

Wesch, D., Lutzker, J. R., Frisch, L., & Dillon, M. M. (1987). Evaluating the impact of a service fee on patient compliance. *Journal of Behavioral Medicine, 10,* 91–101.

Wetter, D. W., Fiore, M. C., Gritz, E. R., Lando, H. A., Stitzer, M. L., Hasselblad, V., et al. (1998). The Agency for Health Care Policy and Research Smoking Cessation Clinical Practice Guideline: Findings and implications for psychologists. *American Psychologist, 53,* 657–669.

Wetzel, F. T., Phillips, F. M., Aprill, C. N., Bernard, T. N., Jr., & LaRocca, H. S. (1997). Extradural sensory rhizotomy in the management of chronic lumbar radiculopathy: A minimum 2-year follow-up study. *Spine, 22,* 2283–2291.

Whincup, P., Cook, D., Papacosta, O., & Walker, M. (1995). Birth weight and blood pressure: Cross sectional and longitudinal relations in childhood. *British Medical Journal, 311,* 773–776.

Whitemore, A. S., Perlin, S. A., & DiCiccio, Y. (1995). Chronic obstructive pulmonary disease in lifetime nonsmokers: Results from NHANES. *American Journal of Public Health, 85,* 702–706.

Whitfield, K. E., Weidner, G., Clark, R., & Anderson, N. B. (2002). Sociodemographic diversity in behavioral medicine. *Journal of Consulting and Clinical Psychology, 70,* 463–481.

Wiens, A. N., & Menustik, C. E. (1983). Treatment outcome and patient characteristics in an aversion therapy program for alcoholism. *American Psychologist, 38,* 1089–1096.

Wiley, J. A., & Camacho, T. C. (1980). Life-style and future health: Evidence from the Alameda County Study. *Preventive Medicine, 9,* 1–21.

Williams, B. K., & Knight, S. M. (1994). *Healthy for life: Wellness and the art of living.* Pacific Grove, CA: Brooks/Cole.

Williams, Paul, & Dickinson, J. (1993). Fear of crime: Read all about it? The relationship between newspaper crime reporting and fear of crime. *British Journal of Criminology, 33,* 33–56.

Williams, P. G., Holmbeck, G. N., & Greenley, R. N. (2002). Adolescent health psychology. *Journal of Consulting and Clinical Psychology, 70,* 828–842.

Williams, P. T. (2001). Health effects resulting from exercise verses those from body fat loss. *Medicine and Science in Sports and Exercise, 33,* S611–S621.

Williams, R. B., Jr. (1989). *The trusting heart: Great news about type A behavior.* New York: Times Books.

Williams, R. B., Jr., Barefoot, J. C., Califf, R. M., Haney, T. L., Saunders, W. B., Pryor, D. B., et al. (1992). Prognostic importance of social and economic resources among medically treated patients with angiographically documented coronary artery disease. *Journal of the American Medical Association, 267,* 520–524.

Williamson, D. A., Thaw, J. M., & Varnado-Sullivan, P. J. (2001). Cost-effectiveness analysis of a hospital-based cognitive-behavioral treatment program for eating disorders. *Behavior Therapy, 32,* 459–470.

Williamson, D. F., & Pamuk, E. R. (1993). The association between weight loss and increased longevity: A review of the evidence. *Annals of Internal Medicine, 119,* 731–736.

Wills, T. A. (1998). Social support. In E. A. Blechman & K. D. Brownell (Eds.), *Behavioral medicine and women: A comprehensive handbook* (pp. 118–128). New York: Guilford Press.

Wilson, G. T., Fairburn, C. C., Agras, W. S., Walsh, B. T., & Kraemer, H. (2002). Cognitive-behavioral therapy for bulimia nervosa: Time course and mechanisms of change. *Journal of Consulting and Clinical Psychology, 70,* 267–274.

Wilson, J. F. (2001, October 29). Pain research comes into its own: Molecular biology may provide answers to relief. *The Scientist, 15*(21), 16–17.

Wilson, R. S., Mendes de Leon, C. F., Barnes, L. L., Schneider, J. A., Bienias, J. L., Evans, D. A., et al. (2002). Participation in cognitively stimulating activities and risk of incident Alzheimer disease. *Journal of the American Medical Association, 287,* 742–748.

Windle, M., & Windle, R. C. (2001). Depressive symptoms and cigarette smoking among middle adolescents: Prospective associations and intrapersonal and interpersonal influences. *Journal of Consulting and Clinical Psychology, 2001, 69,* 215–226.

Wing, R. R., & Polley, B. A. (2001). Obesity. In A. Baum, T. A. Revenson, & J. E. Singer (Eds.), *Handbook of health psychology* (pp. 263–279). Mahwah, NJ: Erlbaum.

Wingard, D. L., Berkman, L. F., & Brand, R. J. (1982). A multivariate analysis of health-related practices: A nine-year mortality follow-up of the Alameda County study. *American Journal of Epidemiology, 116,* 765–775.

Winkleby, M. A., Robinson, T. N., Sundquist, J., & Kraemer, H. C. (1999). Ethnic variation in cardiovascular disease risk factors among children and young adults: Findings from the third National Health and Nutrition Examination survey, 1988–1994. *Journal of the American Medical Association, 281,* 1006–1013.

Winter, R. (1994, September-October). Which pain relievers work best? *Consumers Digest, 33,* 76–79.

Wisborg, K., Kesmodel, U., Henriksen, T. B., Olsen, S. F., & Secher, N. J. (2001). Exposure to tobacco smoke in utero and the risk of stillbirth and death in the first year of life. *American Journal of Epidemiology, 154,* 322–327.

Wise, J. (2000). Largest-ever study shows reduction in cardiovascular mortality. *Bulletin of the World Health Organization, 78,* 562.

Wiseman, C. V., Gray, J. J., Mosimann, J. E., & Ahrens, A. H. (1992). Cultural expectations of thinness in women: An update. *International Journal of Eating Disorders, 11,* 85–89.

Witkin, G., Tharp, M., Schrof, J. M., Toch, T., & Scattarella, C. (1998, June 1). Again: School shooting in Springfield, Oregon. *U.S. News & World Report, 124,* 16–19.

Wofford, J. C. (2001). Cognitive-affective stress response: Effects of individual stress propensity on physiological and psychological indicators of strain. *Psychological Reports, 88,* 768–784.

Wolfgang, M. E. (1957). Victim precipitated criminal homicide. *Journal of Criminal Law and Criminology, 48,* 1–11.

Wolk, A., Manson, J. E., Stampfer, M. J., Colditz, G. A., Hu, F. B., Speizer, F. E., et al. (1999). Long-term intake of dietary fiber and decreased risk of coronary heart disease among women. *Journal of the American Medical Association, 281,* 1998–2004.

Wonderlich, S. A., Brewerton, T. D., Jocic, Z., Dansky, B. S., & Abbott, D. W. (1997). Relationships of childhood sexual abuse and eating disorders. *Journal of the American Academy of Child and Adolescent Psychiatry, 36,* 1107–1113.

Wonderlich, S. A., Wilsnack, R. W., Wilsnack, S. C., & Harris, T. R. (1996). Childhood sexual abuse and bulimic behavior in a nationally representative sample. *American Journal of Public Health, 86,* 1082–1086.

Wood, P. D., Stefanick, M. L., Dreon, D. M., Frey-Hewitt, B., Garay, S. C., Williams, P. T., et al. (1988). Changes in plasma lipids and lipoproteins in overweight men during weight loss through dieting compared with exercise. *New England Journal of Medicine, 319,* 1173–1179.

Woods, S. C., Schwartz, M. W., Baskin, D. G., & Seeley, R. J. (2000). Food intake and the regulation of body weight. *Annual Review of Psychology, 51,* 255–278.

Wright, L. K. (1997). Health behavior of caregivers. In D. S. Gochman (Ed.), *Handbook of health behavior research III: Demography, development, and diversity* (pp. 267–284). New York: Plenum Press.

Writing Group for the Women's Health Initiative Investigators. (2002). Risks and benefits of estrogen plus progestin in healthy postmenopausal women: Principal results from the Women's Health Initiative randomized controlled trial. *Journal of the American Medical Association, 288,* 321–333.

Wu, J. M. (1990). Summary and concluding remarks. In J. M. Wu (Ed.), *Environmental tobacco smoke: Proceedings of the international symposium at McGill University 1989* (pp. 367–375). Lexington, MA: Heath.

Wyden, P. (1965). *The overweight society.* New York: Morrow.

Wylie-Rosett, J. (1998). Diabetes: Medical aspects. In E. A. Blechman & K. D. Brownell (Eds.), *Behavioral medicine and women: A comprehensive handbook* (pp. 623–627). New York: Guilford Press.

Wysocki, T., Harris, M. A., Greco, P., Harvey, L. M., McDonell, D., Danda, C. L. E., et al. (1997). Social validity of support group and behavior therapy interventions for families of adolescents with insulin-dependent diabetes mellitus. *Journal of Pediatric Psychology, 22,* 635–649.

Yaari, S., & Goldbourt, U. (1998). Voluntary and involuntary weight loss: Associations with long term mortality in 9,228 middle-aged and elderly men. *American Journal of Epidemiology, 148,* 546–555.

Yano, E., Wang, Z. M., Wang, X. R., Wang, M. Z., & Lan, Y. J. (2001). Cancer mortality among workers exposed to amphibole-free chrysotile, asbestos. *American Journal of Epidemiology, 154,* 538–543.

Yarnold, P. R., Michelson, E. A., Thompson, D. A., & Adams, S. L. (1998). Predicting patient satisfaction: A study of two emergency departments. *Journal of Behavioral Medicine, 21,* 545–563.

Yates, A., Leehey, K., & Shisslak, C. M. (1983). Running—an analogue of anorexia? *New England Journal of Medicine, 308,* 251–255.

Yi, H., Williams, G. D., & Dufour, M. C. (2001). Trends in alcohol-related fatal traffic crashes, United States, 1977–99. *Alcohol Epidemiologic Data System. Surveillance Report #56.* Rockville, MD: National Institute on Alcohol Abuse and Alcoholism.

Yong, L. C., Brown, C. C., Schatzkin, A., Dresser, C. M., Siesinski, M. J., Cox, C. S., et al. (1997). Intake of vitamins E, C, and A and risk of lung cancer: The NHANES I Epidemiologic Followup Study. *American Journal of Epidemiology, 146,* 231–243.

You, R. X., Thrift, A. G., McNeil, J. J., Davis, S. M., & Donnan, G. A. (1999). Ischemic stroke risk and passive exposure to spouses' cigarette smoking. *American Journal of Public Health, 89,* 572–575.

Young, L. D. (1993). Rheumatoid arthritis. In R. J. Gatchel & E. B. Blanchard (Eds.), *Psychophysiological disorders: Research and clinical applications* (pp. 269–298). Washington, DC: American Psychological Association.

Young, L. R., & Nestle, M. (2002). The contribution of expanding portion sizes to the US obesity epidemic. *American Journal of Public Health, 92,* 246–249.

Young, M. G. (2000, October 30). Recognizing the signs of elder abuse. *Patient Care, 34*(20), 56–80.

Yu, Z., Nissinen, A., Vartiainen, E., Song, G., Guo, Z., Zheng, G., et al. (2000). Associations between socioeconomic status and cardiovascular risk factors in an urban population in China. *Bulletin of the World Health Organization, 78,* 1296–1305.

Zador, P. L., & Ciccone, M. A. (1993). Automobile driver fatalities in frontal impacts: Air bags compared with manual belts. *American Journal of Public Health, 83,* 661–666.

Zakhari, S., & Wassef, M. (1996). *Alcohol and the cardiovascular system.* Bethesda, MD: National Institutes of Health, National Institute on Alcohol Abuse and Alcoholism.

Zautra, A. J. (1998). Arthritis: Behavioral and psychosocial aspects. In E. A. Blechman & K. D. Brownell (Eds.), *Behavioral medicine and women: A comprehensive handbook* (pp. 554–558). New York: Guilford Press.

Zelenko, M., Lock, J., Kraemer, H. C., & Steiner, H. (2000). Perinatal complications and child abuse in a poverty sample. *Child Abuse and Neglect, 24,* 939–950.

Zhang, J., Feldblum, P. J., & Fortney, J. A. (1992). Moderate physical activity and bone density among perimenopausal women. *American Journal of Public Health, 82,* 736–738.

Zhang, Y., Felson, D. T., Ellison, R. C., Kreger, B. E., Schatzkin, A., Dorgan, J. F., et al. (2001). Bone mass and the risk of colon cancer among postmenopausal women: The Framingham Study. *American Journal of Epidemiology, 153,* 31–37.

Zimmerman, M. (1983). Methodological issues in the assessment of life events: A review of issues and research. *Clinical Psychology Review, 3,* 339–370.

Zinberg, N. E. (1984). *Drug, set, and setting: The basis for controlled intoxicant use.* New Haven, CT: Yale University Press.

Zonderman, A. B., Costa, P. T., & McCrae, R. R. (1989). Depression as a risk for cancer morbidity and mortality in a nationally representative sample. *Journal of the American Medical Association, 262,* 1191–1195.

Zorrilla, E. P., Luborsky, L., McKay, J. R., Rosenthal, R., Houldin, A., Tax, A., et al. (2001). The relationship of depression and stressors to immunological assays: A meta-analytic review. *Brain, Behavior, and Immunity, 15,* 199–226.

Zubin, J., & Spring, B. (1977). Vulnerability—a new view of schizophrenia. *Journal of Abnormal Psychology, 86,* 103–127.

Zyazema, N. Z. (1984). Toward better patient drug compliance and comprehension: A challenge to medical and pharmaceutical services in Zimbabwe. *Social Science and Medicine, 18,* 551–554.

Name Index

C

D

H

Subject Index

A

D

E

F

G

H

Q

R

T

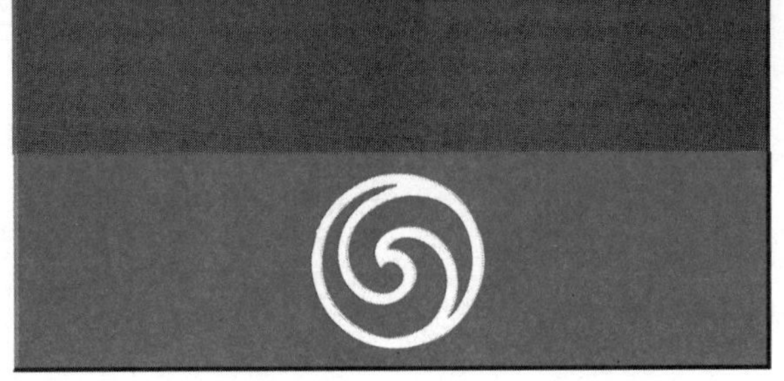

Photo Credits

Chapter 1 Corbis, 8; Corbis, 12; **Chapter 2** Corbis, 29; Jarry Berndt/Stock Boston, 35; **Chapter 3** PhotoDisc, 55; PhotoDisc, 62; Stephen Derr/The Image Bank/Getty Images, Inc., 65; Corbis, 66; Corbis, 67; **Chapter 4** Corbis, 80; Corbis, 82; Bob Dammrich/The Image World, 86; Corbis, 87; PhotoDisc, 92; **Chapter 5** Michael Siluk/The Image Works, 112; Corbis, 113; © Jose Luis Pelac 2, Inc./CORBIS, 114; Corbis, 116; Corbis, 120; **Chapter 6** Corbis, 141; Corbis, 143; Corbis, 145; **Chapter 7** Corbis 161; FPG International/Getty Images, Inc., 168; Corbis, 169; Sepp Seitz/Woodfin Camp & Associates, 171; Corbis, 177; PhotoDisc, 179; Corbis, 181; **Chapter 8** © Michael Keller/CORBIS, 189; PhotoDisc/Getty Images, 198; © Owen Franken/Corbis, 204; **Chapter 9** Hazel Hankin/Stock Boston, 233; Leinwand/Monkmeyer Press, 238; **Chapter 10** Michael Melford/ The Image Bank/ Getty Images, Inc., 261; Michael Siluk/The Image Works, 266; Corbis, 267; Corbis, 273; **Chapter 11** Corbis, 281; Frank Keillor/Jeroboam, 284; Rhoda Sidney/Stock Boston, 295; PhotoDisc, 303; **Chapter 12** Michael Siluk/The Image Works, 314; Corbis, 316; R. S. Uzzell/Woodfin Camp & Associates, 318; Corbis, 322; Corbis, 329; Corbis, 333; **Chapter 13** Penny Tweedy/Tony Stone Images/Getty Images, Inc., 358; Corbis, 359; Corbis, 370; **Chapter 14** Corbis, 389; Courtesy of the U. of Washington School of Medicine, 390; Schneider/Monkmeyer Press, 401; Corbis, 411; **Chapter 15** Wallace Kirkland/Life Magazine, 425; Topham/The Image Works, 433; Corbis, 436; Susan Rosenberg/Photo Researchers, Inc., 443; **Chapter 16** M. Bernsau/The Image Works, 458; Corbis, 474; Corbis, 478; **Chapter 17** Corbis, 486; Paula Lerner/Woodfin Camp & Associates, 492

TO THE OWNER OF THIS BOOK:

I hope that you have found *Health Psychology: An Introduction to Behavior and Health, Fifth Edition* useful. So that this book can be improved in a future edition, would you take the time to complete this sheet and return it? Thank you.

School and address: ____

____

Department: ____

Instructor's name: ____

1. What I like most about this book is: ____

____

____

2. What I like least about this book is: ____

____

____

3. My general reaction to this book is: ____

____

____

4. The name of the course in which I used this book is: ____

____

5. Were all of the chapters of the book assigned for you to read? ______________________

If not, which ones weren't? ____

6. In the space below, or on a separate sheet of paper, please write specific suggestions for improving this book and anything else you'd care to share about your experience in using this book.

____

____

OPTIONAL:

Your name: ______________________________ Date: ________________

May we quote you, either in promotion for *Health Psychology: An Introduction to Behavior and Health, Fifth Edition*, or in future publishing ventures?

Yes: ________ No: ________

Sincerely yours,

Linda Brannon, Jess Feist

FOLD HERE

NO POSTAGE NECESSARY IF MAILED IN THE UNITED STATES

BUSINESS REPLY MAIL

FIRST CLASS PERMIT NO. 34 BELMONT, CA

POSTAGE WILL BE PAID BY ADDRESSEE

ATTN: Michele Sordi, Psychology Editor

WADSWORTH/THOMSON LEARNING
10 DAVIS DRIVE
BELMONT, CA 94002-9801

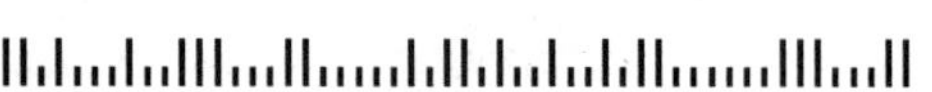

FOLD HERE